Meningococcal Disease

METHODS IN MOLECULAR MEDICINE™

John M. Walker, *Series Editor*

68. Molecular Analysis of Cancer, edited by *Jacqueline Boultwood and Carrie Fidler,* 2002

67. Meningococcal Disease: *Methods and Protocols,* edited by *Andrew J. Pollard and Martin C. J. Maiden,* 2001

66. Meningococcal Vaccines: *Methods and Protocols,* edited by *Andrew J. Pollard and Martin C. J. Maiden,* 2001

65. Nonviral Vectors for Gene Therapy: *Methods and Protocols,* edited by *Mark A, Findeis,* 2001

64. Dendritic Cell Protocols, edited by *Stephen P. Robinson and Andrew J. Stagg,* 2001

63. Hematopoietic Stem Cell Protocols, edited by *Christopher A. Klug and Craig T. Jordan,* 2001

62. Parkinson's Disease: ***Methods and Protocols,*** edited by *M. Maral Mouradian,* 2001

61. Melanoma Techniques and Protocols: ***Molecular Diagnosis, treatment, and Monitoring,*** edited by *Brian J. Nickoloff,* 2001

60. Interleukin Protocols, edited by *Luke A. J. O'Neill and Andrew Bowie,* 2001

59. Molecular Pathology of the Prions, edited by *Harry F. Baker,* 2001

58. Metastasis Research Protocols: ***Volume 2, Cell Behavior In Vitro and In Vivo,*** edited by *Susan A. Brooks and Udo Schumacher,* 2001

57. Metastasis Research Protocols: ***Volume 1, Analysis of Cells and Tissues,*** edited by *Susan A. Brooks and Udo Schumacher,* 2001

56. Human Airway Inflammation: *Sampling Techniques and Analytical Protocols,* edited by *Duncan F. Rogers and Louise E. Donnelly,* 2001

55. Hematologic Malignancies: *Methods and Protocols,* edited by *Guy B. Faguet,* 2001

54. *Mycobacterium tuberculosis* Protocols, edited by *Tanya Parish and Neil G. Stoker,* 2001

53. Renal Cancer: *Methods and Protocols,* edited by *Jack H. Mydlo,* 2001

52. Atherosclerosis: ***Experimental Methods and Protocols,*** edited by *Angela F. Drew,* 2001

51. Angiotensin Protocols, edited by *Donna H. Wang,* 2001

50. Colorectal Cancer: ***Methods and Protocols,*** edited by *Steven M. Powell,* 2001

49. Molecular Pathology Protocols, edited by *Anthony A. Killeen,* 2001

48. Antibiotic Resistance Methods and Protocols, edited by *Stephen H. Gillespie,* 2001

47. Vision Research Protocols, edited by *P. Elizabeth Rakoczy,* 2001

46. Angiogenesis Protocols, edited by *J. Clifford Murray,* 2001

45. Hepatocellular Carcinoma: ***Methods and Protocols,*** **edited by** *Nagy A. Habib,* 2000

44. Asthma: ***Mechanisms and Protocols,*** **edited by** *K. Fan Chung and Ian Adcock,* 2001

43. Muscular Dystrophy: ***Methods and Protocols,*** **edited by** *Katherine B. Bushby and Louise Anderson,* 2001

42. Vaccine Adjuvants: ***Preparation Methods and Research Protocols,*** edited by *Derek T. O'Hagan,* 2000

41. Celiac Disease: ***Methods and Protocols,*** edited by *Michael N. Marsh,* 2000

40. Diagnostic and Therapeutic Antibodies, edited by *Andrew J. T. George and Catherine E. Urch,* 2000

39. Ovarian Cancer: ***Methods and Protocols,*** edited by *John M. S. Bartlett,* 2000

38. Aging Methods and Protocols, edited by *Yvonne A. Barnett and Christopher R. Barnett,* 2000

37. Electrochemotherapy, Electrogenetherapy, and Transdermal Drug Delivery: *Electrically Mediated Delivery of Molecules to Cells,* edited by *Mark J. Jaroszeski, Richard Heller, and Richard Gilbert,* 2000

36. Septic Shock Methods and Protocols, edited by *Thomas J. Evans,* 2000

35. Gene Therapy of Cancer: ***Methods and Protocols,*** edited by *Wolfgang Walther and Ulrike Stein,* 2000

METHODS IN MOLECULAR MEDICINE™

Meningococcal Disease

Methods and Protocols

Edited by

Andrew J. Pollard, MD, PhD

BC Research Institute for Children's and Women's Health, Vancouver, BC Canada

and

Martin C. J. Maiden, PhD

Wellcome Trust Centre for the Epidemiology of Infectious Disease, Oxford, UK

Foreword by

Michael Levin, MD, PhD

Imperial College School of Medicine, St. Mary's Hospital, London, UK

Humana Press **Totowa, New Jersey**

999 Riverview Drive, Suite 208
Totowa, New Jersey 07512
humanapress.com

This publication is printed on acid-free paper. ∞
ANSI Z39.48-1984 (American Standards Institute) Permanence of Paper for Printed Library Materials.

Cover design by Patricia F. Cleary.

Production Editor: Mark J. Breaugh.

For additional copies, pricing for bulk purchases, and/or information about other Humana titles, contact Humana at the above address or at any of the following numbers: Tel.: 973-256-1699; Fax: 973-256-8341; E-mail: humana@humanapr.com; Website: http://humanapress.com

Printed in the United States of America. 10 9 8 7 6 5 4 3 2 1

Library of Congress Cataloging in Publication Data

Main entry under title: Methods in molecular medicine™.

Meningococcal disease: methods and protocols / edited by Andrew J. Pollard and
Martin C.J. Maiden.
p. ; cm. -- (Methods in molecular medicine ; 67)
Companion volume to: Meningococcal vaccines.
Includes bibliographical references and index.

1. Neisseria meningitidis--Laboratory manuals. 2. Meningitis--Molecular
aspects--Laboratory manuals. I. Pollard, Andrew J. II. Maiden, Martin C.J. III.
Meningococcal vaccines. IV. Series.
[DNLM: 1. Meningitis, Meningococcal--diagnosis. 2. Meningitis,
Meningococcal--therapy. WC 245 M5453 2001]
QR82.N4 M46 2001
616.8'2--dc21

ISBN 978-1-61737-221-6 e-ISBN 978-1-59259-149-7

Foreword

Meningococcal septicemia and meningitis continue to be important causes of devastating illness, death, and long-term disability in both developed and resource-poor countries of the world. Few diseases have attracted as much public attention, or are as feared by parents and family members, as well as the medical staff who have to care for affected patients. The unexpected and unpredictable occurrence of the disease in previously healthy children and young adults, its rapid progression, and the frequent occurrence of purpura fulminans with the resulting gangrene of limbs and digits and the requirement for mutilating surgery, have all heightened both public and medical interest in the disease.

Over the past two decades there has been a rapid increase in knowledge of many aspects of meningococcal disease as a result of intensive efforts by workers in many different fields: clinicians have studied the early presenting features and acute pathophysiology of the disorder; clinical scientists have explored the immunopathological mechanisms responsible for disease and have highlighted the important roles played by the host inflammatory response and pro-inflammatory cytokines in mediating damage to blood vessels and organs; microbiologists have developed new diagnostic methods; public health physicians and epidemiologists have improved surveillance techniques with the help of molecular tools provided by bacterial population biologists; and basic scientists have used the powerful new tools in molecular and cell biology to elucidate virulence mechanisms. The paradox of why an organism that begins as a harmless commensal in the majority of the human population, invades the blood stream and brain, and causes devastating illness in a few individuals, appears to be explained by both host and bacterial genetic factors. A major challenge remains to fully link the insights obtained from studying the bacteria to those gained from studying the human host and provide a true picture of the host/pathogen interaction.

Despite the progress that has been made in understanding specific aspects of meningococcal biology and host interactions, it seems likely that the development of improved treatments and an effective vaccine to prevent the disease will depend on novel insights from a range of different disciplines. New tools to treat those affected by the disease are likely to come from an in-depth understanding of the immunopathological mechanisms occurring in acutely ill patients. The identification of novel targets, both for therapeutic interventions and for vaccines, are likely to require detailed understanding of host–pathogen interactions, and elucidation of the components of meningococcus responsible for virulence.

Andrew Pollard and Martin Maiden have brought together some of the leading authorities on meningococcal disease to produce a comprehensive interdisciplinary book describing recent advances and knowledge in a wide range of different fields, which will be an invaluable resource for all those interested in the disease. The linking of basic science, clinical, and epidemiological aspects of the disease will undoubtedly help to broaden understanding of the scientific approach to the study of meningococcal disease. We can all hope that the bringing together of a broad range of different research efforts in this text will ultimately facilitate development of improved treatments and an effective vaccine against this terrible infectious disease.

***Michael Levin,* MD, PhD**

Preface

Neisseria meningitidis is a major cause of morbidity and mortality in childhood in industrialized nations and the organism is responsible for epidemics of disease in Africa and in Asia. Because of its public health impact, meningococcal disease is of interest and importance to clinicians, clinical microbiologists, public health physicians, epidemiologists, and research scientists. In *Meningococcal Disease* we have brought together a series of review and methods-based chapters that provide essential information for diagnosis in the clinical microbiology laboratory, isolate characterization, clinical management, and control of meningococcal disease.

New vaccine initiatives are expected in many countries over the next few years, to control both epidemic and endemic disease, and it is hoped that the information available in this book on surveillance and characterization of meningococcal isolates will be of use in the planning of vaccine strategies. A companion text on *Meningococcal Vaccines* is also available from Humana Press and includes overview chapters and detailed methods for the design and evaluation of meningococcal vaccines.

We are grateful to the many contributors to this text who have provided a series of state-of-the-art chapters for inclusion in this book. We are grateful to the series editor, John Walker, and the staff of Humana Press, for inviting our participation as book editors. We acknowledge the contribution of the many clinicians, microbiologists, and scientists who continue to make a major contribution to the diagnosis, management, surveillance, and control of meningococcal disease around the world.

Andrew J. Pollard, PhD
Martin C. J. Maiden, PhD

Contents

Contributors

Mark Achtman • *Max-Planck Institut für Molekulare Genetik, Berlin, Germany*

Loek van Alphen • *Laboratory of Vaccine Research, National Institute of Public Health and the Environment, Bilthoven, The Netherlands*

Michael A. Apicella • *Department of Microbiology, University of Iowa, Iowa City, IA*

Luisa Arreaza • *Reference Laboratory for Meningococci, National Center for Microbiology, Madrid, Spain*

Sharmila Bakshi • *Department of Paediatrics, University of Oxford, John Radcliffe Hospital, Oxford, UK*

Rosemary A. Barnes • *Department of Medical Microbiology and PHLS, University of Wales College of Medicine, Cardiff, UK*

Albert Bart • *Department of Medical Microbiology, Academic Medical Center, Amsterdam, The Netherlands*

Norman T. Begg • *SmithKline Beecham, Hertsfordshire, UK*

Andrew W. Berrington • *Department of Microbiology and Parasitology, University of Queensland, Brisbane, Australia*

Colin Block • *Department of Clinical Microbiology and Infectious Diseases, Hadassah-University Hospital, Jerusalem, Israel*

Ray Borrow • *Manchester Public Health Laboratory, Withington Hospital, Manchester, UK*

Lucas D. Bowler • *Trafford Centre for Medical Research, University of Sussex, Brighton, UK*

Petter Brandtzaeg • *Department of Pediatrics, Ullevål University Hospital, University of Oslo, Norway*

Keith Cartwright • *Public Health Laboratory, Gloucestershire Royal Hospital, Gloucester, UK*

Dominique A. Caugant • *Department of Bacteriology, National Institute of Public Health, Oslo, Norway*

Ronald Chalmers • *Department of Biochemistry, University of Oxford, UK*

Heike Claus • *Institut für Hygiene und Mikrobiologie, Universität Würzburg, Germany*

W. Terence Coakley • *School of Biosciences, Cardiff University, UK*
Bert H.F. Derkx • *Department of Pediatrics, Academic Medical Center, Amsterdam, The Netherlands*
Marcel van Deuren • *Department of Internal Medicine, University Medical Center, Nijmegen, The Netherlands*
Germie van den Dobbelsteen • *Laboratory of Vaccine Research, National Institute of Public Health and the Environment, Bilthoven, The Netherlands*
Arie van der Ende • *Department of Medical Microbiology, Academic Medical Center, Amsterdam, The Netherlands*
Terje Espevik • *Faculty of Medicine, Norwegian University of Science and Technology, Institute of Cancer Research and Molecular Biology, Trondheim, Norway*
Marino Festa • *Department of Pediatric Intensive Care, The New Children's Hospital, Westmead, Australia*
Hans Fredlund • *Department of Clinical Microbiology & Immunology, Örebro Medical Centre Hospital, Örebro, Sweden*
Matthias Frosch • *Institut für Hygiene und Mikrobiologie, Universität Würzburg, Germany*
Peter C. Giardina • *Department of Microbiology, University of Iowa, Iowa City, IA*
Brad W. Gibson • *Department of Pharmaceutical Chemistry, University of California, San Francisco*
Linda Goodwin • *Division of Molecular and Genetic Medicine, University of Sheffield Medical School, Sheffield, UK*
Stephen J. Gray • *Manchester Public Health Laboratory, Withington Hospital, Manchester, UK*
Ronald de Groot • *Department of Pediatrics, Sophia Children's Hospital, Erasmus Medical Center Rotterdam, The Netherlands*
Malcolm Guiver • *Manchester Public Health Laboratory, Withington Hospital, Manchester, UK*
C. Erik Hack • *Department of Immunopathology, Central Laboratory of the Netherlands Red Cross Blood Transfusion Services, Amsterdam, The Netherlands*
Jan A. Hazelzet • *Department of Pediatrics, Sophia Children's Hospital, Erasmus Medical Center Rotterdam, The Netherlands*
Robert S. Heyderman • *Department of Pathology & Microbiology, School of Medical Sciences, University of Bristol, UK*
Derek W. Hood • *Institute of Molecular Medicine, University of Oxford, UK*
Tom W.J. Huizinga • *Department of Rheumatology, Leiden University Medical Center, Leiden, The Netherlands*

ALEX C. JEFFRIES • *Department of Biology and Biochemistry, University of Bath, UK*
MICHAEL P. JENNINGS • *Department of Microbiology and Parasitology, University of Queensland, Brisbane, Australia*
JENS C. JENSENIUS • *Department of Medical Microbiology and Immunology, University of Aarhus, Denmark*
KEITH A. JOLLEY • *Department of Zoology, University of Oxford, Oxford, UK*
EDWARD B. KACZMARSKI • *Manchester Public Health Laboratory, Withington Hospital, Manchester, UK*
PETER KIERULF • *Department of Clinical Chemistry, Ullevål University Hospital, University of Oslo, Norway*
NIGEL J. KLEIN • *Immunobiology Unit, Institute of Child Health, London, UK*
J. SIMON KROLL • *Department of Pediatrics, Imperial College School of Medicine, London, UK*
BETSY KUIPERS • *Laboratory of Vaccine Research, National Institute of Public Health and the Environment, Bilthoven, The Netherlands*
PAUL R. LANGFORD • *Department of Pediatrics, Imperial College School of Medicine, London, UK*
MICHAEL LEVIN • *Department of Pediatrics, Imperial College School of Medicine, London, UK*
NINA-BEATE LIABAKK • *Faculty of Medicine, Norwegian University of Science and Technology, Institute of Cancer Research and Molecular Biology, Trondheim, Norway*
EGIL LIEN • *Faculty of Medicine, Norwegian University of Science and Technology, Institute of Cancer Research and Molecular Biology, Trondheim, Norway*
IAIN MACINTOSH • *Department of Pediatrics, Imperial College School of Medicine, London, UK*
MARTIN C. J. MAIDEN • *Department of Zoology, University of Oxford, Oxford, UK*
PAOLA MASSARI • *Evans Biomedical Research Center, Boston University School of Medicine, Boston, MA*
GIOVANNA MORELLI • *Max-Planck Institut für Molekulare Genetik, Berlin, Germany*
E. RICHARD MOXON • *Molecular Infectious Diseases Group, Oxford University Department of Pediatrics, Oxford, UK*
SIMON NADEL • *Department of Pediatrics, Imperial College School of Medicine, London, UK*
XAVIER NASSIF • *Laboratoire de Microbiologie, Faculté de Médecine Necker-Enfants Malades, Paris, France*

NORMAN NOAH • *PHLS Communicable Disease Surveillance Centre, London School of Hygiene and Tropical Medicine, London, UK*

PER OLCÉN • *Department of Clinical Microbiology & Immunology, Örebro Medical Centre Hospital, Örebro, Sweden*

REIDUN ØVSTEBØ • *Department of Clinical Chemistry, Ullevål University Hospital, University of Oslo, Norway*

ANDREW J. POLLARD • *BC Research Institute for Children & Women's Health, Vancouver, BC*

ROBERT C. READ • *Division of Molecular and Genetic Medicine, University of Sheffield Medical School, Sheffield, UK*

F. ANDREW I. RIORDAN • *Department of Child Health, Birmingham Heartlands Hospital, Birmingham, UK*

NANCY E. ROSENSTEIN • *Division of Bacterial and Mycotic Diseases, Meningitis and Special Pathogens Branch, National Center for Infectious Diseases, Centers for Disease Control and Prevention, Atlanta, GA*

NIGEL J. SAUNDERS • *Institute of Molecular Medicine, University of Oxford, Oxford, UK*

DAVID SCHEIFELE • *Department of Pediatrics, Division of Infectious and Immunologic Diseases, BC's Children's Hospital, Vancouver, BC*

LAURA SERINO • *Department of Pathology & Microbiology, School of Medical Sciences, University of Bristol, UK*

ANDERS G. SJÖHOLM • *Department of Clinical Microbiology & Immunology, University Hospital of Lund, Lund, Sweden*

MICHAEL A. SOBANSKI • *School of Biosciences, Cardiff University, Cardiff, UK*

JØRGEN STENVIK • *Faculty of Medicine, Norwegian University of Science and Technology, Institute of Cancer Research and Molecular Biology, Trondheim, Norway*

JAMES M. STUART • *Public Health Laboratory, Gloucestershire Royal Hospital, Gloucester, UK*

YAO-HUI SUN • *University Department of Paediatrics, University of Oxford, John Radcliffe Hospital, Oxford, UK*

CHRISTOPH M. TANG • *University Department of Paediatrics, University of Oxford, John Radcliffe Hospital, Oxford, UK*

COLIN R. TINSLEY • *INSERM Unite 411, Faculté de Médecine Necker-Enfants Malades, Paris, France*

LENNART TRUEDSSON • *Department of Clinical Microbiology & Immunology, University Hospital of Lund, Lund, Sweden*

RACHEL URWIN • *Department of Zoology, University of Oxford, UK*

JULIO A. VÁZQUEZ • *Reference Laboratory for Meningococci, National Center for Microbiology, Madrid, Spain*

Mumtaz Virji • *Department of Pathology & Microbiology, School of Medical Sciences, University of Bristol, UK*
Ulrich Vogel • *Institut für Hygiene und Mikrobiologie, Universität Würzburg, Germany*
Anders Waage • *Department of Medicine, Section of Hematology, University Hospital of Trondheim, Trondheim, Norway*
Steven A. R. Webb • *Department of Pediatrics, Imperial College School of Medicine, London, UK*
Elisabeth Wedege • *Department of Vaccinology, National Institute of Public Health, Oslo, Norway*
Jerrold A. Weiss • *Department of Internal Medicine, Division of Infectious Diseases, University of Iowa, Iowa City, IA*
Rudi G. J. Westendorp • *Department of General Internal Medicine and Clinical Epidemiology, Leiden University Medical Center, Leiden, The Netherlands*
Lee Wetzler • *Evans Biomedical Research Center, Boston University School of Medicine, Boston, MA*

1

Microbiology and Laboratory Diagnosis

Keith Cartwright

1. Introduction

1.1. Historical Background

In 1887, Anton Weichselbaum, a Viennese doctor, was the first to report the isolation of meningococci from patients with meningitis *(1)*. Shortly after, came the first description of lumbar puncture in living patients *(2)*, leading to the isolation of meningococci from acute cases of meningitis. Three years later, Kiefer grew meningococci from the nasopharynx of cases of meningococcal disease, and from their contacts *(3)*, a finding of immense significance in advancing understanding of the epidemiology and pathogenesis of the disease. Early serological typing systems demonstrated that there were important differences between meningococci in terms of their virulence *(4)*.

1.2. Meningococcal Carriage and Disease

It is believed that meningococci only occur in humans. They have never been isolated from other animals, possibly owing to their inability to acquire iron from any other than human sources (transferrin and lactoferrin). Their fastidious nature makes it most unlikely that there are any important environmental reservoirs. Meningococci form part of the normal commensal flora and can be isolated from the nasopharynx of approx 10% of individuals overall. Nasopharyngeal carriage is age-dependent, peaking in late teenage and early adulthood at 20–30% or more, but with low prevalence in the young and in the elderly. It is not clear whether acquisition of a new meningococcus in the nasopharynx results in respiratory illness. Meningococci may also be isolated from the urethra and from the rectum from time to time and appear to be capable of causing urethritis.

From: *Methods in Molecular Medicine, vol. 67: Meningococcal Disease: Methods and Protocols*
Edited by: A. J. Pollard and M. C. J. Maiden © Humana Press Inc., Totowa, NJ

Invasion is a rare phenomenon, though probably more frequent than would be suggested by the measured rates of disease. It is well-recognized that a small proportion of young children may present in hospital with a mild febrile illness that resolves rapidly without antibiotic treatment and from whom a meningococcus is subsequently isolated from blood cultures. For both ethical and logistic reasons, blood culture studies of febrile (but otherwise healthy) children in the community are difficult to mount. Were they to be undertaken with large numbers of participants, it seems likely that they would identify at least a small number of febrile children from whose bloodstream a meningococcus could be isolated.

Is it important to confirm the diagnosis in cases of suspected meningococcal infection? The answer must be in the affirmative, both for the optimal management of the patient and his or her contacts, and also for the epidemiological added value. Though meningococci are almost invariably sensitive to penicillin, the exclusion of other causes of meningitis and septicemia remains a key rationale for the full microbiological investigation of both these conditions. Without a detailed understanding of the range of meningococci causing human disease, and the age groups affected, development of effective vaccines is impossible.

1.3. The Changing Pattern of Meningococcal Disease Diagnosis

Diagnostic algorithms in suspected meningococcal infection have changed considerably in the UK over the last 10 years. The drivers have been changes in clinical management and changes in disease epidemiology, allied to technical advances in the laboratory.

In the UK and in other countries where most patients with suspected meningococcal disease present first to a primary care medical practitioner, a substantial and increasing proportion of patients are being treated with a dose of parenteral benzylpenicillin. To date, all but one of the published studies (together with unpublished data) support the efficacy of this early management step. Though beneficial, administration of benzylpenicillin prior to the patient's admission to hospital normally renders blood cultures sterile.

It has been suggested that general practitioners administering benzylpenicillin to patients with suspected meningococcal disease should take blood cultures prior to administering the antibiotic, sending them in to hospital with the patient. This diagnostic step is theoretically possible, but would present a number of logistic difficulties. It is probably not warranted now that good nonculture diagnostic techniques are available (*see* **Subheading 2.1.**).

1.4. Microbiological Investigation as Part of the Early Management of Meningococcal Infection

There is strong evidence to support the view that delay in the active management of meningococcal infection is a major factor increasing the risk of a poor outcome. Studies in various countries have documented some of the reasons for delay in treatment. One of the most frequent reasons for failing to institute prompt treatment is the fear that initiation of antibiotic treatment may adversely affect the microbiological investigations. As a consequence, a patient may arrive in hospital, be subjected to initial clinical evaluation and may be suspected of having meningococcal meningitis. A lumbar puncture may be ordered, and antibiotics withheld pending the results of the lumbar puncture. In a busy pediatric or adult medical unit, this may take an hour or two, or sometimes longer, to arrange. This is unacceptable. As soon as meningococcal infection is suspected, blood cultures should be drawn, a drip set up, and intravenous antibiotics commenced. A lumbar puncture (if deemed appropriate) can then be carried out at the earliest available opportunity. Because it takes at least an hour for antibiotics to begin to arrive in the sub-arachnoid space (even when given by the intravenous route), the chances of isolating a meningococcus (or other bacterium) from the cerebrospinal fluid (CSF) are still high. Even if CSF cultures are negative, the diagnosis may be confirmed by microscopic examination of CSF, by latex agglutination tests, or by amplification of microbial DNA by polymerase chain reaction (PCR).

It is also not widely appreciated that meningococcal DNA is cleared only slowly from the CSF in meningococcal meningitis. If the patient is too unwell or too unstable for lumbar puncture to be contemplated at the time of admission to hospital, and if the diagnosis has not been established within the first 24–48 h, a lumbar puncture is still likely to give a positive PCR result even on d 3 or d 4 of inpatient management. Such a late lumbar puncture will only be needed rarely, but the possibility should be borne in mind.

1.5. Changing Perceptions of Lumbar Puncture

Lumbar puncture is now used less frequently, especially by pediatricians *(5)*. This change in clinical practice has arisen from a combination of concern over its perceived dangers, together with a sense of its lack of contributory value in some situations. Coning, frequently fatal, may occur in about 1% of cases of meningococcal meningitis where lumbar puncture is undertaken, and lumbar puncture may exacerbate hemodynamic instability in a patient verging on the brink of shock. There is also an increasing understanding that analysis of CSF may provide little additional information relevant to the management of the acutely ill patient (especially if fever and a vasculitic rash are present and a diagnosis of meningococcal infection is overwhelmingly likely). Add to this the fact that the results of all initial examinations (protein, glucose, cell count, and Gram-stained smear) may be negative and yet a meningococcus may be grown on the following day from 5–10% of patients *(5)*, and the exercise of caution over the use of lumbar puncture in children is very understandable.

The same is not true in adults with symptoms and signs of meningitis. Here, the epidemiology of bacterial meningitis is very different ***(6)***. A wider range of pathogens is possible, including the pneumococcus, and other more arcane bacteria such as *Listeria monocytogenes*. A few patients with pneumococcal meningitis may have a vasculitic rash and their infection may be confused on clinical grounds with meningococcal meningitis or septicemia. The overriding importance of accurate diagnosis of meningitis in adults is the risk (small as yet in the UK, but substantial in countries such as Spain, France, and South Africa) of true penicillin, or penicillin- and cephalosporin-resistant infection. Lumbar puncture is still the most important investigation in adult patients with suspected bacterial meningitis *(7)*.

2. Specific Clinical Issues Impacting on Microbiological Diagnosis

2.1. Effect of Early Parenteral Antibiotic Treatment on Diagnostic Investigations

In the 1980s, the great majority of patients in the UK with suspected meningococcal meningitis were not treated with benzylpenicillin prior to hospital admission. In such patients (both adults and children), blood cultures were positive in about 50%, and if meningitis was present and a lumbar puncture was undertaken, the CSF would either yield Gram-negative diplococci on the stained smear, or a meningococcus would be isolated on culture in more than 90% of cases.

Alternative diagnostic methods had to be devised to cope with patients with negative blood cultures, and in whom lumbar puncture was contraindicated. Throat swabs have proved of great value in this situation, giving a positive result in up to 50% of patients, a proportion that is largely unaffected by prior benzylpenicillin treatment *(7)*. Per-oral swabs give a better yield than pernasal swabs. If the intention is to isolate a meningococcus, the swab must be plated out as soon as it is obtained. A swab taken in the middle of the night cannot be left to be cultured in the morning.

If a skin rash is present, aspiration of an affected area of skin may yield diplococci on a Giemsa-stained smear, or in a somewhat smaller proportion of cases, a positive culture. Agglutination of latex particles coated with meningococcal serogroup-specific antibodies by meningococci of the homologous serogroup can be made more sensitive by inducing better agglutination by means of ultrasound enhancement.

Demonstration of a rising antimeningococcal antibody titer between acute and convalescent serum samples may also be helpful for epidemiological reasons, though it does not provide information at the time that it is needed for the acute management of the patient.

However, the test that has emerged from the status of a research tool into one of fundamental utility is the detection of meningococcal DNA following its amplification by PCR. In the UK, the Public Health Laboratory Service (PHLS) Meningococcal Reference Unit (MRU) located at the Manchester Public Health Laboratory provides this test. From an initial experimental clinical service in 1996, the service has grown such that there were more than 16,000 requests for meningococcal PCR in 1999. The PCR test can be carried out on peripheral blood or on CSF, and is thought to be specific for meningococcal DNA.

2.2. CSF with Polymorphs but no Organisms Seen or Grown

Another common clinical situation is that in which a febrile child or adult is subjected to lumbar puncture to exclude the possibility of meningitis, and turbid CSF is obtained, in which neutrophils are observed on microscopy and from which no bacteria are grown. Though neutrophils may occasionally predominate in viral meningitis, the presumption is that most such patients have bacterial meningitis. Most will be treated empirically with a third-generation cephalosporin such as cefotaxime or ceftriaxone, but the need to establish (if possible) a more accurate diagnosis lies in the possibility that pneumococci (with the small attendant risk of treatment failure with either penicillin or with cephalosporins) may be the cause of the meningitis.

Antigen-detection tests may be of value here and their sensitivity may be enhanced considerably by the use of ultrasound. Agglutination tests are probably inherently less sensitive than PCR tests. Meningococcal PCR testing of CSF is now widely used in the UK and multiplex PCR tests that will detect DNA from meningococci, pneumococci and from *Haemophilus influenzae* type b are now being evaluated.

2.3. Unusual Presentations of Meningococcal Infection

Patients with meningococcal infection may occasionally present with syndromes other than meningitis or septicemia. Urethritis, conjunctivitis, and pneumonia are all possibilities, as are septic arthritis, endophthalmitis, pericarditis, and other infections of deep, normally sterile, tissues. Isolation of a meningococcus from a normally sterile site is diagnostic, but more difficulty arises in the interpretation of the significance of a meningococcus isolated from a superficial site. Clinical and microbiological judgement may be required, but if there is doubt, and particularly if the meningococcus is present in substantial numbers, and is well-endowed with capsular polysaccharide, the isolate should be treated with a high degree of suspicion. For example, primary meningococcal conjunctivitis should be treated aggressively, because there is a high risk of invasive disease if this is not done. In the US in recent years, there has been an increase in meningãíoccal infections owing to serogroup Y strains, and these may have a particular predilection for the respiratory tract.

Chronic meningococcemia is now very rare, accounting for about 1% of all cases. It is normally diagnosed clinically at first. Blood cultures may need to be repeated frequently before a positive culture is obtained. Meningococcal blood PCR will probably be positive in the periods immediately after live meningococci have been cleared from the bloodstream.

2.3. Clusters

When a sporadic case of suspected meningococcal disease occurs, it is, of course, impossible to say if it will be followed rapidly by another. For this reason (as well as for clinical reasons), all suspected cases of meningococcal disease should be investigated as fully as possible.

There is an ever-present risk that a sporadic case of meningococcal infection may be followed by others in the same family, school, or community. The public-health management of clusters of cases is made much more difficult when the diagnosis is uncertain in one or more of the cases. A typical situation with which public health-medicine specialists have to cope is that in which one or more suspected but unconfirmed cases in a school or other defined community is followed by a confirmed case (or vice versa). Trying to manage the possible cluster in such circumstances is extremely difficult. If one or more of the cases has died, pressure from the community for intervention may be intense, but might not be justified on epidemiological grounds, were good diagnostic information to be available from all cases.

Having an accurate knowledge of the characteristics of the responsible strains is of fundamental value in guiding the management. For example, two or more cases of serogroup C disease occurring within a few days of each other within a defined small community would warrant consideration of the use of vaccine in addition to chemoprophylaxis. This would not apply if the cases were caused by serogroup B strains, or to a mixture of capsular serogroups.

2.4. Postmortem Diagnosis

Because of the aggressive and rapid nature of the infection, some patients with suspected meningococcal infection will die before, or very shortly after arrival in hospital, and before there has been a chance to carry out any investigations. It is the author's experience that a microbiologist is rarely involved in the investigation of such cases, only getting to hear of them many hours, or even days later, by which time chances of a positive culture are remote. Requests for autopsy are often declined by grieving relatives. Blood and/or CSF PCR tests should be of great value in this situation, though they are as yet formally untested. Aspiration, microscopy, culture, and PCR testing of any areas of skin rash are also worth considering.

2.5. The Impact of Changing Epidemiology on Diagnosis

When a patient is suspected of having meningitis, and when there is no microbiological diagnosis, knowledge of the local epidemiology can be of great help in guiding management of both case and contacts. For example, in the UK, the introduction of conjugated Hib vaccines in 1992 has almost eliminated invasive Hib infections in all age groups, and not just in children. The introduction of conjugated meningococcal group C vaccines in November 1999 will result in a rapid fall in the incidence of meningococcal disease owing to this serogroup. Consequently, the relative (though not the absolute) risk of a case of meningitis of unknown etiology proving to be owing to a pneumococcus, with the attendant possibility of penicillin resistance, will rise.

3. The Future

3.1. Nonculture Detection of Meningococci from Throat Swabs

Though it is believed that most, if not almost all invasive meningococcal disease follows initial colonization of the upper respiratory tract, meningococci can only be cultured from throat swabs in about 50% of cases. PCR testing for detection of meningococci in throat swabs is currently under development at the PHLS Meningococcal Reference Unit. It may prove a useful addition to the available range of diagnostic techniques.

3.2. PCR Tests for Penicillin Resistance

Clinical isolates of meningococci remain sensitive to penicillin, despite a small decrease in sensitivity in strains submitted to the England and Wales reference laboratory over the last few years. To date, there have been only a handful of reports of β-lactamase producing meningococci from clinical cases (and no cases of treatment failure owing to this cause) and none of these strains has survived for detailed examination today. Nevertheless, the risk of penicillin resistance remains, with the potential for treatment failure. There would be some value in having available a molecular method for detection of penicillin resistance, and in particular, the capacity to identify β-lactamase producing strains. Such a test could be carried out in conjunction with screening and serogroup-specific PCRs.

3.3. DNA Chips

The pace of development of molecular diagnostics makes it seem increasingly likely that DNA chips for the diagnosis of meningococcal disease (and for a wide range of other meningitis pathogens) will become available within the next few years. As with meningococcal vaccines, their use in developing countries is likely to be restricted by cost factors.

References

1. Weichselbaum, A. (1887) Ueber die aetiologie der akuten meningitis cerebro-spinalis. *Fortschr. Med.* **5,** 573–583, 620–626.
2. Quincke, H. I. (1893) Ueber meningitis serosa. *Samml. Klin. Vort. (Leipzig)* **67,** 655–694.
3. Kiefer, F. (1896) Zur differentialdiagnose des erregers der epidemischen cerebrospinalmeningitis und der gonorrhoe. *Berl. Klin. Woch.* **33,** 628–630.
4. Gordon, M. H. and Murray, E. G. (1915) Identification of the meningococcus. *J. R. Army Med. Corps.* **25,** 411–423.
5. Wylie, P. A. L., Stevens, D. S., Drake III, W., Stuart, J. M., and Cartwright, K. (1997) Epidemiology and clinical management of meningococcal disease in Gloucestershire: retrospective population-based study. *BMJ* **315,** 774–779.
6. Begg, N., Cartwright, K. A. V., Cohen, J., Kaczmarski, E. B., Innes, J. A., Leen, C. L. S., et al. (1999) Consensus statement on diagnosis, investigation, treatment and prevention of acute bacterial meningitis in immunocompetent adults. *J. Infect.* **39,** 1–15.
7. Cartwright, K., Reilly, S., White, D., and Stuart, J. (1992) Early treatment with parenteral penicillin in meningococcal disease. *BMJ* **305,** 143–147.

2

Isolation, Culture, and Identification of Meningococci from Clinical Specimens

Per Olcén and Hans Fredlund

1. Introduction

Humans are the only natural reservoir for meningococci. The appropriate specimens that should be taken for isolation of meningococci are dependent on the clinical question. The most appropriate specimen and/or laboratory techniques for microbiological diagnosis in an acutely sick patient with suspected invasive disease like meningitis/septicemia *(1)* may be quite different from those required for diagnosis of the cause of a local infection in eye, upper respiratory tract, lower respiratory tract, or urogenital tract, or for the study of the carrier state of healthy persons.

Culture still forms the backbone of diagnosis in spite of major improvements in nonculture diagnostic methods (*see* Chapters 3–5), the latter being especially valuable when cultures are "falsely" negative. This can occur for a number of reasons, most often owing to antibiotic treatment before culture, but might also be related to transport media and isolation media. Necropsy tissues and fluids are also particularly difficult *(2,3)*.

Culture is very important because the availability of an isolate growing in the laboratory will allow species designation, antibiotic-susceptibility testing (*see* Chapter 6), and characterization of an isolate for public-health and epidemiological purposes (*see* Chapters 8–22). An evident factor of importance is also that almost every microbiological laboratory can perform cultures for meningococci.

2. Materials (for Diagnostic Sampling Procedures)

In patients with suspected invasive meningococcal disease, it is logical to take cultures from the suspected primary site of infection (throat/nasophar-

From: *Methods in Molecular Medicine, vol. 67: Meningococcal Disease: Methods and Protocols*
Edited by: A. J. Pollard and M. C. J. Maiden © Humana Press Inc., Totowa, NJ

ynx), and sites of septic metastasis (e.g. cerebrospinal fluid [CSF], joint fluid, etc.) in conjunction with blood cultures. Other superficial/local sights should also be considered if clinical signs and symptoms are suggestive (e.g., skin scrapings or aspirate from petechiae or purpuric rash, conjunctiva, middle-ear fluid, secretions from sinuses, sputum, urogenital).

2.1. The Referral Note Accompanying the Sample(s)

Recognition or suspicion of meningococcal disease in the clinical setting requires laboratory confirmation whenever possible as this information can be critical for managing the individual patient, outbreak management, epidemiological purposes, and for vaccine evaluation. Providing the laboratory with appropriate information can aid this process. Besides basic information (patient identification, sample, date, and sender) the clinical data, tests requested, and diagnostic questions can be crucial in directing the optimal handling and reporting of the specimen in the laboratory.

For throat and nasopharyngeal cultures, it is mandatory to request explicitly culture for meningococci. This is most important because many bacterial colonies of the normal flora look the same as meningococci, which can be in a minority. The inclusion of selective culture medium is therefore necessary.

It is also important to inform the laboratory if antibiotics have been given prior to sampling and if any antibiotic treatment is planned, because this will direct appropriate antibacterial-susceptibility testing. The clinicians' contact details should always be available so that information can be directed to the appropriate individual.

2.2. Blood Cultures

A number of blood-culture systems with different indicator systems are in general use. Most of them utilize bottles containing culture media into which the blood is inoculated ***(4,5)***. The manufacturer's instructions should be followed for the use of these blood-culture systems. For meningococci, media with higher concentrations of sodium polyanethol sulfonate (SPS) should be avoided. Any blood-culturing system must be evaluated for its ability to support growth of fastidious bacteria like meningococci.

Detailed descriptions of the procedures for collection of blood for culture is outlined in laboratory methods published by the Centers for Disease Control and Prevention (CDC) in Atlanta, and the World Health Organization (WHO) in Geneva ***(6,7)***. The following general points should be noted:

1. The concentration of meningococci in blood can be low, less than 1 cfu/mL (*see* **ref. *8***). It is therefore important that the cultured blood volume is as large as possible. For smaller children, 1–3 mL is sufficient, whereas 5–10 mL should be recommended from adults.

2. The concentration of meningococci in blood is probably not constant over time. It is therefore recommended that two blood cultures are performed to increase the likelihood of catching live meningococci.
3. In critically ill patients, it is only feasible to take one blood culture, preferably prior to antibiotics. In benign recurrent meningococcaemia blood cultures may have to be repeated several times, preferably at the early phase of chills and fever in order to obtain a positive result.
4. Inoculated blood culture bottles are kept at room temperature until delivery (as fast as possible) to the laboratory.
5. If certified incubators are available at clinics outside the laboratory, the bottles may be kept at 35–37°C to start the growth process before delivery to the laboratory.

2.3. Cerebrospinal Fluid

In patients with signs/symptoms suggesting meningitis/meningoencephalitis, a lumbar puncture is usually performed ***(9)***, providing that there are no absolute contraindications, such as signs of raised intracranial pressure, substantial hemodynamic instability, or known coagulopathy. The concentration of meningococci in CSF varies considerably between patients from 0 up to 10^7 cfu/mL ***(10)***. When antibiotics have been given intravenously for treatment, it can be assumed that meningococci stay alive somewhat longer in CSF than in blood. As a result, lumbar puncture might reasonably be deferred for a few hours until the patient has been fully assessed and contraindications to lumbar puncture excluded. The following general points should be noted:

1. CSF is collected in 3–4 sterile tubes preferably with ≥ 1 mL CSF/tube.
2. Culture bottles can also be inoculated with CSF at the bedside.
3. Examinations are performed for CSF white blood cells, the proportion of polymorphonuclear/mononuclear white blood cells, glucose, protein, lactate (1 tube); microbiological diagnosis (2 tubes) and 1 extra tube, just in case.
4. Transport should be as rapid as possible to the laboratory (minimize "needle to laboratory time") with the sample at room temperature.
5. Trans-isolate (TI) medium ***(11)*** was designed to allow survival of sensitive bacteria in ambient temperature even in tropical settings for long times. In this medium, meningococci can stay alive for weeks after inoculation with infected CSF, thus allowing safe transport from remote areas to diagnostic laboratories far away ***(6,7)***.

2.4. Throat and Nasopharynx

The optimal place from which to take a swab for culture of meningococci in patients and healthy carriers is not known. With good selective culture media, however, it is clear that carriers with or without local symptoms carry meningococci on the tonsils more often than in the nasopharynx with sample taken via the nasal route ***(12)***. Antibiotic activity is decreased on the membranes of the throat and perhaps the upper respiratory tract and meningococci can subsequently survive there ***(13)*** for some hours ***(14)*** in spite of effective treatment of invasive meningococcal disease with high doses of parenteral antibiotics. For this reason, throat cultures should be routinely performed for all cases with suspected meningococcal disease ***(14)***. General observations include:

1. The swab used must be proved to be nontoxic to *Neisseria gonorrhoeae* and meningococci and is often provided with charcoal as the absorbing material for toxic substances.
2. The charcoal destroys most of the quality of direct microscopy (DM) and should subsequently not be used if this is requested.
3. If a swab has to be transported it must be in a high-quality reduced medium, such as different variants of Stuart transport medium ***(15)***, kept and transported at room temperature.
4. In scientific/epidemiological studies of healthy carriers, when it is important to find almost all carriers, direct inoculation on culture media at the bedside and immediate incubation (at least placed in a CO_2 atmosphere), e.g., in a candle jar, is recommended.
5. It has been calculated that 90% of the material on a swab is lost by just putting it in a transport medium ***(12)***. Subsequently, up to 40% of meningococcal carriers can turn out culture-negative when using Stuart transport medium if the sample is kept at room temperature for 24 h before inoculation of culture media, as compared to direct inoculation ***(12)***.
6. It is also well known that taking more than one culture from the same site gives additional yield in the case of hemolytic streptococci ***(16)***. It would be surprising if the situation was different for meningococci.
7. In some studies, it is important to know if several strains of meningococci are carried at the same time (*see* Chapter 19).

2.5. Maculopapular Skin Lesions: Petechiae, Echymoses

Meningococci are well known for their propensity for hematogenous spread, with adhesion/trapping in the periphery, and damage of vessel walls. This is most noticeable in the skin where maculopapular eruptions without pustulation and/or extravasation of blood will give the characteristic picture ranging from single petechiae to extensive cutaneous bleeding. Differential diagnosis concerning the hemorrhagic skin lesions differs from place to place and over time, but disseminated streptococcal disease, measles, hemorrhagic viral diseases, conditions causing thrombocytopaenia, coagulopathies, and vasculitis should always be considered. In patients with dark skin, the manifestations can be difficult to detect and the conjunctiva, oral cavity, hand palms, and foot soles may be the only locations where these lesions can be seen.

Meningococci can be isolated from fresh skin lesions. A high diagnostic sensitivity is reached by direct immunofluorescence (IFL) ***(3)***. Owing to lack of high quality and commercially available IFL conjugates, this method has only rarely reached the status of a routine diagnostic procedure. The number of preserved meningococci is fairly low and Gram staining/methylene blue staining may be used ***(17,18)***. The use of acridine orange (AO) staining ***(19)*** has not been evaluated. Culture from lesions can be helpful. After scraping away the outer epidermis, if possible without causing bleeding, a swab is taken preferably with direct inoculation of culture media. Alternatively, if the lesion is deeper, aspiration may be used with a fine-gauge needle ***(17)***.

2.6. Joint Fluid

Arthritis, usually of a big joint, sometimes results from the systemic spread of meningococci giving signs/symptoms in the acute phase. A so called "reactive arthritis" (sterile) can also be seen after a few days of treatment. In these cases, a diagnostic aspiration of the affected joint is recommended with further handling undertaken as for CSF. Joint fluid could be inoculated into bottles at the bedside, but it is also important to keep some of the fluid in a sterile tube for diagnosis at the laboratory as direct microscopy after Gram and AO staining should be done on the fresh material.

2.7. Other Samples

For other body fluids, the principles are the same as for joint fluid. In cases when very small volumes are aspirated, it is suggested that the material is directly inoculated into a blood-culture bottle. This procedure can include aspiration and reinstallation of a few mL of the broth from the bottle in order to wash out aspirated material from the inside of the needle.

Diagnostic cultures from urethra, cervix and rectum are often taken with a request for *N. gonorrhoeae*. Single patients harbor meningococci ***(20)***, with or without symptoms, probably encountered from the throat (compare gonococci in throat cultures). Meningococci can cause lower respiratory-tract infections and may constitute approx 1% of community-acquired pneumonia in Western countries ***(21,22)***. On rare occasions, meningococci can be isolated from almost any site ***(23)***.

3. Methods for Laboratory Diagnostic Procedures

3.1 Culture Media for Meningococci

Chocolate agar is a rich non-selective medium that is generally used for demanding aerobic bacteria like meningococci, gonococci, and Haemophilus species ***(24,25)***. A formula that is used in accredited clinical diagnostic laboratories has the following constituents: 36 g GC II agar base, 10 g haemoglobin powder, 100 mL horse serum, 10 mL IsoVitalex enrichment, and 900 mL of high-quality water.

This medium can be modified to be fairly selective for meningococci (and gonococci) by addition of a mixture of antibiotics like vancosin - colistin - nystatin (VCN Inhibitor, 10 mL/L of agar). Some laboratories also add trimethoprim. For a detailed presentation of different media, see the CDC/ WHO protocols *(6,7)*.

3.2. Identification of Meningococci by Culture

Plate cultures are inspected after overnight incubation at 35–37°C in humid 5% CO_2 and after 2 d. The broth cultures are inspected daily for turbidity indicating growth or according to the specific suggestions from the manufacturer. If bacterial growth is suspected DM after Gram staining is conducted and two drops of the broth spread on culture media (*see* **Subheading 3.1.**).

Meningococcal colonies are smooth and nonpigmented and, after 18–24 h incubation, 1–2 mm in diameter. From a nonsterile site, the size is dependent on the presence of other competing bacteria. The colonies look the same on chocolate agar medium (nonselective) and selective medium including antibiotics and have a distinctive smell.

Suspected colonies are tested for fast oxidase activity and those giving positive results subjected to Gram staining and microscopy for Gram-negative diplococci. Colonies suspected to be meningococci are subcultured and biochemically tested for degradation of glucose and maltose without degradation of fructose and lactose (ONPG-test) by in house prepared test-plates or commercially available testkits like Rapid NH or api NH. Reference strains for control of all the reactions must always be included. A rapid system which does not require growth but utilizes the preformed enzymes in a heavy suspension can also be used *(26)*. In this system, the individual high-quality sugars are kept in buffer with a pH-indicator. Ready made mixtures can be kept frozen in a mictrotiter format, thus facilitating practical use. Some meningococcal isolates do not degrade maltose in the system used, thus behaving like gonococci *(27)*. In inexperienced hands, these isolates can then be wrongly identified as *N. gonorrhoeae*, a diagnosis that may have serious consequences. On rare occasions, degradation of glucose can be weak or absent.

For problem isolates, additional tests have to be performed, including assays for meningococcal antigens like serogroup/type/subtype, biological requirements, genogroup/type/subtype, or additional genetic methods. Reference laboratories provide essential support in these situations.

3.3. Sensitivity Testing for Antibiotics

Sensitivity testing for antibiotics used for treatment of patients and for prophylaxis (prophylactic treatment) of proven or suspected meningococcal carriers at risk should be performed (*see* Chapter 6). Commonly tested antibiotics are penicillin G, ampicillin, a cephalosporin such as cefotaxime or ceftriaxone, chloramphenicol, rifampicin, and a quinolone. The E-test (AB Biodisk) has proven itself to give reliable MIC values ***(28)*** providing a high-quality medium is used and an experienced technician performs the test. Sulphonamide is seldom used these days for treatment or prophylaxis, but sensitivity/resistance (breakpoint 10 mg/L) is an additional characteristic of an isolate that is used for epidemiological purposes. Tests for β-lactamases with, for example, a chromogen cephalosporin test ***(29)*** should be performed, in spite of the fact that less than 10 such strains have been reported so far in the world ***(30)***.

3.4. Grouping of Meningococci

Serogrouping or genogrouping ***(31–33)*** should be done as soon as possible because this provides valuable information concerning the risk of clusters of cases and the possibility of the use of meningococcal vaccines as a prophylactic tool (*see* Chapter 9). Uncommon groups also indicate possible immune defects, including complement deficiencies, in the host, which can be of importance in the short as well as long perspective.

3.5. Blood Culture

A great number of systems for blood culture are available ***(4,5)***. In a European survey among reference laboratories, the Bactec and the BactAlert systems were predominantly used (European Monitoring Group on Meningococci, 1998). In the laboratory, blood cultures are incubated at 35–37°C for 7–10 d. If there are indications of bacterial growth, a bottle is opened and material taken for DM by Gram stain (*see* below) and eventually AO staining ***(19)***. Tests for meningococcal antigens/DNA can be used on blood-culture material to strengthen the meningococcal suspicion when typical diplococci are seen and also if clinical suspicion is high despite negative cultures (*see* Chapter 4).

One drop of blood-culture material is inoculated on chocolate agar, spread, and incubated at 35–37°C in 5% CO_2-enriched humid atmosphere. The plates are inspected after overnight incubation at 35–37°C in humid 5% CO_2 and after 2 d. In situations with high clinical suspicion of meningococcal bacteremia, the inoculated bottles can be subcultured as mentioned on chocolate medium after 2–4 and 7–10 d despite lack of "signs" of bacterial activity.

3.6. Cerebrospinal Fluid

DM and culture are the main methods used. They are sometimes supplemented by specific nonculture tests, either immediately after receiving the CSF at the laboratory, or when the cultures are negative after 2–3 d in spite of per-

Table 1
Protocol for Laboratory Processing of CSF Samples

Clear CSF (centrifuge if < 1 mL at 600*g* for 10 min)	Turbid CSF (no centrifugation)
1. Microscopy: make two slides for	1. Microscopy make 3–4 slides for
a. Gram staining	a. Gram staining
b. Acridine orange-staining	b. Acridine orange-staining
	c. Slide for teaching/extra
2. Culture	2. Culture
a. Chocolate agar	a. Chocolate agar
b. Anaerobic blood-agar plate for anaerobic incubation	b. Anaerobic blood-agar plate for anaerobic incubation
c. Broth inoculation	c. Broth inoculation
	d. Consider direct inoculation for antibiotic sensitivity testing
	e. Consider optochine test (on blood-agar medium) when suspecting pneumococci
Consider antigen detection	Consider antigen detection
Consider DNA detection	Consider DNA detection

sistent suspicion of meningococcal disease. Some of these methods are described in other chapters of this book and comprise antigen-detection methods including latex- and co-agglutination techniques ***(10)***; direct immunofluorescence with specific conjugates ***(3,10)***; enzyme immunoassays ***(34,35)***; and DNA amplification methods like PCR for different target sequences like the 16S rRNA gene ***(36–38)*** and the *ctrA* gene. A protocol for the laboratory processing of CSF samples is shown in **Table 1**.

3.6.1. Direct Microscopy

1. Apply a drop of CSF on each of the clean microscope slides.
2. Let the drops air dry.
3. Fix by heating in a bunsen burner flame from below.
4. Mark the sample area with a wax crayon or by engraving.
5. Apply Gram and AO stains according to local protocols. Gram staining can be performed as follows:
   a. Flood the slide with crystal violet.
   b. After 1 min wash the slide with water.
   c. Flood the slide with Lugol's iodine.
   d. After 1 min decolorize the slide with 95% alcohol.

e. Wash the slide immediately with water.
f. Counter-stain for at least 15 s with carbol-fuchsin.
g. Wash with water.

The stains may be purchased commercially or prepared according to CDC/WHO ***(6,7)*** or the Clinical Microbiology Procedures Handbook ***(24)***, alt. Manual of Clinical Microbiology ***(25)***.

5. Dry the slides by using filter paper outside the sample area and air dry.
6. Read the Gram-stained slide ×1000 in a high-quality, clean light microscope and the AO-stained slide in a high-quality, clean, and optimally adjusted fluorescent microscope ×400–1000.

AO stain is commercially available and staining is performed by flooding the fixed slide with the solution and washing after 2 min with water. After drying, the slide can be read at a magnification of ×400–1000.

In 60% or more of untreated cases of meningococcal meningitis, Gram-negative diplococci of Neisserial shape can be seen extracellularly and also phagocytosed in neutrophile granulocytes, thus suggesting the diagnosis ***(10)***.

With AO staining, the detection level (expressed as bacterial concentration) can be judged to be 10 times lower as compared to Gram stain, which can be calculated to give a diagnostic sensitivity of at least 70%. AO staining is more easy to read (compared to Gram staining) because Gram-negative bacteria give low contrast to the red-stained debris/protein material commonly seen in meningitis.

The less time there is between LP and slide-making, the better the quality of DM slides. This fact can be used to secure sample quality in field situations by making the slides (without staining) bedside just after LP.

3.6.2. Culture

Culture is performed by placing two drops (about 100 μL) on a high-quality, rich, nonselective solid-agar medium like chocolate agar, spreading the plate, then incubating at 35–37°C in humid 5% CO_2. A candle jar ***(39)*** in 35–37°C is another way to create acceptable incubation conditions in laboratories without CO_2 incubators. Enrichment is achieved by inoculating a ~200 μL of CSF in blood-culture bottles (with nutrient additive owing to lack of the blood) or a broth medium like Müller-Hinton broth for 7–10 d. Just as with blood cultures, blind sub-cultures onto agar could be performed at intervals. It is wise to try to keep some original CSF in the refrigerator/freezer for any further diagnostic procedures.

3.7. Joint Fluid

Owing to high concentration of white blood cells (polymorphonuclear leukocytes dominating) and high protein levels, the Gram-stained samples can be difficult to interpret, especially for Gram-negative bacteria. In these cases, staining with methylene blue *(25)* can be superior owing to less denaturation of the material. The ability of meningococci to stay intact for a while intracellularly after phagocytosis can be helpful in the interpretation. AO staining gives an easier picture than Gram staining and with typical diplococci side by side it is easy to determine the presence of pathogenic Neisseria (do not forget *N. gonorrhoeae*). Culture is performed as for CSF (*see* **Subheading 3.6.**). Joint fluid can, if necessary, be studied further with nonculture methods (*see* Chapters 3 and 4).

3.8. Urogenital Samples

The culture media for gonococci readily allow meningococci to multiply and can cause confusion, both species being rapidly oxidase positive Gram-negative diplococci *(20)*. Growth characteristics (bigger colonies) and species diagnostic tests (sugar degradation or agglutination/co-agglutination tests) will in most cases give clear-cut results, but further characterization is sometimes needed with serological, biological, or genetic methods.

3.9. Reporting of Clinical Isolates

In many countries, meningococcal isolates from normally sterile sites should be reported from the diagnostic laboratories to a National Health Authority and the strains sent for further characterization to a National Reference Laboratory in order to get reliable epidemiological data.

3.10. Storage Meningococcal Isolates

It is often useful to preserve the strains of meningococci in the diagnostic clinical laboratory at either –70°C or freeze-dried for any additional examination in the near or far future *(6,7)*. A reliable medium for storage for many years in –70°C has the following composition: 30.0 g Trypticase soy broth, 3.0 g yeast extract, 0.5 g agar No. 2, 700 mL water (RO), 300 mL horse serum. Mix the first four items. Adjust pH to 7.5 with 2 *M* NaOH. Sterilize at 121°C for 15 min. Allow to cool to +50°C in water bath. Add horse serum and mix. Check pH 7.50 ± 0.1. Dispense in sterile tubes, 2 mL/tube.

3.11. Selective Media

Because of the possibility of meningococcal infection, it is always a good strategy for culture diagnosis to include a very rich nonselective culture medium, such as chocolate agar, for most clinical samples. A high-quality, selective medium like VCN(T) (*see* **Subheading 3.1.**) should be included for culture concerning pathogenic Neisseria from normally non sterile sites and when mixed infections can be suspected. This includes necropsy material.

References

1. van Deuren, M., Brandtzaeg, P., and van der Meer, J. W. M. (2000) Update on meningococcal disease with emphasis on pathogenesis and clinical management. *Clin. Microbiol. Rev.* **13,** 144–166.
2. Danielsson, D., Nathorst-Windahl, G., and Saldén, T. (1971) Use of immunofluorescence for identification of Haemophilus influenzae and Neisseria meningitidis in postmortem human tissue. *Ann. NY Acad. Sci.* **177,** 23–31.
3. Danielsson, D. and Forsum, U. (1975) Diagnosis of Neisseria infections by defined immunofluorescence. Methodologic aspects and applications. *Ann. NY Acad. Sci.* **254,** 334–349.
4. Weinstein, M. P. (1996) Current blood culture methods and systems: clinical concepts, technology, and interpretation of results. *Clin. Inf. Dis.* **23,** 40–46.
5. Mylotte, J. M. and Tayara, A. (2000) Blood cultures: clinical aspects and controversies. *Eur. J. Clin. Microbiol. Infect. Dis.* **19,** 157–163.
6. Centers for Disease Control and Prevention (1998) Laboratory methods for the diagnosis of meningitis caused by Neisseria meningitidis, Streptococcus pneumoniae, and Haemophilus influenzae. Available via Internet http://www.cdc.gov/ncidod/dbmd/diseaseinfo/menigitis_manual.pdf
7. World Health Organization (1999) Laboratory methods for the diagnosis of meningitis caused by Neisseria meningitidis, Streptococcus pneumoniae, and Haemophilus influenzae. WHO/CDS/CSR/EDC/99.7.
8. Cartwright, K. A. V. (ed.) (1995) *Meningococcal disease*. John Wiley and Sons. Chichester, UK.
9. Stephenson, T. (1998) Coning may occur without lumbar puncture being done. *BMJ* **316,** 1015.
10. Olcén, P. (1978) Serological methods for rapid diagnosis of Haemophilus influenzae, Neisseria meningitidis and Streptococcus pneumoniae in cerebrospinal fluid: a comparison of co-agglutination, immunofluorescence and immunoelectrophoresis. *Scand. J. Infect. Dis.* **10,** 283–289.
11. Ajello, G. W., Feeley, J. C., Hayes, P. S., Reingold, A. L., Bolan, G., Broome, C. V., and Phillips, C. J. (1984) Trans-Isolate Medium: a new medium for primary culturing and transport of Neisseria meningitidis, Streptococcus pneumoniae and Heamophilus influenzae. *J. Clin. Microbiol.* **20,** 55–58.
12. Olcén, P., Kjellander, J., Danielsson, D., and Linquist, B. L. (1979) Culture diagnosis of meningococcal carriers. *J. Clin. Path.* **32,** 1222–1225.
13. Abramson, J. S. and Spika, J. S. (1985) Persistence of Neisseria meningitidis in the upper respiratory tract after intravenous antibiotic therapy for systemic meningococcal disease. *J. Infect. Dis.* **151,** 370–371.
14. Cartwright, K., Reilly, S., White, D., and Stuart, J. (1992) Early treatment with parenteral penicillin in meningococcal disease. *BMJ* **305,** 143–147.
15. Gästrin, B., Kallings, L. O., and Marcetic, A. (1968) The survival time for different bacteria in various transport media. *Acta Pathol. Microbiol. Scand.* **74,** 371–380.

16. Kellog, J. A. and Manzella, J. P. (1986) Detection of group A streptococci in the laboratory or physician's office. Culture vs antibody methods. *JAMA* **255,** 2638–2642.
17. van Deuren, M., van Dijke, B. J, Koopman, R. J., Horrevorts, A. M., Meis, J. F., Santman, F. N., et al. (1993) Rapid diagnosis of acute meningococcal infection by needle aspiration of skin lesions. *BMJ* **306,** 1229–1232.
18. Periappuram, M., Taylor, M. R. H., and Keane, C. T. (1995) Rapid detection of meningococci from petechiae in acute meningococcal infection. *J. Infect.* **31,** 201–203.
19. Kronvall, G. and Myhre, E. (1977) Differential staining of bacteria in clinical specimens using acridine orange buffered at low pH. *Acta Pathol. Microbiol. Scand.* **85,** 249–254.
20. Hagman, M., Forslin, L., Moi, H., and Danielsson, D. (1991) Neisseria meningitidis in specimens from urogenital sites. Is increased awareness necessary? *Sex. Transm. Dis.* **18,** 228–232.
21. Koppes, G. M., Ellenbogen, C., and Gebhart, R. J. (1977) Group Y meningococcal disease in United States Air Force recruits. *Am. J. Med.* **62,** 661–666.
22. Weigtman, N. C. and Johnstone, D. J. (1999) Three cases of pneumonia due to Neisseria meningitidis, including serogroup W-135. *Eur. J. Clin. Microbiol. Infect. Dis.* **18,** 456–458.
23. Odegaard, A. (1983) Unusual manifestations of meningococcal infection. A review. *NIPH Ann.* **6,** 59-63.
24. Isenberg, H. D. (ed.) (1992) *Clinical Microbiology Procedures Handbook.* American Society for Microbiology, Washington, DC.
25. Murray, P. R. (ed.) (1999) *Manual of Clinical Microbiology*, 7th ed. ASM Press, Washington, DC.
26. Kellog, D. S. Jr. and Turner, E. M. (1973) Rapid fermentation confirmation of Neisseria gonorrhoeae. *Appl. Microbiol.* **25,** 550–552.
27. Olcén, P., Danielsson, D., and Kjellander, J. (1978) Laboratory identification of pathogenic Neisseria with special regard to atypical strains: an evaluation of sugar degradation, immunofluorescence and co-agglutination tests. *Acta Pathol. Microbiol. Scand.* **86,** 327–334.
28. Gomez-Herruz, P., González-Palacios, R., Romanyk, J., Cuadros, J. A., and Ena, J. (1995) Evaluation of the Etest for penicillin susceptibility testing of Neisseria meningitidis. *Diagn. Microbiol. Infect. Dis.* **21,** 115–117.
29. O'Callaghan, C. H., Morris, A., Kirby, S. M., and Shingler, A. H. (1972) Novel method for detection of β-lactamase by using a chromogenic cephalosporin substrate. *Antimicrob. Agents Chemother.* **1,** 283–288.
30. Bäckman, A., Orvelid, P., Vazquez, J. A., Sköld, O., and Olcén, P. (2000) Complete sequence of a β-lactamase-encoding plasmid in Neisseria meningitidis. *Antimicrob. Agents Chemother.* **44,** 210–212.
31. Orvelid, P., Bäckman, A., and Olcén, P. (1999) PCR identification of a group A Neisseria meningitidis gene in cerebrospinal fluid. *Scand. J. Infect. Dis.* **31,** 481–483.

32. Borrow, R., Claus, H., Guiver, M., Smart, L., Jones, D. M., Kaczmarski, L. B., Frosch, M., and Fox, A. J. (1997) Non-culture diagnosis and serogroup determination of meningococcal B and C infection by a sialyltransferase (siaD) PCR ELISA. *Epidemiol. Infect.* **118,** 111–117.
33. Borrow, R., Claus, H., Chaudhry, U., Guiver, M., Kaczmarski, L. B., Frosch, M., and Fox, A. J. (1998) siaD PCR ELISA for confirmation and identification of serogroup Y and W135 meningococcal infections. *FEMS Microbiol. Lett.* **159,** 209–214.
34. Salih, M. A. M., Ahmed, H. S., Hofvander, Y., Danielsson, D., and Olcén, P. (1989) Rapid diagnosis of bacterial meningitis by an enzyme immunoassay of cerebrospinal fluid. *Epidemiol. Infect.* **103,** 301–310.
35. Salih, M. A. M., Ahmed, A. A., Ahmed, H. S., and Olcén, P. (1995) An ELISA assay for the rapid diagnosis of acute bacterial meningitis. *Ann. Trop. Paediatr.* **15,** 273–278.
36. Rådström, P., Bäckman, A., Qian, N., Kragsbjerg, P., Påhlson, C., and Olcén, P. (1994) Detection of bacterial DNA in cerebrospinal fluid by an assay for simultaneous detection of Neisseria meningitidis, Haemophilus influenzae, and streptococci using a seminested PCR strategy. *J. Clin. Microbiol.* **32,** 2738–2744.
37. Olcén, P., Lantz, P.-G., Bäckman, A., and Rådström, P. (1995) Rapid diagnosis of bacterial meningitidis by a seminested PCR strategy. *Scand. J. Infect. Dis.* **27,** 537–539.
38. Bäckman, A., Lantz, P.-G., Rådström, P., and Olcén, P. (1999) Evaluation of an extended diagnostic PCR assay for rapid detection and verification of bacterial meningitis in CSF and other biological samples. *Mol. Cell Probes* **13,** 49–60.
39. Danielsson, D. and Johannisson, G. (1973) Culture diagnosis of gonorrhoea. A comparison of the yield with selective and non-selective gonococcal culture media inoculated in the clinic and after transport of specimens. *Acta Derm. Venereol. (Stockh)* **53,** 75–80.

3

PCR Diagnosis

Malcolm Guiver and Ray Borrow

1. Introduction

Nonculture diagnosis is of increasing importance in maximizing case ascertainment of disease owing to *Neisseria meningitidis* ***(1)***. In the United Kingdom (UK), greater use of pre-admission antibiotics has lead to a steady decline in the total number of cases confirmed by culture, compared to the number reported to the Office for National Statistics (ONS). In addition, since the introduction of serogroup C oligosaccharide-protein conjugate vaccine ***(2)*** in the UK and its imminent introduction elsewhere, it is necessary to maximize case ascertainment to determine the true level of disease in the population and establish the impact of vaccination programs. Although serodiagnosis is available for confirmation, results are retrospective and often inconclusive ***(1)***. Amplification by polymerase chain reaction (PCR) provides a rapid, highly sensitive, and specific method for detecting meningococcal DNA from clinical samples. A number of assays have been described, some of which provide additional information about serological markers such as serogroup, serotype, and serosubtype ***(3–10)***. The introduction of PCR at the UK Public Health Laboratory Service (PHLS) Meningococcal Reference Unit (MRU) has resulted in a dramatic increase in the number of confirmed cases of meningococcal disease ***(11)***. In 1998 an additional 56% of cases were confirmed by PCR alone compared to those confirmed by culture only.

To take advantage of the sensitivity offered by PCR appropriate, DNA extraction procedures on suitable clinical samples must first be carried out. Protocols for the optimal extraction from cerebrospinal fluid (CSF), ethelyne diamine tetraacetic acid (EDTA) whole blood, plasma, and serum are described here. Evaluation of the Qiagen and Gentra capture column systems described

From: *Methods in Molecular Medicine, vol. 67: Meningococcal Disease: Methods and Protocols*
Edited by: A. J. Pollard and M. C. J. Maiden © Humana Press Inc., Totowa, NJ

in this chapter show that they perform equally well for EDTA blood extraction. However, for CSFs, plasma- and serum-increased sensitivity is achieved by extraction with DNAzol extraction and ethanol precipitation. Alternative capture column methods provide for more reproducible results, reduce the operator variation associated with precipitation methods, and are more readily automated. Although CSF is still the preferred sample for optimal recovery, extraction of meningococcal DNA from an EDTA blood sample offers sensitive detection without the risk associated with lumbar puncture. Plasma and serum samples offer less optimal recovery of meningococcal DNA. A comparison of plasma and EDTA blood samples for the detection of meningococcal DNA for cultured confirmed cases showed 65% were detected using plasma compared to 93% from EDTA blood. It is also worth noting that although PCR can detect nonculturable organisms, an early sample will increase the chances of detection. A recent study of hospitalized cases of meningococcal disease in which serial samples were taken showed that meningococcal DNA could still be detected by PCR 3 d after initiation of antibiotic therapy (unpublished observations).

Some of the first meningococcal PCR assays were based upon the insertion sequence (IS) element IS*1106* ***(7)*** and were adapted to a PCR enzyme-linked immunosorbent assay (ELISA) format to increase specificity and sensitivity for the nonculture confirmation of meningococcal infection ***(8,9)***. IS elements were chosen as gene targets for nonculture diagnosis of bacterial infections owing to the presence of multiple copies within the bacterial genome, which, it was hoped, would increase sensitivity ***(12)***. However, the inherent genetic mobility of these elements ***(13)*** may result in their transfer among species and genera ***(14)*** and, during an evaluation period of the IS*1106* PCR ELISA, a number of false-positive results were caused by organisms other than *N. meningitidis* ***(15)***.

Serosubtype and serotype information may be obtained by amplification and sequence-specific probe detection of either the *porA* or *porB* gene, respectively. Methods for the amplification by PCR of *porA* ***(4)*** and *porB* genes ***(16)*** have been described but, owing to the large amount of sequence variation in these genes, and the correspondingly high numbers of serosubtypes or serotypes, a probe-based system is not advised and sequence-based typing is more appropriate ***(16–19)***.

Amplification of the 16S rRNA gene using conserved nucleotide sequences for detection of all bacterial causes of meningitis has been described ***(5)***. However, contaminating bacterial DNA present in some of the PCR reagents restricts the level of sensitivity achievable with this target ***(20)*** and consequently it is presently not recommended as a suitable target for amplification of bacterial DNA from clinical samples.

In developing PCR assays, we have focused on two gene targets: firstly the *ctrA* gene, which forms part of the capsular biosynthesis locus ***(21)***; and the sialyltransferase gene (*siaD*), which encodes the gene responsible for the polymerization of sialic acid to the polysialic acid chain *(22)*. The meningococcal capsule is a highly conserved virulence factor and the capsular operon includes a gene (*ctrA*) that encodes for a conserved outer-membrane protein (OMP) involved in the transport of the capsular polysaccharide *(21)*. The *ctrA* gene is therefore an ideal target for detection of meningococci by PCR and conserved regions of this gene have therefore been exploited, enabling the amplification of a product from all clinically significant serogroups, thereby providing an initial screening test for all samples. Serogroup-specific sequences within the *siaD* gene have been exploited in designing PCR assays for the identification and discrimination of operons encoding serogroups B, C, Y, and W135 *(10,23)*. A PCR assay has been described for serogroup A, although the authors have no experience with this assay *(24)*.

Using these gene targets, assays have been developed using three detection systems: agarose gel-based detection, PCR ELISA-based detection, and automated amplification and detection using a fluorescent-based PE-ABI Taqman™ system. The first PCR assays described to detect meningococcal DNA were based upon agarose-gel electrophoresis followed by visualization with ethidium bromide and ultraviolet (UV) light *(4–7)*. Agarose gel-based systems offer a low cost option, but they are not suitable for high throughput, are labor-intensive, and are more prone to contamination problems. Sensitivity and specificity can be enhanced by Southern blotting and probe hybridization, but this is a cumbersome and time-consuming procedure.

ELISA-based detection of amplified products using liquid-phase probe hybridization provides equivalent sensitivity and specificity to Southern hybridization *(8)*. The Boehringer-Mannheim PCR ELISA system developed for the detection of meningococcal DNA is in a microtiter plate format, and enables rapid processing and high throughput of samples *(8–10)*. During amplification, the PCR product is labeled with digoxigenin that is subsequently hybridized with a biotin-labeled probe that specifically binds to its complementary sequence. Hybridized probes are immobilized on to streptavidin-coated plates and subsequently detected by anti-digoxigenin peroxidase conjugate and enzyme substrate. Post-PCR processing of amplified products still presents a potential contamination risk. It is therefore recommended to treat PCR reaction mix with uracil DNA glycosylase to reduce the risk of contamination.

Development of the homogeneous TaqMan or 5′-exonuclease assay, which incorporates a fluorescent-labeled probe, enables detection of accumulated product during the amplification process ("real-time PCR"). This assay has been developed as an automated PCR amplification and detection system *(25)*. The PE-ABI 7700 instrument is a closed tube system that eliminates post-PCR processing and consequently virtually eliminates contamination owing to amplified product. The 96-well microtiter format enables high throughput and rapid processing of samples. The TaqMan assay utilizes a dual-labeled fluorescent probe, the 5′ end of which is labeled with one of several reporter dyes such as FAM (6, carboxyfluorescein) and the 3′ end with the fluorescent dye TAMRA (6 carboxy-tetramethylrhodamine) ***(26–29)***. The spatial proximity to the reporter dye quenches the fluorescent emission and during amplification of a specific target sequence the primer is extended towards the probe. The probe is digested by the 5′ exonuclease activity of *Taq* polymerase, releasing the reporter dye and producing a relative increase in fluorescent signal. Automated monitoring of the fluorescent signal is possible using the PE-ABI sequence detection system 7700 during thermal cycling. The monitored reporter signal for a reaction is identified as positive when the fluorescent signal exceeds a background threshold level. Amplification at this point is exponential and has been shown to be the most reliable approach to quantitating input target ***(28–29)***. Taqman assays have been described in the detection of several pathogenic organisms including hepatitis C ***(30)***, Salmonella species ***(31)***, *Listeria monocytogenes* ***(32)***, *Escherichia coli* 0157:H7 ***(33)***, and *Mycobacterium tuberculosis* ***(34)***.

The Taqman *ctrA* assay has been shown to be specific for *N. meningitidis*, whereas the IS*1106* assay gave false-positive results with a number of nonmeningococcal isolates ***(25)***. Sensitivities of the Taqman *ctrA*, IS*1106*, and *siaD* assays, when testing samples from culture-confirmed cases, were found to be 64, 69, and 50%, respectively, for plasma and CSF samples. Using EDTA samples, a sensitivity of 93% for the *ctrA* and 89% for the *siaD* assays was achieved compared to culture-confirmed cases ***(25)***.

The following methods describe nonculture-based PCR detection of meningococcal DNA and serogroup determination from clinical samples. Protocols for DNA extraction from a range of sample types, PCR amplification and detection using low cost agarose gel electrophoresis, a PCR ELISA system, and the fully automated Perkin-Elmer Applied Biosystems (PE-ABI) Taqman Sequence Detection System are described.

2. Materials

2.1. DNA Extraction

2.1.1. DNA Extraction Using DNAzol from Clinical Samples

1. DNAzol Molecular Research Center (MRC) Cincinnati USA (Cat no. DN 127) or Life Technologies, (Cat no 10503-035). Store at room temperature.
2. Polyacryl carrier, MRC (Cat. no. PC-152) Helena Biosciences (Cat no. PC-152). Store at +4°C.
3. 95% ethanol.
4. Aerosol-resistant tips.

5. 1.5-mL Sarstedt tubes with hinged screw cap (Cat no. 72.692.105) or equivalent.
6. Sterile fine-tipped pastets.

2.1.2. Preparation of Positive Amplification Control Material

1. Spectrophotometer capable of measuring optical densities (ODs) at 650 nm.

2.1.3. Preparation of Extraction Controls

1. Human plasma negative for meningococcal DNA.

2.1.4. Extraction of DNA from Whole Blood and Plasma

1. Whole blood extraction kits from Qiagen (Crawley UK, Cat. no. 29104), or:
2. Gentra Systems Capture column kit available from Flowgen (Lichfield UK, Cat. no. D5-0400);
3. Grant Dry block heater available from Flowgen (Cat no. B5-0700). (Gentra capture columns require a heating block that completely covers the column matrix).

2.2. Amplification and Detection by Agarose-Gel Electrophoresis and Ethidium Bromide Staining

2.2.1. Equipment

1. Aerosol-resistant tips.
2. Thermocycler (Perkin-Elmer 9600 thermal cycler or MJ thermal cycler, MJ Research Inc., Watertown, MA, or equivalent).
3. Sterile 200-µL thin-walled PCR tubes (Anachem, Cat. no. SL-7501 or equivalent).
4. Autoclaved 1.5-mL microfuge tubes.
5. UV transilluminator.
6. Gel-electrophoresis tank.

2.2.2. Reagents

1. Agarose.
2. 10X Loading buffer: 50% glycerol, 0.4% bromophenol blue in distilled deionized water.
3. 1X TBE buffer: 100 mL of 10X TBE (Sigma, Cat. no. T4415 or equivalent) and 900 mL distilled deionized water (ddH_2O).
4. 10 mg/mL ethidium bromide (Sigma, Cat. no. E1510 or equivalent) (*see* **Note 1**).
5. Platinum Taq DNA polymerase (Life Technologies, Cat. no. 10966-026). 10X PCR buffer (20 m*M* Tris-HCl, pH 8.4, 500 m*M* KCl) and 50 m*M* $MgCl_2$ are supplied with the enzyme.
6. 10X dNTP solution. Set of dATP, dCTP, dGTP, and dTTP supplied at 100 m*M* each (Boehringer Mannheim, Cat. no. 1 277 049). A solution containing each dNTP at 2 m*M* is prepared by diluting the individual dNTP 1 : 50 (100 µL of each dNTP to a final volume of 5 mL). Aliquot the diluted dNTP mix and store at –20°C.

7. 100 bp molecular weight markers (e.g., Pharmacia).
8. *Xba* I restriction enzyme and 10X reaction buffer (New England Biolabs).

2.2.3. Primers

Primers should be stored in lots at –20°C at a concentration of 20 μ*M*.

2.3. PCR ELISA Detection of Meningococcal DNA

2.3.1. Equipment

1. Perkin-Elmer 9600 thermal cycler or MJ thermal cycler, MJ Research Inc., (Watertown, MA) or equivalent.
2. Sterile 200-μL thin-walled PCR tubes (Anachem, Cat. no. SL-7501 or equivalent).
3. Sterile DNA-free 1.5-mL microfuge tubes.
4. Heated microtiter plate shaker (e.g., Labsystems iEMS shaker with heated lid, Cat. no. 5112220).
5. Microtiter plate washer (e.g., Labsystems Wellwash, Cat. no. 5160 770) (*see* **Note 2**).
6. Microtiter plate reader (e.g., Labsystems Multiskan or similar).

2.3.2. Materials

1. Platinum Taq DNA polymerase (Life Technologies, Cat. no. 10966-026). 10X PCR buffer (20 m*M* Tris-HCl, pH 8.4, 500 m*M* KCl) and 50 m*M* $MgCl_2$ (supplied with the enzyme).
2. 10X Dig labeling Mix plus, Boehringer Mannheim, (Cat. no. 1 835 297) and Uracil DNA glycosylase (supplied with the enzyme; *see* **Note 3**).
3. PCR ELISA (Dig detection) (Boehringer Mannheim, Cat. no. 1636 111).
4. 1.2-mL Microtiter tubes (CamLab, Cat. no. QP/845-F)

2.3.3. Primers and Probes

Primers should be diluted to a concentration of 20 μ*M* and stored in multiple small volumes at –20°C. Primers listed in section **Table 1** for the *ctrA*, *siaD* B, *siaD* C, and *siaD* W135/Y assays are used for PCR ELISA detection. In addition the biotinylated probes listed in **Table 2** are required:

Concentrated probe stocks are stored in multiple small volumes to prevent repeated freeze/thawing. A further working dilution should be made by adjusting the concentration to 750 pmol/mL which is equivalent to a 0.75 μ*M* solution.

2.4. Detection of Meningococcal DNA by PE-ABI TaqMan System

2.4.1. Equipment

1. Microamp PCR 96-well reaction plate, PE-ABI (Cat. no. N801-0560).
2. Microamp optical caps, PE-ABI (Cat. no. N801-0935).

Table 1
Primers for Gel-Based PCR Detection

Gene Target	Primer Direction	Nucleotide Sequence of Primer
ctrA	Forward	5′- GCT GCG GTA GGT GGT TCA A -3′
ctrA	Reverse	5′-TTG TCG CGG ATT TGC AAC TA-3′
siaD C	Forward	5′-GCA CAT TCA GGC GGG ATT AG-3′
siaD C	Reverse	5′-TCT CTT GTT GGG CTG TAT GGT GTA-3′
siaD B	Forward	5′-CTC TCA CCC TCA ACC CAA TGT C-3′
siaD B	Reverse	5′-TGT CGG CGG AAT AGT AAT AAT GTT-3′
siaD W-135/Y	Forward	5′- CAA ACG GTA TCT GAT GAA ATG CTG GAA G 3′
siaD W-135/Y	Reverse	5′ -TTA AAG CTG CGC GGA AGA ATA GTG AAA T 3′

Table 2
Additional Primers for PCR ELISA

Gene Target	Nucleotide Sequence of Primer
ctrA	5′ biotin-CAT TGC CAC GTG TCA GCT GCA CAT-3′
siaD B	5′ biotin-CAA TGG TGG AAA ACA CTG AAA TG-3′
siaD C	5′ biotin-TGG ACT GAC ATC GAC TTC TAT TG-3′
siaD Y	5′ biotin- CTA ATC ATG ACA TCT CAA AGC GAA GGC-3′
siaD W-135	5′ biotin-TGA TCA TGA CAT CAG AAA GTG AGG GAT T 3′

3. Aerosol-resistant tips.
4. 0.5-mL PCR tubes, Anachem (Cat. no. M-1516/1000) or equivalent.
5. Microamp optical caps, PE-ABI (Cat. no. N801-0935).
6. Microamp capping tool, PE-ABI (Cat. no. N801-0438).

2.4.2. Materials

1. Sterile water.
2. Taqman Universal Master Mix, PE-ABI (Cat. no. 4304447). (TaqMan(tm) Universal Master mix contains AmpliTaq gold, 5 m*M* $MgCl_2$, Uracil DNA glycosylase and dNTPs.)

2.4.3. Primers and Probes

Taqman probes require HPLC purification. Primer and probe for the *ctrA* assay are the same as those used for agarose and PCR ELISA detection described in **Subheadings 2.2.3.** and **2.3.2.** Primers and probe sequences for

Table 3
Primers for Use with the PE-ABI TaqMan System

Gene Target	Primer Direction	Nucleotide Sequence of Primer
siaD B	Forward	5′- TGC ATG TCC CCT TTC CTG A-3′
	Reverse	5′- AAT GGG GTA GCG TTG ACT AAC AA-3′
	TaqMan	5′ FAM-TGC TTA TTC CTC CAG CAT GCG CAA A-3′
siaD C	Forward	5′- TGC TTA TTC CTC CAG CAT GCG CAA A-3′
	Reverse	5′- TGA GAT ATG CGG TAT TTG TCT TGA AT-3′
	TaqMan	5′ FAM- TTG GCT TGT GCT AAT CCC GCC TGA-3′

the *siaD* B and C TaqMan assays are listed in **Table 3** and are different to those described for the agarose and PCR ELISA based detection. Stocks of primers and probes should be stored at –20°C in small volumes to reduce freeze/thawing of these reagents to a minimum. 10X concentrations should be prepared from the concentrated stocks and stored at –20°C. Fluorescent-labeled probes are light-sensitive and exposure to light should be minimized.

3. Methods

3.1. DNA Extraction

Depending on the sample to be extracted for PCR, different methodologies are required (*see* **Note 4**). Clinical samples may be transported to the testing laboratory unfrozen as long as the sample is received within 4 d.

3.1.1. DNA Extraction from CSF and Sera Using DNAzol

DNAzol is a guanidinium isothiocyanate-based DNA extraction medium available from Molecular Research Centre Ltd. The protocol has been adapted for use in the extraction of bacterial and viral DNA from cultures, CSFs, plasma, and serum samples. Aerosol-resistant tips must be used throughout the procedure. Aliquot DNAzol solution in 10–20 mL volumes in sterile universals and stored and room temperature.

1. Prepare an appropriate amount of extraction solution by pipetting 1 mL of DNAzol for every sample to be extracted into a sterile universal. Add 10 µL of polyacryl carrier for every 1 mL of DNAzol solution. Mix the solution thoroughly.
2. Using a 1-mL Gilsen pipet add 1 mL of extraction solution to a labeled 1.5 mL capacity hinged cap Sarstedt tube. Include a negative and positive control for each extraction series. A positive extraction control should be included in every

run. A negative extraction control should be included after every fifth sample tested (*see* **Subheading 3.1.3.**).

3. Pipette 100 μL of CSF, plasma, or serum into an appropriately labeled tube containing DNAzol extraction solution. Close caps and vortex the tubes thoroughly and incubate at room temperature for 10 min.
4. Pipette 500 μL of ethanol into each of the samples and control tubes. Close caps and mix each tube and leave at room temperature for 10 min. Spin in a microfuge at 12,000*g* for 10 min at +18°C.
5. Remove the supernatant using a fine-tipped sterile pastet being careful not to disturb the pellet and discard in to a universal. Waste should be stored for appropriate professional disposal.
6. Add 1 mL of 95% ethanol to each tube, close the cap, and mix to dislodge the pellet. Spin the tubes for 5 min at 12,000*g* at +18°C. Remove the supernatant and discard.
7. Re-centrifuge the tubes for 10 s at 12,000*g* and carefully remove any residual ethanol with a pipet tip.
8. Resuspend the pellet in 50 μL of sterile injectable water. Allow the pellet to resuspend for at least 10 min. Extracts may be stored at +4°C for 1–2 d, and at –20°C for long-term storage.

3.1.2. Preparation of Positive Amplification-Control Material

1. Plate cultures of serogroups B, C, W-135, and Y *N. meningitidis* grown on blood agar and incubate at +37°C overnight in an atmosphere of 5% CO_2.
2. In a Class 2 microbiological safety cabinet, prepare a suspension of each culture in 2 mL of sterile distilled water, using approx 4–5 colonies.
3. Transfer each suspension to a spectrophotometer cuvet and read its OD at 650 nm with a cuvet of path length of 10 mm. Cover the open top of cuvet if the spectrophotometer is outside a microbiological safety cabinet.
4. To standardize the meningococcal suspension to an OD of 0.1, the concentration of the suspension is adjusted as in the following example: if the OD were 0.670 take 0.1 mL of the meningococcal suspension and add to 0.57 mL of sterile water.
5. Dilute each suspension to by 1:1000 by first adding 10 μL to 990 μL of sterile water then add 100 μL of the 1:100 dilution to 900 μL of sterile water. This produces a suspension that contains approx 1000 cfu/mL.
6. Boil the suspension for 15 min and cool before dividing into 20 μL samples. Store at –20°C.

3.1.3. Preparation of Extraction Controls

1. Follow the procedure for the preparation of amplification controls (**Subheading 3.1.2.**) to **step 4.**
2. Dilute the bacterial suspension to 1:100 by adding 100 μL to 9.9 mL of sterile water. Add the 10 mL of bacterial suspension to 90 mL of plasma or serum negative for *N. meningitidis* by PCR analysis. Divide into 200 μL samples and store at –20°C.

Table 4
PCR Reaction Mixture Used in the Gel-Based Electrophoresis Method (*see* Subheading 3.2.)

Reagent	Volume for 1 reaction (μL)	Final concentration
Sterile distilled water	30.1	
10X buffer	5	1X
dNTP mix (2 m*M* each)	5	0.2 m*M*
Forward primer	1.25	0.5 μ*M*
Reverse primer	1.25	0.5 μ*M*
Platinum Taq polymerase (5 U/μL)	0.4	2 U
$MgCl_2$ (50 m*M*)	2	2 m*M*

3. Store a similar batch of PCR negative plasma or serum samples without adding the *N. meningitidis* suspension to be used as a negative extraction control.

3.1.4. Extraction of DNA from Whole Blood and Plasma

Commercially available whole-blood extraction kits are available from Qiagen or Gentra Systems Capture column kit from Flowgen. Gentra capture columns require a heating block that completely covers the column matrix. Both systems extract from 200 μL of whole blood. The manufacturers' protocols should be followed. Both protocols generate a final eluate of 200 μL. These methodologies do not co-purify PCR inhibitors (*see* **Note 5**).

3.2. Amplification and Detection by Agarose-Gel Electrophoresis and Ethidium-Bromide Staining

Amplification by PCR and detection by agarose-gel electrophoresis can be carried out using the primers described in **Table 4**. Note that the same primers are used for the amplification of serogroups W-135 and Y, and that *Xba* I restriction digest following amplification is carried out to distinguish these serogroups.

3.2.1. PCR Amplification

The reaction mix contains Platinum Taq polymerase, which is inactive prior to heating to +95°C, and therefore enables a "hot-start" PCR to be carried out.

1. Preparation of reaction mix. Prepare a batch of PCR reaction mix and add the appropriate forward and reverse primers for the relevant gene target. Prepare two more PCR reaction mixes than the number of samples and controls to be tested to allow for pipetting loss. Divide into samples of 45 μL volumes and store in 200 μL PCR reaction tubes.
2. Template addition. Add 5 μL of extracted DNA, or negative or positive control sample to the 45 μL of PCR reaction mix.

3. Cycling conditions. For amplification of the *ctrA* gene sequence the thermal cycling conditions are as follows: 95°C for 2 min followed by 45 cycles of 95°C for 15 s, 60°C for 30 s and 72 for 1 min, and a final extension of 72°C for 5 min. For amplification of the *siaD* B, C and W135/Y sequences thermal cycling are: 95°C for 2 min followed by 45 cycles of 95°C for 20 s, 58°C for 40 s and 72°C for 1 min, and a final extension step of 72°C for 1 min.
4. Restriction digest of W135/Y PCR products. To distinguish between serogroups W135 and Y the amplified product is cut with the restriction endonuclease *Xba* I. To 7 µL of the PCR product add 1 µL of *Xba* I, 2 µL of 10X buffer (New England Biolabs), and incubate at +37°C for 2 h.

3.2.2. PCR Product Detection

1. For detection of *ctrA* PCR products prepare a 3.5% agarose gel in 1XTBE containing 0.5 µg/mL of ethidium bromide. For examination of *siaD* B, C, and W135/Y amplified products prepare a similar gel containing 2% agarose. For safety purposes, add ethidium bromide after the gel has melted and cooled.
2. Add 1 µL of 10X loading buffer to 10 µL of the PCR products and load gel. Include 100 bp size markers. Electrophoresis is carried out by applying 100 volts constant voltage until the bromophenol blue dye marker has migrated towards the end of the gel. Following electrophoresis, examine the gel using a UV transilluminator.
3. Following electrophoresis examine the gel using a UV transilluminator. For the *ctrA* primer set an amplified product of 111 bp is expected. For the siaD B and the *siaD* C assays amplified products of 457 bp and 442 bp are expected, respectively. *Xba* I digests of the amplified *siaD* sequence from serogroup Y meningococci produce two fragments of 438 and 260 bp. Serogroup W135 *siaD* sequence is not restricted by *Xba* I and the intact amplified product remains at the predicted 698 bp.

3.3. PCR ELISA Detection of Meningococcal DNA

3.3.1. PCR Amplification and Digoxigenin Labeling

1. Preparation of reaction mix. Prepare a batch of PCR reaction mix (*see* **Table 5**) and add the appropriate forward and reverse primers for the relevant gene target. Prepare two more PCR reaction mixes than the number of samples and controls to be tested. Aliquot 45 µL volumes into 200-µL PCR reaction tubes.
2. Template addition. Add 5 µL of extracted DNA, negative and positive control to the 45 µL of PCR reaction mix. Amplification is carried out as described in **Subheading 3.2.1., Step 3**, except that an additional incubation steps of 50°C for 2 min is carried out at the beginning for all assays. This allows the UNG included in the PCR ELISA to inactivate any potentially contaminating PCR product.

3.3.2. PCR ELISA Detection

All reagents required for the ELISA-based detection, except the biotinylated probe, are provided in the Boehringer Mannheim PCR ELISA kit. The digoxigenin-labeled PCR products are denatured and subsequently hybridized

Table 5
PCR Reaction Mixture Used in PCR ELISA (*see* Subheading 3.3.)

Reagent	Volume for 1 reaction (μL)	Final concentration
Sterile distilled water	28.1	
10X buffer	5	1X
Forward primer (20 μ*M*)	1.25	5 μ*M*
Reverse primer (20 μ*M*)	1.25	5 μ*M*
Platinum Taq polymerase (5 U/μL)	0.4	2 U
$MgCl_2$ (50 m*M*)	2	2 m*M*
10X dig labeling mix plus	5	1X
Uracil DNA glycosylase (1 U/μL)	2	2 U

to their respective biotinylated probe. For the *siaD* W-135/Y assay, the serogroup-specific biotinylated probes are reacted separately with samples of the same amplified product.

1. Set out an appropriate number of microtiter tubes in the 96-place rack (*see* **Note 6**). Carefully pipet 20 μL of denaturation solution to the base of each of the tubes, then pipet 20 μL of the digoxigenin-labeled PCR product and mix by pipetting up and down 2–3 times. For the *siaD* W-135/Y assay, prepare duplicate tubes of denatured PCR product for each sample. Leave at room temperature for 10 min.
2. During this period prepare the probe solution. Biotinylated probes are stored as undiluted stocks and as diluted aliquots at a concentration of 750 pmol/mL. Prepare hybridization solution by adding 10 μL of the 750 pmol/mL probe stock to 1 mL of the hybridization buffer (solution 4, blue cap). For each specimen and control tested, 210 μL probe in hybridization buffer is required. Prepare probe solution to the nearest whole number of mL required. For example, for 40 PCR samples prepare 9 mL of probe solution by adding 90 μL of 750 pmol/mL probe stock to 9 mL of hybridization solution 4.
3. After 10 min denaturation, add 210 μL of diluted probe to each of the microtiter tubes. Using a multichannel pipet, transfer 200 μL to streptavidin-coated microtiter strips. For the *siaD* W-135/Y assay, add the diluted serogroup Y probe to one of the denatured PCR products and W-135 diluted probe to the other. Cover wells with adhesive plate sealer and incubate in shaking incubator for 1 h at +37°C.
4. Wash the plate 5 times using a microtiter plate washer. Prepare wash buffer by adding 1 wash tablet (bottle 5) to 2 L of distilled water. Store at +4°C.
5. Add 200 μL of dilute conjugate to each well and incubate for 30 min at +37°C in a shaking incubator. Conjugate is supplied freeze-dried and should be prepared at least 15 min before use by adding 250 μL of distilled water to each of the vials. For use, reconstituted conjugate is diluted 1 in 100 in conjugate diluent buffer (vial 6, red cap). Dilute only enough for the number of wells required plus one.

Table 6
PCR Reaction Mixture Used in the TaqMan PCR Method

Reagent	Volume for 1 reaction (μL)	Final concentration
Universal master mix	12.5 μL	1X
Forward primer (2 μ*M*)	2.5 μL	0.2 μ*M*
Reverse primer (2 μ*M*)	2.5 μL	0.2 μ*M*
TaqMan probe (1 μ*M*)	2.5 μL	0.1 μ*M*
Sterile distilled water	3.0 μL	
Total	23 μL	

For example, for 40 wells prepare working strength conjugate for 41 wells by adding 82 μL of conjugate to 8.2 mL of conjugate buffer.

6. Wash the plate 5 times as before.
7. Add 200 μL of substrate to each well. Seal with adhesive plate sealer and incubate in microtiter plate shaker for 30 min at +37°C. Substrate is prepared by adding 1 substrate tablet (vial 9) to 5 mL of substrate diluent (bottle 8, green cap). Allow 5 min for tablets to dissolve.
8. Read the plate using an ELISA plate reader at 405 nm with a reference filter of 492 nm.
9. Samples with OD readings equal to or greater than twice the OD of the negative extract control are considered positive.

3.4. Amplification and Detection of Meningococcal DNA by PE-ABI TaqMan System

Refer to the "User Manual" for detailed description of the operation of the ABI 7700 system.

1. TaqMan PCR reaction mix. Prepare a batch of PCR reaction mix (*see* **Table 6**) and add the appropriate forward and reverse primers and the TaqMan probe for the relevant gene target. Prepare two more PCR reaction mixes than the number of samples and controls to be tested. Aliquot 23 μL volumes into the microtiter reaction plate.
2. Template addition. Pipette 2 μL of extracted samples and controls into the appropriate wells. Include a negative and a positive amplification control for each run (*see* **Subheadings 3.1.2.** and **3.1.3.** for preparation of controls).
3. Cycling conditions. The microwell plate is placed into the thermal cycler of the PE-ABI ABI 7700 and subjected to the following thermocycling parameters: 50°C for 2 min, 95°C for 10 min, followed by 45 cycles of 95°C for 15 s and 60°C for 1 min. These are the default settings for the thermal cycling parameters. Note the default setting for the number of cycles has to be changed to 45 for each run. The sample volume of 25 μL should be selected but can be saved as a default setting.

4. Result analysis. Examine the control amplification plots to validate the run. The efficiency of the extraction procedure can be assessed by recording the cycle-number amplification was detected (Ct value) of the positive extraction control. The typical cycle number at which a positive extraction control batch is detected can be determined. Detection of amplification occurring later in the thermocycling profile indicates problems during the extraction process leading to reduced sensitivity. Similarly, the efficiency of the amplification process can be determined by examining the cycle number at which the amplification control is detected as positive.

4. Notes

1. This agent is a mutagen and should be stored in a contained area. It should only be handled with gloves and disposed of with the appropriate safety measures (e.g., charcoal-based columns) ***(35)***.
2. A microtiter plate washer is not essential and adequate washing can be achieved by using a multi-channel pipet to add washing buffer. Alternative microtiter plate-heated shakers may be used; however, the heated lid facility of the Labsystems iEMS shaker, which eliminates condensation on the underside of the plate sealer, avoiding cross-contamination between wells, is preferred.
3. PCR is an extremely powerful technique that can suffer from cross-contamination especially from amplified products. Every precaution should be taken to minimize this risk. Amplification reactions should be prepared in a DNA-free environment that is in an area separate from the analysis of the amplified products. Use of aerosol-resistant pipet tips is recommended. Automated closed tube systems such as the TaqMan reduce the contamination risk to a minimum. Additional precautions to reduce this risk are employed, such as pre-incubation of PCR reaction mixes with uracil DNA glycosylase. Amplification is carried out with deoxyuridine triphosphate (dUTP) instead of deoxythymidine triphosphate (dTTP). Uracil-glycosidic bonds in DNA containing dUTP are hydrolyzed by UNG, creating abasic sites from which Taq DNA polymerase cannot extend ***(36)***. The PCR ELISA and the TaqMan both include UNG treatment as a precaution against contamination. The agarose-based assay described has not been developed with UNG treatment. UNG treatment can be include but will involve optimization of the assay with dUTP instead of dTTP.
4. In addition to the samples that are suitable for detection of meningococcal DNA, we have had success in extracting joint aspirates, pus, and pleural effusions using the DNAzol protocol. A sample of CSF and/or EDTA blood should also be analyzed in addition to these samples.
5. Substances that can reduce or inhibit the PCR reaction may lead to false-negative results. There are a number of approaches to determine if inhibitors are present by demonstrating the potential for PCR amplification to occur in negative samples. A co-purified human genomic housekeeping-gene target (e.g., β-actin) can be used or an unrelated DNA sequence may be added to the amplification reaction. PE-ABI provide an exogenous internal control reagent (Cat. no. 4308323) for use with the Taqman system, which allows PCR inhibition to be detected. Low concentrations of primers are used to avoid competing with ampli-

fication of the meningococcal target. The control sequence is detected using a VIC-labeled probe that can be distinguished from meningococcal FAM-labeled probe. A survey of clinical samples received for meningococcal PCR and extracted using protocols described here was performed and revealed that no PCR inhibitors were present *(24)*.

6. Denaturation of the digoxigenin-labeled PCR product can be carried out in microfuge tubes, however transfer to PCR ELISA microtiter plate strips using a multichannel pipet is possible using the microtiter tubes and rack from Camlab, which is more efficient, especially if a large number of samples are tested.

Acknowledgments

The authors would like to thank Ian Feavers (NIBSC, South Mimms, Potters Bar, Herts, UK) for critically reviewing this chapter.

References

1. Kaczmarski, E. B. (1997) Meningococcal disease in England and Wales: 1995. *Commun. Dis. Rep. Rev.* **7,** R55–R91.
2. Chief Medical Officer, Chief Nursing Officer, Chief Pharmaceutical Officer (1999) *Introduction of Immunisation Against Group C Meningococcal Infection.* Department of Health, London.
3. Kristiansen, B., Ask, E., Jenkins, A., Fermer, C., Radström, P., and Skold, O. (1991) Rapid diagnosis of meningococcal meningitis by polymerase chain reaction. *Lancet* **337,** 1568–1579.
4. Saunders, N. B., Zollinger, W. D., and Rao, V. B. (1993) A rapid and sensitive PCR strategy employed for amplification and sequencing of *porA* from a single colony forming unit of *Neisseria meningitidis*. *Gene* **137,** 153–162.
5. McLaughlin, G. L., Howe, D. K., Biggs, D. R., Smith, A. R., Ludwinski, P., Fox, B. C., et al. (1993) Amplification of rDNA loci to detect and type *N. meningitidis* and other eubacteria. *Mol. Cell. Probes* **7,** 7–17.
6. Rådström, P., Bäckman, A., Qian, N., Kragsbjerg, P., Påhlson, C., and Olcén, P. (1994) Detection of bacterial DNA in CSF by assay for simultaneous detection of *N. meningitidis*, *H. influenzae*, and Streptococci using a seminested PCR Strategy. *J. Clin. Microbiol.* **32,** 2738–2744.
7. Ni, H., Knight, A. I., Cartwright, K. A. V., Palmer, W. H., and McFadden, J. (1992) Polymerase chain reaction for diagnosis of meningococcal meningitis. *Lancet* **340,** 1432–1434.
8. Davison, E., Borrow, R., Guiver, M., Kaczmarski, E. B., and Fox, A. J. (1996) The adaptation of the IS*1106* PCR to a PCR ELISA format for the diagnosis of meningococcal infection. *Serodiagn. Immunother. Infect. Dis.* **8,** 51–56.
9. Newcombe, J., Cartwright, K. A. V., Palmer, W. H., and McFadden, J. (1996) PCR of peripheral blood for diagnosis of meningococcal disease. *J. Clin. Microbiol.* **34,** 1637–1640.
10. Borrow, R., Claus, H., Guiver, M., Smart, L., Jones, D. M., Kaczmarski, E. B., Frosch, M., and Fox, A. J. (1997) Non-culture diagnosis and serogroup determi-

nation of meningococcal B and C infection by a sialyltransferase (*siaD*) PCR ELISA. *Epidemiol. Infect.* **118,** 1111–1123.
11. Kaczmarski, E. B., Ragunathan, P. L., Marsh, J., Gray, S. J., and Guiver, M. (1998) Creating a national service for the diagnosis of meningococcal disease by polymerase chain reaction. *Commun. Dis. Public Health* **1,** 54–56.
12. Zhou, L., Hui, F. M., and Morrison, D. A. (1995) Characterisation of IS*1167*, a new insertion sequence in *Streptococcus pneumoniae. Plasmid* **33,** 127–138.
13. Hernandez Perez, M., Fomukong, N. G., Hellyer, T., Brown, I. N., and Dale, J. W. (1994) Characterisation of IS*1110*, a highly mobile genetic element from *Mycobacterium avium. Mol. Microbiol.* **12,** 717–724.
14. Mulcahy, G. M., Kaminski, Z. C., Albanese, E. A., Sood, R., and Pierce, M. (1996) IS*6110*-based PCR methods for the detection of *Mycobacterium tuberculosis. J. Clin. Microbiol.* **34,** 1348–1349.
15. Borrow, R., Guiver, M., Sadler, F., Kaczmarski, E. B., and Fox, A. J. (1998) False positive diagnosis of meningococcal infection by the IS*1106* PCR ELISA. *FEMS Microbiol. Lett.* **162,** 215–218.
16. Urwin, R., Kaczmarski, E. B., Guiver, M., Fox, A. J., and Maiden, M. C. J. (1998) Amplification of the meningococcal *porB* gene for non-culture serotype characterisation. *Epidemiol. Infect.* **120,** 257–262.
17. Russell, J. E., Maiden, M. C. J., and Feavers, I. M. (1998) Molecular analysis of antigenic variation within the *porA* gene of disease causing *Neisseria meningitidis* isolated in the United Kingdom, in *Eleventh International Pathogenic Neisseria Conference* (Nassif, X., Quentin-Millet, J., and Taha, M.-K., eds.). EDK, Paris, p. 281.
18. Sacchi, C. T., Lemos, A. P., Whitney, A. M., Solari, C. A., Brandt, M. E., Melles, C. E., et al. (1998) Correlation between serological and sequencing analyses of the PorB outer membrane protein in the *Neisseria meningitidis* serotyping system. *Clin. Diagn. Lab. Immunol.* **5,** 348–354.
19. Arhin, F. F., Moreau, F., Coulton, J. W., and Mills, E. L. (1998) Sequencing of porA from clinical isolates of *Neisseria meningitidis* defines a subtyping scheme and its genetic regulation. *Can. J. Microbiol.* **44,** 56–63.
20. Corless, C. E., Guiver, M., Borrow, R., Edwards-Jones, V., Kaczmarski, E. B., and Fox, A. J. (2000) Contamination and sensitivity issues with a 'real-time' universal 16S rRNA PCR. *J. Clin. Microbiol.* **38(5),** 1747–1752.
21. Frosch, M., Müller, D., Bousset, K., and Müller, A. (1992) Conserved outer membrane protein of *Neisseria meningitidis* involved in capsule expression. *Infect. Immun.* **60,** 798–803.
22. Frosch, M., Weisgerber, C., and Meyer, T. F. (1989) Molecular characterisation and expression in *Escherichia coli* of the gene complex encoding the polysaccharide capsule of *Neisseria meningitidis* group B. *Proc. Natl. Acad. Sci. USA* **86,** 1669–1673.
23. Borrow, R., Claus, H., Chaudhry, U., Guiver, M., Kaczmarski, E. B., Frosch, M., and Fox, A. J. (1998) *SiaD* PCR ELISA for confirmation and identification of

serogroup Y and W135 meningococcal infections. *FEMS Microbiol. Lett.* **159,** 209–214.

24. Orvelid, P., Backman, A., and Olcen, P. (1999). PCR identification of the group A *Neisseria meningitidis* gene in cerebrospinal fluid. *Scand. J. Infect. Dis.* **31,** 481–483.
25. Guiver, M., Borrow, R., Marsh, J., Gray, S. J. Kaczmarski, E. B., Howells, D., et al. (2000). Evaluation of the applied biosystems automated TaqMan PCR system for the detection of meningococcal DNA. *FEMS Immunol Med Microbiol.* **28,** 173–179.
26. Lee, L. G., Connell, C. R., and Bloch, W. (1993) Allelic discrimination by nick-translation PCR with fluorogenic probes. *Nucleic Acids Res.* **21,** 3761–3766.
27. Livak, K. J., Flood, S. J., Marmaro, J., Giusti, W., and Deetz K. (1995) Oligonucleotides with fluorescent dyes at opposite ends provide a quenched probe system useful for detecting PCR product and nucleic acid hybridization. *PCR Methods. Appl.* **4,** 357–362.
28. Gibson, E. M., Heid, C. A., and Williams, P. M. (1996) A novel method for real time quantitative RT-PCR. *Genome Res.* 6, 995–1001.
29. Heid, C. A., Stevens, J., Lival, J., and Williams, M. J. (1996) Real time quantitative PCR. *Genome Res.* **6,** 986–994.
30. Morris, T., Robertson, B., and Gallagher, M. (1996) Rapid reverse transcription-PCR detection of hepatitis C virus RNA in serum by utilising the Taqman fluorogenic detection system. *J. Clin. Microbiol.* **34,** 2933–2936.
31. Chen, S., Yee, A., Griffiths, M., Larkin, C., Yamashiro, C. T., Behari, R., et al. (1997) The evaluation of a fluorogenic polymerase chain reaction assay for the detection of Salmonella species in food commodities. *Intl. J. Food Microbiol.* **35,** 239–250.
32. Bassler, H. A., Flood, S. J., Livak, K. J., Marmaro, J., Knorr, R., and Batt, C. A. (1995) Use of a fluorogenic probe in a PCR-based assay for the detection of *Listeria monocytogenes*. *App. Environ. Microbiol.* **61,** 3724–3728.
33. Oberst, R. D., Hays, M. P., Bohra, L. K., Phebus, R. K., Yamashiro, C. T., Paszko-Kolva, C., et al. (1998) PCR-based DNA amplification and presumptive detection of *Escherichia coli* 0157:H7 with an internal fluorogenic probe and the 5′ nuclease (Taqman) assay. *Appl. Environ. Microbiol.* **64,** 3389–3396.
34. Desjardin, L. E., Chen, Y., Perkins, M. D., Teixeira, L., Cave, M. D., and Eisenach, K. D. (1998) Comparison of the ABI 7700 system (Taqman) and competitive PCR for quantification of IS*6110* DNA in sputum during treatment of tuberculosis. *J. Clin. Microbiol.* **36,** 1964–1968.
35. Hengen, P. N. (1994) Disposal of ethidium bromide. *Trends Biochem. Sci.* **19,** 257–258.
36. Longo, M. C., Berninger, M. S., and Hartley, J. L. (1990). Use of DNA uracil DNA glycosylase to control carry-over contamination in polymerase chain reaction. *Gene* **93,** 125–128.

4

Detection of Meningococcal Antigen by Latex Agglutination

Michael A. Sobanski, Rosemary A. Barnes, and W. Terence Coakley

1. Introduction

Meningococcal meningitis and septicemia are serious infections with significant morbidity and mortality. A sensitive affordable test is required to provide evidence of meningococcal disease at the earliest opportunity to improve local management and give early warning of potential outbreaks of disease. Culture of organisms is considered the gold standard for diagnosis but is slow (24 h or more) and increasingly influenced by prior antibiotic treatment. Recently, the development of polymerase chain reaction (PCR) has improved diagnosis but this sensitive assay is costly, is not available at most primary care institutions and is not feasible for developing countries. Conventional latex agglutination (LA) enables rapid detection of bacterial antigen in cerebrospinal fluid (CSF) *(1,2)* and can also be used to test specimens of blood *(3,4)* or urine *(5)* and for serogroup determinations on primary cultures *(6,7)*. We discuss here test-card agglutination and also describe a new technique based upon LA in an ultrasonic standing wave that retains the speed of direct antigen testing while significantly increasing sensitivity.

1.1. Test-Card Latex Agglutination

The polystyrene microspheres employed (typically 0.2–1 µm in diameter) in conventional test-card agglutination have been coated with antibody that reacts with the group-specific capsular polysaccharides of *Neisseria meningitidis* serogroups A, B, C, Y, and W135. Antibody-coated microspheres cross-linked by antigen form agglutinates large enough to be visualized with

From: *Methods in Molecular Medicine, vol. 67: Meningococcal Disease: Methods and Protocols*
Edited by: A. J. Pollard and M. C. J. Maiden © Humana Press Inc., Totowa, NJ

the naked eye, against a "contrasting" background on a test card or glass slide *(2)*. LA can be used by nonspecialist laboratories with minimal specimen preprocessing. Several commercial kits are available containing latex reagents that differentiate between the most common meningococcal serogroups encountered, thus choice of kit is determined by the geographical variation of prevalent strains. Two meningococcal reagents are available from Abbott-Murex (Wellcogen), the first coated with polyclonal antibody (PAb) to meningococcal serogroups A, C, Y, and W135 and the second coated with monoclonal antibody (MAb) specific for meningococcal serogroup B and *Escherichia coli* K1 *(8)*. The Pastorex meningitis kit (from Bio-Rad, formerly Sanofi Diagnostics) contains separate, color-coded microspheres that differentiate between meningococcal groups B, C, and A infection plus a single combined reagent specific for groups Y and W135. Both the Slidex meningite (bioMerieux) and Directigen™ (Becton Dickinson) meningitis kits enable differentiation between serogroup A, B, and C disease.

1.1.1. Sensitivity and Specificity

It has long been established that LA is more sensitive than counter-current immuno-electrophoresis ***(1,2,5,9,10)*** or coagglutination ***(11)*** and has been shown to be equally sensitive to reverse passive haemagglutination ***(10)*** and radioimmunoassay ***(9)***. LA has proved to be extremely effective for identifying serogroups of cultured meningococci ***(6,7)***; however, the published values for the sensitivity of conventional agglutination testing in CSF vary considerably, with values ranging from 11–95 % for "in house" assays and 32–96% for commercial kits (*see* **Table 1**). Although antigen detection in CSF is generally more sensitive, there can be some usefulness in testing blood ***(16)*** and even concentrated urine ***(17)***; although the lower concentration of antigens present makes testing these fluids inherently less sensitive. Meningococcal disease in its most serious form of sepsis without meningitis accounts for up to 40% of all disease cases. CSF is an inappropriate specimen in this condition; moreover, lumbar puncture is contraindicated in severely ill patients.

Specificity is influenced by method of specimen collection ***(18,19)*** and also sample processing ***(20)***. In clinical studies, the specificity of meningococcal-antigen detection by LA in CSF, ranged from 96–100% ***(2,8,10,15)***. Cross-reactivity has been demonstrated among isolates of *N. meningitidis*, and *E. coli*, *Bacillus pumilis*, and *Moraxella nonliquefaciens* ***(21–23)***. Antigenic similarities between *N. meningitidis* B and *E. coli* K1 polysaccharide ***(24)*** is considered useful in that *E. coli* K1 is a likely cause of bacterial sepsis in neonates ***(25)***.

1.1.2. Clinical Utility

Although most workers consider that LA on CSF is a useful adjunct to other microbiological investigations ***(7,15,17)*** and recommend routine use, some

Table 1
Sensitivity of Detection of Meningococcal Antigen in CSF, Blood, or Urine from Patients with Culture-Proven Disease and from Culture-Negative Patients with a Clinical Diagnosis of Meningococcal Disease

Body Fluids	Sensitivity in culture-proven case	Sensitivity in patients with a clinical diagnosis	Latex reagents used	Reference
CSF	96–32%	44–27%	Commercial	***(3,11–16)***
	95–11%	57–29%	In house	***(1,2,4,9,10)***
Serum	60–36%	22%	Commercial	***(3,16)***
Conc. urine	56–31%	10%	Commercial	***(16,17)***

believe its role to be beneficial only in antibiotic-treated patients ***(26)*** or where no microbiological evidence of infection exists ***(13,27)***. The simplicity of the test is in its favor ***(1)***. Other workers have demonstrated that the test was no more sensitive than Gram stain ***(14,12,28)*** and suggest its use only where Gram staining fails to confirm infection ***(12,19,27)***. Staining confirms the presence of diplococci but cannot indicate causative serogroups. Some authors are of the opinion that bacterial antigen detection does not provide useful information in clinical practice ***(19,29)*** and has little influence on patient care ***(19,27)***.

The cost of antigen testing where other laboratory indications are positive makes nonselective routine screening controversial ***(19,27)***. Moreover, in one study, utilizing antigen detection in urine, false-positive reactions owing to contamination by skin and perineal flora led to inappropriate clinical interventions ***(19)***. It has been suggested that cost could be reduced by restricting latex testing to cases where no organism is identified and to patients with abnormal CSF leucocyte counts ***(27,30,31)***. This represents an absolute indication and as such LA tests on CSF should be available in all routine diagnostic laboratories. This suggestion takes no account of other potential benefits such as preliminary serogroup information that could affect management of patients and their contacts.

1.2. Ultrasound-Enhanced LA

Recently, the speed and sensitivity of antigen detection by LA has been improved by performing assays in a noncavitating ultrasonic standing-wave field ***(32,33)***. Antibody-coated latex particles suspended in the wave are subjected to physical forces that promote formation of aggregates by increasing particle–particle contact and hence agglutination in the presence of antigen ***(34)***. Ultrasound-enhanced LA has been applied to detection of soluble and particulate antigen of bacterial, fungal, and viral origin ***(33,35–39)*** with sensi-

Table 2
Diagnostic Particle Agglutination Tests Enhanced by Standing-Wave Ultrasound

Analyte	Method	Enhancement
Meningococcal (group A, B, C, Y, W135) polysaccharide	LA (Murex)	32–64-fold sensitivity increase
Pneumococcal polysaccharide	LA (Murex)	16-fold sensitivity increase
E. coli O157 polysaccharide	LA (Oxoid)	1024-fold sensitivity increase
Aspergillus galactomannan	LA (Bio-Rad)	1024-fold sensitivity increase
Candida mannan	LA (Bio-Rad)	250-fold sensitivity increase
C-reactive protein	LA (Microgen)	256-fold sensitivity increase
Rotavirus outer-coat antigen	LA (bioMerieux)	16-fold sensitivity increase
Anti-CMV antibodies	LA (CMVScan, Becton Dickinson)	32-fold test-time reduction
Hepatitis B surface antigen	Hemagglutination (Wellcome)	23-fold test-time reduction

tivity increases in the order of 100-fold greater than that achievable through conventional test-card latex agglutination testing (*see* **Table 2**). The latex suspension (diluted eightfold) and test specimen are mixed and exposed to a 4.5 MHz radial standing-wave field within a glass capillary held on the axis of a tubular ultrasonic transducer *(33)*. Suspended latex particles experience physical forces that act to localize particles at submillimetre separations (half an acoustic wavelength). Following treatment the sample is expelled onto a nonadsorbing surface and stirred lightly to disturb aggregated particles not bridged by antibody-antigen interaction. Shearing forces are required but must not be so great that they separate antigen cross-linked beads. The sample is examined microscopically for agglutination.

Exposure of Wellcogen latex reagents for detection of meningococcal capsular polysaccharide (in buffer) to standing-wave ultrasound gave sensitivity enhancements of up to 64-fold in comparison to standard agglutination *(38)* raising the possibility of using serum rather than CSF for antigen detection. Similar enhancements were observed with test particles for detection of meningococcal antigen from both bioMerieux and Sanofi LA kits (unpublished observations) and with Phadebact (Boule Diagnostics) staphylococcal co-agglutination test reagents *(38)*. Detection of *N. meningitidis* serogroup polysaccharide in clinical samples has been possible with increased sensitivity in comparison to the test-card method and without nonspecific reactivity *(16,38,40)*. Recent studies showed that the number of cases of meningococcal disease identified using ultrasound enhanced agglutination rose fivefold in comparison to conventional LA and was complementary in-use to PCR assays ***(41,42)*** for detection of meningococci ***(40)***. In 90 patients with clinically diagnosed meningococcal disease, the sensitivities of culture, ultrasonic immunoassay, test-card LA, the meningococcal specific (*ctrA*) PCR and the serogroup-specific (*siaD*) PCR assays were 28, 50, 10, 67, and 48%, respectively. In a subset of cases with microbiologically confirmed disease (26 patients) the relative sensitivities rose to 76, 19, 88, and 69% for ultrasound enhanced, conventional LA, *ctrA* PCR and *siaD* PCR assays, respectively. There was good agreement between the results obtained with PCR and the enhanced latex assay and no discrepancies were observed when both assays provided serogroup characterization.

1.2.1. Prognostic Value

The serum antigen titer had been shown to bear some relationship to clinical outcome ***(43,44)***. However, the poor sensitivity of conventional assays for polysaccharide antigen has limited the prognostic value of antigen measurement. In recent work, serum antigen concentration has been estimated using ultrasonic immunoassay by titration and serial testing of antigen-positive specimens ***(45)***. Further refinement of the correlation between antigen level and outcome may result from investigation of the dependence of antigen concentration on the time interval since antibiotic administration. Ultrasound enhancement is not only cost-effective and convenient for countries that lack the resources needed for culture or PCR facilities ***(40)*** but could otherwise be used to provide serogroup confirmation and prognostic information rapidly following hospital admission.

Instructions for performing test-card LA and ultrasonic immunoassay are presented together with photographs and light micrographs of clinical specimens tested by both methods to assist operator interpretation of results.

2. Materials

2.1. Sample Preparation

1. Sterile microcentrifuge tubes and fixed-speed microfuge (14,000*g*).
2. Sterile syringes (2 mL) (Becton Dickinson, Oxford, UK) and sterile Microlance® 3 (23 G) needles (Becton Dickinson).
3. 0.2-µm Millex-GS (cellulose acetate/nitrate mixed esters) Millipore filters (Sigma, Poole, UK).
4. 0.1 *M* di-sodium ethylenediamine tetraacetic acid (EDTA) pH 7.0.

2.2. Latex Agglutination

Several commercial kits for detection of meningococcal antigen are available. The discussion here is confined largely to the use of reagents from the Wellcogen bacterial antigen kit (Murex-Abbott Diagnostics Ltd., Dartford,

UK) for direct detection of meningococcal polysaccharide in body fluids. Other commercial kits will be referred to where methods diverge significantly from those described for the Wellcogen kit.

2.2.1. Kit Reagents

Kit reagents should be stored at 4°C for the duration of the recommended kit shelf life (*see* **Note 1**).

1. *N. meningitidis* serogroup B/*E. coli* K1 test latex reagent.
2. *N. meningitidis* serogroup ACYW135 test latex reagent.
3. Control latex suspensions, similar to the two meningococcal test latexes, coated with antibody against *Bordetella bronchiseptica*.
4. Freeze dried polyvalent meningococcal capsular polysaccharide positive control reconstituted in sterile phosphate-buffered saline (PBS) containing preservative (145 m*M* NaCl, 5 m*M* phosphate, 0.1% sodium azide, pH 7.4).
5. Test cards, mixing sticks.

2.2.2. Ultrasound Enhanced Latex Test

1. Test and control meningococcal latex reagents diluted 1/8 in PBS (containing 0.1% sodium azide).
2. Serially diluted positive control meningococcal antigen made in PBS (containing 0.1% sodium azide).
3. 2-mm internal diameter round glass capillary (transferpipettor) tubes (Fisher Scientific, Loughborough, UK) (*see* **Note 2** and **Subheading 2.3.**).
4. A 2-mL syringe (Becton Dickinson, Oxford, UK) attached to a piece of 2-mm bore silicone rubber tubing (Fisher Scientific) approx 30 mm in length to form an airtight seal on the glass capillary.
5. 0.2-mm pathlength rectangular cross-section glass microslides (Camlab, Cambridge, UK).
6. Mixing sticks (of the type used with many test-card kits).

2.3. Ultrasonic Equipment

The ultrasound apparatus has been described extensively in the literature *(32,33)*. Essentially, a lead zirconate titanate tubular transducer (PCA4; Morgan Matroc, Wrexham, UK), with a fundamental thickness resonance frequency of 1.5 MHz, is mounted as illustrated in **Fig. 1**. The transducer encloses a reservoir which is filled with distilled water up to a level of about 1 mm from the transducer's upper edge. A locating well at the base of the reservoir and a central hole in the lid of the chamber hold the glass capillary (containing the test sample) on the axis of the transducer in the high acoustic pressure region of the sound field *(33)*. The transducer is driven at 4.5 MHz at an output power of about 3 watts (VA) by applying voltage to the inner and outer electroded walls of the transducer. A recently developed compact voltage generating

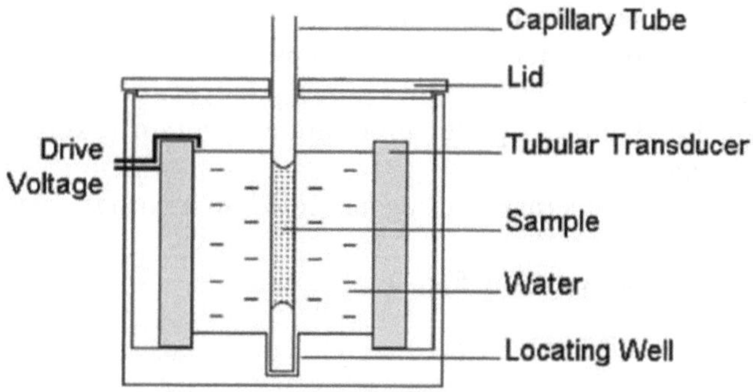

Fig. 1. A schematic cross-section of the ultrasonic chamber showing the tubular transducer and water to couple ultrasound to the on-axis capillary. The transducer was 20 mm in height with a wall thickness of 1.9 mm and an internal diameter of 31.5 mm.

device (Immunosonic, Electro-Medical Supplies, Wantage, UK) is now commercially available.

The light micrographs presented and the guidance discussed here aim to inform operator interpretation of the test and are based on our experiences using in-house test equipment (where the transducer is driven by the output of an RF amplifier [ENI model 240L, ENI, NY] using a Hewlett-Packard 33120A frequency synthesizer). Conclusions are consistent with observations, now made routinely here, using the Immunosonic prototype equipment (*see* **Note 2**). Representative fields of view were captured using a Leica Q500MC image-analysis system and depict images as viewed microscopically under the ×10 objective (Adobe Photoshop software and image analysis were used for presentation purposes only).

3. Methods

3.1. Sample Preparation

Where practicable, collect specimens immediately and store at 4°C until testing (separate plasma from whole blood before storage to avoid hemolysis). Sample processing is required for both conventional LA and ultrasonic immunoassay to liberate bound antigen from immunocomplexes and to eliminate cross-reactive material that could potentially compromise test specificity ***(20,46)***. Processed specimens may be stored at –20°C but must be centrifuged (at 14,000*g*) for 5 min before testing (*see* **Note 3**).

3.1.1. Serum or Plasma

1. To one volume of serum/plasma (*see* **Note 4**), add three volumes of 0.1 *M* EDTA in a heat resistant tube.

2. Heat in a boiling water bath for 5 min.
3. Allow to cool and transfer the boiled sample using a wide-bore pipet tip to a microfuge tube.
4. Centrifuge for 5 min to pellet precipitated protein (using a fixed-speed microcentrifuge).
5. Carefully draw the supernatant using a needle into a syringe so as not to disturb the precipitate.
6. Clarify by filtration (*see* **Note 5**).

3.1.2. CSF

1. Transfer samples to heat-resistant microcentrifuge tubes and boil for 5 min.
2. Allow to cool and centrifuge the specimen for 5 min in a microfuge.
3. Aspirate supernatant into a second tube using a needle and syringe and filter if sample is of sufficient volume (*see* **Note 5**).

3.2. LA Test

3.2.1. Test-Card Procedure

The sample should be of sufficient volume for testing with both meningococcal test latexes and the appropriate control reagent if agglutination is observed. If a negative control is required, it should be examined alongside the agglutinated test specimen. The Wellcogen kit instructions recommend simultaneous execution of test and control experiments.

1. Shake latex suspensions before use, preferably using a vortex mixer.
2. Holding the dropper bottle vertically, place one drop of each meningococcal test latex reagent (approx 40 μL) (and controls, volume permitting) onto a separate reaction circle on the surface of the test card.
3. Place an equal volume (*see* **Note 6**) of processed test specimen (using a pipet) adjacent to each drop of latex reagent within the same reaction circle.
4. Spread the droplet using a mixing stick to form a pool of reaction mixture that covers the area of the reaction circle (using a separate mixing stick for each test).
5. Manually rotate the test card using a rocking motion for exactly 3 min. During this time observe each reaction circle at reading distance for agglutination in the pool of reactants (agglutination can occur within seconds in high antigen concentrations).

3.2.2. Interpretation of Results

Score a sample as positive if clear agglutination is visible within 3 min of mixing the test latex and the test sample without agglutination occurring in the control latex reagent with the same patient specimen. The appearance of results using the test card method (*see* **Note 7**) and using a slide agglutination format (*see* **Note 8**) are shown in **Figs. 2** and **3**, respectively. Agglutination of both meningococcal test latexes with the same patient specimen should be disregarded.

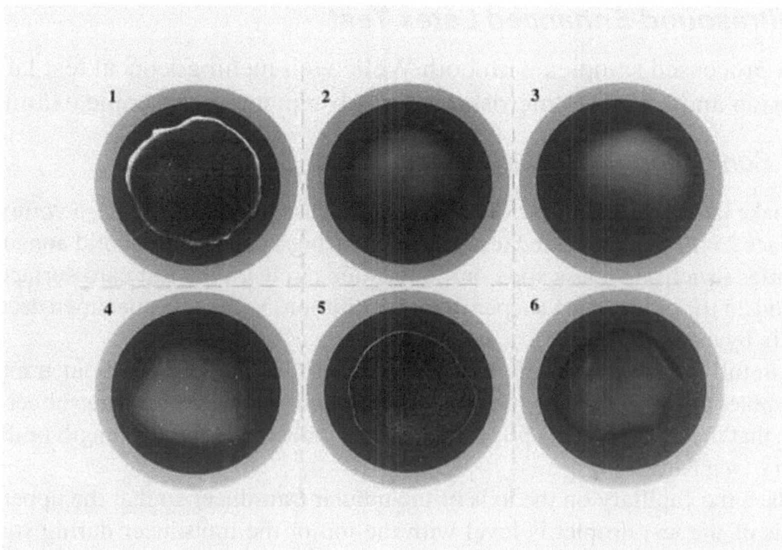

Fig. 2. Specimens from two patients with microbiologically confirmed meningococcal infection tested using Wellcogen test-card latex agglutination. Patient 1 (group C infection) tested with (1) *N. meningitidis* ACYW135 test reagent (+ve); (2) *N. meningitidis* B/*E. coli* K1 test reagent (–ve); (3) *N. meningitidis* ACYW135 control reagent (–ve). Patient 2 (group B infection) tested with (4) *N. meningitidis* ACYW135 test reagent (–ve); (5) *N. meningitidis* B/*E. coli* K1 test reagent (+ve); (6) *N. meningitidis* B/*E. coli* K1 control reagent (–ve).

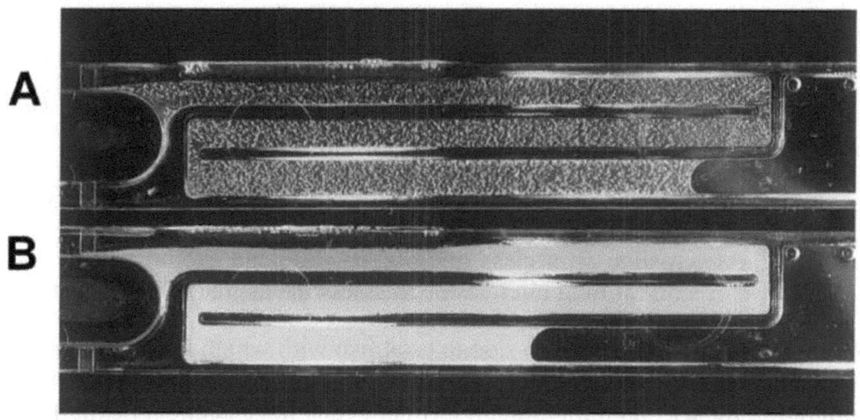

Fig. 3. Pastorex latex agglutination test on CSF from a patient with culture-confirmed meningococcal group B infection. The upper slide **(A)** shows positive agglutination with the *N. meningitidis* B/*E. coli* K1 test reagent. The lower slide **(B)** shows the same CSF specimen tested with the *N. meningitidis* B/*E. coli* K1 control reagent (–ve reaction).

3.3. Ultrasound-Enhanced Latex Test

Test processed samples with both Wellcogen meningococcal test latexes in succession and set aside microslides for subsequent microscopic examination.

3.3.1. Sonication Procedure

1. Shake latex suspensions (diluted 1/8) before use, preferably using a vortex mixer.
2. Place 25 µL of a processed test specimen (using a pipet) onto a solid nonadsorbing surface such as a glass slide or the reaction circle on the test card surface.
3. Add 25 µL of test latex suspension (1/8 dilution) to the test-specimen droplet and mix by aspiration.
4. Carefully draw the 50 µL test droplet into the capillary (without trapping air bubbles) using a syringe (attached to the capillary via 2 mm bore rubber tubing) so that the test droplet is positioned approx halfway along the length of the capillary (*see* **Note 2**).
5. Place the capillary on the axis of the tubular transducer so that the upper meniscus of the test droplet is level with the top of the transducer during sonication (**Fig. 1**). When inserting the capillary through the lid ensure that the lower end of the capillary is held by the locating well (applied pressure on the syringe maintains droplet position).
6. Sonicate for 60 s.
7. Remove the capillary from the transducer assembly slowly and carefully so as not to disturb the sonicated droplet (particle aggregates should be visible within the droplet *see* **Note 9**).
8. Expel droplet slowly (applying pressure on the syringe) onto a solid nonadsorbing surface.
9. Stir the sonicated droplet with 3–4 rotations using a mixing stick. It is important that the same level of stress is applied to each test sample to ensure experimental consistency (*see* **Note 10**).

3.3.2. Microscopy and Interpretation

1. Draw the test droplet into a 200-µm pathlength glass microslide by capillary action (*see* **Note 11**).
2. Place the microslide on a glass microscope slide and examine under the ×10 objective of a bright field microscope to assess the degree of agglutination.

Compare microslides side-by-side to establish with which latex reagent (if any) agglutination occurs ***(47)***. If clear agglutination is observed throughout the entire length of the microslide with a given test latex, test the specimen using the corresponding control latex to check specificity. Score the sample as positive if the agglutination seen with the test latex is clearly greater than any residual background clumping observed with the control reagent (*see* **Note 12**). The difference between a negative and a positive result with meningococcal latexes following sonication and the difference in appearance between the agglutinated test and control latex is shown in **Fig. 4** (*see* **Note 13**). Agglutination of both meningococcal test latexes with the same patient specimen or agglutination of test and control latexes (*see* **Fig. 5**) should be disregarded (*see* **Note 14**).

3.3.3. Estimation of Blood Antigen Level

Ultrasound-enhanced agglutination can provide a rapid prognostic indicator by sensitive measurement of serum antigen concentration *(45)*.

1. Make a doubling dilution series in PBS (containing sodium azide) using the processed blood sample (positive for meningococcal polysaccharide using ultrasound enhancement).
2. Test each serial dilution using the appropriate test latex reagent only (repeat testing with the control latex is unnecessary).
3. Continue serial dilution and testing using the test reagent until agglutination is no longer discernible (*see* **Fig. 6**). The titer obtained in this manner reflects the level of antigen present in the original blood sample (*see* **Note 15**).

In patients where specific features of meningococcal sepsis are absent and meningococcal antigen is not detected by ultrasound enhancement, the use of other test latexes (e.g., Murex *Streptococcus pneumoniae*, *Streptococcus* group B, or *Haemophilus influenzae*) and urine testing (*see* **Note 16**) should be considered *(47)*. Knowledge of patient details and clinical guidance can aid interpretation.

4. Notes

1. Latex suspensions should be checked for deterioration by using polyvalent positive control (contained in the kit) in place of the test sample and inspected for aggregation (autoagglutination) before use. The positive control should be reconstituted according to the manufacturer's instructions using sterile PBS containing 0.1% sodium azide as preservative. Definite agglutination should be obtained with the test latex reagents.
2. A 1-mm internal dimension square glass capillary (microcell) tube (Vitrocom Inc., NJ, USA) is used with the commercially available sonication equipment.
3. Degradation of antigen in CSF has been reported following storage at –20°C *(8)* and even short-term storage in air (at 37°C) has been shown to have a detrimental effect on LA *(48)*.
4. Hemolyzed or hyperlipidemic blood specimens are not recommended for use by test-card manufacturers and are unsuitable for ultrasound-enhanced testing. Serum or plasma specimens are obtained from fresh whole blood by centrifugation.
5. For filtration a minimum volume of 300 µL is required. Use a 19-G needle to draw the supernatant into a syringe without disturbing precipitated protein. Remove needle and attach a Millex-GS filter to syringe.
6. In our experience, reducing the volume of latex reagent used in the test-card procedure (from 40 to 25 µL) saves reagent and is useful when only small speci-

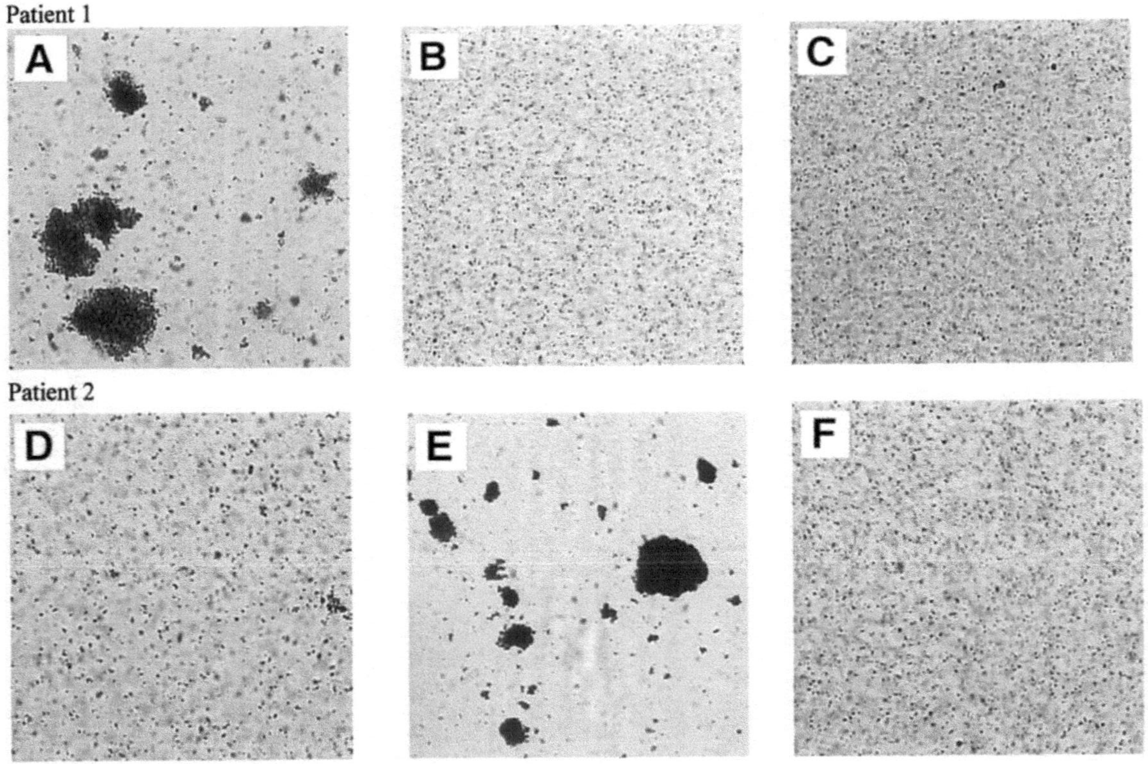

Fig. 4. Serum from two patients with confirmed meningococcal disease tested using ultrasound-enhanced latex agglutination with Wellcogen reagents. Patient 1 (group C infection) tested with **(A)** *N. meningitidis* ACYW135 test reagent (+ve); **(B)** *N. meningitidis* B/*E. coli* K1 test reagent (–ve); **(C)** *N. meningitidis* ACYW135 control reagent (–ve). Patient 2 (group B infection) tested with **(D)** *N. meningitidis* ACYW135 test reagent (–ve); **(E)** *N. meningitidis* B/*E. coli* K1 test reagent (+ve); **(F)** *N. meningitidis* B/*E. coli* K1 control reagent (–ve).

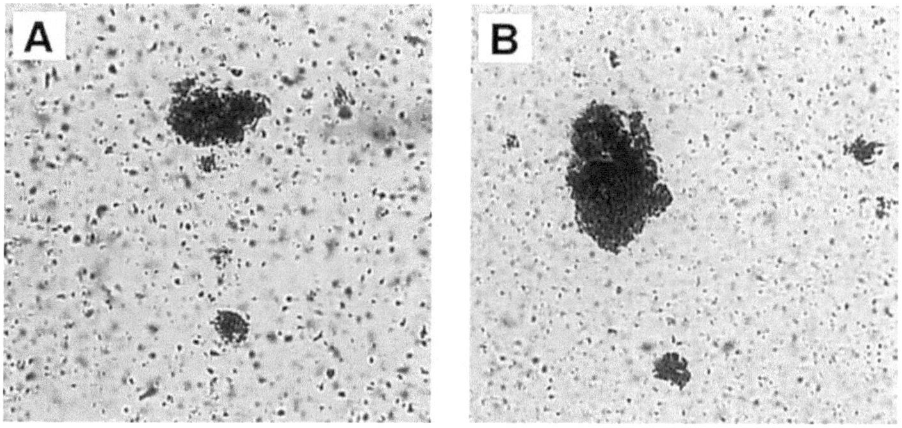

Fig. 5. Ultrasonic testing of serum from a patient with confirmed meningococcal group C disease showing nonspecific reactivity. **(A)** Wellcogen *N. meningitidis* ACYW135 test latex (+ve); **(B)** Wellcogen *N. meningitidis* ACYW135 control latex (+ve).

men volumes are available. Removing the dropper from the neck of the dispensing bottle allows latex suspension to be manipulated using standard pipet tips.

7. **Fig. 2** shows the test-card results obtained in two patients both with confirmed meningococcal disease (patient 1 was confirmed as meningococcal group C infection by *SiaD* PCR and culture; patient 2 was culture-positive for meningococcal group B). In serum obtained from patient 1, the *N. meningitidis* ACYW135 test latex agglutinated (**Fig 2.1**) but the serogroup B test latex and the *N. meningitidis* ACYW135 control reagent did not, indicating the presence of either group A, C, Y, or W135 polysaccharide. Likewise, in CSF from patient 2, agglutination of the *N. meningitidis* B/*E. coli* K1 test latex (**Fig. 2.5**) and negative reactions elsewhere indicated the presence of meningococcal group B or *E. coli* K1 polysaccharide. The Wellcogen Bacterial Antigen Kit instruction booklet (Murex, 1995) advises, "As a general rule a positive result with Wellcogen *N. meningitidis* B/*E. coli* K1 against a neonatal specimen suggests *E. coli* K1 infection; with older patients, meningococcus group B is more likely." The opaque appearance of the sample in a negative reaction is seen in **Fig. 2.2** and **2.4**. Negative reactions with test latexes indicate that antigen, if present, was below the threshold required for cross-linking of latex particles.
8. It is noteworthy that the Pastorex *N. meningitidis* serogroup B/*E. coli* K1 test is not performed on a test card but using a slide that draws a sample along a channel by capillarity. Here, an equal volume of reagent and test specimen are first dropped into a mixing well and drawn into a track to allow better visualization of fine agglutination (over a 10-min period) when positive (**Fig. 3**). In our experience, this procedure offers at most a twofold increase in sensitivity (of antigen detection in buffer) compared with other commercial test-card methods.

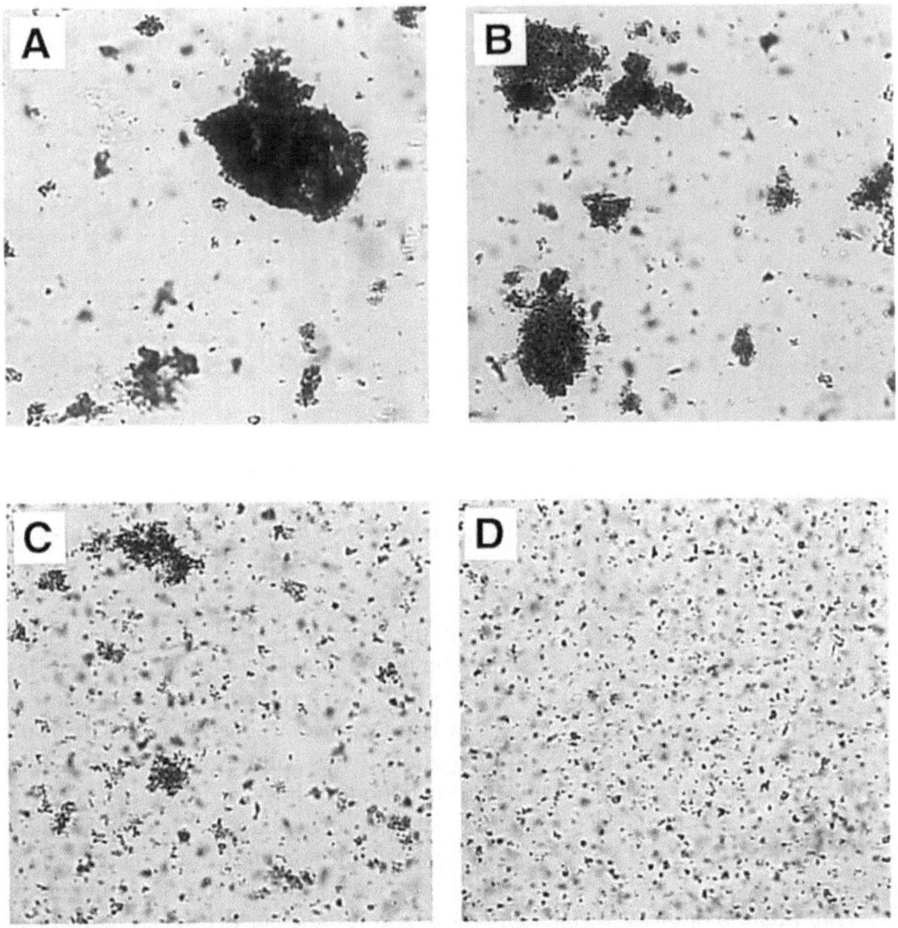

Fig. 6. Serial dilution and ultrasonic testing of sera from a patient (confirmed meningococcal group C infection) with the Wellcogen *N. meningitidis* ACYW135 test latex in **(A)** undiluted serum (+ve); **(B)** serum diluted 1/16 (+ve); **(C)** serum diluted 1/32 (*weak* +ve); **(D)** serum diluted 1/64 (negative reaction).

9. In many cases, a positive sample can be identified by eye on expulsion of the treated droplet from the capillary.
10. The stress required is the amount necessary to dissociate nonspecific clumps formed with negative controls (but not true agglutinates formed in the presence of antigen) following sonication. This stress level should be routinely applied to both controls and test samples on expulsion from the capillary. Stirring is necessary to dissociate aggregates formed by acoustic forces where no antigen-antibody cross-bridging occurs.

11. Rapid sample uptake can introduce shearing forces and, to keep extraneous stresses consistent, the microslide should be held at an angle of about 60° to the perpendicular.
12. Direct comparison of the agglutinated test reagent and the negative control latex (examination of adjacent microslides) facilitates identification of positive samples. It is important for operators to familiarize themselves with the typical appearance of test reagents as viewed microscopically in negative patient specimens as this serves to avoid sample overreading *(47)*.
13. **Figure 4** shows ultrasound results obtained using serum from two patients in whom meningococcal disease was suspected and where in each case, conventional LA had failed to detect antigen. In patient 1, significant agglutination was observed with the *N. meningitidis* ACYW135 test latex (**Fig. 4A**) but not with the *N. meningitidis* B/*E. coli* K1 test latex (**Fig. 4B**) or subsequently with the *N. meningitidis* ACYW135 control reagent (**Fig. 4C**). In patient 2, significant agglutination occurred with the *N. meningitidis* B/*E. coli* K1 test latex (**Fig. 4E**), whereas agglutination did not occur using either the *N. meningitidis* ACYW135 test latex (**Fig. 4D**) or the appropriate control (**Fig. 4F**). Ultrasound enhancement therefore detected serum antigen from one of the meningococcal groups A, C, Y, or W135 in patient 1 and antigen from either *N. meningitidis* group B or *E. coli* K1 in patient 2, in agreement with results obtained microbiologically. (Patient 1 was culture negative but the causative agent was confirmed as *N. meningitidis* group C by *SiaD* PCR on blood (specimens obtained at a different time were also test-card positive) patient 2 was culture confirmed and meningococcal *CtrA* PCR positive.) The meningococcal B/*E. coli* K1 test particles are typically monodisperse (**Fig. 4B**), in contrast to the appearance of small particle aggregates often present in the meningococcal ACYW135 test latex (**Fig. 4D**).
14. Infrequently, as in any immunoagglutination-based test, nonspecific reactions can occur. When aggregates form as a result of nonspecific agglutination, similar clumping occurs in test and control latexes and the sample should be scored as non-interpretable. **Figure 5** shows an example of a patient serum sample (subsequently confirmed as serogroup C disease by culture) tested ultrasonically (test-card LA was negative) in which the *N. meningitidis* ACYW135 test latex agglutinated but on subsequent testing of the control latex, the degree of clumping with both reagents was judged to be similar. Consequently, the result was non-interpretable owing to nonspecific reactions. Nonspecific clumping can sometimes be distinguished from true agglutinates because they are labile and have a diffuse appearance *(47)*. In our experience, nonspecific reactions are rarest in monoclonal-based tests (e.g., the *N. meningitidis* B/*E. coli* K1 test latex).
15. **Figure 6** demonstrates serial testing of antigen-positive serum from a patient with confirmed meningococcal C infection (by *SiaD* PCR on blood). In this example, agglutination was still discernible at a 1/32 dilution (**Fig. 6C**) but was not observed at a 1/64 dilution of serum (**Fig. 6D**). In sonicated specimens with a high antigen concentration, large agglutinates with well-defined edges are clearly visible throughout the whole length of the microslide (**Fig. 6A**). The background

particle density increases with decreasing antigen concentration as less particles are cross-linked and therefore involved in clump formation (**Fig. 6C**).

16. Samples of urine are boiled (5 min), centrifuged (using a fixed speed microcentrifuge) for 5 min and clarified by filtration (*see* **Note 5**). Urine pH can be adjusted to 8.0 (to minimize nonspecific agglutination reactions and aid interpretation) prior to centrifugation ***(38,49)***. Boiled urine samples of <8-mL volume may be concentrated using a Minicon® B-15 concentrator (Amicon Corp., UK).

Acknowledgments

This work was supported by the Meningitis Research Foundation and in part the Biotechnology and Biological Sciences Research Council (BBSRC) Analytical Biotechnology Initiative.

References

1. Severin, W. P. J. (1972) Latex agglutination in the diagnosis of meningococcal meningitis. *J. Clin. Path.* **25,** 1079–1082.
2. Leinonen, M. and Herva, E. (1977) The latex agglutination test for the diagnosis of meningococcal and *Haemophilus influenzae* meningitis. *Scand. J. Infect. Dis.* **9,** 187–191.
3. Ingram, D. L., Pearson, A. W., and Occhiuti, A. R. (1983) Detection of bacterial antigens in body fluids with the Wellcogen *H. Influenzae* b, *S. pneumoniae* and *N. meningitis* (ACYW135) LATs. *J. Clin. Microbiol.* **18,** 1119–1121.
4. Kaldor, J., Asznowicz, R., and Buist, D. G. P. (1977) Latex agglutination in diagnosis of bacterial infections, with special reference to patients with meningitis and septicemia. *Am. J. Clin. Pathol.* **68,** 284–289.
5. Requejo, H. I. Z., Nascimento, C. M. P. C., and Fahrat, C. K. (1992) Comparison of counterimmunoelectrophoresis, latex agglutination and bacterial culture for the diagnosis of bacterial meningitis using urine, serum and cerebrospinal fluid samples. *Braz. J. Med. Biol. Res.* **25,** 357–367.
6. Van Der Ende, A., Schuurman, I. G. A., Hopman, C. T. P., Fijen, C. A. P., and Dankert, J. (1995) Comparison of commercial diagnostic tests for identification of serogroup antigens of *N. meningitidis*. *J. Clin. Microbiol.* **33,** 3326–3327.
7. Williams, R. G. and Hart, C. A. (1988) Rapid identification of bacterial antigen in blood cultures and cerebrospinal fluid. *J. Clin. Pathol.* **41,** 691–693.
8. Krambovitis, E., McIllmurray, M. B., Lock, P. A., Holzel, H., Lifely, M. R., and Moreno, C. (1987) Murine monoclonal antibodies for detection of antigens and culture identification of *Neisseria meningitidis* group B and *Escherichia coli* K1. *J. Clin. Microbiol.* **25,** 1641–1644.
9. Leinonen, M. and Kayhty, H. (1978) Comparison of counter-current immunoelectrophoresis, latex agglutination and radioimmunoassay in detection of soluble capsular polysaccharide antigens of *Haemophilus influenzae* type b and *Neisseria meningitidis* of groups A or C. *J. Clin. Pathol.* **31,** 1172–1176.

10. Rai, G. P., Kumar, P., Phadke, S., Chandran, C. P., and Belapurkar, K. M. (1996) Detection of *N. meningitidis* antigen in cerebrospinal fluid by reverse pasive haemagglutination assay. *Biomed. Lett.* **54,** 87–95.
11. Dirks-Go, S. I. S. and Zanen, H. C. (1978) Latex agglutination, counterimmunoelectrophoresis, and protein A co-agglutination in diagnosis of bacterial meningitis. *J. Clin. Pathol.* **31,** 1167–1171.
12. Finlay, F. O., Witherow, H., and Rudd, P. T. (1995) Latex agglutination testing in bacterial meningitis. *Arch. Dis. Childhood* **73,** 160–161.
13. Muller, P. D., Donald, P. R., Burger, P. J., and Van Der Horst, W. (1989) Detection of bacterial antigens in cerebrospinal fluid by a latex agglutination test in "septic unknown" meningitis and serogroup B meningococcal meningitis. *S. Afr. Med. J.* **76,** 214–215.
14. Mein, J. and Lum, G. (1999) CSF bacterial antigen detection tests offer no advantage over Gram's stain in the diagnosis of bacterial meningitis. *Pathology* **31,** 67–69.
15. Camargos, P. A. M., Almeida, M. S., Cardoso, I., Filho, G. L., Filho D. M., Martins, J. I., et al. (1995) Latex particle agglutination test in the diagnosis of *Haemophilus influenzae* type b, *Streptococcus pneumoniae* and *Neisseria meningitidis* A and C meningitis in infants and children. *J. Clin. Epidemiol.* **48,** 1245–1250.
16. Barnes, R. A., Jenkins, P., and Coakley, W. T. (1998) Preliminary clinical evaluation of meningococcal disease and bacterial meningitis by ultrasonic enhancement. *Arch. Dis. Childhood* **78,** 58–60.
17. Al-Wali, W. and Hughes, C. (1998) Urine antigen detection can be quicker than PCR in the diagnosis of meningococcal disease. *J. Hosp. Infect.* **40,** 326–328.
18. D'Amato, R. F., Hochstein, L., and Fay, E. A. (1990) False positive latex agglutination test for *Neisseria meningitidis* group A and Y caused by povidone-iodine antiseptic contamination of cerebrospinal fluid. *J. Clin. Microbiol.* **28,** 2134–2135.
19. Perkins, M. D., Mirrett, S., and Reller, L. B. (1995) Rapid bacterial antigen detection is not clinically useful. *J. Clin. Microbiol.* **33,** 1486–1491.
20. Weinberg, G. A. and Storch, G. A. (1985) Preparation of urine samples for use in commercial latex agglutination tests for bacterial antigens. *J. Clin. Microbiol.* **21,** 899–901.
21. Robbins, J. B., Myerowitz, R. L., Whisnant, J.K., Argaman, M., Schneerson, R., Handzel, Z. T., and Gotschlich, E. C. (1972) Enteric bacteria cross-reactive with *Neisseria meningitidis* groups A and C and *Diplococcus pneumoniae* types I and III. *Infect. Immun.* **6,** 651–656.
22. Vann, W. F., Liu, T. Y., and Robbins, J. B. (1976) *Bacillus pumilus* polysaccharide cross-reactive with meningococcal group A polysaccharide. *Infect. Immun.* **13,** 1654–1662.
23. Bovre, K., Bryn, K., Closs, O., Hagen, N., and Oddvar Froholm, L. (1983) Surface polysaccharide of *Moraxella non-liquefaciens* identical to *Neisseria meningitidis* group B capsular polysaccharide. *NIPH Ann.* **6,** 65–73.
24. Fallon, R. J. and McIllmurray, M. B. (1976) *Escherichia coli* K1. *Lancet* 201.

25. Sarff, L. D., McCracken, G. H., Schiffer, M. S., Glode, M. P., Robbins, J. B., Orskov, I., and Orskov, F. (1975) Epidemiology of *Escherichia coli* K1 in healthy and diseased newborns. *Lancet* 1099–1104.
26. Alkmin, M. D. G. A., Melles, C. E. A., and Landgraf, I. M. (1995) Contribution of latex agglutination test for the diagnosis of pretreated meningitis. *Serodiagn. Immunother. Infect. Disease* **7,** 141–142.
27. Maxson, S., Lewno, M. J., and Schutze, G. E. (1994) Clinical usefulness of cerebrospinal fluid bacterial antigen studies. *J. Pediatrics* **125,** 235–238.
28. Narchi, H. (1997) CSF bacterial antigen detection testing in the diagnosis of meningitis. *Ann. Saudi Med.* **17,** 101–103.
29. Forward, K. R. (1988) Prospective evaluation of bacterial antigen detection in cerebral spinal fluid in the diagnosis of bacterial meningitis in a predominantly adult hospital. *Diagn. Microbiol. Infect. Dis.* **11,** 61–63.
30. Feuerborn, S. A., Capps, W. I., and Jones, J. C. (1992) Use of latex agglutination testing in diagnosing pediatric meningitis. *J. Fam. Practice* **34,** 176–179.
31. Kiska, D. L., Jones, M. C., Mangum, M. E., Orkiszewski, D., and Gilligan, P. H. (1995) Quality assurance study of bacterial antigen testing of cerebrospinal fluid. *J. Clin. Microbiol.* **33,** 1141–1144.
32. Grundy, M. A., Bolek, W. E., Coakley, W. T., and Benes, E. (1993) Rapid agglutination testing in an ultrasonic standing wave. *J. Immunol. Methods* **165,** 47–57.
33. Grundy, M. A., Moore, K., and Coakley, W. T. (1994) Increased sensitivity of diagnostic latex agglutination tests in an ultrasonic standing wave field. *J. Immunol. Methods* **176,** 169–177.
34. Coakley, W. T. (1997) Ultrasonic separations in analytical biotechnology. *TIBtech.* **15,** 506–511.
35. Grundy, M. A., Barnes, R. A., and Coakley, W. T. (1995) Highly sensitive detection of fungal antigens by ultrasound-enhanced latex agglutination. *J. Med. Vet. Mycol.* **33,** 201–203.
36. Ellis, R. W., Hastings, J. G. M., and Sobanski, M. A. (1998) Enhancement of rotavirus latex detection by ultrasonic standing wave treatment (abstract). *J. Infection* **36,** A12.
37. Thomas, N. E. and Coakley, W. T. (1996) Measurement of antigen concentration by an ultrasound enhanced latex immunoagglutination assay. *Ultrasound Med. Biol.* **22,** 1277–1284.
38. Jenkins, P., Barnes, R. A., and Coakley, W. T. (1997) Detection of meningitis antigens in buffer and body fluids by ultrasound-enhanced particle agglutination. *J. Immunol. Methods* **205,** 191–200.
39. Gualano, M. P., Grundy, M. A., Coakley, W. T., Parry, S. H., and Stickler, D. J. (1995) Ultrasound-enhanced latex agglutination for the detection of bacterial antigens in urine. *Br. J. Biomed. Sci.* **52,** 178–183.
40. Gray, S. J., Sobanski, M. A., Kaczmarski, E. B., Guiver, M., Masrsh, W. J., Borrow, R., et al. (1999) Ultrasound enhanced latex immunoagglutination and PCR as complementary methods for non-culture-based confirmation of meningococcal disease. *J. Clin. Microbiol.* **37,** 1797–1801.

41. Borrow, R., Claus, H., Guiver, M., Smart, L., Jones, D. M., Kaczmarski, E. B., et al. (1997) Nonculture diagnosis and serogroup determination of meningococcal B and C infection by a sialyltransferase (*siaD*) PCR ELISA. *Epidemiol. Infect.* **118,** 111–117.
42. Kaczmarski, E. B., Ragunathan, P. L., Marsh, J., Gray, S. J., and Guiver, M. (1998) Creating a national service for the diagnosis of meningococcal disease by polymerase chain reaction. *Comm. Dis. Public Health* **1,** 54–56.
43. Edwards, E. A. (1971) Immunologic investigations of meningococcal disease I. Group-specific *Neisseria meningitidis* antigens present in the serum of patients with fulminant meningococcemia. *J. Immunol.* **106,** 314–317.
44. Feldman, W. E. (1977) Relation of concentrations of bacteria and bacterial antigen in cerebrospinal fluid to prognosis in patients with bacterial meningitis. *N. Engl. J. Med.* **296,** 433–435.
45. Sobanski, M. A., Barnes, R. A., Gray, S. J., Carr, A. D., Kaczmarski, E. B., O'Rourke, A., et al. (2000) Measurement of serum antigen concentration by ultrasound enhanced immunoassay and correlation with clinical outcome in meningococcal disease. *Eur. J. Clin. Microbiol.* **19,** 260–266.
46. Doskeland, S. O. and Berdal, B. P. (1980) Bacterial antigen detection in body fluids: methods for rapid antigen concentration and reduction of nonspecific reactions. *J. Clin. Microbiol.* **11,** 380–384.
47. Sobanski, M. A., Gray, S. J., Cafferkey, M., Ellis, R. W., Barnes, R. A., and Coakley W. T. (1999) Meningitis antigen detection: interpretation of agglutination by ultrasound-enhanced latex immunoassay. *Br. J. Biomed. Sci.* **56,** 239–246.
48. Cunniffe, J. G., Whitby-Strevens, S., and Wilcox, M. H. (1996) Effect of pH changes in cerebrospinal fluid specimens on bacterial survival and antigen test results. *J. Clin. Pathol.* **49,** 249–253.
49. Harrison, L. H., Steinhoff, M. C., Sridharan, G., Castelo, A., Khallaf, N., Ostroff, S. M., and Arthur, R. R. (1996) Monovalent latex agglutination reagents for the diagnosis of nonmeningitic pneumococcal infection. *Diagn. Microbiol. Infect. Dis.* **24,** 1–6.

5

Meningococcal Serology

Stephen J. Gray, Ray Borrow, and Edward B. Kaczmarski

1. Introduction

Meningococcal serology has been mainly used over the last 20 years in the field of vaccinology, to evaluate candidate vaccines and quantify individuals' immune responses. With the increasing usage of pre-admission antibiotic treatment *(1)*, nonculture diagnostic methods such as polymerase chain reaction (PCR) (Chapter 3), antigen detection (Chapter 4), and serology have become important tools. Nonculture diagnosis of meningococcal disease is rapidly becoming of equal importance for the confirmation of meningococcal infection as the isolation of *Neisseria meningitidis* organisms *(2)*. This has occurred at a time when accurate case ascertainment of meningococcal disease has become a crucial aspect of assessing effectiveness of the recently introduced serogroup C polysaccharide-protein conjugate vaccine in the UK *(3)*. *N. meningitidis* polysaccharide vaccines have been available for over 20 years *(4)* and evaluation of candidate vaccines and assessment of levels of antibody requires accurate and reproducible assays.

Antibody responses to these capsular polysaccharide vaccines have been measured by a number of serological methods including hemagglutination *(5)*, immunofluorescence *(6)*, radial immunodiffusion *(7)*, latex agglutination (*see* Chapter 4), opsonizing antibody (*see* Meningococcal Vaccines, edited by A. J. Pollard and M. C. J. Maiden, Humana Press), complement-fixing antibody *(8)*, bactericidal antibody (*see* Meningococcal Vaccines, edited by A. J. Pollard and M. C. J. Maiden, Humana Press), radioimmunoassay (RIA) *(9)*, and enzyme-linked immunosorbent assay (ELISA). Meningococcal serogroup A and C polysaccharide vaccines were licensed using data obtained by RIA and bactericidal assays. Of those procedures that are quantitative, only RIA and

From: *Methods in Molecular Medicine, vol. 67: Meningococcal Disease: Methods and Protocols*
Edited by: A. J. Pollard and M. C. J. Maiden © Humana Press Inc., Totowa, NJ

ELISA accurately measure antibody levels within the small serum volumes usually available from infants and young children.

The main format for meningococcal serology over the last 20 years has been based on the ELISA. The ELISA format has been preferentially chosen because it is safe, simple, sensitive, reproducible, and specific. In the past, the radiolabeled antigen-binding assay has been used for quantification of levels of antibody to meningococcal polysaccharide ***(10)*** but the radiolabeled antigen-binding assay has been shown to be subject to inconsistencies in the method and intensity of antigen radiolabeling ***(11)***. Results, however, have been shown to correlate well with radiolabeled antigen-binding assay data in studies of *Haemophilus influenzae* type b ***(12,13)***.

Negatively charged polysaccharides, such as meningococcal capsular components, do not easily adsorb to polystyrene from which microtiter plates are manufactured. Thus, various methods have been used to increase binding of the polysaccharide to the microtiter plate. These methods have included: capture antibodies ***(14)***, coupling the polysaccharide to tyramine ***(15)***, coupling the polysaccharide to poly-L-lysine ***(16–18)***, biotinylation ***(19)***, and mixing with methylated human serum albumin ***(18,20,21)***.

Much attention has been focused upon standardized assays to evaluate meningococcal polysaccharide and conjugate vaccines in order to avoid the problems with comparing results generated among laboratories as occurred with *H. influenzae* type b ***(11,22,23)***. Multi-center comparisons of ELISAs have resulted in the acceptance of the use of standardized assays for serogroup A ***(21)*** and C ***(24)***. These assays may be adapted to discriminate between meningococcal serogroups for nonculture serogroup confirmation.

The use of a poly-L-lysine ELISA for measurement of antibodies against meningococcal serogroups B and C polysaccharide has been described ***(11,25)*** and illustrates the use of ELISA in trying to improve surveillance of meningococcal disease. Care must be taken, however, with the use of poly-L-lysine in an ELISA owing to nonspecific binding of some human sera ***(16,20)***. Methylated human serum albumin is now recommended in preference to poly-L-lysine because it has been shown to give better reproducibility and higher resulting titers ***(18)***.

Attention has also been focused on the class of antibody responses to meningococcal polysaccharides ***(25)***. For serogroup C, both IgG and IgM antibodies have been demonstrated following disease ***(25,26)***. Serogroup C-specific antibodies are also induced following oropharyngeal carriage of serogroup C meningococci ***(27)*** or following vaccination with serogroup C polysaccharide ***(4)*** or conjugate ***(28)*** vaccines. By drawing upon UK experience with a large age-stratified serological survey conducted in England and Wales by the Public Health Laboratory Service (PHLS) Meningococcal Reference Unit (MRU) on samples collected in 1996–1997, it was possible to calculate an appropriate cut-off for unvaccinated individuals. For vaccinated individuals, limited antibody-persistence data are available from infants and children under 5 yr of age enabling the calculation of a cut-off for this age group.

To date, conflicting results have been reported on the human isotype responses and duration of responses to serogroup B polysaccharide. Studies have shown the presence of serogroup B IgM isotype antibodies in healthy individuals ***(16,29)***, whereas others have shown these to be absent ***(30)***. Low levels of serogroup B polysaccharide-specific IgG have been detected in sera from healthy individuals ***(16)*** but not in convalescent sera from patients recovering from serogroup B disease ***(25)***. Antibody isotype responses following serogroup B infection are largely of the IgM isotype ***(16,25,30)***. Serogroup A- and C-specific antibodies may be quantified (in an ELISA format) utilizing a standard reference serum ***(31)*** but there is no such reference serum currently available for serogroup B-specific antibodies. Few studies have been published on the age-related responses to serogroup B polysaccharide, the persistence of those antibodies after disease, or the seroprevalence of serogroup B-specific antibodies in the general population. In-house assays are often used ***(25,32,33)***, employing different criteria to differentiate serogroups B and C.

The case confirmation of serogroup A disease is not required in most developed countries but a serogroup A-specific polysaccharide ELISA has been described for quantification of antibodies following vaccination with serogroup A polysaccharide vaccines ***(21)***. This assay may be modified as for serogroup C, but the authors' experience with this assay is for the measurement of immune responses following vaccination rather than confirming cases of serogroup A disease.

Outer-membrane vesicle (OMV)-based ELISAs have largely been utilized to evaluate meningococcal OMV-based vaccines ***(34)*** and have been employed by some workers to confirm meningococcal disease in the absence of a positive culture result ***(32,33,35)***. In our laboratory, the OMV assay is used only as a screen to which positives are forwarded for the serogroup B and C polysaccharide ELISAs. Care must be taken with interpretation of positives owing to the oropharyngeal carriage of meningococci or other *Neisseria* species (often commensal) inducing antibodies that may cross-react and may indeed be protective against meningococcal disease ***(27)***. *N. meningitidis* carriage without clinical disease may induce both IgG and IgM isotype antibodies ***(36)***.

This chapter describes an OMV screening assay from which positives may be subjected to the serogroups B and C ELISA. Reasonably accurate interpretative criteria (cut-offs) are available now for serogroup C but not serogroup B anti-polysaccharide antibodies, though the assay described can be used to give an indication of the likelihood of recent serogroup B disease.

The microbiological confirmation of the diagnosis of acute meningococcal disease is by traditional microscopy, culture, antigen detection, and increasingly by DNA detection using PCR-based methods. Meningococcal serology can be a useful adjunct for corroborative evidence but by its nature is a retrospective investigation. We believe serological evidence alone is not suitable to define cases of meningococcal disease without strong clinical evidence. Ideally the serological tests should be performed on paired sera, the convalescent sample having been taken at least 10 d after onset. Single, convalescent samples taken within 6 wk after onset may provide useful results. Clinical details (including meningococcal vaccine history) and date of onset of symptoms are crucial for appropriate interpretation.

The methods to be described within this chapter include: a meningococcal OMV ELISA assay (*see* **Subheadings 2.1.** and **3.1.**), which measures the level of anti-OMV IgG and IgM isotype in cases of suspected or confirmed meningococcal disease to determine acute infections and screen samples for testing in the meningococcal polysaccharide-specific ELISA assays; preparation of methylated human serum albumin (*see* **Subheadings 2.2.** and **3.2.**), as required for the serogroup C polysaccharide-specific IgG ELISA (*see* **Subheadings 2.3.** and **3.3.**), adapted from the method of Gheesling et al. *(25)* (*see* **Subheading 3.3.**); modified assays for serogroup B polysaccharide-specific total Ig (*see* **Subheading 3.4.**); and serogroup A polysaccharide-specific IgG (*see* **Subheading 3.5.**).

2. Materials

2.1. OMV ELISA Assay

2.1.1. Equipment

1. Centrifuge-Sorvall RC28S centrifuge (Dupont) or equivalent. With F-28/13 rotor and appropriate polypropylene centrifuge tubes or equivalent.
1. Sonicator: MSE Soniprep 150 with probe and glass sonication vessels.
2. Shaking environmental incubator, model G25 (New Brunswick Scientific Co.) or equivalent.
3. Ballotini solid-glass soda balls (4.7–5.3 mm diameter) (Jencons plc., Cat. no. 136-024) or equivalent.
4. Microtiter plates: Falcon MicroTest 111, 96-well, flat-bottom well, (Becton Dickinson, Cat. no. 3912) or equivalent.
5. Falcon MicroTest 111, flexible lids, (Becton Dickinson, Cat. no. 3913) or equivalent.
6. ELISA washer: SkanWasher 300, version B (Skatron) or equivalent.
7. Spectrophotometer: Titertek Multiskan MCC (Type 341) or equivalent.
8. PPN Tubes (ICN, Cat. no. 61-226-C2) or equivalent.
9. PPN tubeholder-96 W/Cover (ICN, Cat. no. 61-225-00).
10. 250-mL flasks (4102 Erlenmeyer flasks, polymethylpentene, Nalgene Labware, Cat. no. 4109-0250) or equivalent.

2.1.2. Reagents

1. Goat anti-human IgG peroxidase conjugate, (Sigma, Cat. no. A6029), stored at –20°C in single-use volumes.
2. Goat anti-human IgM peroxidase conjugate, (Sigma, Cat. no. A8650), stored at +4°C in single-use volumes.
3. Columbia blood agar plates (containing 5% horse blood) (Oxoid, Cat. no. CM331) or equivalent.
4. BCA protein assay kit (Pierce and Warriner, Cat. no. 2322522) or equivalent.
5. Sodium deoyxcholate, ($C_{24}H_{39}O_4Na$, BDH, Cat. no. 43035) or equivalent.
6. Trizma base [Tris(hydroxymethyl)aminomethane], ($C_4H_{11}NO_3$, Sigma, Cat. no. T8524) or equivalent.
7. Ethylenediaminetetraacetic acid (EDTA), ($C_{10}H_{16}N_2O_8$, Amresco, Cat. no. AO/0105) or equivalent.
8. Tween 20, polyoxyethylenesorbitan monolaurate, (Sigma, Cat. no. P1379) or equivalent.
9. Bovine serum albumin (BSA), Fraction V (Sigma, Cat. no. A7906) or equivalent.
10. Phosphate-buffered saline (PBS) tablets (Oxoid, Cat. no. BR14M) or equivalent.
11. Dried skimmed milk powder, "Marvel" (Premier Beverages, Knighton, Adbaston, Stafford UK) or equivalent.
12. Normal goat serum (Sigma, Cat. no. G6767) or equivalent.
13. Sodium carbonate (Na_2CO_3, Fisons, Cat. no. S/2920/60) or equivalent.
14. Sodium bicarbonate, ($NaHCO_3$, Sigma, Cat. no. S8875) or equivalent.
15. Dibasic sodium phosphate (Na_2HPO_4, Sigma, Cat. no. S0876) or equivalent.
16. Citric acid ($C_6H_8O_7.H_2O$, Sigma, Cat. no. C7129) or equivalent.
17. OPD (O-Phenylenediamine dihydrochloride) substrate tablets ($C_6H_8N_2.2HCl$, Sigma, Cat. no. P8287) or equivalent.
18. Hydrogen peroxide (30%), (H_2O_2, Merck, Cat. no.101284N) or equivalent.
19. Sulfuric acid 2.5 *M*, (H_2SO_4, Merck, Cat. no. 19167) or equivalent.
20. Phenylmethylsulfonyl fluoride (PMSF) (Sigma, Cat. no. P7626) or equivalent.
21. Propan-2-ol (C_3H_8O, Merck, Cat. no. 10224) or equivalent.

2.1.3. Buffers

1. Deoxycholate buffer: 0.1 *M* Trizma base, pH 8.5, 0.01 *M* EDTA, 0.5% (w/v) sodium deoxycholate. Warm the sodium deoxycholate to dissolve. Store the buffer at room temperature.
2. Bicarbonate buffer, pH 9.6: 15 m*M* Na_2CO_3, 35 m*M* $NaHCO_3$. Use sterile double-distilled water and adjust to pH 9.6, store at +4°C for use within 2 wk.
3. Serum and conjugate buffer (SC): Phosphate buffered saline (PBS) containing: 0.05% (v/v) Tween 20, 1% (w/v) Dried skimmed-milk powder, 5% (v/v) normal goat serum. Make up the buffer as required, do not store longer than 2 d at +4°C.
4. Substrate buffer (for peroxidase enzyme): 0.2 *M* Na_2HPO_4, 0.1 *M* citric acid, 0.02% H_2O_2 (30%), 2 m*M* OPD. (To make 25 mL: immediately before use dissolve 10 mg OPD [1 tablet] in 25 mL of substrate buffer made using sterile distilled water followed by the addition of 4 µL of 30% hydrogen peroxide).

2.1.4. Sera

1. Test sera. Perform the test on paired sera, the convalescent sample having been taken at least 14 d after onset. Single, convalescent samples taken within 6 wk after onset may provide useful results. On receipt in the laboratory, transfer the test sera to 1.5-mL sterile plastic vials, for storage at –20°C prior to testing. Where possible storage at –80°C is preferred. The OMP ELISA assay described in **Subheading 3.1.4.** allows for the testing of 38 sera (in duplicate).
2. Positive control serum (P). The positive control reagent is a pool of several clinical serum samples that were found to be high positives within the OMP ELISA assay. Aliquots (20 µL) are stored at –20°C or if possible –80C.
3. Negative control (N). The negative control serum is from a single individual with a nonreactive OMP ELISA result.

2.2. mHSA Preparation for Polysaccharide-Specific IgG ELISA

The mHSA is prepared in accordance with Mandell and Hershey *(38)* and Carlone et al. *(21)*. Refer to local safety procedures (EEC Risk and COSHH assessments) before starting this procedure.

2.2.1. Equipment

1. Protective exhaust-fume hood, Astecair or equivalent.
2. Magnetic stirrer.
3. Glass universal containers (without rubber liners in lid).
4. Centrifuge, (MSE Mistral 2000 or equivalent).
5. "Gyrovap," centrifuge evaporation unit with solvent trap, (Howe) or equivalent.
6. Freeze-drying apparatus.

2.2.2. Reagents

1. Human albumin: Fraction V, 96-99% albumin (Sigma, Cat. no. A-1653) or equivalent.
2. Methanol (CH_3OH, Sigma, Cat. no. M3641) or equivalent.
3. Hydrochloric acid, concentrated 12 *M* (HCl, Merck, Cat. no. 101125) or equivalent.
4. Ether ($(C_2H_5)_2O$, Merck, Cat. no. 10483) or equivalent.
5. Phosphorous pentoxide (P_2O_5, Merck, Cat. no. 33170) or equivalent.

2.3. Serogroup C Polysaccharide-Specific IgG ELISA

2.3.1. Equipment

1. Flat-bottom, 96-well polystyrene microtitration plates (Cat. no. M129B, Dynex Technologies Ltd.) or equivalent.
2. Titertek plate sealers, pressure-sensitive film (Cat. no. 77-400-05, ICN) or equivalent.

3. Automatic ELISA plate washer, SkanWasher 300 version B (Skatron) or equivalent.
4. Titertek multiskan ELISA reader, model MCC (type 340) or equivalent.
5. Automated multi-channel electronic pipet (Roche Diagnostics).

2.3.2. Reagents

1. Polysaccharide antigen. Lyophilized *N. meningitidis* serogroup C polysaccharide produced by BioMerieux available from NIBSC (National Institute for Biological Standards and Control, South Mimms, UK). Alternative sources of *N. meningitidis* serogroup C polysaccharide may include other meningococcal polysaccharide-vaccine manufacturers.

   Reconstitute the polysaccharide to 25 mg/mL in pyrogen-free water and store in 50-μL volumes at –20°C to avoid repeated freezing and thawing.
2. Methylated human serum albumin (mHSA). The mHSA is prepared in accordance with Mandell and Hershey ***(38)*** and Carlone et al. ***(21)*** as described in **Subheading 3.2.1.** Known amounts (approx 0.1 g) are stored freeze-dried at +4°C. The mHSA is re-hydrated with sterile pyrogen-free water to yield a stock solution of 10 mg/mL. Stored at +4°C , the mHSA solution should be used within 3 mo.
3. Monoclonal antibody (MAb) to Human IgG Fc PAN (1,2,3,4) HRP conjugated (Stratech Scientific Ltd., Cat. no.6043HRP) or equivalent. Alternative conjugates are described (*see* **Note 8**).
4. Polyoxyethylene 23 lauryl ether, Brij-35 detergent 30% solution, ($C_{12}E_{23}$, Sigma, Cat No. 430AG-6) or equivalent.
5. PBS tablets, (Oxoid, Cat. no. BR14M) or equivalent.
6. Newborn bovine serum (NBBS) (ICN, Cat no. 29-121-54), divided into 20-mL amounts and stored at –20°C.
7. Pyrogen-free water for injections BP (Phoenix Pharmaceuticals Ltd.) or equivalent.
8. Dibasic sodium phosphate (Na_2HPO_4, Sigma, Cat. no. S0876) or equivalent.
9. Citric acid ($C_6H_8O_7.H_2O$, Sigma, Cat. no. C7129) or equivalent.
10. 3,3′,5,5 ′-tetramethylbenzidine dihydrochloride, TMB substrate tablets (1 mg), ($C_{16}H_{20}N_2.2HCl$, Sigma, Cat. no.T3405) or equivalent.
11. Hydrogen peroxide, 30% solution (H_2O_2, BDH, Cat. no. 101284N) or equivalent.
12. 0.2 *M* sulfuric acid, (H_2SO_4, BDH, Cat. no.19815 4Y) or equivalent.

2.3.3. Sera

2.3.3.1. Test Sample Selection

Most sera tested for serogroup C-specific polysaccharide antibody are from subjects with a high suspicion of meningococcal disease. Unfortunately the anti-polysaccharide antibody assay to be described has limited throughput (four test sera per ELISA plate). To target suitable material the PHLS MRU has used the OMV assay described in this chapter to choose reactive samples for the detection of serogroup C polysaccharide-specific IgG antibodies. Ideally the paired sera should be tested on the same plate.

2.3.3.2. Standard Reference Serum (for Antibody Quantification)

The international standard reference serum for *N. meningitidis* serogroup A and C polysaccharide antibody is a donor human serum pool designated CDC 1992 ***(31)*** available from NIBSC and CDC (Atlanta, GA). The total serogroup C anti-capsular IgG antibody concentration is 24.1 μg/mL. For use re-hydrate each vial with 1 mL of pyrogen-free water and distribute in 50 μL amounts for long-term storage at –80°C. Dilute the CDC 1992 serum 1/75 in the SC buffer ready for addition to the plate. (Diluted 1:1 in the plate, the initial dilution of the standard reference calibration curve is 1/150 (*see* plate template, **Note 1**). It is worthwhile checking the standard curve and adjusting the starting dilution if titers are tending towards either the lower or upper asymptote.

2.3.3.3. Internal Quality-Control Serum

A post-vaccination "immune serum" is used as the ELISA assay quality-control serum. Dilute the quality-control serum in SC buffer to yield optical densities in the high, middle, and low portions of the standard reference calibration curve. Stock working solutions of the three quality-control dilutions are prepared, aliquoted, and frozen at –80°C.

2.3.3.4. Test-Sample Preparation

The sera are single convalescent (or paired acute and convalescent samples) that have been stored at –20°C or if possible –80°C. Dilute the test sera 1/25 in SC buffer prior to addition to the plates.

2.3.4. Buffers

1. Antigen (polysaccharide) coating buffer: 10 m*M* PBS, pH 7.4, made with pyrogen-free water.
2. Wash buffer: 10 m*M* PBS, pH 7.4, containing 0.1% (v/v) Brij-35, using double-distilled water.
3. Blocking buffer: 10 m*M* PBS, pH 7.4, containing 5% (v/v) NBBS, using double-distilled water. (0.1% Brij-35 may be added to the block buffer and will not affect the background OD).
4. Serum and conjugate buffer (SC): 10 m*M* PBS, pH 7.4, containing 5% (v/v) NBBS, 0.1% Brij-35, using double-distilled water.
5. TMB substrate buffer: 24 m*M* citric acid, pH 5.0, 50 m*M* Na_2HPO_4, 0.02% H_2O_2 (30%), 31 m*M* TMB. (To make 10 mL: add 1 mg tablet of TMB to 2.57 mL of 0.2 *M* dibasic sodium phosphate, 2.43 mL of 0.1 *M* citric acid, and 5.0 mL of double-distilled water. Then add 2 μL hydrogen peroxide [30%].)

6. Computer software: "ELISA" for Windows version 1.07 data analysis software (provided by CDC), 4-parameter logistic curve model ***(39)***.

2.4. Serogroup B Polysaccharide-Specific Antibody ELISA

All equipment and reagents are the same as for serogroup C IgG ELISA except for:

1. Serogroup B polysaccharide: If a source of purified serogroup B polysaccharide is available, this may be used, or alternatively *E. coli* K1 capsular polysaccharide
2. Serogroup control serum: This may be a serum from a culture proven case of serogroup B meningococcal infection but a pooled serum is preferable. Sera with levels of serogroup B-specific antibody that are at least 3 times higher than the mean found in healthy subjects, in specimens taken 2–6 wk after clinical presentation are regarded as indicative of recently having encountered serogroup B meningococci. At the PHLS MRU, the positive control pool of sera was assigned an arbitrary value of 3400 AU/mL after comparison with the serogroup C control, CDC 1992.
3. Conjugates: For serogroup B total Ig antibody use a pool of IgG, IgM, and IgA conjugates (*see* **Note 7**) as a low level of IgG isotype antibody is induced in response to serogroup B polysaccharide ***(16,25,30)***.

2.5. Serogroup A Polysaccharide-Specific IgG ELISA

Materials for the are identical to those the described serogroup C polysaccharide-specific IgG ELISA (*see* **Subheading 2.3.**) except for the following:

1. Serogroup A polysaccharide: Can be obtained from NIBSC or various meningococcal polysaccharide vaccine manufacturers.
2. CDC1992 standard reference serum. The serogroup A polysaccharide-specific IgG = 91.8 μg/mL, whilst the level of total meningococcal polysaccharide-specific Ig = 135.8 μg/mL ***(31)***.

3. Methods

3.1. Preparation of Meningococcal OMV ELISA Antigen

3.1.1. Safety Considerations

Local safety requirements must be followed. EU countries require COSHH assessment for all procedures. All manipulations of the *N. meningitidis* isolates that may generate aerosols **must** be carried out in a microbiological safety cabinet to give operator protection.

3.1.2. N. meningitidis *Isolates for Pooled OMV Antigen Preparation*

The choice of the *N. meningitidis* isolates to be used for the OMV preparation is based on epidemiological surveillance of the predominant disease-causing phenotypes (serotype and serosubtypes).

3.1.3. Meningococcal OMV Preparation for OMV ELISA Assay (37)

Steps 1–3 must be performed in a microbiological safety cabinet.

1. Sub-culture each of the selected *N. meningitidis* organisms onto a single Columbia blood-agar plate (containing 5% horse blood) and incubate for 18 h at 37°C in a 5% CO_2 atmosphere.
2. Following incubation, inoculate each isolate on to 20 Columbia blood-agar plates and re-incubate as described in **Step 1**.
3. Remove the growth from the agar plates by scraping the surface with a clean glass microscope slide, into 30 mL of deoxycholate buffer.
4. Transfer the *N. meningitidis* suspension into a 250-mL polymethylpentene conical flask containing 20 solid-glass balls (5-mm diameter). Seal the flask with a screw-capped lid. Then place each flask in two polythene bags inside a sealed container and carry to a shaking environmental incubator.
5. Carefully but securely attach the polythene-covered flasks to the base plate of the shaking incubator. Set the incubator at 60°C and 300 rpm for 30 min to separate the OMVs from the whole cells.
6. Remove the whole cells by transferring the suspension to 10-mL polypropylene centrifuge tubes and centrifugation at 20,000*g* for 30 min at +4°C (using a Sorvall RC28S with a F-28/13 rotor or equivalent).
7. Following centrifugation transfer the supernatant by gentle aspiration into a clean 10-mL polypropylene centrifuge tube (and discard the pellet). Centrifuge the supernatant again at 100,000*g* for 60 min at +4°C.
8. Discard the second supernatant and re-suspend the pellet (OMVs) in 0.5 mL of sterile distilled water.
9. Transfer the re-suspended pellet to a glass sonication vessel and sonicate with 3 bursts of 10 s duration using the probe attached to a MSE Soniprep 150 (or equivalent).
10. Quantify the OMV (antigen) preparation using a BCA protein assay kit (or equivalent) and adjust to a protein concentration of 400 μg/mL.
11. Combine the OMVs from each strain in the ratio 1 : 1 : 1 to produce a "universal" OMV antigen reagent for the meningococcal OMV ELISA assay. The mixed antigen (OMVs) allows the detection of antibodies to the selected serotype and sero-subtypes. If the OMVs are retained separately individual OMV antigens can be used to determine antibody responses against each specific isolate.
12. Whether individual or mixed preparations are made, store the OMVs at –20°C. Samples of 100 μL can be stored for a maximum of 1 yr. Proteolysis of the OMV preparations may be retarded by the addition of 40 μg/mL of PMSF dissolved in propan-2-ol.

3.1.4. Meningococcal OMV ELISA Assay Method

This is a semi-automated alternative method for OMV ELISA assay (*see* **Note 3**).

1. Add 100 μL of the OMV antigen at 1/1000 dilution in bicarbonate buffer (*see* **Note 4**) to all wells (columns 1 → 12) of two flat-bottomed microtiter plates and

incubate the plates overnight at +4°C. One plate is required for IgG and the other plate for IgM isotype antibody detection.
2. Wash the plates 5 times with 200 µL of wash buffer. This stage is best suited for an automated whole plate washer such as the Skatron washer (or equivalent).
3. Block the nonspecific binding sites by the addition of 200 µL of freshly prepared 3% (w/v) BSA in PBS to all wells.
4. Incubate the plates for 1 h at +37°C.
5. Wash the plates 5 times with 200 µL of wash buffer.
6. Prepare 1/100 sample dilutions of the 38 test serum and controls prior to testing by the addition of 10 µL serum to 990 µL SC buffer. Mix the diluted samples and add 100 µL to both the IgM and IgG plates (in duplicate) to the wells of a pair of columns as indicated in the plate template (*see* **Note 4**). Add the diluted positive (P) and negative control (N) sera in 3 sets of duplicates distributed throughout the plate (*see* **Note 4**).
7. Incubate the plates for 2 h at +37°C.
8. Wash the plates 5 times with 200 µL of wash buffer.
9. Add 100 µL of the anti-human IgG peroxidase conjugate at 1/1000 dilution in SC buffer to all the wells of the IgG plate. Similarly, add 100 µL of the anti-human IgM peroxidase conjugate at 1/1000 dilution to the IgM plate.
10. Re-incubate the plates for 2 h at +37°C.
11. Wash the plates 5 times with 200 µL of wash buffer.
12. Prepare the OPD substrate solution immediately prior to use and add 100 µL to each well of both the IgG and IgM plates. Incubate the plates at room temperature for 12 min.
13. Stop the color reaction by the addition of 50 µL of 2.5 *M* sulfuric acid to each well. Read the OD at 492 nm on a Titertek Multiskan MCC (Type 341) spectrophotometer or equivalent, blanking the plate OD readings on column 1.

3.1.5. Calculation of EIU for OMV ELISA Assay

For both the IgG and the IgM plates subtract the mean OD of the reagent blank column 1 from each of the test and control wells. Calculate the mean values for the Positive and Negative controls and use in the following equation:

$$\text{The cut-off} = [\text{Negative OD}/(\text{Positive OD} - \text{Negative OD})] \times 100$$

Calculate the mean value for each test sample and compare with the cut-off value.

Calculate the test sera result in EIU (Enzyme Immunoassay Units) as follows:

$$\text{EIU} = [(\text{Test OD} - \text{Negative OD}) / (\text{Positive OD} - \text{Negative OD})] \times 100$$

If the test sample EIU < than cut-off value the result is positive. If the test sample EIU > than the cut-off the result is negative.

3.1.6. Interpretation of OMV ELISA Assay Results

It is necessary to consider both the IgM and IgG isotype antibody values in relation to the onset date of meningococcal disease (for both acute and convalescent sera where possible). Documenting seroconversion (either by demonstrating a change in antibody level or by showing a change in antibody isotype from IgM to IgG) is indicative of an acute episode of meningococcal disease. For a more detailed interpretation of results, OMV-assay characteristics, and recommendations, refer to **Notes 5, 6, and 7**, respectively.

3.1.7. Troubleshooting OMV ELISA Assay

1. If a reduction of positive to negative range is detected between assay runs, *see* **Note 3**.
2. If variable optical densities (ODs) are detected between assay runs, *see* **Note 9**.

3.2. mHSA Preparation for Polysaccharide-Specific IgG ELISA

The mHSA is prepared in accordance with Mandell and Hershey *(38)* and Carlone et al. *(21)*. Refer to local laboratory safety procedures before starting this procedure (e.g., Risk and COSHH assessments in the UK). An appropriate chemical fume hood **must** be used for the solvent washes and manipulations.

3.2.1. mHSA Preparation Method

1. In chemical fume cabinet (exhaust protective), add 5 g of human albumin to 500 mL of methanol. (The bottle is kept dark by wrapping in aluminum foil).
2. Add 4.2 mL of concentrated (12 *M*) hydrochloric acid and a magnetic stirrer to the albumin solution.
3. Tightly seal the bottle and leave stirring for 3 d in the fume hood.
4. Distribute the mixture in 20 mL amounts in glass universals (the internal rubber seals having been removed) and then centrifuge at 1614*g* for 5 min.
5. Open the universal containers in the fume hood and remove the supernatant using 10-mL plastic pipets and discard the waste solvent in accordance with local regulations.
6. Add 15 mL of methanol to the retained precipitate before re-centrifugation at 1614*g* for 5 min.
7. Discard the supernatants, wash the precipitates again in 15 mL methanol, and re-centrifuge at 1614*g* for 5 min.
8. Wash the precipitates twice with 15 mL of ether and centrifuge twice at 1614*g* for 5 min. (A glass pipet should be used for the removal of the ether.)
9. After the final ether wash, leave the tubes with the lids off in the fume hood for approx 30 min to evaporate the remaining ether.
10. Transfer the cleaned precipitates (mHSA) into suitable glass tubes and dry under vacuum in a centrifuge for 20 min (using a "Gyrovap" centrifuge evaporation unit or equivalent).

11. Transfer the mHSA to freeze-drying ampoules and placed them in a –80°C freezer overnight before freeze-drying the following night in the presence of phosphorus pentoxide. Cap and weigh the vials. Calculate the approximate weight for each mHSA-containing vial by subtraction of the mean weight of several empty capped vials. Store the freeze-dried mHSA vials at +4°C. (Date of expiration is not known but material is still effective after 5 yr).

3.3. Serogroup C Polysaccharide-Specific IgG ELISA Assay

This method is adapted from that described by Gheesling et al. *(25)*.

3.3.1. Serogroup C Polysaccharide-Specific IgG ELISA Assay Method

Day 1: Preparation of microtiter plates prior to serum testing.

1. Coat microtiter plates (Immulon 2 plates or equivalent) with a mixture of mHSA at a final concentration of 5 μg/mL and serogroup C meningococcal polysaccharide at a final concentration of 5 μg/mL using 10 m*M* PBS, pH 7.4. (To coat a single plate with polysaccharide antigen, 15 mL of the mHSA-meningococcal serogroup C polysaccharide mixture is required.)
2. Add 7.5 mL of 10 m*M* PBS, pH 7.4, to two new and sterile plastic containers. To one container add 3 μL of the serogroup C polysaccharide. To the other container add 7.5 μL of mHSA (from stock 10 mg/mL) and a magnetic stirring bar.
3. Place the mHSA PBS mixture on a magnetic stirrer and then add the polysaccharide mixture slowly drop-wise (while stirring), using a sterile disposable plastic pipette (or using clean glass burette for larger volumes).
4. Add 100 μL of the mHSA-polysaccharide mixture to each well of the plate using a sterile reservoir.
5. Cover the plates with plastic film and incubate at +4°C overnight. Plates can be stored for use up to 14 d after preparation.

Day 2: Serum testing.

6. After overnight incubation wash the antigen-coated plate 5 times with 200 μL of wash buffer using an automated plate washer (SkanWasher or equivalent).
7. Blot the plates vigorously on absorbent paper.
8. Add 200 μL of blocking buffer to each well.
9. Seal the plates with plastic film and incubate at room temperature for 1 h. The plates can be kept at room temperature for several hours whilst the test sera and controls are prepared.
10. Dilute the CDC 1992 serum 1/75 (*see* **Subheading 2.3.3.2.**) in the SC buffer ready for addition to the plate. Diluted 1 : 1 in the plate, the initial dilution of the standard reference calibration curve is 1/150 (*see* **Note 1**).
11. Dilute the QC serum with SC buffer to yield ODs within the high, middle, and low range of the standard reference serum calibration curve.

12. Dilute the samples for serogroup C IgG antibody determination 1/25 in SC buffer before addition to the microtiter plates.
13. Decant the blocking buffer from a single plate (do not decant and add sera to multiple plates as antibody binding to the antigen occurs rapidly, before the dilution series are made).
14. Blot the plate vigorously on absorbent towel.
15. Fill the plate wells, except column 12 (used for quality-control dilutions) with 100 μL of SC buffer (*see* **Note 1**).
16. Add 100 μL of the quality-control samples to plate wells A12-B12 (high), C12-D12 (middle), and E12-F12 (low).
17. Add 100 μL SC buffer to plate wells G12-H12 for use as conjugate control (Blank).
18. Add 100 μL of the 1/75 dilution standard reference serum to the calibration series (*see* **Note 9**).
19. Mix the contents of plate wells A1, A2, and A3 five times. Transfer 100 μL of the contents of plate wells A1, A2, and A3 to plate wells B1, B2, and B3 and mix five times. Continue with the same procedure until complete transfer of 100 μL of the contents of wells G1, G2, and G3 to plate wells H1, H2, and H3.
20. Mix the contents of plate wells H1, H2, and H3, and then discard 100 μL from these wells.
21. Dispense the patient sera (4 sera per plate, 8 twofold serial dilutions, in duplicate) into the microtiter plate as follows: dispense the prepared 1/25 dilution (2X) of the first test patient serum into plate wells A4 and B4 (100 μL per well). Dispense the 1/25 dilution of the second, third, and fourth patient sera into plate wells C4 and D4, E4, and F4, and G4 and H4, respectively. Mix the contents of plate wells A5-H5 (column 5) 5 times using an automated multi-channel pipet with 8 tips. Continue the mixing and dilution procedure through plate wells A11–H11. (To test 16 patient sera, a two-dilution modification of the microtiter plate layout has been utilized *see* **Note 10**).
22. Discard 100 μL of the contents of plate wells A11–H11 to adjust the volume to 100 μL.
23. Seal the plate and incubate overnight at +4°C.

Day 3: Serum testing continued.

24. Wash each plate 5 times with wash buffer and blot the plate vigorously on absorbent paper.
25. Add 100 μL of 1/2000 dilution of human IgG Fc PAN monoclonal antibody in SC buffer to each well.
26. Seal the plate and incubate at room temperature for 2.5 h. (It is recommended to check each batch of conjugate for the optimal dilution.)
27. Immediately before use prepare an appropriate amount of substrate solution by adding one TMB tablet to 10 mL of substrate buffer (*see* **Subheading 2.2.4.5.**).
28. Wash each plate 5 times with wash buffer and blot the plate vigorously on absorbent paper.

29. Add 100 µL of the TMB substrate to each well and incubate the plates at room temperature for 30 min.
30. Add 100 µL of 0.2 *M* sulfuric acid to each well to stop the color reaction.
31. Read the plates at 450 nm in the spectrophotometer (Multiskan). Adjust the OD readings to take account of the blank wells G12 and H12. Store the data electronically for analysis in the ELISA program.

3.3.2. Validation of Data for Serogroup C Polysaccharide-Specific IgG ELISA

The assay validation (based on Plikaytis et al., **ref. *40***) is designed for vaccine evaluation but is applicable to sero-diagnosis and demonstrates the quality of results that can be obtained with the described assay.

1. Check:
   a. for the conformity of the assay standard reference curve compared with previous assay standard reference curves, and
   b. that the assay standard reference curve correlation r^2 value is at least 0.990. Any plate that does not satisfy these checks should be repeated.
2. Quality control: Check that each dilution of the quality control (high, middle, low) has a within dilution CV ≤15% and that each within-assay coefficient of variance (CV) of the dilutions of the quality control is ≤15%. Also that each dilution of the quality controls (high, middle, low) as well as the mean of all three dilutions of the quality control is within ±2 SD of its established mean. Repeat the assay of any plate whose quality controls do not satisfy the checking criteria. (Occasionally a quality-control result will be within ±3 SD of its established mean).
3. Check that each within dilution average OD for an unknown (after subtraction of the average OD of the blank wells) is ≥ the average OD of the blank wells of the assay. If no unknown within dilution average OD (after subtraction of the average OD of the blank wells) is ≥ the average OD of the blank wells of the assay, report the antibody level of that unknown as being less than the lower limit of detectable for that assay.
4. Check that each within dilution average OD for an unknown is ≤95% of the average OD of the upper limit of the working area of the standard-reference calibration. Do not accept any within dilution average OD that does not satisfy this check.
5. Check that each within dilution CV for an unknown is ≤15%:
   a. if all or the majority of the within dilution calculated data for an unknown have CVs >15%, re-test the unknown;
   b. if one of the two results for a particular dilution of an unknown is not calculated while the other is calculated, do not accept either result;
   c. if only the 1/50 dilution of an unknown is accepted, signify on the report of that unknown that a 1/50 dilution was used and report the 1/50 antibody level for that unknown as its final result;

   d. if only the 1/3,200 and 1/6,400 dilutions of an unknown are accepted, re-test that unknown using dilution series starting at 1/100.
6. Check that the within assay CV for an unknown is ≤20%:
   a. If two or more of the within dilution results for an unknown are accepted, the ODs of the accepted data increases with increasing serum concentration and the within assay CV is >20%, signify on the report of that unknown that it is nonparallel to the assay standard-reference curve and if the initial 1/50 dilution gives a OD of >0.5 record the median antibody level for that unknown as its final result; if the OD of the initial 1/50 dilution is <0.5 take the first (1/50) dilution;
   b. If two or more of the within dilution results for an unknown are accepted, the ODs of the accepted data does not increase with increasing serum concentration and the within assay CV is >20%, re-test the unknown.
7. Check that the OD of each of the blank wells is <0.1. Re-test the samples if the OD ≥0.1.

3.3.3. Data Analysis for Serogroup C Polysaccharide-Specific IgG ELISA

1. Capture the ELISA OD readings from the Titertek multiskan MCC 340 (or equivalent) by Multiscan Auto Read Version 5.0 software and process by "ELISA" version 1.07 data analysis software package (provided by CDC), 4-parameter logistic curve model ***(39)***. (*See* "Program ELISA—User's Manual".)
2. Use the calibration factor for total IgG antibody in the CDC 1992 control sera = 24.1 µg/mL if that standard calibration serum is used. The results are for total IgG antibody to serogroup C polysaccharide and expressed in µg/mL.

3.3.4. Interpretation of Results

Serogroup C polysaccharide-specific IgG antibody levels following a clinical case are usually in the range 15.0–100 µg/mL within 6 wk after clinical presentation. Antibody levels of ≥15 µg/mL in specimens taken 2–6 wk after clinical presentation are regarded as indicative of recent serogroup C meningococcal infection in patients not recently vaccinated with meningococcal polysaccharide. For a more detailed evaluation of the assay characteristics and recommendations, *see* **Notes 11** and **12**, respectively.

3.4. Serogroup B Polysaccharide-Specific Total Antibody ELISA Method

Because no internationally recognized standard-reference serum or antigen is available, in-house reagents must be produced (*see* **Subheading 2.4.**). The assay procedure is the same as described for the serogroup C polysaccharide-specific IgG ELISA with the use of the alternative conjugates (*see* **Note 2**) and an in-house defined serogroup B specific control serum (*see* **Subheading 2.4.2.**).

3.4.1. Calculation of Serogroup B Polysaccharide-Specific Total Antibody

Calculate the concentration of serogroup B polysaccharide antibody by using the "ELISA" data analysis software package (provided by CDC) as described for serogroup C but using an in-house serogroup B calibration serum. At the PHLS MRU, the positive control pool of sera was assigned an arbitrary value of 3400 AU/mL after comparison with CDC1992 (the serogroup C calibration serum).

For serogroup B ELISA results interpretation and assay characteristics, *see* **Note 13**.

3.5. Serogroup A Polysaccharide-Specific IgG ELISA Method

The assay procedure, results calculation and validation is essentially that used for determining antibody levels to serogroup C polysaccharide-specific IgG (*see* **Subheadings 3.3.1.**, **3.3.2.**, ***(21)***) with following exceptions:

1. Use serogroup A polysaccharide to coat the plates.
2. The starting dilution of the CDC 1992 standard serum should be 1/350, therefore a 1/175 2X dilution is made prior to adding to the microtiter plate.
3. For serogroup assay results interpretation, *see* **Note 14**.

4. Notes

1. Serogroup C polysaccharide-specific IgG ELISA plate template (*see* **Fig. 2**).
2. Alternative conjugates for serogroup C polysaccharide total antibody quantification. The IgG peroxidase conjugate listed here may be used as an alternative to the described MAb Human IgG Fc PAN (1,2,3,4) HRP conjugated in the specific IgG ELISA or together with IgA and IgM for total antibody quantification but the specificity of these conjugates is generally lower than the MAb. If total serogroup C Ig is calculated the value of the CDC 1992 standard reference serum = 32.1 μg/mL.
   a. Anti-human IgA conjugate (α-chain specific) peroxidase (Sigma, Cat. no. A7032) or equivalent.
   b. Anti-human IgG conjugate (γ-chain specific) peroxidase (Sigma, Cat. no. A6029) or equivalent.
   c. Anti-human IgM conjugate (γ-chain specific) peroxidase (Sigma, Cat. no. A6907) or equivalent.
3. Alternative protocol for semi-automated screening meningococcal OMP assay. The meningococcal OMV ELISA as used at the PHLS MRU, makes use of an automatic sample handler (Kemble, Lifescreen Ltd., Johnson & Johnson) and an automatic enzyme-immunoassay processor (Omni, Launch Diagnostics) with appropriate wash buffer. OMV antigen and TMB substrate preparation are similar to that previously described (*see* **Subheadings 3.1.3.** and **2.3.4., item 5**, respectively).

	1	2	3	4	5	6	7	8	9	10	11	12
A	B	P	N									
B	L	P	N									
C	A											
D	N											
E	K				P	N						
F					P	N						
G											P	N
H											P	N

Fig. 1. The mean OD for column 1 (A1-H1) is the reagent Blank. The wells A1-H1 are not used for test or control sera. Test and control sera are added to the plate as indicated ≠2 → 12 (A2-H12). The controls (positive = P and negative = N) must be added to the 12 positions indicated on each plate. Please note that alternative software analysis packages may require a different template.

4. Meningococcal OMV ELISA assay microtiter plate template (*see* **Fig. 1**).
5. Interpretation of OMV ELISA assay. The OMV antigen will contain cell membrane components other than OMPs including lipooligosaccharide and will therefore detect IgM and IgG isotype antibodies directed against these antigens; however, the nonspecific quality of the antigen preparation may be of advantage in widening the range of meningococci that can be detected. The illness-onset date and clinical details are essential (as for interpretation of any serological assay) and particularly so with meningococci where carriage and chronic disease are well documented. It is necessary to consider both the IgM and IgG isotype antibody values in relation to the onset date of meningococcal disease (for both acute and convalescent sera where possible). Documenting seroconversion (either by demonstrating a change in antibody level or by showing a change in antibody isotype from IgM to IgG) is indicative of an acute episode of meningococcal disease. The nonspecific nature of the antigen preparation and the fact that approx 10% of the population may be carrying *N. meningitidis* organisms and mounting an antibody response as a result with no obvious clinical disease can cause interpretation

Table 1
OMV IgM Assay Results for Patients With or Without Clinical Meningococcal Disease

OMV ELISA result	Clinical and laboratory diagnosis		
	+	–	Total
+	59	12	71
–	3	298	301
Total	62	310	372

Sensitivity, 95%; Specificity, 96%. Positive predictive value (PPV), 83%; Negative predictive value (NPV), 99%.

Table 2
OMV IgM Assay for Patients from a Study of Possible Meningococcal Disease

OMV ELISA result	Clinical and laboratory diagnosis		
	+	–	Total
+	42	26	68
–	2	38	40
Total	44	64	108

Sensitivity, 95%; Specificity, 60%. Positive predictive value, 61%; Negative predictive value, 95%

problems. In rapidly fatal cases of meningococcal infection, the OMV assay is unhelpful, as circulating OMVs from whole or disrupted organisms will bind any circulating IgM antibodies in vivo. PCR and antigen-detection tests are likely to be more useful in this instance in the absence of positive culture results.

6. OMV ELISA assay characteristics. The OMV ELISA has been evaluated in a number of studies, where performance characteristics were assessed using specimens from laboratory-proven cases, blood-transfusion donors, and antenatal patients. Using specimens from patients with no evidence of meningococcal disease, in the OMV IgG assay, 42 (13.6%) of 310 sera tested had levels above the threshold limit giving a specificity of 86.4%. The OMV IgM assay gave reactivity in 12 (4%) of the sera tested giving a specificity of 96%. Because of its superior performance, the IgM reactivity was used in subsequent analysis (*see* **Table 1**).

   These performance characteristics, however, are not matched when applied to a series of specimens including acute and convalescent specimens from patients with clinical presentation including rash, a proportion of which are caused by illnesses other than meningococcal infection (*see* **Table 2**) with the specificity and PPV in particular being adversely affected.

7. Further interpretation of results and recommendations: The disappointing performance of the OMV ELISA in terms of specificity and PPV when applied in the clinical situation needs to be set against acceptable sensitivity and NPV. This assay cannot be used as a single diagnostic test for meningococcal infection. Indeed the demonstration that clinical cases and asymptomatic carriers can show equivalent responses in all serological and functional assays (assessed in this laboratory and elsewhere) indicates that, at best, sero-reactivity can only be used to help support a suspicion of meningococcal infection based on the clinical presentation. The high sensitivity and NPV of the OMV ELISA mean that this assay, which it is possible to automate and thus screen high throughput, can be used to indicate which of the submitted specimens can most gainfully be tested for presence of serogroup-specific polysaccharide antibodies. Any sera that are nonreactive are unlikely to have demonstrable antibody to meningococcal polysaccharide. The convalescent test sera are generally positive for OMV IgG (>50 EIU), whereas the acute sera (or plasma) are tested for polysaccharide antibodies if they had high positive (>100 EIU) OMV IgM and IgG responses.
8. Reduction of positive to negative range. If the OMV positive control (P) shows reduced OD all batch numbers and expiry dates should be checked. The bicarbonate buffer and OMV antigen concentration should also be checked. Make and check the pH of a fresh batch of bicarbonate buffer as it deteriorates after 2 wk. Titrate the antigen to determine the optimal dilution for the maximum range between the positive and negative. It is recommended that a new batch of OMV antigen be prepared each year to maintain the quality of the assay. (For OMV antigen storage details, *see* **Subheading 3.1.3., step 12**).
9. Variable optical density of positive controls between assays. Maintain constant substrate-incubation conditions. Check all reagents but particularly the substrate tablets and hydrogen peroxide solution. It is recommended that the hydrogen peroxide solution is stored at +4°C and replaced every 3 mo.
10. Alternative two-dilution assay for serogroup C polysaccharide-specific IgG ELISA. The 16-sera per plate are tested in duplicate at two dilutions 1/50 and 1/500 requiring a specific "ELISA" Program template to calculate the concentrations of antibody. The initial (1/50) dilution is made by adding 10 μL of sera to 490 μL of SC buffer, which is then diluted to 1/500.
    a. Decant SC buffer from plate and blot the plate vigorously on absorbent towel.
    b. Load the patient sera dilutions (100 μL) into the plate after careful mixing to wells column ≠4 → 11).
    c. Add the standard reference calibration curve, quality controls and blanks, and dilute as described previously. Cover the plates and incubate overnight at +4°C.
    d. Use the peroxidase conjugates for total antibody (pooled anti-human IgG, IgA, and IgM) at a final dilution of 1/1000 for each in SC buffer are in the assay. Process the plates as described previously using TMB substrate and spectrophotometer reading.
11. Characteristics of serogroup C polysaccharide-specific IgG ELISA. Accurate quantification of anti-polysaccharide antibody can be used to infer disease likelihood

	1	2	3	4	5	6	7	8	9	10	11	12
A	↓ REF. STD CDC 1992			PATIENT # 1 – 8 TWO-FOLD SERIAL DILUTIONS IN DUPLICATE (A4 & B4, A5 & B5, etc.) →								HIGH
B	↓ 8x TWO-FOLD SERIAL			" " " " " →								HIGH
C	↓ DILUTIONS IN TRIPLICATE			PATIENT # 2 - (C4 & D4, C5 & D5, etc.) →								MID
D	↓ (A1-H1, A2-H2, A3-H3)			" " " " " →								MID
E	↓			PATIENT # 3 - (E4 & F4, E5 & F5, etc.) →								LOW
F	↓			" " " " " →								LOW
G	↓			PATIENT # 4 - (G4 & H4, G5 & H5, etc.) →								BLK
H	↓			" " " " " →								BLK

Fig. 2. The serogroup C polysaccharide-specific IgG ELISA microtiter plate layout above allows the testing of 4 unknown patient sera for the accurate quantification of polysaccharide antibody compared to the standard calibration curve. Blank wells are indicated in G12 and H12. Quality control sera (high, middle, and low) are included to facilitate the validation of results (*see* **Subheading 3.2.2.**). (To test 16 patient sera a modification to the above microtiter plate layout for use in the "ELISA" program was made, *see* **Note 12**).

in the spectrum of patient age ranges. The serogroup C polysaccharide-specific antibody ELISA has been evaluated. Experience with material from culture proven cases seen at the MRU and from studies in healthy subjects, shows that antibody levels following a clinical case are usually in the range 15.0–100 μg/mL within 6 wk after clinical presentation. The lower limit defined here is approx 5 times the mean level seen in sera of patients in whom meningococcal infection has been excluded. Antibody levels of ≥15 μg/mL in specimens taken 2–6 wk after clinical presentation are regarded as indicative of recent serogroup C meningococcal infection in patients who have not been recently vaccinated with meningococcal polysaccharide (including meningococcal serogroup C conjugate vaccine). When applied to a series of specimens (including acute and convalescent specimens) from patients

Table 3
Serogroup C IgG ELISA Results for Patients with Clinical Presentation of Possible Meningococcal Disease (Including Rash)

C polysaccharide ELISA result	Clinical and laboratory diagnosis		
	+	–	Total
+	13	2	15
–	3	62	65
Total	16	64	80

Sensitivity, 81%; Specificity, 97%. Positive predictive value, 87%; Negative predictive value, 95%.

with clinical presentation including rash, a proportion of which were owing to etiologies other than meningococcal infection, the serogroup C ELISA had the characteristics shown in **Table 3**.

12. Recommendations for interpretation of serogroup C polysaccharide-specific IgG ELISA: As with the OMP ELISA, the C polysaccharide assay cannot be used as a definitive diagnostic test for meningococcal infection because cases and asymptomatic carriers can show equivalent and overlapping levels of response. At best, sero-reactivity can only be used to help support a suspicion of meningococcal infection based on the clinical picture. Demonstrating seroconversion in a patient with a compatible clinical syndrome reinforces the diagnostic significance.

    Although sensitivity and PPV are sub-optimal, the high specificity means that when a positive result is obtained, the serogroup C ELISA provides useful supporting indication of likely cause of disease for individual cases and, more importantly, in clusters where culture and PCR tests fail to provide laboratory evidence of infection. It is well-recognized that infants and young children have poorer immunological responses to polysaccharide antigens than older individuals and in these younger patients, lower antibody levels may be seen following infection.

    Tests for serogroup C antibody are being used in the enhanced monitoring of infection during the phased introduction of meningococcal C conjugate vaccine in the UK population. Cases reactive in the PHLS MRU screening PCR test (*ctrA* PCR; *see* Chapter 3) that fail to react in the serogroup B, C, Y, or W135 PCR assays (*siaD* PCRs; *see* Chapter 3) have acute and convalescent specimens collected, which are tested in parallel and the results interpreted according to the following criteria:

    Serogroup C antibody result interpretation in patients with a clinical presentation suggestive of serogroup C disease: Following paired sera testing a >fourfold rise in IgG antibody to C polysaccharide between the acute and convalescent sera, the latter with a concentration of specific IgG antibody of greater than 3 μg/mL is regarded as being highly suggestive of recent serogroup C meningococcal

Table 4
Serogroup B Total Ig ELISA Results for Patients with Clinical Presentation of Possible Meningococcal Disease (Including Rash)

B polysaccharide ELISA result	Clinical and laboratory diagnosis		
	+	–	Total
+	19	5	24
–	10	59	69
Total	29	64	93

Sensitivity, 66%; Specificity, 92%. Positive predictive value, 79%; Negative predictive value, 86%.

infection. For a single convalescent serum sample with a serogroup C-specific IgG level of ≥15 μg/mL in an unvaccinated child under 10 yr of age or ≥32 μg/mL in an unvaccinated individual ≥10 yr of age is regarded as indicating recent serogroup C meningococcal infection. The levels represent >2 SD (i.e., the upper 2.5% of the population) above the age specific geometric mean titer (GMT) found in a large age-stratified serological survey conducted in England and Wales by the MRU on samples collected by PHLS laboratories in 1996–1997. Single high-titer criteria in vaccinated individuals are more difficult to define because they will be dependent on time since vaccination and age. Based on limited antibody-persistence data from infants and children followed up in PHLS trials, the criterion of ≥15 μg/mL would be >2 SD above the GMT 6 mo post-MCC vaccination for those under 5 yr of age. No single high-titer criteria are proposed for older vaccinated individuals.

13. Interpretation of serogroup B polysaccharide total antibody ELISA results: Serological responses following serogroup B cases are typically lower than those seen following serogroup C disease, generally falling in the range 1,000–4,000 AU/mL. Studies of antibody isotype response following serogroup B infection have shown that most of the antibody produced is IgM and in some cases the peak level may be achieved within 10 d of presentation. When applied to a series of specimens including acute and convalescent specimens from patients with clinical presentation including rash, a proportion of which are caused by illnesses other than meningococcal infection the serogroup B ELISA had the characteristics shown in **Table 4**.

As with the OMV and serogroup C polysaccharide assays, the serogroup B ELISA cannot be used as a definitive diagnostic test for meningococcal infection because cases and asymptomatic carriers can show equivalent and overlapping levels of response. At best, sero-reactivity provides laboratory support when there is suspicion of meningococcal infection based on the clinical picture. Demonstrating seroconversion in a patient with a compatible clinical syndrome bolsters the diagnostic significance.

Sensitivity, PPV and NPV for the serogroup B ELISA are not as high as for the serogroup C ELISA however when positive this assay provides useful supporting indication of likely cause of disease for individual cases and in clusters of infection where culture and PCR tests fail to provide laboratory evidence. It is well-recognized that serogroup B meningococci cross-react with *E. coli* KI ***(41)***. Serogroup B polysaccharide is known to be an intrinsically poor immunogen in infants, and young children in general have poorer immunological responses to polysaccharide antigens than older individuals following infection. Performing both serogroup B and C assays in parallel usually gives a mutually exclusive result.

14. Interpretation of serogroup A polysaccharide-specific IgG ELISA. This assay is essentially a modification of Carlone et al. used for determining antibody levels to serogroup C polysaccharide ***(21)***. Antibody responses following serogroup A disease in different age groups have not been previously reported therefore guidelines cannot be given. This would also vary considerably by country depending on the prevalence of serogroup A disease. Care must be taken in that other bacterial species have polysaccharide structures similar to serogroup A polysaccharide and may induce cross-reacting antibodies ***(42,43)***.

Acknowledgments

The authors would like to thank George Carlone, Cheryl Elie, and Patricia Holder (CDC, Atlanta, GA) for their comments on the content of this chapter.

References

1. Cartwright, K., Reilly, S., White, D., and Stuart, J. (1992) Early treatment with parenteral penicillin in meningococcal disease. *BMJ* **305,** 1484.
2. Kaczmarski, E. B. (1997) Meningococcal disease in England and Wales: 1995. *Commun. Dis. Rep. Rev.* **7,** R55–R59.
3. Chief Medical Officer, Chief Nursing Officer, Chief Pharmaceutical Officer (1999). Department of Health, London. *Introduction of Immunisation Against Group C Meningococcal Infection.*
4. Gotschlich, E. C., Goldschneider, I., and Artenstein, M. S. (1969) Human immunity to the meningococcus. IV. Immunogenicity of group A and group C meningococcal polysaccharides in human volunteers. *J. Exp. Med.* **129,** 1367–1384.
5. Jones, D. M. and Tobin, B. M. (1972) Incidence of haemagglutinating antibodies to meningococci in north-west England. *J. Clin. Path.* **25,** 955–958.
6. Mitchell, M. S., Rhoden, D. L., and Marcus, B. B. (1966) Immunofluorescence techniques for demonstrating bacterial pathogens associated with cerebrospinal meningitis. 3. Identification of meningococci from the nasopharynx of asymptomatic carriers. *Am. J. Epidemiol.* **83,** 74–85.
7. German, G. P., Chernokhvostova, E. V., Vengerǒv, Y. Y., Smirnova-Muiusheva, M. A., Mishina, A. I., Chernysheva, T. F., et al. (1977) Serum immunoglobulin levels in various forms of meningococcal infection and in meningococcus carriers. *J. Hyg. Epidemiol. Microbiol. Immunol.* **21,** 341–349.

8. Haeney, M. R., Thompson, R. A., Faulkner, J., Mackintosh, P., and Ball, A. P. (1980) Recurrent bacterial meningitis in patients with genetic defects of terminal complement components. *Clin. Exp. Immunol.* **40,** 16–24.
9. Monto, A. S., Brandt, B. L., and Artenstein, M. S. (1973) Response of children to *Neisseria meningitidis* polysaccharide vaccines. *J. Infect. Dis.* **127,** 394–400.
10. Brandt, B. L., Wyle, F. A., and Artenstein, M. S. (1972) A radioactive antigen-binding assay for *Neisseria meningitidis* polysaccharide antibody. *J. Immunol.* **108,** 913–920.
11. Anderson, P., Insel, R. A., Porcelli, S., and Ward, J. I. (1987) Immunochemical variables affecting radioantigen-binding assays of antibody to *Haemophilus influenzae* type b capsular polysaccharide in childrens' sera. *J. Infect. Dis.* **156,** 582–590.
12. Lagergard, T., Trollfors, B., Claesson, B. A., Schneerson, R., and Robbins, J. B. (1988) Comparison between radioimmunoassay and direct and indirect enzyme-linked immunosorbent assays for determination of antibodies against *Haemophilus influenzae* type b capsular polysaccharide. *J. Clin. Microbiol.* **26,** 2554–2557.
13. Phipps, D. C., West, J., Eby, R., Koster, M., Madore, D. V., and Quataert, S. A. (1990) An ELISA employing a *Haemophilus influenzae* type b oligosaccharide-human serum albumin conjugate correlates with the radioantigen binding assay. *J. Immunol. Methods* **135,** 121–128.
14. Basta, M. T., Russell, H., Guirguis, N. I., Hafez, K., and El Kholy, A. (1982) Enzyme-linked immunosorbent assay for determination of human antibodies to group C meningococcal polysaccharide. *Proc. Soc. Exp. Biol. Med.* **169,** 7–11.
15. Barra, A., Schulz, D., Aucouturier, P., and Preud'homme, J. L. (1988) Measurement of anti-*Haemophilus influenzae* type b capsular polysaccharide antibodies by ELISA. *J. Immunol. Methods.* **115,** 111–117.
16. Leinonen, M. and Frasch, C. E. (1982) Class-specific antibody response to group B *Neisseria meningitidis* capsular polysaccharide: use of polylysine precoating in an enzyme-linked immunosorbent assay. *Infect. Immun.* **38,** 1203–1207.
17. Messina, J. P., Hickox, P. G., Lepow, M. L., Polara, B., and Venezia, R. A. (1985) Modification of a direct enzyme-linked immunosorbent assay for the detection of immunoglobulin G and M antibodies to pneumococcal capsular polysaccharide. *J. Clin. Microbiol.* **21,** 390–394.
18. Akinwolere, O. A., Kumararatne, D. S., Bartlett, R., Goodall, D. M., and Catty, D. (1994) Two enzyme linked immunosorbent assays for detecting antibodies against meningococcal capsular polysaccharides A and C. *J. Clin. Pathol.* **47,** 405–410.
19. Diaz Romero, J. and Outschoorn, I. (1993) Selective biotinylation of *Neisseria meningitidis* group B capsular polysaccharide and application in an improved ELISA for the detection of specific antibodies. *J. Immunol. Methods.* **160,** 35–47.
20. Arakere, G. and Frasch, C. E. (1991) Specificity of antibodies to O-acetyl-positive and O-acetyl-negative group C meningococcal polysaccharides in sera from vaccinees and carriers. *Infect. Immun.* **59,** 4349–4356.
21. Carlone, G. M., Frasch, C. E., Siber, G. R., Quataert, S., Gheesling, L. L., Turner, S. H., et al. (1992) Multicenter comparison of levels of antibody to the *Neisseria*

meningitidis group A capsular polysaccharide measured by using an enzyme-linked immunosorbent assay. *J. Clin. Microbiol.* **30,** 154–159.

22. Greenberg, D. P., Ward, J. I., Burkart, K., Christenson, P. D., Guravitz, L., and Marcy, S. M. (1987) Factors influencing immunogenicity and safety of two *Haemophilus influenzae* type b polysaccharide vaccines in children 18 and 24 months of age. *Pediatr. Infect. Dis. J.* **6,** 660–665.
23. Ward, J. I., Greenberg, D. P., Anderson, P. W., Burkart, K. S., Christenson, P. D., Gordon, L. K., et al. (1988) Variable quantitation of *Haemophilus influenzae* type b anticapsular antibody by radioantigen binding assay. *J. Clin. Microbiol.* **26,** 72–78.
24. Gheesling, L. L., Carlone, G. M., Pais, L. B., Holder, P. F., Maslanka, S. E., Plikaytis, B. D., et al. (1994) Multicenter comparison of *Neisseria meningitidis* serogroup C anti-capsular polysaccharide antibody levels measured by a standardised enzyme-linked immunosorbent assay. *J. Clin. Microbiol.* **32,** 1475–1482.
25. Anderson, J., Berthelsen, L., and Lind, I. (1997) Measurment of antibodies against meningococcal capsular polysaccharides B and C in an enzyme-linked immunosorbent assays: towards an improved surveillance of meningococcal disease. *Clin. Diag. Lab. Immunol.* **4,** 345–351.
26. Käyhty, H., Jousimies Somer, H., Peltola, H., and Mäkelä, P. H. (1981) Antibody response to capsular polysaccharides of groups A and C *Neisseria meningitidis* and *Haemophilus influenzae* type b during bacteremic disease. *J. Infect. Dis.* **143,** 32–41.
27. Goldschneider, I, Gotschlich, E. C., and Artenstein, M. S. (1969) Human immunity to the meningococcus II. Development of natural immunity. *J. Exp. Med.* **129,** 1327–1348.
28. Costantino, P., Viti, S., Podda, A., Velmonte, M. A., Nencioni, L., and Rappuoli, R. (1992). Development and phase 1 clinical testing of a conjugate vaccine against meningococcus A and C. *Vaccine* **10,** 691–698.
29. Devi, S. J., Robbins, J. B., and Schneerson, R. (1991) Antibodies to poly[(2-8)-alpha-N-acetylneuraminic acid] and poly[(2-9)-alpha-N-acetylneuraminic acid] are elicited by immunization of mice with *Escherichia coli* K92 conjugates: potential vaccines for groups B and C meningococci and *E. coli* K1. *Proc. Natl. Acad. Sci. USA* **88,** 7175–7179.
30. Griffiss, J. M. (1995) Mechanisms of host immunity, in *Meningococcal Disease* (Cartwright, K. A. V., ed.) John Wiley and Sons, London, pp. 35–70.
31. Holder, P. K., Maslanka, S., Pais, L. B., Dykes, J., Plikaytis, B. D., and Carlone, G. M. (1995) Assignment of *Neisseria meningitidis* serogroup A and C class-specific anticapsular antibody concentrations to the new standard reference serum CDC1992. *Clin. Diagn. Lab. Immunol.* **2,** 132–137.
32. Jones, D. M. and Kaczmarski, E. B. (1993) Meningococcal infections in England and Wales: 1992. *Commun. Dis. Rep. Rev.* **3,** R129–R131.
33. Wall, R., Gray, S. J., Borrow, R., Sutcliffe, E., Smart, L. E., Fox, A. J., and Kaczmarski, E. B. (1996) Assessment of serological response to meningococcal

outer membrane proteins and capsular polysaccharide in the diagnosis of meningococcal infection, in *Abstracts of the Tenth International Pathogenic Neisseria Conference*, Baltimore, MD, (Zollinger, W. D., Frasch, C. E., Deal, C. D., eds.), 1996, pp. 536–537.
34. Zollinger, W. D., Mandrell, R. E., Griffiss, J. M., Altieri, P., and Berman, S. (1979) Complex of meningococcal group B polysaccharide and type 2 outer membrane proteins immunogenic in man. *J. Clin. Invest.* **63,** 836–848.
35. Saunders, N. B., Shoemaker, D. R., Brandt, B. L., and Zollinger, W. D. (1997) Confirmation of suspicious cases of meningococcal meningitis by PCR and enzyme-linked immunosorbent assay. *J. Clin. Microbiol.* **35,** 3215–3219.
36. Kremastinou, J., Tzanakaki, G., Pagalis, A., Theodondou, M., Weir, D. M., and Blackwell, C. C. (1999) Detection of IgG and IgM to meningococcal outer membrane proteins in relation to carriage of *Neisseria meningitidis* or *Neisseria lactamica. FEMS Immunol. Med. Microbiol.* **24,** 73–78.
37. Borrow R., Fox A. J., and Jones D. M. (1997) The immune response to a *N. meningitidis* 200 kDa surface exposed protein following carriage and disease. *Serodiagn. Immunother. Infect. Dis.* **8,** 179–184.
38. Mandell, J. D. and Hershey, A. D. (1960) A fractionating column for analysis of nucleic acids. *Anal. Biochem.* **1,** 66–77.
39. Plikaytis, B. D., Turner, S. H., Gheesling, L. L., and Carlone, G. M. (1991) Comparisons of standard curve-fitting methods to quantitate *Neisseria meningitidis* group A polysaccharide antibody levels by enzyme-linked immunosorbent assay. *J. Clin. Microbiol.* **29,** 1439–1446.
40. Plikaytis, B. D., Holder, P. F., Pais, L. B., Maslanka, S. E., Gheesling, L. L., and Carlone, G. M. (1994) Determination of parallelism and nonparallelism in bioassay dilution curves. *J. Clin. Microbiol.* **32,** 2441–2447.
41. Kasper, D. L., Winklehake, J. L., Zollinger, W. D., Brandt, B. L., and Artenstein, M. S. (1973) Immunochemical similarities between polysaccharide antigens of *Escherichia coli* 07:K1(L):NM and group B Neisseria meningitidis. *J. Immunol.* **110,** 262–268.
42. Robbins, J. B., Scheerson, R., Liu, T. Y., Schiffer, M. S., Schiffman, G., Myerowitz, R. C., et al. (1974) Cross-reacting bacterial antigens and immunity to disease caused by encapsulated bacteria, in *The Immune System and Infectious Disease* (Neter, E., and Milgrom, F., eds.), S. Karger, AG, Basel, pp. 218–241.
43. Guirguis, N., Schneerson, R., Bax, A., Egan, W., Robbins, J. B., Shiloach, J., et al. (1985) *Escherichia coli* K51 and K93 capsular polysaccharides are crossreactive with the group A capsular polysaccharide of *Neisseria meningitidis*. Immunochemical, biological, and epidemiological studies. *J. Exp. Med.* **162,** 1837–1851.

6

Antibiotic Susceptibility Testing

Colin Block

1. Introduction

At the start of the Third Millennium, consensus has yet to be reached regarding the best techniques for meningococcal susceptibility testing and their standardization. Worse, there is no general agreement as to the definition of resistance, or perhaps more accurately, nonsusceptibility, to antibiotics of clinical importance. Even such widely known organizations such as the National Committee for Clinical Laboratory Standards (NCCLS) and other national and regional bodies have not seriously tackled the meningococcus to date. The reasons behind this are several:

1. There is uncertainty as to the clinical significance of reduced susceptibility to certain agents. Reports of treatment failure have been few and solid data are lacking ***(1–6)***. Failures of chemoprophylaxis have also been reported, although this has been associated with easily detected high levels of resistance to rifampicin, for example *(7)*.
2. Different drugs may have different clinical applications (therapy or chemoprophylaxis) with different antibacterial objectives (elimination from tissues, blood, and cerebrospinal fluid (CSF) in disease, and eradication from the pharynx in prevention).
3. There is lack of uniformity in the selection of drugs to be tested. Laboratories of different kinds in different geographical regions perform different types of tests.

The result has been a huge variation in the range of test categories, the methods used to perform them, and the breakpoints or definitions used in their interpretation and the issuing of reports.

From: *Methods in Molecular Medicine, vol. 67: Meningococcal Disease: Methods and Protocols*
Edited by: A. J. Pollard and M. C. J. Maiden © Humana Press Inc., Totowa, NJ

Table 1
Breakpoints in Use by Reference Laboratories for Susceptibility of *N. meningitidis* to Penicillin and Rifampicin

Susceptibility breakpoints (mg/L)	Number of laboratories using breakpoint	
	Penicillin	Rifampicin
≤0.003	2	—
≤0.06	13	1
≤0.13	3	2
≤0.25	1	—
≤0.5	1	2
≤1.0	1	9
≤2.0	—	2
≤4.0	—	2
No. of laboratories responding	21	18

1.1. The Need for Uniformity

A survey of reference laboratories carried out in 1999 for the European Monitoring Group on Meningococci (EMGM) revealed extensive differences in methods and breakpoint values. In addition to 21 European laboratories, centers in Australia, Iceland, Israel, Russia, and the United States also contributed data. Thirteen of the 26 respondents used the Etest as their primary test method, 7 deployed the disk diffusion test, 2 laboratories each used agar dilution or broth microdilution, and 1 each macrodilution or agar breakpoints. Fourteen variations of five well-known media formulations were in use. Breakpoint definitions for susceptibility categories were inconsistent as well. Examples for penicillin and rifampicin are given in **Table 1.**

One upshot of all this is that much of the vast quantities of data being produced in different centers cannot reliably be compared. Another consequence of the lack of agreed-upon methodology concerns diagnostic microbiology laboratories and their role in susceptibility testing of meningococci. Most such laboratories will be hospital-based. Should these laboratories be testing at all? This depends on the environment in which a clinical microbiology laboratory operates. A good way to illustrate this is to ask how important it is to have a quick result. In an area where access to a reference laboratory is limited, and resistance to the drug used for chemoprophylaxis is known to occur, it may be essential to perform the test immediately in order to support the public-health response to a case of meningococcal disease or an outbreak.

1.2. Selecting a Method

Methods that have been used are disk diffusion, broth dilution, agar dilution, Etest (AB Biodisk, Solna, Sweden), partly automated methods, β-lactamase detection, and molecular methods. Despite several studies that have tried to optimize disk-diffusion testing ***(8–10)***, especially for the detection of reduced sensitivity to penicillin, convincing arguments have been put forward that this method should not be recommended ***(11,12)***. There are insufficient data regarding kit-based semi-automated methods to support their use.

Routine β-lactamase detection is currently probably not essential, considering that strains producing such enzymes have been encountered extremely rarely, in Canada ***(13)***, South Africa ***(14)***, and Spain ***(15,16)***. Recently, the plasmids encoding these TEM-1 β-lactamases in two epidemiologically related Spanish isolates have been sequenced ***(17)***. β-lactamase testing should be mandatory for strains with unusually high minimal inhibitory concentrations (MICs) for penicillin G. The MICs of the Canadian and South African isolates were reported to be 256 mg/L, while the first Spanish isolate had a penicillin MIC of 8 mg/L ***(18)***. The related disease and carrier isolates from the second Spanish report also had relatively modest MICs of 2 mg/L ***(16)***. Testing for β-lactamase production is a simple procedure, usually carried out using a chromogenic cephalosporin, and will not be discussed further here.

Molecular detection of drug resistance has not as yet come into regular service in reference laboratories. Activity in this area has involved penicillin ***(19–21)*** and rifampicin ***(22)***, but further work will be required before techniques such as PCR diagnosis of resistance become a practical option.

MIC determinations remain the methods of choice, the agar dilution or broth microdilution being recommended as suitable for reference work. Tests should be selected on the basis of a number of considerations:

1. The use to which susceptibility data will be put, e.g., a) clinical or public health decision-making for individual events, b) research or comparison with data from other sources;
2. Reference laboratory or clinical diagnostic laboratory;
3. Workload, staffing, support, etc., and
4. Cost.

2. Materials

2.1. Antibiotics

1. Only powders that have been assayed and are identified by generic names and lot numbers, and are labeled with expiry dates and potency per mg of powder should be obtained (*see* **Note 1**).

2. Penicillin (benzylpenicillin), a third-generation cephalosporin (e.g., ceftriaxone or cefotaxime), a fluoroquinolone (e.g., ciprofloxacin or ofloxacin) and rifampicin would comprise an appropriate minimal list of drugs for testing (*see* **Note 2**).
3. Powders should be stored desiccated at –20°C or lower, or according to the manufacturer's instructions.
4. Prepare stock solutions for storage at a minimum concentration of 1,280 mg/L. Place convenient volumes in small plastic vials suitable for freezing at –60°C or lower (*see* **Note 3**). Calculate the weight of powder or volume required according to the following formulae:

weight (mg) = volume (mL × required concentration (mg/L)/assay potency (μg/mg)

or

volume (mL) = weight (mg) × assay potency (μg/mg) /required concentration (mg/L)

All the aforementioned drugs except rifampicin should be dissolved and diluted in sterile distilled water. Further dilution for use may be done in broth medium if required. Rifampicin should be dissolved in absolute methanol and diluted further in sterile distilled water.

5. For Etest, *see* **Subheading 2.2.3.**

2.2. Media (*see* Note 4)

2.2.1. Agar Dilution

1. Mueller-Hinton agar supplemented with 5% whole defibrinated sheep blood (*see* **Subheading 2.2.4.**) is an acceptable medium (*see* **Note 5**). For testing sulphonamides, lysed horse blood should be substituted for sheep blood.
2. The dry powder is available from many suppliers and should be shown to be acceptable by complying with recommendations of a reputable organization such as the NCCLS *(23)*.
3. The sheep blood formulation of the product selected should support good growth of *N. meningitidis* and at the least should yield MIC results within the limits for recommended quality-control organisms (*see* **Subheading 2.3.**) *(24,25)*.

2.2.2. Broth Microdilution

1. Cation-adjusted Mueller-Hinton broth (CAMHB) with 5% lysed horse blood is a good choice (*see* **Subheading 2.2.4.** and **Note 7**). This medium is currently used by the Centers for Disease Control and Prevention (CDC), Atlanta, GA. (Dr. F.C. Tenover, personal communication). The NCCLS suggestion for this medium is to use 2–5% lysed horse blood *(24,25)*. This formulation, with lysed horse blood, is appropriate for testing sulphonamides, subject to appropriate quality-control measures.
2. Mueller-Hinton broth is available from many suppliers and may be purchased as either a dry powder or a prepared medium. The medium may conveniently be purchased pre-adjusted to yield correct concentrations of calcium and magne-

sium ions. Instructions for adjusting media with inadequate concentrations of Ca^{2+} and Mg^{2+} are given in the NCCLS document M7-A5 ***(24)*** (*see* **Note 8**).
3. The finished medium should support good growth of *N. meningitidis* and at the least should yield acceptable results with recommended quality-control organisms (*see* **Subheading 2.3.**) in performance of antimicrobial susceptibility testing ***(24)***.

2.2.3. Etest

1. The manufacturer of Etest (AB Biodisk, Sweden) currently recommends Mueller-Hinton agar supplemented with 5% sheep blood (in **Subheading 2.2.1.**) or 1% hemoglobin + 1% Isovitalex ***(26)***. It should be noted that the German study (*see* **Note 5**) found that Mueller-Hinton agar with Isovitalex alone failed to support the growth of 4.5% of their 110 strains ***(27)***.
2. The manufacturer requires that the depth of the agar for the Etest should be 4 ± 0.5mm.
3. Etest strips of the desired antibiotics should be purchased with due attention to expiration dates and shelf life, and stored according to the manufacturer's instructions. Strips should have MIC scales that span the selected interpretative breakpoints for *N. meningitidis*.

2.2.4. Blood for the Media

1. Care must be exercised in selecting suppliers for sheep and horse blood. Products should be shown to be sterile and free of antimicrobial substances before preparing media for the above tests.
2. Horse blood should be lysed by repeated freezing and thawing under sterile conditions. It is useful to aseptically mix the lysate with sterile distilled water in equal volumes. Because the reaction mixture has to be clear to allow reading of the wells, the diluted lysate may be clarified by high-speed centrifugation before adding the appropriate quantity to achieve the 5% working dilution.

2.2.5. Organism Storage

1. Sterile 20% or 30% glycerol should be available in aliquots suitable for mixing 1:1 with heavy meningococcal suspensions in Tryptic Soy Broth (TSB). TSB is available from many suppliers, ready-made or as dry powder.
2. Aliquots of the mixture are frozen in sterile cryopreservation vials at –70°C. Suitable vials are available from many suppliers.
3. A medium used for freeze-drying, made up of TSB + 6% lactose (C. E. Frasch, personal communication), has successfully maintained meningococcal cultures at –70°C for many years at the Israel National Center for Meningococci.

2.3. Reference Organisms

1. The following selections from the NCCLS recommendations ***(24)*** may be used for controlling the MIC procedure:

Table 2
Reference Etest QC Ranges for *N. meningitidis* serogroup C ATCC 13102

Agent	MIC Range
Penicillin G	0.016–0.064
Cefotaxime	0.002–0.004
Ceftriaxone	<0.002
Chloramphenicol	0.25–1
Ciprofloxacin	0.002–0.008
Doxycycline	0.032–0.25
Rifampicin	0.008–0.064
Sulphadiazine	0.25–1
Trimethoprim/sulphamethoxazole	0.008–0.064

   a. For penicillin: *Staphylococcus aureus* ATCC 29213 and *Enterococcus faecalis* ATCC 29212. *S. aureus* ATCC 25923 has been added for the Etest ***(28)***.
   b. For ceftriaxone: *Escherichia coli* ATCC 25922.
   c. For rifampicin: *S. aureus* ATCC 29213 and *E. faecalis* ATCC 29212.
   d. For ciprofloxacin or other fluoroquinolone: *S. aureus* ATCC 29213 and *E. coli* ATCC 25922 or *Pseudomonas aeruginosa* ATCC 27853.
2. Although no consensus yet exists as to meningococcal strains for quality control, the following have been used in various studies:
   a. *N. meningitidis* serogroup C ATCC 13102. This strain is now recommended for the Etest by the manufacturer in a 1999 draft application sheet. Reference MIC values (quality-control ranges) in mg/L are shown in **Table 2**.
   b. *N. meningitidis* serogroup B ATCC 13090 (CIP 104218). This strain is recommended by the NCCLS for media QC ***(29)***.
   c. *N. meningitidis* serogroup A ATCC 13077 (NCTC 10025).
3. Sources: The organisms mentioned above may be obtained from the American Type Culture Collection (ATCC), the National Collection of Type Cultures (NCTC) in the UK, the Pasteur Institute Collection (CIP) in France, other national collections, and some commercial suppliers.

2.4. Barium Sulphate Turbidity Standard

1. Barium chloride: 1.175% [w/v] $BaCl_2 \cdot 2H_2O$.
2. Sulfuric acid: 0.36 N H_2SO_4 - 1% [v/v].

2.5. The Inoculator for the Agar Dilution Test

Manually or electrically operated devices are commercially available (e.g., Mast Diagnostics, Bootle, Merseyside, UK). These consist essentially of a set of inoculating pins, mounted on a plate, which deliver 1–2 μL volumes to the agar surface. The pins pick up a volume of the suspension from a set of wells filled with the adjusted inoculum. These wells are usually provided in a metal or plastic (Teflon®) block.

3. Methods

3.1. Inoculum Preparation

The aim of standardizing the preparation of inocula is to minimize the effect of variations in inoculum density on interpretation of the results. A widely agreed-upon means of limiting such variation is to use a turbidity standard (0.5 McFarland), most often in the form of a barium-sulphate suspension.

3.1.1. Preparation of Turbidity Standard

1. Add 0.5 mL of the $BaCl_2$ solution to 99.5 mL of the sulphuric acid working solution while stirring. The suspension should yield an optical density (OD) of 0.08–0.1 at 625 nm.
2. Add suitable aliquots to tubes of the same dimensions as those used for preparing the bacterial suspension. These tubes must be sealed and stored in the dark. Tubes should be replaced each 3–4 wk, unless their turbidity has been shown to be unchanged.
3. Mix tubes on a vortex mixer before use, to achieve an even suspension. Discard tubes in which aggregated particles have appeared.

3.1.2. Inoculum Preparation

The method used by almost all reference laboratories polled in the EMGM survey was the so-called direct colony suspension method. The following procedure is acceptable:

1. Make a suspension in sterile, normal saline from meningococcal colonies grown for 18–24 h on a nonselective medium.
2. Adjust the suspension to match the 0.5 McFarland standard, either visually or using a spectrophotometer. A good method for visual matching is to observe the tubes in good light against a background such as a white paper or card printed with parallel black lines.
3. Each laboratory should determine and monitor the colony-count equivalent at this turbidity by periodically performing plate counts on suspensions made using one of the standard strains of *N. meningitidis* mentioned in **Subheading 2.3.**

3.2. Agar Dilution Method

This method is especially suited to the testing of large numbers of isolates. Antibiotic dilutions are prepared in agar in a series of plates, on each of which a large number of test organisms may be inoculated simultaneously using a multipoint inoculator. References strains are included in each set of inocula.

3.2.1. Preparation of Plates (see **Note 6***)*

1. Preparation of the antibiotic dilutions:
   a. Prepare a doubling dilution series of the antibiotics in sterile distilled water. The dilution scale is selected to span the interpretative breakpoints used for each drug. The volume prepared is determined by the amount of agar to be used for each dilution (*see* **Step 1c**). Calculate the dilutions on the basis that 1 part of antibiotic solution is added to 9 parts of molten agar.
   b. Prepare the agar according to the manufacturer's instructions. After autoclaving in convenient containers (e.g., Erlenmeyer flasks) in volumes appropriate for the number of plates of each concentration to be poured, the agar is held at 48–50°C in a water bath and the sheep blood and antibiotic solutions added aseptically.
   c. Mix the agar, blood, and antibiotic solution well and pour Petri dishes, on a levelled table, to a depth convenient for the method of inoculation (some multipoint devices require a minimum height of the agar surface to produce satisfactory contact with the inoculating pins). The volume required per plate will also depend on the size of the plate, and should be determined empirically.
   d. The pH of the prepared medium should be between 7.2 and 7.4.
2. Plate storage: If not used immediately, store plates at 2–8°C in sealed plastic bags. For reference work, the NCCLS recommends storage up to 5 d. The antibiotics suggested for testing (*see* **Subheading 2.1.**) are not known to be particularly labile in storage, so that each laboratory might wish to determine its own optimal storage times for reference or routine work. Because reference strains are included in each run, over the full dilution range, deterioration of the plates should not go undetected.

3.2.2. Inoculation Adjustment and Preparation for Inoculation

1. The inoculum of each organism placed on the plate should be as close as possible to 10^4 colony forming units (cfu)/spot. Each laboratory should calculate the required adjustment of the 0.5 McFarland suspension according to their counts made of these suspensions as outlined in **Subheading 3.1.2.**
2. Place a sufficient volume in each well of the inoculum block to permit adequate pick-up by the pins during the entire process of inoculation.
3. A convenient way to ensure correct orientation of the plate for reading is to fill one well in the inoculum block (e.g., the upper left-hand well) with India Ink instead of with a bacterial suspension.
4. Streak a sample of each inoculum on blood agar for overnight incubation in 5% CO_2 as a purity check. In situations where variability in inoculum densities is a problem, it may be necessary to perform abbreviated colony counts on the inocula to detect significant deviations from the desired 10^4 per spot.

3.2.3. Preparing the Plates for Inoculation

1. Bring the plates to room temperature before inoculation.
2. Check the agar surfaces for excess moisture. Plates may be dried by holding them with lids partly open in a laminar flow hood or incubator for 20–30 min.
3. Arrange the plates to be inoculated in convenient stacks as follows: an antibiotic-free plate first (viability and purity control), then the dilution series of the particular antibiotic, and finally, a second antibiotic-free plate (to control for contamination and excessive drug "carry-over" during the inoculation process).

3.2.4. Inoculating the Plates

1. Operate the inoculating device according to its design. The inoculation process should begin as soon as possible after final inoculum adjustment. The NCCLS recommends an optimal limit of 15 min for regular nonfastidious bacteria ***(24)***.
2. Leave the plates to stand at room temperature for a few minutes to allow absorption of the fluid from the inoculum, before being inverted and placed in the incubator.
3. Because the meningococcus is potentially hazardous to laboratory staff, a detailed written procedure for decontamination of the inoculation equipment should be provided by each laboratory and personnel compliance strictly monitored.

3.2.5. Controls

Control strains appropriate for each drug tested should be selected (*see* **Subheading 2.3.**) and included in each run. The results should be monitored and corrective action taken according to laboratory policy.

3.3. Broth Microdilution Method

3.3.1. Preparation of Plates (see **Note 6***)*

Preparation of the antibiotic dilutions:

1. Prepare appropriate doubling dilutions in CAMHB from stock solutions in sterile test tubes in 10-mL volumes. The dilution scale is selected to span the interpretative breakpoints used for each drug.
2. Dispense the resulting dilutions into sterile U-bottomed microdilution plates (*see* **Note 9**) in one of two ways. If inoculation of the wells is to be performed with a device that delivers a very small volume of bacterial suspension (no more than 10% of the volume in the well), then 0.1 mL of the antibiotic solution is added to each well at its final reaction concentration. If the inoculum is to be added by pipet in a volume of 0.05 mL, then 0.05 mL of the antibiotic solution is added at twice the final reaction concentration.
3. Use 8- or 12-well series depending on the number of dilutions required. Each plate should have at least 1 growth-control well and 1 uninoculated well. This arrangement suits plates in which only one antibiotic is tested. A second layout (favored by laboratories testing few isolates) might be to have different antibiot-

ics on the same plate. In this case, each row would require a growth-control well and a sterility check (uninoculated well).

4. Seal plates in plastic bags and keep frozen at –20°C or less. If plates are to be kept for months before use, –60°C or less is required. There should be no problem with stability of the antibiotics recommended earlier. Investigators wishing to use additional agents (especially carbapenems) will have to adjust storage times for frozen plates accordingly. Sufficient plates should be frozen to allow for quality control performance weekly (or with each run if plates are used more infrequently).
5. Do not store plates in self-defrosting freezers (sublimation of the ice results in increases in drug concentrations), and thawed plates must not be refrozen.

3.3.2. Inoculum Adjustment and Preparation for Inoculation

1. Prepare 0.5 McFarland suspensions of test and control organisms by the direct colony suspension method (*see* **Subheading 3.1.2.**).
2. Small (0.005 mL) or large (0.05 mL) inocula for each well will be selected depending on the manner in which the antibiotic solutions were prepared (*see* **Subheading 3.3.1., Step 2**).
3. The final inoculum density in each well should be 5 × 10^5 cfu/mL, so that each laboratory should calculate the required adjustment according to its counts of 0.5 McFarland suspensions (as in **Subheadings 3.1.1.** and **3.1.2.**).
4. Reservoirs for the suspensions: If single pipets are to be used, suspensions may be left in test tubes. If multi-channel pipets are to be used, choose appropriate reservoirs according to the layout of the plate.
   a. Laboratories testing small numbers of isolates might well prefer to place several different antibiotics on each plate. In this case, only one organism will be inoculated on each plate and a single-compartment reservoir will suffice (*see* **Subheading 3.3.1., Step 3**). A drawback of this layout is that a second plate might be needed to run the control strains.
   b. If the plate contains only one antibiotic in all the rows, a multi-compartmented reservoir suitable for the pipet will be required. If the small 0.005 mL inoculum is used, a microwell plate will be suitable.

3.3.3. Inoculation

1. Thaw frozen plates and allow to come to room temperature.
2. Within 15 min of preparation of the inoculum, inoculate each well except the sterility control wells with 0.005 mL or 0.05 mL of suspension as appropriate.
3. Purity check: streak samples of the inoculum on blood agar for overnight incubation.
4. Inoculum density check: Dilute 0.05 mL taken from the growth control well in 10 mL (1 : 1000) sterile broth or normal saline, and perform a surface count using 0.1 mL spread evenly on a blood-agar plate. A count of 50 cfu/mL would reflect an inoculum density of 5 × 10^5/mL.
5. Seal or cover each plate before incubation.

3.3.4. Controls

Control strains appropriate for each drug tested should be selected (*see* **Subheading 2.3.**) and included in each run. The results should be monitored and corrective action taken according to laboratory policy.

3.4. Incubation Conditions

There is general agreement that incubation in a CO_2-enriched environment is desirable, because not all strains of *N. meningitidis* will grow well in room air, and a proportion of strains will not grow at all. The current NCCLS recommendation calls for incubation in 5% CO_2 at 35°C for 24 h *(25)*.

3.5. End-Point Determination and Interpretation

3.5.1. Agar-Dilution Method

The lowest drug dilution at which complete inhibition of growth is observed is the MIC. It is recommended to ignore the occasional single colony appearing in a spot. This is consistent with the view that the endpoint is determined by inhibition of more than 99.9% of the inoculum of 10^4 cfu/spot. A fine film may be deposited at the site of the inoculum, which should also be ignored. Other phenomena such as paradoxical growth at some of the higher concentrations, or persistent growth of a small number of colonies after clear inhibition at the MIC, should be resolved by checking the identity of the growth and repeating the test.

3.5.2. Broth-Dilution Method

The growth control should show a button of growth at least 2 mm in diameter, or definite turbidity. The MIC is the lowest concentration that completely inhibits growth in the wells. If sulphonamides are tested, there may be a small amount of growth. The MIC should be determined by estimating which well represents 80% reduction in growth when compared with the growth control.

3.5.3. Interpretation

In the absence of generally agreed MIC breakpoints for *N. meningitidis*, the MIC value should be reported. The method used to determine the MIC should be included in the report. The clinical significance of the MIC values should be interpreted in consultation between the reference laboratory and the party interested in the results, e.g., when the use of a drug is contemplated for chemoprophylaxis. A rifampicin MIC of greater than 256 mg/L would unquestionably denote resistance *(7)*, whereas values of 0.25–1 mg/L would require careful evaluation in taking a decision to use rifampicin or an alternative agent *(30)*.

3.6. Etest

The Etest has found favor with a number of laboratories, the convenience of its use being its chief advantage. A number of studies have reported on its reliability ***(10,26,31–34)***, although it should not be regarded as a reference method. Pascual et al. have shown the susceptibility of the method to variations in in vitro conditions *(28)*.

When epidemiological circumstances demand urgent results, e.g., in areas where rifampicin resistance is relatively frequent, some advantage may be gained by direct estimation of the MIC. This test involves spreading cerebrospinal fluid (CSF) directly onto a suitable agar surface and applying Etest strips. This procedure should be attempted only when Gram-negative diplococci are readily visible in the CSF film. The test will give information on high-order resistance to drugs used for chemoprophylaxis. In all such cases, MIC determinations should be repeated using a proper inoculum before results are finalized and reported.

3.6.1. Performance of the Test and End-Point Estimation

The Etest is a commercial system and should be carried out according to the manufacturer's instructions.

3.6.2. Adaptation to the Conventional MIC Scale

The Etest scale does not follow the usual convention of doubling dilutions based on 1 mg/L (e.g., 16, 8, 4, 2, 1, 0.5, 0.25, 0.125, 0.0625). This is of little consequence unless readings are to be compared with MICs determined by agar- or broth-dilution, in which case Etest readings should be rounded up to the next conventional value as necessary (e.g., 0.094 mg/L would be read as 0.125 mg/L, 0.38mg/L as 0.5 mg/L, and so on).

3.7. Comment on Safety

Studies of the antimicrobial susceptibilities of *N. meningitidis* may involve work with large numbers of cultures, with potential exposure to large numbers of bacteria. In recent years evidence has accumulated that an appreciable risk of laboratory-acquired meningococcal infection exists for laboratory personnel working with the organism ***(35–39)***. Such infections have been attended by a significant case-fatality ratio. Acute viral infection may be an important risk factor ***(40)***.

A policy for preventing such infections should be adopted by each laboratory, and would ideally be founded on the following principles:

1. Awareness of the risks and factors contributing to them.
2. Attention to detail. Meticulous care in handling cultures should be actively promoted, and proficiency and knowledge of personnel monitored.

3. Containment and personal protective equipment (PPE). Any work with multiple meningococcal cultures or large volumes of viable meningococci, especially when aerosol-producing procedures are employed, should be carried out in a biological safety cabinet. The need for PPE will depend on the availability and type of safety cabinet. At the least, gloves should be worn (and used correctly!), with eye and face protection deployed as appropriate. An acceptable procedure should be developed in each laboratory, based, for example, on the Standard Precautions advocated in the USA ***(41,42)***. Another excellent source is the booklet: Biosafety in Microbiological and Biomedical Laboratories (BMBL), which is available in print and on the internet ***(43,44)***.
4. Personnel with acute respiratory infections should not be permitted to handle meningococcal cultures.
5. Immunization. Despite the limitations of currently available vaccines, active immunization of personnel chronically exposed to *N. meningitidis* should be considered. Care should be taken to ensure that personnel are aware of the imperfect nature of the protection, in order to discourage excessive reliance on immunization.
6. A procedure should be adopted for reporting and action in the case of mishaps. This should include a policy determining the indications for and manner of chemoprophylaxis.

3.8. Comment on Changing Information

The field of antimicrobial susceptibility testing is constantly evolving. This results in frequent adjustments to published recommendations and guidelines, for example, the NCCLS publishes annual updates of tables and recommended procedures, and its standards are periodically revised or new standards added. Investigators should familiarize themselves with available resources, especially regarding such organizations as the NCCLS (located on the internet at http://www.nccls.org), the European Committee on Antimicrobial Susceptibility Testing (Eucast), the British Society for Antimicrobial Chemotherapy (http://www.bsac.org.uk), Swedish Reference Group for Antibiotics (http://www.ltkronoberg.se/ext/raf/RAFENG/SRGA.HTM), and others.

4. Notes

1. Care must be exercised in the choice of suppliers of antibiotic powders. Apart from the drug manufacturers, a number of commercial and other sources are available (e.g., Sigma). Pharmaceutical formulations for administration to patients should not be used.
2. Choice of antibiotics for testing will undoubtedly vary somewhat in accordance with regional differences in prescribing practices for therapy and chemoprophylaxis. However, in view of the lack of agreed-upon interpretative criteria and testing methods, it would be wise to limit the range of drugs tested (for reporting) to those currently in use or useful as epidemiological markers (sulphonamides). Chloramphenicol would be appropriate in areas where the drug is likely to be

used, especially in view of the recently reported high-level resistance *(45)*. Newer agents that have been evaluated for chemoprophylaxis, such as azithromycin, may need to be added to the list if early promising results are borne out *(46)*. No doubt, newer fluoroquinolones will come under scrutiny, especially because reduced sensitivity to ciprofloxacin has already been observed *(47)*.

3. Practical procedures for the storage and handling of powders, and the preparation of stock and working solutions are given in detail in the NCCLS methods *(24)* and tables *(25)*.
4. The ability of media to support adequate growth and to yield consistent results have been central difficulties preventing agreement on uniform methods. Therefore in making choices, laboratory directors should try to evaluate batches of media prior to purchase. This will be much simpler for large reference laboratories, which receive large numbers of strains and which have developed collections of meningococci. Although no generally agreed-upon battery of meningococci is available, using regular Gram-positive and Gram-negative quality-control reference strains for evaluating susceptibility test performance may not be appropriate for this purpose. Smaller reference laboratories or clinical laboratories will likely be working with media chosen for more general testing purposes, so that in each case adequate growth on the test medium should be a minimum requirement, and referral to a larger laboratory for confirmation of results will be required. In accordance with accepted quality-assurance practice, records of manufacturers and lot identification data will allow the accumulation of useful information regarding sources of good materials, customer service, and so on.
5. Several different media are in regular use in reference centers all over the world. It is clear from the literature that supplemented or enriched media best support meningococcal growth, the debit side being that consistently higher MICs may be the result, as has been documented in Germany for GC agar *(27)*. The medium favored by this author is Mueller-Hinton agar supplemented with 5% whole sheep blood. This is also currently recommended by the NCCLS *(24,25)*.
6. The reader is referred to the appropriate NCCLS document for practical guidance in preparing antibiotic dilutions in the chosen agar or broth media *(25)*. There is no doubt that the local experience of each laboratory will determine the manner of the work to a large degree.
7. Broth dilution tests are much less frequently encountered in reference laboratory practice. Macrodilution tests using similar conditions, are also infrequently used, but might be tempting for clinical laboratories that encounter *N. meningitidis* very infrequently because they can be performed without maintaining a routine system for MIC determination. In this latter case, confirmation of results by a reference laboratory will be required.
8. The need for cation-adjustment of Mueller-Hinton Broth has not been established for *N. meningitidis*. CAMHB is commonly available as a medium for testing MICs in many laboratories.
9. Sterile microdilution trays are available from many commercial sources. U-bottomed wells are preferred.

References

1. Bardi, L., Badolati, A., Corso, A., and Rossi, M. A. (1994) Failure of the treatment with penicillin in a case of *Neisseria meningitidis* meningitis. *Medicina. (B. Aires.)* **54,** 427–430.
2. Turner, P. C., Southern, K. W., Spencer, N. J. B., and Pullen, H. (1990) Treatment failure in meningococcal meningitis. *Lancet* **335,** 732–733.
3. Casado-Flores, J., Osona, B., Domingo, P., and Barquet, N. (1997) Meningococcal meningitis during penicillin therapy for meningococcemia. *Clin. Infect. Dis.* **25,** 1479.
4. Contoyiannis, P. and Adamopoulos, D. A. (1974) Penicillin-resistant *Neisseria meningitidis*. *Lancet* **i,** 462.
5. Perez-Trallero, E., Aldamiz-Echeverria, L., and Perez-Yarza, E. G. (1990) Meningococci with increased resistance to penicillin. *Lancet* **335,** 1096.
6. Luaces, C. C., Garcia, G. J., Roca, M. J., and Latorre, O. C. (1997) Clinical data in children with meningococcal meningitis in a Spanish hospital. *Acta Paediatr.* **86,** 26–29.
7. Yagupsky, P., Ashkenazi, S., and Block, C. (1993) Rifampicin-resistant meningococci causing invasive disease and failure of chemoprophylaxis. *Lancet* **341,** 1152–1153.
8. Campos, J., Mendelman, P. M., Sako, M. U., Chaffin, D. O., Smith, A. L., and Saez-Nieto, J. A. (1987) Detection of relatively penicillin G-resistant *Neisseria meningitidis* by disk susceptibility testing. *Antimicrob. Agents Chemother.* **31,** 1478–1482.
9. Campos, J., Trujillo, G., Seuba, T., and Rodriguez, A. (1992) Discriminative criteria for *Neisseria meningitidis* isolates that are moderately susceptible to penicillin and ampicillin. *Antimicrob. Agents Chemother.* **36,** 1028–1031.
10. Nicolas, P., Cavallo, J. D., Fabre, R., and Martet, G. (1998) Standardization of the *Neisseria meningitidis* antibiogram. Detection of strains relatively resistant to penicillin. *Bull. WHO* **76,** 393–400.
11. Tenover, F. C. (1993) Antimicrobial susceptibility testing of *Neisseria meningitidis*. *Clin. Microbiol. Newsl.* **15,** 37–38.
12. Block, C., Davidson, Y., and Keller, N. (1998) Unreliability of disc diffusion test for screening for reduced penicillin susceptibility in *Neisseria meningitidis*. *J. Clin. Microbiol.* **36,** 3103–3104.
13. Dillon, J. R., Pauze, M., and Yeung, K.-H. (1983) Spread of penicillinase-producing and transfer plasmids from the gonococcus to *Neisseria meningitidis*. *Lancet* **i,** 779–781.
14. Botha, P. (1988) Penicillin-resistant *Neisseria meningitidis* in Southern Africa. *Lancet* **i,** 54.
15. Fontanals, D., Pineda, V., Pons, I., and Rojo, J. C. (1989) Penicillin-resistant beta-lactamase producing *Neisseria meningitidis* in Spain. *Eur. J. Clin. Microbiol. Infect. Dis.* **8,** 90–91.
16. Vazquez, J. A., Enriquez, A. M., De la, F. L., Berron, S., and Baquero, M. (1996) Isolation of a strain of beta-lactamase-producing *Neisseria meningitidis* in Spain. *Eur. J. Clin. Microbiol. Infect. Dis.* **15,** 181–182.

17. Backman, A., Orvelid, P., Vazquez, J. A., Skold, O., and Olcen, P. (2000) Complete sequence of a beta-lactamase-encoding plasmid in *Neisseria meningitidis*. *Antimicrob. Ag. Chemother.* **44,** 210–212.
18. Roy, C., Tirado, M., Reig, R., Hermida, M., Fontanals, D., Esteva, C. , and Vidal, R. (1989) Type TEM beta-lactamase activity in a *Neisseria meningitidis* strain. *Enferm. Infecc. Microbiol. Clin.* **7,** 206–209.
19. Spratt, B. G., Zhang, Q., Jones, D. M., Hutchison, A., Brannigan, J. A., and Dowson, C. G. (1989) Recruitment of a penicillin-binding protein gene from *Neisseria flavescens* during the emergence of penicillin resistance in *Neisseria meningitidis*. *Proc. Natl. Acad. Sci. USA* **86,** 8988–8992.
20. Spratt, B. G., Bowler, L. D., Zhang, Q. Y., Zhou, J., and Smith, J. M. (1992) Role of interspecies transfer of chromosomal genes in the evolution of penicillin resistance in pathogenic and commensal *Neisseria* species. *J. Mol. Evol.* **34,** 115–125.
21. Maggs, A. F., Logan, J. M., Carter, P. E., and Pennington, T. H. (1998) The detection of penicillin insensitivity in *Neisseria meningitidis* by polymerase chain reaction. *J. Antimicrob. Chemother.* **42,** 303–307.
22. Abadi, F. J., Carter, P. E., Cash, P., and Pennington, T. H. (1996) Rifampin resistance in *Neisseria meningitidis* due to alterations in membrane permeability. *Antimicrob. Ag. Chemother.* **40,** 646–651.
23. National Committee for Clinical Laboratory Standards (1996) *Evaluating Production Lots of Dehydrated Mueller-Hinton Agar.* Approved Standard M6-A. NCCLS, Wayne, PA.
24. National Committee for Clinical Laboratory Standards (2000) *Methods for Dilution Antimicrobial Susceptibility Tests for Bacteria that Grow Aerobically.* Approved Standard M7-A5. 5th ed. NCCLS, Wayne, PA.
25. National Committee for Clinical Laboratory Standards (2000) *MIC Testing: Supplemental Tables M100-S10* NCCLS, Wayne, PA.
26. Marshall, S. A., Rhomberg, P. R., and Jones, R. N. (1997) Comparative evaluation of etest for susceptibility testing *Neisseria meningitidis* with eight antimicrobial agents. An investigation using U.S. Food and Drug Administration regulatory criteria. *Diagn. Microbiol. Infect. Dis.* **27,** 93–97.
27. Geiss, H. K., Geiss, M., Heller, J., Sonntag, A., and Sonntag, H. G. (1995) Evaluation of five different agar media for antimicrobial susceptibility testing of *Neisseria meningitidis*. *Med. Microbiol. Lett.* **4,** 263–267.
28. Pascual, A., Joyanes, P., Martinez-Martinez, L., Suarez, A. I., and Perea, E. J. (1996) Comparison of broth microdilution and E-test for susceptibility testing of *Neisseria meningitidis*. *J. Clin. Microbiol.* **34,** 588–591.
29. National Committee for Clinical Laboratory Standards (1996) *Quality Assurance for Commercially Prepared Microbiological Culture Media:* M22-A2. 2nd ed. NCCLS, Wayne, PA.
30. Darouiche, R., Perkins, B., Musher, D., Hamill, R., and Tsai, S. (1990) Levels of rifampin and ciprofloxacin in nasal secretions: correlation with MIC90 and eradication of nasopharyngeal carriage of bacteria. *J. Infect. Dis.* **162,** 1124–1127.

31. Gomez-Herruz, P., Gonzalez-Palacios, R., Romanyk, J., Cuadros, J. A., and Ena, J. (1995) Evaluation of the Etest for penicillin susceptibility testing of *Neisseria meningitidis*. *Diagn. Microbiol. Infect. Dis.* **21,** 115–117.
32. Hughes, J. H., Biedenbach, D. J., Erwin, M. E., and Jones, R. N. (1993) E test as susceptibility test and epidemiologic tool for evaluation of *Neisseria meningitidis* isolates. *J. Clin. Microbiol.* **31,** 3255–3259.
33. Perez-Trallero, E., Gomez, N., and Garcia-Arenzana, J. M. (1994) E test as susceptibility test for evaluation of *Neisseria meningitidis* isolates. *J. Clin. Microbiol.* **32,** 2341–2342.
34. Koeck, J. L., Cavallo, J. D., Fabre, R., Crenn, Y., Chapalain, J. C., and Meyran, M. (1994) Value of the E-test for the determination of the susceptibility to antibiotics of *Neisseria meningitidis*. *Pathol. Biol. (Paris)* **42,** 465–467.
35. Anon. (1991) Laboratory-acquired meningococcemia: California and Massachusetts. *Morb. Mortal. Wkly. Rep.* **40,** 46–55.
36. Anon. (1992) Laboratory-acquired meningococcal infection. *Commun. Dis. Rep. CDR Wkly.* **2,** 39.
37. Bhatti, A. R., DiNinno, V. L., Ashton, F. E., and White, L. A. (1982) A laboratory-acquired infection with *Neisseria meningitidis*. *J. Infect.* **4,** 247–252.
38. Paradis, J. F. and Grimard, D. (1994) Laboratory-acquired invasive meningococcus: Quebec. *Can. Commun. Dis. Rep.* **20,** 12–14.
39. Guibourdenche, M., Darchis, J. P., Boisivon, A., Collatz, E., and Riou, J. Y. (1994) Enzyme electrophoresis, sero- and subtyping, and outer membrane protein characterization of two *Neisseria meningitidis* strains involved in laboratory-acquired infections. *J. Clin. Microbiol.* **32,** 701–704.
40. Cartwright, K. A., Jones, D. M., Smith, A. J., Stuart, J. M., Kaczmarski, E. B., and Palmer, S. R. (1991) Influenza A and meningococcal disease. *Lancet* **338,** 554–557.
41. Garner, J. S. and Hospital Infection Control Practices Advisory Committee (1996) Guideline for isolation precautions in hospitals. *Infect. Control Hosp. Epidemiol.* **17,** 53–80.
42. Garner, J. S. and Hospital Infection Control Practices Advisory Committee (1996) Guidelines for Isolation Precautions in Hospitals. Centers for Disease Control and Prevention: Prevention Guidelines. http://aepo-xdv-www.epo.cdc.gov/wonder/PrevGuid/p0000419/p0000419.htm
43. Centers for Disease Control and Prevention and National Institutes of Health (1999) Biosafety in Microbiological and Biomedical Laboratories. http://www.cdc.gov/od/ohs/biosfty/bmbl4/bmbl4toc.htm
44. Centers for Disease Control and Prevention and National Institutes of Health. (1999) *Biosafety in Microbiological and Biomedical Laboratories*, 4th ed. U.S. Department of Health and Human Services, U.S. Government Printing Office, Washington, DC.
45. Galimand, M., Gerbaud, G., Guibourdenche, M., Riou, J. Y., and Courvalin, P. (1998) High-level chloramphenicol resistance in *Neisseria meningitidis*. *N. Engl. J. Med.* **339,** 868–874.

46. Girgis, N., Sultan, Y., Frenck, R. W. J., El-Gendy, A., Farid, Z., and Mateczun, A. (1998) Azithromycin compared with rifampin for eradication of nasopharyngeal colonization by *Neisseria meningitidis. Pediatr. Infect. Dis. J.* **17,** 816–819.
47. Kaczmarski, E. B., Gray, S. J., Carr, A. D., and Mallard, R. H. (1999) Antimicrobial agent susceptibility of clinical *Neisseria meningitidis* isolates from England and Wales (Abstract No. 2103). *Abstracts of the 39th Interscience Conference of Antimicrobial Agents and Chemotherapy.* Amer. Soc. for Microbiol., Washington, D.C.

7

Molecular Approach for the Study of Penicillin Resistance In *Neisseria meningitidis*

Luisa Arreaza and Julio A. Vázquez

1. Introduction

1.1. Evolution of Penicillin Resistance in Neisseria meningitidis

Neisseria meningitidis was previously considered extremely susceptible to penicillin, with most isolates showing minimal inhibitory concentrations (MICs) of ≤ 0.06 µg/mL. However, meningococcal isolates with decreased susceptibility to penicillin have been reported from asymptomatic carriers from as long ago as 1964 ***(1)***. Since then, meningococcal clinical isolates with decreased susceptibility to penicillin have been widely described in different countries, with MICs between 0.12 µg/mL to 1 µg/mL ***(2–9)***.

Meningococcal isolates with low-level resistance to penicillin have been named "moderately penicillin resistant" or strains with "decreased susceptibility," but the tendency now is to refer them as "moderately susceptible strains" (Pen^{ms}) because of their uncertain clinical significance. In fact, only two treatment failures associated with Pen^{ms} meningococci have been reported ***(10,11)***.

Nowadays MICs are similar to those found several years ago, with most of the Pen^{ms} strains showing an MIC of 0.12 µg/mL or 0.25 µg/mL ***(12)***, and for this reason this drug is still regarded as the antimicrobial agent of choice for treating meningococcal disease ***(13,14)***.

Although, microbiologically, it is considered first-line therapy, penicillin is infrequently the initial antimicrobial agent for meningococcal disease treatment in developed countries, because of the possibility of alternate diagnoses and better penetration into cerebrospinal fluid (CSF) broad-spectrum cephalosporins (e.g., ceftriaxone) are recommended ***(15)***.

From: *Methods in Molecular Medicine, vol. 67: Meningococcal Disease: Methods and Protocols*
Edited by: A. J. Pollard and M. C. J. Maiden © Humana Press Inc., Totowa, NJ

Several studies have demonstrated that Pen^{ms} meningococcal strains also show an increase in the MICs of narrow-spectrum cephalosporins but no differences or very slight increase have been observed for broad-spectrum cephalosporins such as cefotaxime and ceftriaxone *(16)*.

1.2. Genetic Basis of Moderate Susceptibility to Penicillin in N. meningitidis

Resistance to penicillin in meningococci is owing, at least in part, to the production of altered forms of penicillin-binding-protein (PBP) 2 that have decreased affinity for this drug *(17,18)*. The PBPs are bacterial enzymes that are essential for peptidoglycan synthesis. PBPs are targets for β-lactams antibiotics, which form permanent antibiotic-PBP complexes, preventing the normal cross-linking of the peptide chains of peptidoglycan resulting in cell death. Altered PBPs have a reduced affinity for the β-lactam and increased drug concentrations are required for their in vitro inhibition.

Altered forms of the PBP2 are owing to the expression of different alleles of the *penA* gene that encodes for that protein. So, although *penA* genes from fully susceptible strains appear highly uniform in sequence, those from Pen^{ms} are quite diverse, showing mosaic structures such that very conserved areas alternate with highly diverse regions *(19)*. Principally this diversity results from blocks of nucleotide sequence within the *penA* gene that are up to 23% divergent from the susceptible isolates. The meningococcus is naturally competent for transformation, and for this reason it is possible that these blocks of DNA have been acquired by horizontal genetic exchange involving *penA* genes from closely related species. The throat commensals *Neisseria flavescens*, *Neisseria mucosa*, and *Neisseria lactamica* are likely candidates as they appear more resistant to penicillin than *N. meningitidis* *(20–24)*.

Further support for the theory that replacement of the *penA* gene of meningococci with those from the intrinsically resistant *Neisseria* species can result in decreased susceptibility to penicillin has been obtained by the demonstration that the chromosomal DNA from those species can transform penicillin-susceptible isolates of *N. meningitidis* to increased resistance to penicillin *(24,25)*. The mechanism is likely to be the result of different and separate recombination events because many different mosaic *penA* alleles have been found in Pen^{ms} meningococci *(26)*.

Although modification of the normal PBP2 is the major cause of decreased susceptibility to penicillin in meningococci, high-level resistant meningococcal strains owing to β-lactamase production have been described in the literature. To date there have been four reports of resistance in meningococcal strains associated with this mechanism *(27–30)*. The β-lactamase gene is borne in a plasmid and conjugation is thought to be the most common way in which plasmids are transferred *(31)*. The role of *Neisseria gonorrhoeae* as reservoir for the mobilization of plasmid-encoded β-lactamase has been demonstrated recently. Complete sequencing of β-lactamase-encoding-plasmids in two different meningococcal strains have shown that they are almost identical with the pJD5 and pJD4 gonococcal plasmids. These results imply that these plasmids might have been picked up from a gonococcus in vivo *(32)*.

1.3. Population Structure of Moderately Susceptible Meningococci Strains

The frequency of Pen^{ms} meningococcal strains increased rapidly in Spain from 0.4% in 1985 to 42.6% in 1990. It was thought initially that these strains were derived from one or a few resistant isolates. Several analyses of the genetic structure meningococcal in populations have been carried out *(16,33)*. These studies demonstrated a similar genetic diversity among both fully suceptible (Pen^{s}) and Pen^{ms} isolates. Apparently, moderate susceptibility to penicillin did not appear in a new clone distinct from those already established. It is possible that the mechanism of resistance appeared in more than one line and further spreading took place by genetic interchange.

Previous studies have suggested a possible association between C:2b phenotype and the moderate susceptibility to penicillin. This fact could explain the high frequency of Pen^{ms} meningococci strains in Spain, where in the last few years the majority of meningococcal disease cases have been produced from strains showing that antigenic expression *(34)*.

Fortunately, MICs are still at a similar level to those found several years ago, as mentioned earlier *(12)*. Additional changes, perhaps in others PBPs, as has been described in gonococci, would be necessary to determine high level of resistance to penicillin *(35)*.

1.4. PCR: A Tool for the Detection of Moderately Susceptible Meningococcal Strains?

In cases of meningococcal disease, antibiotic therapy must be started as early as possible because delay in commencing antibiotic therapy may increase the mortality rate *(36,37)*. For this reason, it is often impossible to recover meningococcal strains from the patients and it is necessary to use nonculture techniques, such as polymerase chain reaction (PCR)-based methods if a certain diagnosis is to be made. These methods are also becoming increasingly important for the detection of antibiotic resistance.

To date the detection of Pen^{ms} meningococcal strains by a simple PCR protocol has not been described, although several studies have been done *(38)*.

Although the mechanism of resistance to penicillin in meningococci was described several years ago, there are few studies in which the *penA* gene sequence is analyzed. Restriction fragment-length polymorphism (RFLP) profiles have been used to analyze the diversity of the *penA* gene in large collections of Pen^{ms} meningococcal strains *(39)*. This method has limitations because identity of RFLP pattern does not necessarily indicate the identity of nucleotide sequence. For this reason, it is important to sequence the *penA* gene in Pen^{ms} strains belonging to different hipervirulent clones and so try to determine the most frequent mosaicism and possible relationships between specific mutations and MIC to penicillin. This information would be very useful for the design of a simple PCR protocol that could be regarded as a valid method for identifying Pen^{ms} meningococcal strains.

2. Materials

2.1. Growth of Bacteria and Preparation of DNA Template for PCR

1. Sterile distilled water.
2. Blood-agar plates.

2.2. Buffers and Stock Solution for PCR

All components of PCR reactions should be prepared in sterile deionized water dedicated to PCR. This can be obtained commercially.

1. Deionized distilled water.
2. PCR buffer (10X stock): 100 m*M* Tris-HCl, pH 8.3, 500 m*M* KCl. Commercially available from *Taq* polymerase manufacturer.
3. $MgCl_2$: 25 m*M* stock solution.
4. dATP, dCTP, dGTP, dTTP: each at 10 m*M*. Minimize freeze-thawing.
5. Primers: A 50 μ*M* solutions of each primer in sterile desionized water. Store frozen in small volumes.
   GCup2: 5′-TTTGCACACGTCATCGGATTTAC-3′
   GCdown3: 5′-TCGTGAATTCGGGGATATAACTGCGGCCGTC-3′
6. *Taq* DNA polymerase: 5 U/μL (Perkin-Elmer).

2.3. Agarose Gel

1. Agarose: Type II, Medium E.E.O (Sigma)
2. Electrophoresis buffer: Tris-Borate EDTA 10X: 0.9 *M* Tris base, 0.9 *M* boric acid, 0.02 *M* Na_2EDTA.
3. Sample loading buffer: 0.25% bromophenol blue, 50% glycerol, 50% TE Buffer (10 m*M* Tris-HCl, 1 m*M* EDTA, pH 8.0).
4. DNA markers: Ready Load 1kb DNA Ladder (Gibco-BRL), which is suitable for DNA fragments from 500 bp to 12 kb.
5. Ethidium bromide (EB). *Caution:* EB is a powerful mutagen and potential carcinogen. Always wear gloves when handling the solid or liquids containing the chemical, and dispose of appropriately.

2.4. Agarose Gel Electrophoresis

1. Electrophoresis tank, gel frame, well-former and tape as appropiate for system in use.
2. Power supply.
3. UV transillumінator and camera. *Caution:* Suitable eye and skin protection should be worn when working with UV.

2.5. Purifying PCR Products

2.5.1. Method I

1. Polyethylene glycol 8000.
2. NaCl.
3. 70% ethanol: store at –20°C.
4. Sterile H_2O.

2.5.2. Method II

1. Low-gelling temperature agarose.
2. Quiaquick Gel Extraction Kit (Quiagen).
3. Isopropanol.
4. Sterile H_2O.

2.6. DNA Sequencing

2.6.1. PCR

1. BigDye Terminator Cycle Sequencing v2.0 Ready Reaction (PE Biosystems).
2. Sterile H_2O.
3. Primers.
   GCup2: 5′-TTTGCACACGTCATCGGATTTAC-3′
   GCdown3: 5′-TCGTGAATTCGGGGATATAACTGCGGCCGTC-3′
   Fo: 5′-TATACCGCACTGACGCACGAC-3′
   Ro: 5′-GCCGTCGTGCGTCAGTGC-3′

2.6.2. Purifying PCR Products

1. 100% Ethanol: store at –20°C.
2. 70% Ethanol: store at –20°C.
3. Sterile H_2O.

2.6.3. Electrophoresis

Automatic sequencer.

3. Methods

3.1. Growth of Bacteria and Preparation of DNA Template for PCR

1. Grow meningococci on blood agar at 37°C in a 5% CO_2 atmosphere.
2. Remove cells from agar plates using a swab and suspend in 1000 μL of sterile distilled water.

3. Suspensions are boiled for 10 min, chilled, and centrifuged for 10 min at 14,000*g* (*see* **Notes 1 and 2**).

3.2. Amplification of penA Gene

The PCR protocol allows amplification of a 1.4 kb region of the *penA* gene (from codon 183–187 bp downstream of the coding region). The first fragment of this gene (~600 pb) is highly conserved in Pen^s and Pen^{ms} meningococcal strains, so we do not consider it necessary to analyze it.

3.2.1. Preparation of Reaction Mixes (see Note 3)

1. Add 5 µL of the supernatant of each sample into numbered, thin-walled PCR tubes (*see* **Note 4**).
2. Prepare a master mix for the PCR reaction. The volumes of each component are dependent on the number of individual reactions to be prepared. The followings components are added to a separate tube (volumes are given per reaction).
3. H_2O 66.5 µL
   $MgCl_2$ 6 µL (25 m*M* stock = 1.5 m*M* final conc.)
   10X Reaction Buffer 10 µL
   dNTP mix 8 µL (2 µL of each 10 m*M* dNTP)
   PCR primer (GCup2) 2 µL (50 µ*M* primer stock = 1 µ*M* final conc.)
   PCR primer (GCdown3) 2 µL (50 µ*M* primer stock = 1 µ*M* final conc.)
   Taq polymerase 0.5 µL (2.5 U of enzyme)
   Total 95 µL
4. Immediately aliquot the reaction mix to each tube of template taking great care to avoid cross-contamination. The simplest way is to use a separate pipet tip for each transfer (*see* **Note 5**).
5. Place the tubes into the thermal cycler and close the lid.

3.2.2. Cycling Conditions

Step 1 95°C 3 min
Step 2 94°C 1 min
Step 3 62°C 1 min
Step 4 72°C 2 min
Step 5 Repeat steps 2, 3, and 4 a further 29 times
Step 6 72°C 7 min
Step 7 4°C

3.2.3. Analysis of PCR Products

After cycling, check that amplification was successful by running 5 µL of each reaction on an agarose gel, with size standards.

1. Prepare a 0.8% agarose gel in 0.5X Tris-borate EDTA (TBE) buffer (*see* **Notes 6** and **7**). Add ethidium bromide into the agarose gel at concentrations of ~0.5 µg/mL.

2. Add 2 μL of loading dye to 5 μL of the PCR product in the wells of a microtiter plate. Load the samples into the wells of the gel. Load DNA markers to at least one well, flanking the sample wells.
3. Run the gel in 0.5X TBE at 10 V/cm until the bromophenol blue dye has migrated approx 4/5 the length of the gel.
4. Photograph the gel using an UV transilluminator to visualize the DNA bands.

3.3. Purifying PCR Products

Before sequencing the amplified DNA it is necessary to remove all the dNTPs and primers from the amplified DNA. Both, dNTPs and primers can be removed by different methods.

3.3.1. Method I (see **Note 8**)

1. Transfer the contents of each PCR tube into a labeled 1.5-mL Eppendorf tubes.
2. Add 60 μL of 20% PEG-2.5 *M* NaCl to each tube and mix.
3. Incubate for 15 min at 37°C.
4. Pellet the PCR products by spinning in a centrifuge at maximum speed for 20 min.
5. Discard the supernatant and wash the DNA pellet by adding 0.5 mL of 70% EtOH and spin at maximum speed for a further 5 min.
6. Discard the supernatant and dry pellets in the vacuum dryer.
7. Resuspend the dried PCR products in 20–30 μL sterile H_2O. Store at –20°C.

3.3.2. Method II

1. Prepare a 0.8% agarose gel in 0.5X TBE Buffer. In this case we use low melting-temperature agarose. Add ethidium bromide into the agarose gel at concentrations of ~0.5 μg/mL (*see* **Note 9**).
2. Mix the PCR product with loading buffer (~5 μL), load onto the gel and carry out electrophoresis at 4°C to ensure that the gel does not melt during the run.
3. Examine the gel by ultraviolet (UV) light and locate the band of interest.
4. Using a scalpel or razor blade and cut out a slice of agarose containing the band of interest and transfer it to a clean, disposable plastic tube.
5. Elute DNA from agarose using Quiaquick Gel Extraction Kit (Quiagen) according the instructions provided by the manufacturer.

3.4. Gel Electrophoresis of Purified PCR Product

1. Prepare a 0.8% agarose gel in 0.5X TBE Buffer. Add ethidium bromide into the agarose gel at concentrations of ~0.5 μg/mL
2. Load 1 μL of sample plus 1 μL of loading buffer in each well. Use as markers appropriate restriction digests of known quantities of the original DNA.

3.5. DNA Sequence Determination

3.5.1. Cycle Sequencing

1. Add between 1 and 5 μL of purified PCR product into thin-walled PCR tube (*see* **Note 10**).

2. Dilute the 50 μ*M* stock solution of sequencing primer 1:10 with sterile distilled H_2O.
3. Add 1 μL of the diluted sequencing primer into each tube (*see* **Note 11**).
4. Add 4 μL of the BigDye Ready Reaction Termination Mix into each tube.
5. Complete with sterile distilled water until a final volume of 10 μL.
6. Place the tubes in the thermal cycler and close the lid.
7. Cycling conditions

Step 1	94°C	3 min
Step 2	96°C	10 s
Step 3	50°C	5 s
Step 4	60°C	4 min
Step 5	Repeat steps 2, 3, and 4 a further 24 times	
Step 7	4°C	

3.5.2. Purification of PCR Products

Unincorporated dye terminators must be completely removed before the samples can be analyzed by electrophoresis. Excess dye terminators in sequencing reactions obscure data in the early part of the sequence and can interfere with base calling. Any method that removes dNTPs and primers should work.

In our laboratory purifying is done by ethanol precipitation according the following protocol (*see* **Note 12**)

1. Transfer the contents of each PCR tube into labelled 1.5-mL Eppendorf tubes.
2. Add 30 μL of sterile distilled water and 60 μL of 95% EtOH and vortex briefly to mix.
3. Keep the Eppendorfs on ice for 10 min.
4. Spin the tubes for 20 min at maximum speed. Immediately after spinning, remove the supernatant using a pipet.
5. Wash the pellet by adding 500 μL of 70% EtOH to each tube. Spin again at maximum speed for 10 min.
6. Remove as much of the EtOH as possible (pour and then use a pipet tip) and dry the pellets in the vacuum dryer (*see* **Note 13**).

3.5.3. Electrophoresis

For information on how to perform sample electrophoresis on the automatic sequencers, refer to the manuals provided by the manufacturer.

3.6. Data Analyses

The DNA sequence is translated into amino acid sequence using the DNA Star program (DNA Star Inc, Madison, WI). If several sequences (from different strains) are available then a multiple alignment should be done (e.g., using Jotun Hein Method).

4. Notes

1. Extended boiling reduces the amount of final PCR product, presumably by destroying the DNA.
2. This very simple method of preparing PCR templates works very well in the authors' experience and avoids the need for more complex protocols, such as those involving DNA extraction.
3. A master PCR reaction mix should be prepared, allowing for control reactions and pipetting inaccuracies.
4. Remember to set up a negative PCR control, which consists of reaction components and water instead of template DNA.
5. Reaction products must not contaminate stock reaction components or they will act as templates in any reactions set up using the contaminated component solutions yielding misleading results. Contamination can be minimized following some rules: always use clean, sterile pipet tips for each reaction component; establish separate areas for handling of reaction components and products; use positive-displacement pipets and tips to prevent aerosols; use commercially obtained sterile distilled water and use aliquotted batches of dNTPs, primers, and PCR reaction buffers.
6. To prepare a 0.8% agarose gel, add 0.8 g of agarose to 100 mL of 0.5X TBE buffer in a flask. Cover the flask with foil to prevent evaporation and boil to dissolve the agarose. Allow the agarose to cool to about 55–60°C, then seal the ends of a gel tray with tape and pour the agarose into it. Position a comb with the required number of teeth to form wells and allow the gel to set.
7. It is important to use the same batch of electrophoresis buffer in both the electrophoresis tank and the gel. Small differences in ionic strength or pH create can affect the mobility of DNA fragments.
8. This is the protocol that we normally use. However, when more than one PCR product is amplified (it happens rarely) it would be recommended to use the second protocol (Method II).
9. This is the agarose in which hydroxyethil groups have been introduced into the polysaccharide chain. This modification causes the agarose to gel at ~30°C and to melt at approx 65°C. These characteristics have been used to develop a simple technique for the recovery of DNA from gels.
10. The amount of PCR product to use in sequencing will depend on the purity of the PCR product. The authors recommend ~250 ng. If your purified PCR product is not concentrated enough and you need to add more than 5 μL, you have to concentrate it. You can do this according the following protocol:
    a. Mix the PCR product with 100% ethanol (2.5 mL of ethanol per mL of sample) plus 3 *M* sodium acetate (0.1 mL of 3 *M* sodium acetate per mL of sample).
    b. Place the Eppendorfs on ice for 10 min.
    c. Spin the tubes for 10 min at maximum speed. Immediately after spinning, remove the supernatant using a pipet.
    d. Wash the pellet by adding 250 μL of 70% EtOH to each tube. Spin again at maximum speed for 2 min.

e. Remove as much of the alcohol as possible (pour and then use a pipet tip) and dry the pellets in the vacuum dryer.
f. Resuspend the dried PCR products in 5 µL sterile H_2O.

11. The internal primers have been designed (in order to avoid sequencing mistakes) using DNA Star Program. Because the sequencing fragment shows mosaicism in Pen^{ms} strains, it might be necessary sometimes to design new primers.
12. This method of purification is cheaper and faster, although removes less of the unincorporated dye-labeled terminators than others methods. For this reason, it can obscure data at the beginning of the sequence.
13. The dried pellets can be stored at –20°C until you are ready to load them onto a sequencing gel.

References

1. Martin, J. E., Sammuels, S. B., Peacok, W. L., and Thayer, J. D. (1964) *Neisseria gonorrhoeae* and *Neisseria meningitidis* sensitivity to spectomycin, lincomycin and penicillin G. *Antimicrob. Agents Chemother.* **5,** 366–368.
2. Sáez-Nieto, J. A., Vázquez, J. A., and Marcos, C. (1990) Meningococci moderately resistant to penicillin. *Lancet* **336,** 54.
3. Sutcliffe, E. M., Jones, D. M., El-Sheikh, S., and Percival, A. (1988) Penicillin insensitive meningococci in the UK. *Lancet* **i,** 657–658.
4. Tzanakaki, G., Blackwell, C. C., Kremastinau, J., Kallergi, C., Kouppari, G., and Weir, D. M. (1992) Antibiotic sensitivities of *Neisseria meningitidis* isolates from patients and carriers in Greece. *Epidemiol. Infect.* **108,** 449–455.
5. Enting, R. H., Spanjaard, L., van de Beek, D., Hensen, E. F., de Gans, J., and Dankert, J. (1996) Antimicrobial susceptibility of *Haemophilus influenzae*, *Neisseria meningitidis* and *Streptococcus pneumoniae* isolates causing meningitis in The Netherlands, 1993–1994. *J. Antimicrob. Chemother.* **38,** 777–786.
6. Woods, C. R., Smith, A. L., Wasilauskas, B. L., Campos, J., and Givner, L. B. (1994) Invasive disease caused by *Neisseria meningitidis* relatively resistant to penicillin in North Carolina. *J. Infect. Dis.* **170,** 453–456.
7. Blondeau, J. M., Ashton, F. E., Isaacson, M., Yaschuck, Y., Anderson, C., and Ducasse, G. (1995) *Neisseria meningitidis* with decreased susceptibility to penicillin in Saskatchewan, Canada. *J. Clin. Microbiol.* **33,** 1784–1786.
8. Block, C., Davidson, Y., Melamed, E., and Keller, N. (1993) Susceptibility of *Neisseria meningitidis* in Israel to penicillin and other drugs of interest. *J. Antimicrob. Chemother.* **32,** 166–168.
9. Rosenstein, N. E., Stocker, S. A., Popovic, T., Tenover, F. C., and Perkins, B. A. (2000) Antimicrobial resistance of *Neisseria meningitidis* in the United States, 1997. The Active Bacterial Core surveillance (ABCs) Team. *Clin. Infect. Dis.* **30,** 212–213.

10. Bardi, L., Badolati, A., Corso, A., and Rossi, M. A. (1994) Failure of the treatment with penicillin in a case of *Neisseria meningitidis* meningitis. *Medicina (Buenos Aires)* **54,** 427–430.
11. Turner, P. C., Southern, K. W., Spencer, N. J., and Pullen, H. (1990) Treatment failure in meningococcal meningitis. *Lancet* **335,** 732–733.
12. Arreaza, L., de la Fuente, L., and Vázquez., J. A. (2000) Antibiotic susceptibility patterns of *Neisseria meningitidis* isolates from patients and asymptomatic carriers. *Antimicrob. Agents Chemother.* **44,** 1705–1707.
13. Cartwright, K. A. and Ala'Aldeen, D. A. (1997) *Neisseria meningitidis*: clinical aspects. *J. Infect.* **34,** 15–19.
14. Quagliarello, V. J. and Scheld, W. M. (1997). Treatment of bacterial meningitis. *N. Engl. J. Med.* **336,** 708–716.
15. Peltola, H., Anttila, M., and Renkonen, O. V. (1989) Randomised comparison of chloramphenicol, ampicillin, cefotaxime and ceftriaxone for childhood bacterial meningitis. *Lancet* **i,** 1281–1287.
16. Sáez-Nieto, J. A., Luján, R., Berrón, S., Campos, J., Viñas, M., Fusté, C., et al. (1992) Epidemiology and molecular basis of penicillin resistant *Neisseria meningitidis* in Spain: a five year history (1985–1989). *Clin. Infect. Dis.* **14,** 394–402.
17. Spratt, B. G. (1994) Resistance to antibiotics mediated by target alterations. *Science* **264,** 388–393.
18. Dowson, C. G., Coffey, T. J., and Spratt, B. G. (1994) Origin and molecular epidemiology of penicillin-binding-protein-mediated resistance to beta-lactam antibiotics. *Trends Microbiol.* **2,** 361–366.
19. Maiden, M. C. J. (1998) Horizontal genetic exchange, evolution, and spread of antibiotic resistance in bacteria. *Clin. Infect. Dis.* **27(Suppl.1),** S12–S20.
20. Spratt, B. G., Zhang, Q. Y., Jones, D. M., Hutchison, A., Brannigan, J. A., and Dowson, C. G. (1989) Recruitment of a penicillin-binding protein gene from *Neisseria flavescens* during the emergence of penicillin resistance in *Neisseria meningitidis*. *Proc. Natl. Acad. Sci. USA* **86,** 8988–8992.
21. Spratt, B. G., Bowler, L. D., Zhang, Q. Y., Zhou, J., and Smith, J. M. (1992) Role of interspecies transfer of chromosomal genes in the evolution of penicillin resistance in pathogenic and commensal *Neisseria* species. *J. Mol. Evol.* **34,** 115–125.
22. Pérez Castillo, A., Pérez Castillo, A. M., Luján, R., and Sáez Nieto, J. A. (1994) Comparison of *penA* (PBP2) gene sequences of *Neisseria mucosa* moderately resistant to penicillin (pen^r) and *Neisseria meningitidis* (pen^r and pen^s) strains. *Rev. Esp. Quimioter* **7,** 228–237.
23. Luján, R., Zhang, Q. Y., Sáez-Nieto, J. A., Jones, D. M., and Spratt, B. G. (1991) Penicillin resistant isolates of *Neisseria lactamica* produced altered forms of penicillin binding protein 2 that arose by interspecies gene transfer. *Antimicrob. Agents Chemother.* **35,** 300–304.

24. Sáez-Nieto, J. A., Luján, R., Martínez-Suárez, J. V., Berrón, S., Vázquez, J. A., Viñas, M., and Campos, J. (1990) *Neisseria lactamica* and *Neisseria polysaccharea* as possible sources of meningococcal beta-lactam resistance by genetic transformation. *Antimicrob. Agents Chemother.* **34,** 2269–2272.
25. Bowler, L. D., Zhang, Q. Y., Riou, J. Y., and Spratt, B. G. (1994) Interspecies recombination between the *penA* genes of *Neisseria meningitidis* and commensal *Neisseria* species during the emergence of penicillin resistance in *N. meningitidis*: natural events and laboratory simulation. *J. Bacteriol.* **176,** 333–337.
26. Zhang, Q. Y., Jones, D. M., Sáez-Nieto, J. A., Pérez Trallero, E., and Spratt, B. G. (1990) Genetic diversity of penicillin-binding protein 2 genes of penicillin-resistant strains of *Neisseria meningitidis* revealed by fingerprinting of amplified DNA. *Antimicrob. Agents Chemother.* **34,** 1523–1528.
27. Botha, P. (1988) Penicillin resistant *Neisseria meningitidis* in southern Africa. *Lancet* **i,** 54.
28. Dillon, J. R., Pauze, M., and Yeung, K. H. (1983) Spread of penicillinase-producing and transfer plasmids from the gonococcus to *Neisseria meningitidis*. *Lancet* **i,** 779–781.
29. Fontanals, D., Pineda, V., Pons, I., and Rojo, J. C. (1989) Penicillin-resistant beta-lactamase producing *Neisseria meningitidis* in Spain. *Eur. J. Clin. Microbiol. Infect. Dis.* **8,** 90–91.
30. Vázquez, J. A., Enriquez, A. M., de la Fuente, L., Berrón, S., and Baquero, M. (1996) Isolation of a strain of beta-lactamase producing *N. meningitidis* in Spain. *Eur. J. Clin. Microbiol. Infect. Dis.* **15,** 181–182.
31. Roberts, M. C. and Knapp, J. S. (1988) Transfer of β-lactamase plasmids from *Neisseria gonorrhoeae* to *Neisseria meningitidis* and commensal *Neisseria* species by the 25.2 megadalton conjugative plasmid. *Antimicrob. Agents Chemother.* **32,** 1430–1432.
32. Bäckman, A., Orvelid, P., Vázquez J. A., Sköld, O., and Olcén, P. (2000) Complete sequence of a β-lactamase-encoding plasmid in *Neisseria meningitidis*. *Antimicrob. Agents Chemother.* **44,** 210–212.
33. Berrón, S. and Vázquez, J. A. (1994) Increase in moderate penicillin resistance and serogroup C in meningococcal strains isolated in Spain. Is there any relationship? *Clin. Infect. Dis.* **18,** 161–165.
34. Fernández, S., Arreaza, L., Santiago, I., Malvar, A., Berrón, S., Vázquez, J. A., et al. (1999). Carriage of a new epidemic strain of *Neisseria meningitidis* and its relationship with the incidence of meningococcal disease in Galicia, Spain. *Epidemiol. Infect.* **123,** 349–357.
35. Dougherty, T. J. (1986) Genetic analysis and penicillin-binding protein alterations in *Neisseria gonorrhoeae* with chromosomally mediated resistance. *Antimicrob. Agents Chemother.* **30,** 649–652.
36. Cartwright, K., Strang, J., Gossain, S., and Begg, N. (1992) Early treatment of meningococcal disease. *Br. Med. J.* **305,** 774.

37. van Deuren, M., Brandtzaeg, P., and van der Meer, J. W. (2000) Update on meningococcal disease with emphasis on pathogenesis and clinical management. *Clin. Microbiol. Rev.* **13,** 144–166.
38. Maggs, A. F., Logan, J. M. J., Carter, P. E., and Pennigton, T. H. (1998) The detection of penicillin insensitivity in *Neisseria meningitidis* by polymerase chain reaction. *J. Antimicrob. Chemother.* **42,** 303–307.
39. Campos, J., Fusté, M. C., Trujillo, G., Sáez-Nieto, J. A., Vázquez, J. A., Lorén, J. G., et al. (1992) Genetic diversity of penicillin-resistant *Neisseria meningitidis*. *J. Infect. Dis.* **166,** 173–177.

8

Overview: Epidemiology, Surveillance, and Population Biology

Martin C. J. Maiden and Norman T. Begg

1. Introduction

A combination of data obtained by classical epidemiological techniques with insights gained from the analysis of the population biology of *Neisseria meningitidis* have proved to be critical in understanding the spread of meningococcal disease. This is a consequence of the natural history and evolution of this bacterium, which, despite its fearsome reputation as an aggressive pathogen *(1)*, is ordinarily a harmless commensal inhabitant of the nasopharynx of adult humans *(2)*. Further, it has been established that "natural," (that is to say, carried) populations of meningococci are highly diverse, with a minority of genotypes (the "hyperinvasive lineages") being responsible for the majority of disease *(3)*. Finally, it is known that distinct hyperinvasive lineages tend to be associated with particular epidemiological manifestations of meningococcal disease *(4)* and some are especially associated with severe disease (the "hypervirulent" lineages) *(5)*. These complexities have important implications for public-health interventions, as different disease epidemiologies, caused by genetically diverse meningococci, require distinct approaches to public-health management. For example, the public-health response necessary to combat large-scale meningococcal-disease outbreaks in Africa *(6)* is different from that required during an institutional disease outbreak in Europe and North America, and prolonged geographical outbreaks in these countries require a different response again *(7)*. In recognition of the importance of the multi-disciplinary approach necessary to establish these insights, this section contains chapters ranging from outbreak management through surveillance and isolate characterization techniques to phylogenetic methods. Together the chapters provide

From: *Methods in Molecular Medicine, vol. 67: Meningococcal Disease: Methods and Protocols*
Edited by: A. J. Pollard and M. C. J. Maiden © Humana Press Inc., Totowa, NJ

the methodologies necessary for monitoring, understanding, and reacting to the spread of meningococcal disease.

2. Meningococcal Epidemiology

As discussed in Chapters 18 and 21, meningococcal disease is a global problem that occurs in all human populations studied. This is presumably a reflection of widespread distribution of carried meningococci throughout the world. The ubiquity of the disease, however, is accompanied by variation in its epidemiology in different countries. There is a general pattern of a background level of endemic disease interspersed by unpredictable epidemics, but within this pattern the precise epidemiology of meningococcal disease in any particular time and place is dependent on a number of factors, with the genetic lineages of meningococci circulating in the carrier state having a major influence on disease rates. Indeed, meningococcal outbreaks often occur when a new lineage is introduced into a susceptible population for the first time (*see* Chapter 18).

The occurrence of meningococcal disease in epidemics has been recognized for nearly 200 years ***(8)***, although it is intriguing for a disease with such prominent clinical features that the first probable description of a meningococcal disease outbreak was as late as 1805, when Vieusseux described an epidemic of cerebrospinal meningitis in Geneva, Switzerland. A major advance in meningococcal disease epidemiology came during World War I, when it was established that army recruit camps were at risk from meningococcal disease outbreaks, especially during periods of overcrowding, which were accompanied by high rates of carriage of meningococci. The vulnerability of military recruits continues to this day and has proved to be a major motivator for research into the development of meningococcal vaccines. A number of other factors that predispose individuals to meningococcal carriage, disease, or both have since been identified, including passive smoking, recent influenza infection, hereditary complement deficiencies, and asplenia; these are discussed briefly in Chapter 22.

A further milestone was the development of the serological typing of meningococci ***(9)***, which led to the recognition of different capsules of the organism ***(10)***, and later to the immunological characterization of the highly diverse subcapsular antigens ***(11)***. The serological techniques that played such an important part in the development of meningococcal biology are described in Chapter 9. The differential serological properties of capsules of different chemical composition is the basis of the serogrouping system for meningococci and the genetical basis for these differences, which has been established, are discussed in Chapter 13. Molecular studies of the expression of one of the most important subcapsular antigens for pathogenesis, the lipopolysaccharide (sometimes referred to as lipooligosaccharide in the meningococcus) are described in Chapter 14.

Of the 13 recognized serogoups, only 5—serogroups A,B,C, Y, and W-135—are associated with disease ***(1)***, implicating the capsules defined by these serogroups as major virulence determinants. Serogroup A meningococci caused the disease outbreaks in the First and Second World Wars, but meningococci expressing this serogroup have not caused significant disease in Western Europe and North America since then ***(12)***. These meningococci, however, continue to be a major cause of disease in Asia and Africa, especially in the "meningitis belt" of the Sahel region of sub-Saharan Africa, which was defined in a seminal monograph by Lapeyssonnie in 1963 ***(13)***. The epidemiology of meningococcal disease in this region has since been extensively studied and is discussed in Chapter 21. It is characterized by explosive, localized epidemics that invariably occur in the dry winter months (the harmattan) and that often appear and wane over a period of a few weeks. Although most epidemics in the meningitis belt are caused by serogroup A strains, more localized serogroup C epidemics also occur ***(14)***.

Two serogroup A lineages, known as subgroup I and subgroup III, have been responsible for successive pandemics of meningococcal disease, which have spread from Asia to Africa and on some occasions beyond ***(15–17)***. These outbreaks remain the most serious manifestation of meningococcal disease, with attack rates as high as 1,000 cases per 100,000 during intense epidemics. In the latest outbreak in Africa during 1996, which was caused by subgroup III, meningococci a total of 109,580 cases and 11,717 deaths were recorded in Nigeria alone ***(18)***. The annual Haj pilgrimage to Mecca has been associated with outbreaks of serogroup A disease, notably the spread of serogroup A; subgroup III organisms in 1987 ***(19)***. During 2000, members of the ET-37 complex expressing serogroup W135 capsules have spread by this means ***(20)*** as well. Some of these outbreaks are discussed in Chapters 20–22.

In the Americas (Chapter 22), Europe (Chapter 20), and Australasia ***(21)***, meningococcal disease occurs at substantially lower rates and is more common in winter than in summer, this seasonal pattern being particularly marked in the Northern hemisphere. In these areas, the annual incidence of meningococcal disease is usually between 1 and 10 per 100,000 population, with localized outbreaks occurring from time to time, where attack rates may rise to as high as 50–100 per 100,000. In addition, some geographic areas experience elevated incidence of disease, or hyperendemics, over a period of several years. Attack rates are usually highest in children under 5 yr of age and there is sometimes a smaller, second peak in disease incidence in teenagers. During outbreaks, the age distribution can change, with a shift toward older children and young adults. The majority of disease is caused by meningococci expressing serogroup B or C capsules, with disease caused by serogroup B organisms generally the most common. Disease outbreaks caused by meningococci expressing each of the disease-associated capsules have been described, although they are commonly caused by organisms expressing a serogroup C capsule. During the 1990s, serogroup C meningococcal disease outbreaks occurred in several countries, including Canada *(5)*, the UK *(22)*, Spain *(23)*, and the Czech Republic *(24)*. Serogroup Y infections have emerged as a significant cause of morbidity in the US in the last few years (*see* Chapter 22), and other serogroups may sometimes predominate (for example, serogroup A infections are common in Russia *[25]*). The case-fatality rate is usually about 10%, although it may be higher, particularly during outbreaks.

The application of multi-locus enzyme electrophoresis (MLEE, described in Chapter 18) for analysis of genetic relatedness and monoclonal antibodies (MAbs) for the improved characterization of subcapsular protein antigens enabled the underlying epidemiology of meningococcal disease to be elucidated. In a groundbreaking study, Dominique Caugant and colleagues established that meningococcal populations were genetically highly diverse, indeed they were the most diverse bacterial population examined up to that time *(26)*. These data permitted the categorization of the many genotypes into lineages. Although the members of these lineages clearly shared a recent common ancestor, there was much genetic diversity even within a given lineage, leading to the concept of the clonal complex, a group of related strains that had begun to diverge. Examination of the serological properties of the individual complexes established that serological classification of meningococci could be misleading as genetically related organisms could be antigenically diverse. This high diversity and the mobility of variants by horizontal genetic exchange has important implications for the development and introduction of vaccines against this organism.

In practical terms, the application of these techniques enabled the global tracking of particular hyperinvasive meningococci, such as the members of the ET-5 complex *(27)*. It is now well-established that a few clonal complexes cause most meningococcal disease *(28)* and that these change over time. Often increases in disease incidence accompany the introduction of a new lineage (clonal complex) into a given human population. The epidemic spread of different lineages is discussed in Chapter 18. More precise characterization of isolates also enabled the diversity of carried meningococci to be identified and established that the disease-associated meningococci were a minority component of the meningococcal population as a whole *(29)*.

The advent of nucleotide-sequence determination for the characterization of bacterial genes, which is described in Chapters 11 and 12, have provided more precise identification of genetic and antigenic variants. Nucleotide-sequence data also provided a wealth of evidence to suggest that diverse and dynamic nature of meningococcal populations was at least in part a consequence of the transformable nature of the organism. *Neisseria* are competent for transformation throughout their growth cycle and high rates of carriage presumably provide many instances of co-colonization, which permit horizontal genetic exchange within and among lineages and among the different species of meningococci ***(30)***. In addition, it is now clear that antigenic diversity is being continually generated in several surface proteins, presumably driven by immune selection ***(31)***. Some of the phylogenetic techniques that are employed to establish and measure the genetic diversity of meningococci are discussed in Chapter 23.

Molecular techniques that enable the comparison of genetically and pathogenically distinct meningococci, for both epidemiological and research purposes, are becoming ever more sophisticated. A particularly exciting prospect is the ability to compare whole genomes. The first technique that was able to achieve this was pulsed-field gel electrophoresis (PFGE) ***(32)***, a technique that permits the resolution of whole chromosomes on an agarose gel. This has been used to map meningococcal chromosomes and also in outbreak investigation to identify relationships among isolates and identify outbreak strains, and is discussed in Chapter 10. An alternative approach to the comparison of meningococcal genomes, representational difference analysis, is discussed in Chapter 16. This technique enables the gene content of different meningococci to be compared. Perhaps the most dramatic contribution of molecular techniques to the study of the meningococcus was the determination of two complete genomes for different meningococci a serogroup A subgroup IV-1 ***(33)*** and an ET-5 complex isolate ***(34)***, genome sequencing and annotation are described in Chapter 15. The prospect of ever more detailed comparisons of meningococcal genomes associated with particular pathogenic and epidemiological characteristics, provides a tantalizing prospect for an incremental improvement in our understanding of the epidemiology of meningococcal disease.

3. Public-Health Responses to Meningococcal Disease

In many industrialized countries, the investigation and control of an outbreak of meningococcal disease is one of the most challenging tasks for a public-health practitioner. An outbreak usually occurs without warning; predictions about its evolution are difficult if not impossible, and the reaction of the public, the media, and sometimes health professionals is often irrational and even hysterical. Moreover, the evidence base for control measures is weak, so it can be difficult to justify action taken. For this reason, control policies vary greatly from country to country. The level of intervention will depend on many factors, including the setting of the outbreak, the organism responsible, the resources available, and the level of public concern. The investigation and management of outbreaks is considered in Chapter 17. Carriage studies are often helpful in outbreak investigations; their planning and execution in both outbreak and nonoutbreak situations is described in Chapter 19. Further, high-quality surveillance of meningococcal disease and appropriate carriage studies backed up by accurate characterization are all critical to inform control strategies.

The surveillance of meningococcal disease is much more challenging in developing countries where resources for case ascertainment and investigation are limited. Most cases will be clinically diagnosed without laboratory confirmation, and disease incidence is usually based on estimates derived from ad hoc studies. The surveillance of meningococcal disease in developing countries is considered in Chapter 21. In developed countries, surveillance is usually based on both notifications of clinically diagnosed cases and laboratory reports. The level of case ascertainment is generally high, particularly where meningococcal disease is perceived as a significant problem, and therefore all potential cases are investigated. In recent years, notification data and laboratory data have become increasingly divergent *(35)*. The surveillance of meningococcal disease has been greatly enhanced by the advent of nonculture-based diagnostic techniques, especially detection of meningococcal DNA, the techniques for which have been discussed in Chapter 3. At the individual country level, the number of cases of meningococcal disease may be too small to provide robust information. International surveillance schemes can add public-health value by pooling data from several countries; an example of an international scheme is described in Chapter 20.

Vaccines against the meningococcus are the subject of a companion volume to this text, *Meningococcal Vaccines*, also published Humana Press, and will be discussed only briefly here. Childhood vaccination at the population level would be an effective policy for meningococcal disease control; however, there is as yet no comprehensive meningococcal vaccine that is effective from early childhood *(36)*. Meningococcal disease-surveillance data show that, in principle, the formulation of vaccines against the meningococcus should be relatively straightforward to develop and implement. Possession of one of the five disease-associated capsules (corresponding to serogroups A, B, C, Y, and W-135) is an absolute requirement for pathogenesis and it was established in the late 1960s that vaccines against meningococcal capsules can protect against infection *(37)*. Consequently, a five-valent vaccine would protect against all meningococcal disease. Unfortunately, the plain polysaccharide vaccines are ineffective in infants and may induce tolerance in older age groups. The development of protein-polysaccharide vaccines overcame these problems, rendering polysaccharide vaccines effective in stimulating amnestic responses, even in small children. While such vaccines are a realistic prospect from serogroups A, C , Y, and W-135, problems remain for the development of protein-conjugate serogroup B polysaccharide vaccines, owing to its particularly poor properties as an immunogen ***(36)***. These are very likely to be related to its chemical and immunological identity to host polysaccharides ***(38)***, raising regulatory issues if vaccines to this antigen were developed. Attempts to develop comprehensive protein-based vaccines have been frustrated by the high variability of these proteins and the mobility of genes encoding variants by horizontal genetic exchange. A number of large-scale trials or population-scale interventions with partial meningococcal vaccines have been undertaken ***(39,40)*** or are currently being planned and the long-term effect of such introductions will have to be carefully monitored using many of the techniques described in this section.

4. Conclusions

Meningococcal epidemiology is intimately related to the complex natural history of this intriguing organism. The meningococcus has evolved numerous mechanisms that enable it to survive as an obligate inhabitant of human mucosal surfaces, mostly as a harmless commensal. Despite recent advances made in our understanding of meningococcal biology, many of which have been achieved by combining epidemiological and molecular approaches, there are many mysteries surrounding meningococcal populations; for example, why are meningococcal populations so diverse? Of particular concern is our lack of understanding of the dynamics of meningococcal populations and the effects of the introduction of vaccines that do not offer comprehensive protection against meningocococcal disease. It is probable that further advances are also likely to depend on an integrated and multidisciplinary approach. The ultimate challenge is to translate this understanding into comprehensive and effective public-health interventions.

References

1. Peltola, H. (1983) Meningococcal disease: still with us. *Rev. Infect. Dis.* **5,** 71–91.
2. Broome, C. V. (1986) The carrier state: *Neisseria meningitidis*. *J. Antimicrob. Chemother.* **18(Suppl. A),** 25–34.
3. Caugant, D. A., Froholm, L. O., Sacchi, C. T., and Selander, R. K. (1991) Genetic structure and epidemiology of serogroup B *Neisseria meningitidis*, in *Neisseriae 1990* (Achtman, M., Kohl, P., Marchal, C., Morelli, G., Seiler, A., and Thiesen, B., eds.), Walter de Gruyter, Berlin, pp. 37–42.
4. Maiden, M. C. J. and Feavers, I. M. (1995) Population genetics and global epidemiology of the human pathogen *Neisseria meningitidis*, in *Population Genetics of*

Bacteria (Baumberg, S., Young, J. P. W., Wellington, E. M. H., and Saunders, J. R., eds.), Cambridge University Press, Cambridge, UK, pp. 269–293.
5. Whalen, C. M., Hockin, J. C., Ryan, A., and Ashton, F. (1995) The changing epidemiology of invasive meningococcal disease in Canada, 1985 through 1992. Emergence of a virulent clone of *Neisseria meningitidis*. *JAMA* **273,** 390–394.
6. Hart, C. A., Cuevas, L. E., Marzouk, O., Thomson, A. P., and Sills, J. (1993) Management of bacterial meningitis. *J. Antimicrob. Chemother.* **32(Suppl. A),** 49–59.
7. Begg, N. (1995) Outbreak management, in *Meningococcal Disease* (Cartwright, K. A. V., ed.), John Wiley and Sons, Chichester, UK, pp. 286–305.
8. Cartwright, K. A. V. (1995) *Meningococcal Disease.* John Wiley & Sons, Chichester, UK.
9. Branham, S. E. (1953) Serological relationships among meningococci. *Bact. Rev.* **17,** 175–188.
10. Vedros, N. A. (1987) Development of meningococcal serogroups, in *Evolution of Meningococcal Disease*; vol. II (Vedros, N. A., ed.), CRC Press Inc., Boca Raton, FL, pp. 33–37.
11. Frasch, C. E., Zollinger, W. D., and Poolman, J. T. (1985) Serotype antigens of *Neisseria meningitidis* and a proposed scheme for designation of serotypes. *Rev. Infect. Dis.* **7,** 504–510.
12. Moore, P. S. and Broome, C. V. (1994) Cerebrospinal meningitis epidemics. *Sci. Am.* **271,** 24–31.
13. Lapeyssonnie, L. (1963) La meningite cerebrospinale en Afrique. *Bull. WHO* **28(Suppl.),** 53–114.
14. Schwartz, B., Moore, P. S., and Broome, C. V. (1989) Global epidemiology of meningococcal disease. *Clin. Microbiol. Rev.* **2,** s118–s124.
15. Achtman, M. (1991) Clonal properties of meningococci from epidemic meningitis. *Trans. R. Soc. Trop. Med. Hyg.* **85(Suppl. 1),** 24–31.
16. Achtman, M. (1990) Molecular epidemiology of epidemic bacterial meningitis. *Rev. Med. Microbiol.* **1,** 29–38.
17. Wang, J.-F., Caugant, D. A., Li, X., Hu, X., Poolman, J. T., Crowe, B. A., and Achtman, M. (1992) Clonal and antigenic analysis of serogroup A *Neisseria meningitidis* with particular reference to epidemiological features of epidemic meningitis in China. *Infect. Immun.* **60,** 5267–5282.
18. Mohammed, I., Nasidi, A., Alkali, A. S., Garbati, M. A., Ajayi-Obe, E. K., Audu, K. A., et al. (2000) A severe epidemic of meningococcal meningitis in Nigeria, 1996. *Trans. R. Soc. Trop. Med. Hyg.* **94,** 265–270.
19. Moore, P. S., Harrison, L. H., Telzak, E. E., Ajello, G. W., and Broome, C. V. (1988) Group A meningococcl carriage in travelers returning from Saudi Arabia. *JAMA* **260,** 2686–2689.
20. Popovic, T., Sacchi, C. T., Reeves, M. W., Whitney, A. M., Mayer, L. W., Noble, C. A., et al. (2000) Neisseria meningitidis serogroup W135 isolates associated with the ET- 37 complex [letter]. *Emerg. Infect. Dis.* **6,** 428–429.

21. Hansman, D. (1983) Meningococcal disease in South Australia: incidence and serogroup distribution 1971–1980. *J. Hyg.* **90,** 49–54.
22. Kaczmarski, E. B. (1997) Meningococcal infections in England and Wales. *Communi. Dis. Rep. Rev.* **7,** R55–R59.
23. Barquet, N., Domingo, P., Cayla, J. A., Gonzalez, J., Rodrigo, C., Fernandez-Viladrich, P., et al. (1999) Meningococcal disease in a large urban population (Barcelona, 1987–1992): predictors of dismal prognosis. Barcelona Meningococcal Disease Surveillance Group. *Arch. Intern. Med.* **159,** 2329–2340.
24. Krizova, P., Musilek, M., and Kalmusova, J. (1997) Development of the epidemiological situation in invasive meningococcal disease in the Czech Republic caused by emerging *Neisseria meningitidis* clone ET-15/37. *Cent. Eur. J. Public Health* **5,** 214–218.
25. Kremastinou, J., Tzanakaki, G., Velonakis, E., Voyiatzi, A., Nickolaou, A., Elton, R. A., et al. (1999) Carriage of *Neisseria meningitidis* and *Neisseria lactamica* among ethnic Greek school children from Russian immigrant families in Athens. *FEMS Immunol. Med. Microbiol.* **23,** 13–20.
26. Caugant, D. A., Mocca, L. F., Frasch, C. E., Froholm, L. O., Zollinger, W. D., and Selander, R. K. (1987) Genetic structure of *Neisseria meningitidis* populations in relation to serogroup, serotype, and outer membrane protein pattern. *J. Bacteriol.* **169,** 2781–2792.
27. Caugant, D. A., Froholm, L. O., Bovre, K., Holten, E., Frasch, C. E., Mocca, L. F., et al. (1987) Intercontinental spread of *Neisseria meningitidis* clones of the ET-5 complex. *Antonie van Leeuwenhoek J. Microbiol.* **53,** 389–394.
28. Maiden, M. C. J., Bygraves, J. A., Feil, E., Morelli, G., Russell, J. E., Urwin, R., et al. (1998) Multilocus sequence typing: a portable approach to the identification of clones within populations of pathogenic microorganisms. *Proc. Natl. Acad. Sci. USA* **95,** 3140–3145.
29. Caugant, D. A., Kristiansen, B. E., Froholm, L. O., Bovre, K., and Selander, R. K. (1988) Clonal diversity of *Neisseria meningitidis* from a population of asymptomatic carriers. *Infect. Immun.* **56,** 2060–2068.
30. Maiden, M. C. J. (1993) Population genetics of a transformable bacterium: the influence of horizontal genetical exchange on the biology of *Neisseria meningitidis. FEMS Microbiol. Lett.* **112,** 243–250.
31. Gupta, S., Maiden, M. C. J., Feavers, I. M., Nee, S., May, R. M., and Anderson, R. M. (1996) The maintenance of strain structure in populations of recombining infectious agents. *Nat. Med.* **2,** 437–442.
32. Bygraves, J. A. and Maiden, M. C. J. (1992) Analysis of the clonal relationships between strains of *Neisseria meningitidis* by pulsed field gel electrophoresis. *J. Gen. Microbiol.* **138,** 523–531.
33. Parkhill, J., Achtman, M., James, K. D., Bentley, S. D., Churcher, C., Klee, S. R., et al. (2000) Complete DNA sequence of a serogroup A strain of *Neisseria meningitidis* Z2491. *Nature* **404,** 502–506.

34. Tettelin, H., Saunders, N. J., Heidelberg, J., Jeffries, A. C., Nelson, K. E., Eisen, J. A., et al. (2000) Complete genome sequence of *Neisseria meningitidis* serogroup B strain MC58. *Science* **287,** 1809–1815.
35. Carrol, E. D., Thomson, A. P., Shears, P., Gray, S. J., Kaczmarski, E. B., and Hart, C. A. (2000) Performance characteristics of the polymerase chain reaction assay to confirm clinical meningococcal disease. *Arch. Dis. Child* **83,** 271–273.
36. Pollard, A. J. and Levin, M. (2000) Vaccines for prevention of meningococcal disease. *Pediatr. Infect. Dis. J.* **19,** 333–444.
37. Gotschlich, E. C., Goldschneider, I., and Artenstein, M.S. (1969) Human immunity to the meningococcus IV. Immunogenicity of group A and group C meningococcal polysaccharides. *J. Exp. Med.* **129,** 1367–1384.
38. Finne, J., Leinonen, M., and Makela, P.H. (1983) Antigenic similarities between brain components and bacteria causing meningitis: implications for vaccine development and pathogenesis. *Lancet* **ii,** 355–357.
39. Bjune, G., Closs, O., Froholm, L. O., Gronnesby, J. K., Hoiby, E. A., and Nokleby, H. (1991) Design of clinical trials with an outer membrane vesicle vaccine against systemic serogroup B meningococcal disease in Norway. *NIPH. Ann.* **14,** 81–91.
40. de Moraes, J. C., Perkins, B. A., Camargo, M. C., Hidalgo, N. T., Barbosa, H. A., Sacchi, C. T., et al. (1992) Protective efficacy of a serogroup B meningococcal vaccine in Sao Paulo, Brazil. *Lancet* **340,** 1074–1078.

9

Serological Characterization

Betsy Kuipers, Germie van den Dobbelsteen, Elisabeth Wedege, and Loek van Alphen

1. Introduction

Immunoassays employ a range of methods to detect and quantify antigens or antibodies and to study the composition of antigens. This chapter describes four useful immunoassays for serological characterization of antigens of *Neisseria meningitidis*: whole-cell enzyme-linked immunosorbent assay (ELISA); dot blot, colony blot, and immunoblot. Serological characterization of *N. meningitidis* antigens is valuable for epidemiological studies as well as for identifying immunologically important antigens in vaccine development ***(1,2)***. Typing of *N. meningitidis* is based on the immunological detection of specific epitopes on the outer-membrane proteins (OMP) and lipopolysaccharides (LPS) ***(3)***, and panels of monoclonal antibodies (MAbs) have been developed by several laboratories to refine the serological classification system ***(4–8)***. Differences in capsular polysaccharides determine the meningococcal serogroup, whereas the serotypes and serosubtypes are based on antigenic differences of the PorB OMP and PorA OMP, respectively ***(3)***. The PorA protein contains two variable loops (VR1 and VR2), each of which determine a distinct set of serosubtypes. Thus the serosubtypes of an isolate can include two independent designations ***(9–11)***. Variation in the oligosaccharide moiety of the LPS determines the immunotype, and more than one epitope can be present in the same population of a single isolate ***(6,12)***. In the current typing scheme the classification is given as [serogroup] : [serotype] : [serosubtype] : [immunotype], e.g., B : 15 : P1.7,16 : L3,7,9.

Each of these characters can be determined using specific MAbs in a whole-cell ELISA ***(4,6,13,14)***. Briefly, plates are coated with bacteria, incubated with

From: *Methods in Molecular Medicine, vol. 67: Meningococcal Disease: Methods and Protocols*
Edited by: A. J. Pollard and M. C. J. Maiden © Humana Press Inc., Totowa, NJ

MAbs of known specificities and detected by enzyme-labeled secondary antibody followed by a substrate reaction. Meningococci can also be typed by dotting the bacterial suspensions on nitrocellulose (NC)-filters followed by incubation with specific MAbs and enzyme-labeled secondary antibodies ***(14–18)***. Dot blotting can be regarded as a miniaturized ELISA, except that the substrates for enzyme detection are insoluble products immobilized on NC-filters. Dot blotting requires less expensive equipment, and smaller volumes of primary and secondary antibodies, than the ELISA method and all incubations are performed at room temperature. The typing results in ELISA and dot blotting are generally equivalent ***(14,18)*** except for a few serotype 4 MAbs that have low sensitivity in ELISA ***(19,20)***.

There are certain limitations with the current serological-typing system, as 15–20% of the isolates are recorded as nontypable for one or more determinant. There are a number of reasons for this: the surface structure may not react with the current panel of MAbs, or the determinant epitopes may be absent owing to phase variation or mutations ***(15,21,22)***. More universal DNA sequence-based methods have been developed for typing *N. meningitidis* using polymerase chain reaction (PCR) of epitope regions (*see* Chapter 11) ***(23,24)***. Nevertheless, serological classification still provides valuable information for defining variation among meningococcal antigens, especially because these techniques are sensitive and can be performed easily, rapidly, and reproducibly in routine laboratories ***(13)***.

Phase-variable expression of antigens and antigenic variation are common properties of *N. meningitidis* ***(15,21,22,25)***. For research and vaccine development, various laboratories are constructing new variants of meningococci ***(26)***. A useful technique for the selection of phase variants, transformed or mutated bacteria is colony blot, because single colonies of a particular phenotype can be identified readily ***(27–30)***. Briefly, agar plates containing colonies are covered with NC membranes, resulting in transfer of part of the bacterial colonies to the membrane. The antigens retain their antigenicity on blot and are readily accessible to antibodies. Single bacterial colonies can be picked up from the reincubated master cultures after comparing them with their color-developed colony blots. A double-staining method has been developed to visualize all colonies, thereby simplifying the identification of a negative colony among a large number of positive colonies. After streaking and retesting, pure cultures are obtained with the desired phenotypic characteristic. The effect of transformations and/or mutations on the expression of certain outer-membrane components can be quantified in whole cell ELISA.

The final technique described in this chapter is immunoblotting, in which whole bacterial suspensions or preparations containing outer-membrane complexes/vesicles (OMC/OMV), separated on a sodium dodecyl sulfate (SDS)-gel, are transferred to a support membrane and probed with antibodies *(17,18,31,32)*. Immunoblotting combines the selectivity of gel electrophoresis with the specificity of immunoassays, allowing individual proteins in complex mixtures to be detected and analyzed. The effect of a mutation or transformation can be visualized at the protein level. An important factor that determines the success of an immunoblotting procedure is the nature of the epitopes recognized by the antibodies. Standard SDS-polacrylamide gel electrophoresis (PAGE) techniques involve denaturation of the antigen sample, so only antibodies that recognize nonconformational epitopes are likely to bind unless renaturating agents are used (*see Meningococcal Vaccines*, edited by A. J. Pollard and M. C. J. Maiden, also available from Humana Press).

2. Materials

2.1. Whole-Cell ELISA

2.1.1. Equipment

1. Microtiter 96-well plates (e.g., Immulon II, Dynatech Laboratories).
2. Plate washer (e.g., PW96 SLT Labinstruments).
3. Multi-channel pipet and disposable pipet tips.
4. Incubator at 37°C.
5. Microtiter plate reader with 450-nm filter (e.g., EL312, Bio-Tek instruments) and corresponding software (e.g., KinetiCalc).

2.1.2. Reagents

1. Bacterial suspensions (*see* **Note 1**) in PBS + 0.02% sodium azide with an optical density (OD) at 620 nm adjusted to 0.08–0.1
2. Phosphate-buffered saline (PBS): 0.01 *M* phosphate, 0.154 *M* NaCl, pH 7.2. Dissolve 1.37 g $Na_2HPO_4.2H_2O$, 0.32 g $NaH_2PO_4.H_2O$, and 9.0 g NaCl in 1 L deionized water.
3. PBS-T: PBS + 0.1% (w/v) Tween 80.
4. PBS-T-MP: PBS + 0.1% (w/v) Tween 80 + 0.5 % (w/v) milk powder (e.g., Protifar, Nutricia). Prepare 30 min before use.
5. Washing solution (WS): deionized water + 0.03–0.05% (w/v) Tween 80.
6. MAbs specific for meningococcal antigens (*see* **Table 1**).
7. Horseradish peroxidase (HRP)-labeled anti-mouse IgG (e.g., Southern Biotechnology Associates [SBA] 1030-05) (*see* **Note 2**).
8. Substrate (prepare not longer than 30 min before use): Dilute buffer A 10 times with deionized water and add per 10 mL of this buffer 100 µL of solution B and 4 µL of solution C.
   a. 10X acetate/citrate buffer (1.1 *M*): dissolve 9.02 g sodium acetate anhydrous in 100 mL deionized water, adjust pH to 5.5 with saturated citric acid.

Table 1
Characteristics of *N. meningitidis* Antigens and References to Specific Monoclonal Antibodies

Antigen	Typing	M.W. in kD (SDS-PAGE)	References
Capsular polysaccharide	Serogroup	>200	***(5,14,36,37)***
Class 1 OMP (PorA)[a]	Serosubtype	41–43	***(13,16,18)***
Class 2 OMP (PorB)[a]	Serotype	37–40	***(13,15,17,18)***
Class 3 OMP (PorB)[a]	Serotype	34–37	***(13,15,17,18)***
Class 4 OMP (rmp)		33–34	***(38,39)***
Class 5 OMP (Opa/Opc)		27–31	***(7,25)***
NspA		18	***(8,40)***
Lipopolysaccharide	Immunotype	4	***(6,41,42)***
Iron-regulated proteins		37,70,80,100	***(31,43,44)***

[a]Providers of MAbs anti-PorA and PorB are: NIBSC, PO Box 1193, Blanche Lane, South Mimms Potters Bar, Herts, EN6 3QG, UK: and SVM, PO Box 457, 3720 AL Bilthoven, The Netherlands.

b. TMB solution: Dissolve 250 mg 3,3′, 5,5′ tetramethylbenzidine (e.g., Sigma T-2885) in 25 mL 96% ethanol (Store at room temperature protected from light for not longer than 2 mo).
c. Hydrogen peroxide 30% (H_2O_2).

9. Sulphuric acid 2 *M*: Add 109 mL concentrated sulphuric acid to 891 mL deionized water.

2.2. Dot blotting

2.2.1. Equipment

1. NC membranes (Bio-Rad, 0.45 µm).
2. Pipets with disposable tips, graduated pipets.
3. Incubation trays (8-well trays with lids, e.g., Acutran™ from Schleicher & Schuell) and suitable plastic boxes.
4. Horizontal rotator.
5. Suction pump.
6. Pen that can be used to write on NC-filters, flat forceps, soft pencil, scalpel, ruler, glass or plastic plates of dimensions approx 15 × 20 cm.

2.2.2. Reagents

All reagents are stored at +4°C if not otherwise stated.

1. Whole-cell suspensions (*see* **Note 1**) of test strains and a set of reference strains (**ref.** ***3***) adjusted to an OD of about 0.2 at 650 (e.g., Spectronic 20). The density of the test strains should be in the same range as for the reference strains.
2. PBS, pH 7.2 (*see* **Subheading 2.1.2.**).

3. Blocking buffer; 3% bovine serum albumin (BSA) in PBS.
4. 0.05 *M* sodium acetate buffer, pH 5.0 (*see* **Subheading 2.3.2.**)
5. 3-amino-9-ethyl-carbazole (AEC) in dimethylformamide (Toxic) (*see* **Subheading 2.3.2.**).
6. Hydrogen peroxide 30% (Caustic).
7. Peroxidase-conjugated rabbit anti-mouse Ig (e.g., DAKO A/S, Denmark).
8. MAbs specific for meningococcal antigens as shown in **Table 1**.

2.3. Colony Blotting

2.3.1. Equipment

1. Nitrocellulose membranes (e.g., Protan BA 85/20, 82 mm diameter, 5 mm grid, Schleicher & Schuell).
2. Flat forceps.
3. Containers with lid.
4. Shaking water bath.
5. Petri dishes, 85-mm diameter (e.g., Greiner).
6. Horizontal rotator.
7. Incubator at 37°C with 5% CO_2 and humid atmosphere.
8. Bacteriological loops.

2.3.2. Reagents

1. Bacterial suspension of about 10^4 CFU/mL (*see* **Note 1**) in PBS.
2. Washing solution (WS) 0.01 *M* Tris, 0.154 *M* NaCl: Dissolve 1.2 g Tris-(hydroxymethyl)-aminomethane and 9.0 g NaCl in 1 L deionized water, adjust to pH 7.4 with 6 *M* HCl.
3. WS-T: washing solution + 0.5 % (w/v) Tween 80.
4. WS-T-MP: Washing solution + 0.5 % (w/v) Tween 80 + 0.5 % (w/v) milk powder (e.g., Protifar, Nutricia). Prepare 30 min before use.
5. MAbs specific for meningococcal antigens (*see* **Table 1**).
6. Conjugates (*see* **Note 2**):
   a. Alkaline phosphatase (AP)-labeled anti-mouse IgG 1, 2a, 2b, 3 (e.g., SBA 1070-04, 1080-04, 1090-04, 1100-04).
   b. HRP-labeled anti-mouse IgG 1, 2a, 2b, 3 (e.g., SBA 1070-05, 1080-05, 1090-05, 1100-05).
7. Substrates (prepare fresh):
   Remark: These agents are irritating/toxic; handle with gloves and put waste in special containers for toxic chemicals.
   a. For AP-conjugates: Dissolve 1 BCIP/NTB tablet (Sigma B-5655) in 10 mL deionized water.
   b. For HRP-conjugates: Add to 47.5 mL acetate buffer (A) 2.5 mL AEC/DMF (B) and 25 µL 30% H_2O_2.
      A. 0.05 M acetate buffer, pH 5.0: Add 74 mL of 0.2 N acetic acid (11.55 mL glacial acetic acid/L) and 176 mL 0.2 M sodium acetate (27.2 g sodium acetate trihydrate/ L) to 750 mL deionized water.

B. AEC/DMF: Dissolve 10 tablets 3-amino-9-ethyl-carbazole (AEC) (Sigma A-6926) in 25 mL dimethylformamide (DMF).This solution is stable at +4°C for 3 mo.

8. Translucent agar plates suitable for growing meningococci (e.g., GC plates).

2.4. Immunoblotting

2.4.1. Equipment

1. 12% gels for separation of proteins and 16% gels for separation of LPS (*see Meningococcal Vaccines*, edited by A. J. Pollard and M. C. J. Maiden, Humana Press and **ref. *[33]***).
2. NC membranes (e.g., Protan BA83 Schleicher & Schuell [0.2 μm]).
3. Flat forceps.
4. Filter papers (e.g., Bio-Rad laboratories).
5. Electroblotter and power supply (e.g., Ancos, Denmark).
6. Containers with lid.
7. Mini-incubation trays (e.g., Bio-Rad laboratories) or Petri dishes (e.g., Greiner).
8. Horizontal rotator.

2.4.2. Reagents

1. Bacterial suspension (*see* **Note 1**) in PBS + 0.02% Na-azide with OD at 620 nm adjusted to 1.0 or OMV/OMC preparations with a protein concentration of ±1 mg/mL.
2. Low molecular-weight protein marker (e.g., Pharmacia 17-0446-01)
3. Staining and destaining reagents for protein gels (e.g., Coomassie blue) or LPS gels (silver stain).
4. Blotbuffer: 0.025 *M* Tris, 0.192 *M* glycine, 20% ethanol, pH 8.3. Dissolve 3.0 g Tris- (hydroxymethyl)-aminomethane, 14.4 g glycine in 800 mL deionized water, add 200 mL ethanol (pH should be 8.3, do not adjust).
5. WS-T: *see* **Subheading 2.3.2.**
6. WS-T-MP: *see* **Subheading 2.3.2.**
7. Mouse MAbs specific for meningococcal antigens (*see* **Table 1**).
8. Conjugates (*see* **Note 2**):
   a. Alkaline phosphatase (AP)-labeled anti-mouse IgG (e.g., SBA 1030-04).
   b. HRP-labeled anti-mouse IgG (e.g., SBA 1030-05).
9. Substrates (prepare fresh): *see* **Subheading 2.3.2.**
10. Protein dye (e.g., Aurodye forte, Amersham RPN 490).

3. Methods

3.1. Whole-Cell ELISA

1. Coating of ELISA plates: Dispense 100 μL of the bacterial suspensions (OD_{620nm} 0.08–0.1) per well (mix well before use). For typing of a single strain coating of one well for each MAb is sufficient. For quantification of outer-membrane anti-

gens coat at least a row of eight wells with one strain for each MAb. Control plates should be coated with (reference) strains with known types and/or amount of expression of certain proteins or LPS. Place the plates without lid in an incubator at 37°C until evaporation is complete. During all incubation steps the plates are placed straight and separate (not stacked) in the incubator. Covered coated plates can be stored at room temperature or at 37°C for 1 yr (avoid moisture).
2. Wash the plates at least 3 times with washing solution, 200 µL/well (*see* **Note 3**).
3. Make a stock solution of MAbs in PBS-T sufficient for maximal binding as described by the supplier. For typing add 100 µL of each MAb stock solution to one well of each coated strain. For quantification of outer-membrane components, prepare threefold serial dilutions from the MAb stock solutions in accordance with the number of coated wells per strain (eight or more) and add 100 µL of the MAb dilutions per well.
4. Place the plates covered with a lid or plate sealer in an incubator of 37°C for 1 h.
5. Wash the plates at least 3 times with washing solution, 200 µL/well.
6. Dilute the anti-mouse IgG-HRP conjugate in PBS-T-MP as recommended by the supplier and add 100 µL of the conjugate solution to all wells.
7. Place the plates covered with lid or plate sealer in an incubator of 37°C for 1 h.
8. Wash the plates at least 3 times with washing solution, 200 µL/well.
9. Add TMB-substrate to all wells, 100 µL/well. Stop the staining reaction (blue) after 10 min by adding 2 *M* sulphuric acid (yellow)
10. Read the OD of the formed yellow color at 450 nm.
11. The strain is considered positive for a type if the OD of the test strain is more than 50% of the OD of the positive control strain. Quantitative analysis: for both test and control strains, calculate the dilution of the MAb at which the OD reaches 50% of the maximal OD for that particular MAb. Compare the "titres" of the test strains with those of the control strains with known amount of the antigens.

3.2. Dot Blotting

Use gloves and/or forceps when handling the NC-strips. All steps are performed at room temperature.

1. Mark a suitable area of the NC-filter with soft pencil lines 1 cm apart; then cut off vertical strips of dimensions 0.5 × 10 cm. Align them on a suitable plate and label the NC-strips in the top square. Dot 2 µL of the relevant reference isolate suspension in the middle of the next pencil-outlined square and 2 µL of the test isolates successively onto each of the other squares. Make an identical set of dotted strips for each of the MAbs to be used with the corresponding reference strain in the top square. Take care that each strain has the same position on every set of strips.
2. Dry the strips for 15 min or more.
3. Fill the wells of the incubation trays with 2 mL blocking buffer (*see* **Note 4**). Transfer the strips to the wells and incubate them for 30 min with gentle shaking. The strips have to be fully wetted by the blocking buffer.

4. Add the MAbs (in 1 : 10 dilution) directly to the blocking solution (*see* **Note 5**). Depending on the supplier of the MAb, the final dilutions may range from 1 : 10 up to 1 : 500,000 (*see* **Note 6**).
5. Put the lid on the trays and incubate overnight with gentle shaking (*see* **Note 7**).
6. Next morning, remove the antibody solutions from the strips by using a pipet tip connected to a suction pump or similar devise. Rinse the tip with water between each set of strips that were incubated with different MAbs to prevent transfer of the MAbs.
7. Add not more than 2 mL PBS per well and incubate for about 5 min with shaking. Remove as described in **step 6**.
8. Repeat the washing procedure twice.
9. Dilute the peroxidase-labelled antibody in a suitable volume of blocking buffer. Use 1 : 1,000 dilution for the serogrouping MAbs and 1 : 2,000 dilution for the PorA and PorB specific MAbs. Add 0.5–2 mL of the diluted secondary antibodies to the wells and incubate for 2 h with shaking (*see* **Note 7**). Take care that the strips are fully wetted.
10. Wash twice with PBS as described in **steps 6**, **7**, and **8**.
11. Transfer all strips that were incubated with one MAb to a suitable box, wash them for some minutes with 0.05 *M* sodium acetate buffer and discard the solution.
12. Mix 25 mL sodium acetate buffer with 1 mL AEC in DMF and add to the strips. Incubate for a few minutes, and add 15 µL hydrogen peroxide. For each MAb, stain until distinct red dots are observed for the reference strain, this will usually take 2–10 min.
13. Rinse the strips in water, align them flat on a plate, and tilt the plate slightly to dry the strips at room temperature. Grade the staining intensity of each dot visually relative to the color presented by the reference strain as positive, weak, or negative (*see* **Note 8**). A permanent record can be obtained by photography, video camera with a video printer or gel scanner, the latter method is less suitable for many strips. File the strips in a plastic pocket protected from light.

3.3. Colony Blotting

1. To obtain separate colonies, spread 100 µL of a bacteria suspension of 10^4 cfu/mL in PBS on 10 numbered agar plates (*see* **Note 1**).
2. Incubate 16–18 h in a 37°C incubator with 5% CO_2 at a humid atmosphere.
3. Label the required number of membranes and mark them nonsymmetrically with three small lines on the edge.
4. Overlay a membrane on each agar plate (try to avoid air bubbles and don't move the membrane after it has touched the plate). Indicate on the bottom of the plate where the marks on the membrane are situated so that they can be re-oriented later.
5. Remove the membranes from the plates after 2–3 min with a forceps and collect them in a container half-filled with WS-T (5–10 membranes per container). Return the agar plates to the incubator for at least 4 h.

6. Inactivate the bacteria on the membranes in the covered containers for 1 h in a water bath at 56°C while gently shaking.
7. Empty the containers in a waste bottle and rinse the membranes twice by adding about 100 mL WS-T, shaking briefly, and pouring the fluid into the same waste bottle.
8. Transfer the membranes to separate Petri dishes, add 10 mL WS-T and incubate for another 15 min on a horizontal rotator at room temperature.
9. In order to identify positive colonies or colonies with a high expression of a certain antigen (for example after transformation) incubate the membranes with 10 mL WS-T containing one MAb with the desired specificity. A double-staining method is recommended for picking up a negative colony between a large number of positive colonies. Incubate with the appropriate combination of two MAbs (with different IgG isotype; *see* **Note 2**). In this way, for example, a colony that is negative for Opc protein but still has the L3 immunotype can be recognized.
10. Incubate for 1 h on a horizontal rotator.
11. Rinse three times: pipet 10 mL WS-T on the membrane, shake briefly, and discard the washing fluid after each step.
12. Perform a blocking step to prevent nonspecific binding of conjugate: add 10 mL WS-T-MP to each membrane and incubate for 15 min on a horizontal rotator (*see* **Note 9**).
13. For single staining: remove the blocking reagent and add 10 mL AP-conjugate in WS-T-MP per membrane. For double staining: mix two conjugates with different label: AP-labeled for detecting positive colonies (example: anti-IgG isotype of the used anti-Opc MAb) and HRP-labeled for detecting a common antigen present on all colonies (e.g., anti-IgG isotype of the used anti-L3 MAb).
14. Incubate for 1 h on a horizontal rotator.
15. Rinse as described in **step 11** and perform two more washing steps with 10 mL deionized water.
16. Add 5 mL AP substrate (BCIP/NTB) to all membranes and incubate until dark purple spots are visible and/or the fluid starts to color (5–10 min).
17. Remove the substrate and rinse two times with 10 mL deionized water as described in **step 11** (discard the substrate and the first rinse in a container for toxic chemicals).
18. If double staining add 5 mL HRP substrate (AEC) to all membranes and incubate until red spots are clearly visible and/or the fluid starts to color (5–10 mins).
19. Perform the same washing procedure as described in **step 17**.
20. Compare the stained membranes with the corresponding agar plates (mirrored) and locate the colony of interest on the agar plate. Membranes can be dried between filter paper and the image kept protected for light in a file for several years.
21. Pick the selected colonies from the agar plate with a bacteriological loop, spread on a pre-warmed agar plate, and incubate for 16–18 h in an incubator at 37°C with 5% CO_2 in a humid atmosphere.
22. If a single colony was picked, perform the same colony-blotting procedure on the following day as a control.

23. Store the bacteria at –80°C for further use and, if desired, perform gel electrophoresis (and immunoblotting) to check the protein composition of the isolated bacteria.

3.4. Immunoblotting

1. Separate proteins and LPS of bacterial suspensions (20 μL/slot) or OMV/OMC (5 μL/slot) on SDS-polyacrylamide gels. When testing several samples for the presence of one particular protein antigen or LPS type, all samples are loaded on the same gel. If only one isolate is to be tested for different proteins or LPS, the same sample is loaded multiple times on the gel. Include a low molecular-weight marker on each gel.
2. Blot immediately after gel electrophoresis to NC membranes.
3. Transfer the membranes separately to suitable containers with lids and rinse them twice with 10 mL WS-T and discard the washing solution. Add 10 mL WS-T to each membrane and incubate (shaking) for 15 min in a waterbath at 56°C to remove SDS from the membrane. Rinse again twice with WS-T. After this step, membranes can be stored between filter paper at –20°C for at least a year.
4. Immunoassay: Cut a small strip from the membrane where the molecular weight marker is situated and stain this strip with a protein dye as described by the supplier (e.g., Aurodye). Cut the remaining part of the membrane in strips with one or more samples and put them in incubation trays with MAbs appropriately diluted in WS-T. Adjust the volume of the MAb solution to the size of the incubation tray and take care that during all incubation steps the membrane strips are completely covered with fluid.
5. Incubate at room temperature for 1 h on a horizontal rotator.
6. Rinse three times with WS-T and discard the washing solution.
7. Perform a blocking step to prevent nonspecific binding of conjugate by incubating the membranes for 15 min in WS-T-MP on a horizontal rotator (*see* **Note 9**)
8. Dilute the AP or HRP-conjugate as described by the supplier in WS-T-MP.
9. Incubate at room temperature with the same volume as used for the incubation with the MAbs (*see* **step 4**) for 1 h on a horizontal rotator.
10. Rinse three times as described in **step 6** with WS-T and twice with deionized water.
11. To visualize MAb binding, incubate the membranes with the appropriate substrate: BCIP/NTB for AP-conjugate (dark purple) or AEC for HRP-conjugate (red) (*see* **Subheading 3.3.**) to visualize the binding of the MAbs.
12. Rinse the membranes three times with deionized water and dry the membrane between filter papers. Take a photograph or make a photocopy and/or keep the membranes protected from light in a file.
13. Judge the tested samples for the presence (in high or low amount) or absence of certain proteins and/or LPS by comparing the stained bands on the membrane.

4. Notes

1. Bacteria are cultured on agar plates for 18–20 h in a 37°C incubator with a 5% CO_2 humid atmosphere to obtain bacteria in the same growth phase. Bacteria are streaked on to the plates in such a way as to ensure that separate colonies are

present after culturing. The following day, suspensions are made by taking at least 100 separate colonies from the plates with a sterile swab and dispersing them in 5 mL PBS with 0.02% Na-azide (vortex vigorously). For whole-cell ELISA, dot blotting, and immunoblotting, the bacteria have to be heat-inactivated at 56°C in a water bath (at least 30 min for volumes ≤5 mL, extend inactivation time to 1 h for larger volumes and store the suspensions at +4°C). For colony blotting, the suspensions (in PBS without Na-azide) are immediately measured at 620 nm, the density is adjusted to 0.25 (±10^9 cfu/mL), and diluted 100,000 times with PBS to get a suspension of ±10^4 cfu/mL.

2. For anti-mouse-IgG conjugates, it is important that the labeled antibodies bind with equal affinity to all IgG isotypes. Colony blotting with the double-staining procedure is only possible if all anti-IgG isotype conjugates are highly specific. For all tests, determine a conjugate dilution where specific binding is maximal and background (nonspecific) binding is minimal.
3. If a plate washer is not available, washing of ELISA plates can be carried out by using a multi-channel pipet or a plastic squirt bottle. Take care that all fluid is completely removed from the wells after each incubation and washing step, by turning the plate upside down above the sink and shaking the plates out on a dry cloth.
4. The minimum incubation volume for 1 strip is 0.5 mL. Up to four strips with about 40 dotted samples can be incubated in a total volume of 2 mL. Leave an empty well in the incubation trays between each set of strips that are incubated with different MAbs.
5. When many isolates are to be tested, it is advisable to first analyze them with MAbs against the most prevalent PorA and PorB types. Thereafter, the negative samples can be examined with the remaining typing MAbs. Isolates that remain negative can then be analyzed with PCR method.
6. Typing MAbs can be used in much higher dilution in dot-blotting than in ELISA.
7. If necessary, the procedure can be performed in a shorter time by reducing the incubation times with the primary and secondary antibodies to 2 and 1 h, respectively. Alternatively, where speed is essential, for some MAbs it is possible to use a 2-h incubation of the blocked strips in a mixture of the MAb and the secondary antibody *(34)* followed by direct staining. Even though the background is higher compared to the standard method, distinct dots are obtained. In both cases, the amounts of the primary and secondary antibodies are doubled compared to the standard incubation.
8. As described in **Subheading 1.**, weak or no reactions may be caused by the choice of MAbs used, phase variation, or mutations. For PorA and PorB, SDS-PAGE of the whole-cell suspensions will reveal the expression of no or low protein levels. Variants may be detected by small changes in molecular weights of the immunoractive bands after immunoblotting *(35)* or by low or no binding on immunoblots compared to dot blots. A single colony taken up in a small volume of PBS-azide can also be typed on dot-blots.
9. Blocking steps should be carried out to prevent nonspecific binding. Tween 80 and BSA are very effective at blocking residual binding capacity of ELISA plates

and NC membranes after coating and blotting, respectively. The nonspecific binding occurs particularly in the second incubation step (conjugate), but can be prevented successfully with milk powder.

References

1. Scholten, R. J., Bijlmer, H. A., Poolman, J. T., Kuipers, B., Caugant, D. A., Van Alphen, L., Dankert, J., and Valkenburg, H. A. (1993) Meningococcal disease in The Netherlands, 1958–1990: a steady increase in the incidence since 1982 partially caused by new serotypes and subtypes of *Neisseria meningitidis. Clin. Infect. Dis.* **16,** 237–246.
2. Poolman, J. T. (1996) Bacterial outer membrane protein vaccines. The meningococcal example. *Adv. Exp. Med. Biol.* **397,** 73–77.
3. Frasch, C. E., Zollinger, W. D., and Poolman, J. T. (1985) Serotype antigens of *Neisseria meningitidis* and a proposed scheme for designation of serotypes. *Rev. Infect. Dis.* **7,** 504–510.
4. Poolman, J. T. and Abdillahi, H. (1988) Outer membrane protein serosubtyping of *Neisseria meningitidis. Eur. J. Clin. Microbiol. Infect. Dis.* **7,** 291–292.
5. Nato, F., Mazie, J. C., Fournier, J. M., Slizewicz, B., Sagot, N., Guibourdenche, M., Postic, D., and Riou, J. Y. (1991) Production of polyclonal and monoclonal antibodies against group A, B, and C capsular polysaccharides of *Neisseria meningitidis* and preparation of latex reagents. *J. Clin. Microbiol.* **29,** 1447–1452.
6. Scholten, R. J., Kuipers, B., Valkenburg, H. A., Dankert, J., Zollinger, W. D., and Poolman, J. T. (1994) Lipo-oligosaccharide immunotyping of *Neisseria meningitidis* by a whole-cell ELISA with monoclonal antibodies. *J. Med. Microbiol.* **41,** 236–243.
7. Danelli, M. G., Batoreu, N. M., Lacerda, M. D., Ferreira, C. R., Cardoso, J. D., Peralta, J. M., and Frasch, C. E. (1995) Surface antigen analysis of group B *Neisseria meningitis* outer membrane by monoclonal antibodies: identification of bactericidal antibodies to class 5 protein. *Curr. Microbiol.* **31,** 146–151.
8. Cadieux, N., Plante, M., Rioux, C. R., Hamel, J., Brodeur, B. R., and Martin, D. (1999) Bactericidal and cross-protective activities of a monoclonal antibody directed against *Neisseria meningitidis* NspA outer membrane protein. *Infect. Immun.* **67,** 4955–4959.
9. McGuinness, B., Barlow, A. K., Clarke, I. N., Farley, J. E., Anilionis, A., Poolman, J. T., and Heckels, J. E. (1990) Deduced amino acid sequences of class 1 protein (PorA) from three strains of *Neisseria meningitidis*. Synthetic peptides define the epitopes responsible for serosubtype specificity. *J. Exp. Med.* **171,** 1871–1882.
10. van der Ley, P., Heckels, J. E., Virji, M., Hoogerhout, P., and Poolman, J. T. (1991) Topology of outer membrane porins in pathogenic Neisseria spp. *Infect. Immun.* **59,** 2963–2971.
11. Maiden, M. C., Suker, J., McKenna, A. J., Bygraves, J. A., and Feavers, I. M. (1991) Comparison of the class 1 outer membrane proteins of eight serological reference strains of *Neisseria meningitidis. Mol. Microbiol.* **5,** 727–736.

12. Jennings, M. P., Srikhanta, Y. N., Moxon, E. R., Kramer, M., Poolman, J. T., Kuipers, B., and van der Ley, P. (1999) The genetic basis of the phase variation repertoire of lipopolysaccharide immunotypes in *Neisseria meningitidis. Microbiology* **145,** 3013–3021.
13. Poolman, J. T., Kriz-Kuzemenska, P., Ashton, F., Bibb, W., Dankert, J., Demina, A., Froholm, L. O., Hassan-King, M., Jones, D. M., and Lind, I. (1995) Serotypes and subtypes of *Neisseria meningitidis*: results of an international study comparing sensitivities and specificities of monoclonal antibodies. *Clin. Diagn. Lab. Immunol.* **2,** 69–72.
14. Rosenqvist, E., Wedege, E., Hoiby, E. A., and Froholm, L. O. (1990) Serogroup determination of Neisseria meningitidis by whole-cell ELISA, dot-blotting and agglutination. *APMIS* **98,** 501–506.
15. Sacchi, C. T., Lemos, A. P., Whitney, A. M., Solari, C. A., Brandt, M. E., Melles, C. E., Frasch, C. E., and Mayer, L. W. (1998) Correlation between serological and sequencing analyses of the PorB outer membrane protein in the *Neisseria meningitidis* serotyping system. *Clin. Diagn. Lab. Immunol.* **5,** 348–354.
16. Sacchi, C. T., Lemos, A. P., Brandt, M. E., Whitney, A. M., Melles, C. E., Solari, C. A., Frasch, C. E., and Mayer, L. W. (1998) Proposed standardization of *Neisseria meningitidis* PorA variable-region typing nomenclature. *Clin. Diagn. Lab. Immunol.* **5,** 845–855.
17. Zollinger, W. D., Moran, E. E., Connelly, H., Mandrell, R. E., and Brandt, B. (1984) Monoclonal antibodies to serotype 2 and serotype 15 outer membrane proteins of *Neisseria meningitidis* and their use in serotyping. *Infect. Immun.* **46,** 260–266.
18. Wedege, E., Hoiby, E. A., Rosenqvist, E., and Froholm, L. O. (1990) Serotyping and subtyping of *Neisseria meningitidis* isolates by co-agglutination, dot-blotting and ELISA. *J. Med. Microbiol.* **31,** 195–201.
19. Wedege, E., Caugant, D. A., Froholm, L. O., and Zollinger, W. D. (1991) Characterization of serogroup A and B strains of *Neisseria meningitidis* with serotype 4 and 21 monoclonal antibodies and by multilocus enzyme electrophoresis. *J. Clin. Microbiol.* **29,** 1486–1492.
20. Urwin, R., Feavers, I. M., Jones, D. M., Maiden, M. C., and Fox, A. J. (1998) Molecular variation of meningococcal serotype 4 antigen genes. *Epidemiol. Infect.* **121,** 95–101.
21. Feavers, I. M., Fox, A. J., Gray, S., Jones, D. M., and Maiden, M. C. (1996) Antigenic diversity of meningococcal outer membrane protein PorA has implications for epidemiological analysis and vaccine design. *Clin. Diagn. Lab. Immunol.* **3,** 444–450.
22. van der Ende, A., Hopman, C. T., Zaat, S., Essink, B. B., Berkhout, B., and Dankert, J. (1995) Variable expression of class 1 outer membrane protein in *Neisseria meningitidis* is caused by variation in the spacing between the -10 and -35 regions of the promoter. *J. Bacteriol.* **177,** 2475–2480.
23. Maiden, M. C., Bygraves, J. A., McCarvil, J., and Feavers, I. M. (1992) Identification of meningococcal serosubtypes by polymerase chain reaction. *J. Clin. Microbiol.* **30,** 2835–2841.

24. Feavers, I. M., Suker, J., McKenna, A. J., Heath, A. B., and Maiden, M. C. (1992) Molecular analysis of the serotyping antigens of *Neisseria meningitidis*. *Infect. Immun.* **60,** 3620–3629.
25. Achtman, M., Wall, R. A., Bopp, M., Kusecek, B., Morelli, G., Saken, E., and Hassan-King, M. (1991) Variation in class 5 protein expression by serogroup A meningococci during a meningitis epidemic. *J. Infect. Dis.* **164,** 375–382.
26. van der Ley, P., van der Biezen, J., and Poolman, J. T. (1995) Construction of *Neisseria meningitidis* strains carrying multiple chromosomal copies of the porA gene for use in the production of a multivalent outer membrane vesicle vaccine. *Vaccine* **13,** 401–407.
27. Schneider, H., Hammack, C. A., Apicella, M. A., and Griffiss, J. M. (1988) Instability of expression of lipooligosaccharides and their epitopes in Neisseria gonorrhoeae. *Infect. Immun.* **56,** 942–946.
28. van der Ley, P. and Poolman, J. T. (1992) Construction of a multivalent meningococcal vaccine strain based on the class 1 outer membrane protein. *Infect. Immun.* **60,** 3156–3161.
29. van der Ley, P., van der Biezen, J., Hohenstein, P., Peeters, C., amd Poolman, J. T. (1993) Use of transformation to construct antigenic hybrids of the class 1 outer membrane protein in *Neisseria meningitidis*. *Infect. Immun.* **61,** 4217–4224.
30. Moran, E. E., Brandt, B. L., and Zollinger, W. D. (1994) Expression of the L8 lipopolysaccharide determinant increases the sensitivity of *Neisseria meningitidis* to serum bactericidal activity. *Infect. Immun.* **62,** 5290–5295.
31. Pettersson, A., Kuipers, B., Pelzer, M., Verhagen, E., Tiesjema, R. H., Tommassen, J., and Poolman, J. T. (1990) Monoclonal antibodies against the 70-kilodalton iron-regulated protein of *Neisseria meningitidis* are bactericidal and strain specific. *Infect. Immun.* **58,** 3036–3041.
32. Rouppe van der Voort, E., van der Ley, P., van der Biezen, J., George, S., Tunnela, O., van Dijken, H., Kuipers, B., and Poolman, J. (1996) Specificity of human bactericidal antibodies against PorA P1.7,16 induced with a hexavalent meningococcal outer membrane vesicle vaccine. *Infect. Immun.* **64,** 2745–2751.
33. Lesse, A. J., Campagnari, A. A., Bittner, W. E., and Apicella, M. A. (1990) Increased resolution of lipopolysaccharides and lipooligosaccharides utilizing tricine-sodium dodecyl sulfate-polyacrylamide gel electrophoresis. *J. Immunol. Methods* **126,** 109–117.
34. Lee, N., Yang, J. S., and Testa, D. (1988) A simplified high speed multicolor immunoblotting method. *Anal. Biochem.* **175,** 30–34.
35. Wedege, E., Dalseg, R., Caugant, D. A., Poolman, J. T., and Froholm, L. O. (1993) Expression of an inaccessible P1.7 subtype epitope on meningococcal class 1 proteins. *J. Med. Microbiol.* **38,** 23–28.
36. Bitter-Suermann, D. and Roth, J. (1987) Monoclonal antibodies to polysialic acid reveal epitope sharing between invasive pathogenic bacteria, differentiating cells and tumor cells. *Immunol. Res.* **6,** 225–237.

37. Hurpin, C. M., Carosella, E. D., and Cazenave, P. A. (1992) Bactericidal activity of two IgG2a murine monoclonal antibodies with distinct fine specificities for group B *Neisseria meningitidis* capsular polysaccharide. *Hybridoma* **11,** 677–687.
38. Munkley, A., Tinsley, C. R., Virji, M., and Heckels, J. E. (1991) Blocking of bactericidal killing of *Neisseria meningitidis* by antibodies directed against class 4 outer membrane protein. *Microb. Pathog.* **11,** 447–452.
39. Rosenqvist, E., Musacchio, A., Aase, A., Hoiby, E. A., Namork, E., Kolberg, J., et al. (1999) Functional activities and epitope specificity of human and murine antibodies against the class 4 outer membrane protein (Rmp) of *Neisseria meningitidis. Infect. Immun.* **67,** 1267–1276.
40. Martin, D., Cadieux, N., Hamel, J., and Brodeur, B. R. (1997) Highly conserved *Neisseria meningitidis* surface protein confers protection against experimental infection. *J. Exp. Med.* **185,** 1173–1183.
41. Gu, X. X., Tsai, C. M., and Karpas, A. B. (1992) Production and characterization of monoclonal antibodies to type 8 lipooligosaccharide of *Neisseria meningitidis. J. Clin. Microbiol.* **30,** 2047–2053.
42. Verheul, A. F., Kuipers, A. J., Braat, A. K., Dekker, H. A., Peeters, C. C., Snippe, H., and Poolman, J. T. (1994) Development, characterization, and biological properties of meningococcal immunotype L3,7,(8),9-specific monoclonal antibodies. *Clin. Diagn. Lab. Immunol.* **1,** 729–736.
43. Ala'Aldeen, D. A., Davies, H. A., and Borriello, S. P. (1994) Vaccine potential of meningococcal FrpB: studies on surface exposure and functional attributes of common epitopes. *Vaccine* **12,** 535–541.
44. Pettersson, A., van der Ley, P., Poolman, J. T., and Tommassen, J. (1993) Molecular characterization of the 98-kilodalton iron-regulated outer membrane protein of *Neisseria meningitidis. Infect. Immun.* **61,** 4724–4733.

10

Pulsed-Field Gel Electrophoresis

Mark Achtman and Giovanna Morelli

1. Introduction

DNA molecules in an agarose matrix elongate and migrate toward the anode when exposed to an electric field. An agarose matrix represents a highly irregular network with pores of various dimensions, large open areas, and regions with different densities. During electrophoresis, migration will be retarded by obstructions that prevent sieving by size and result in "end-on" migration as if through a sinuous tube ("reptation" *[1]*). The limit of resolution is reached when the radius of gyration of the linear DNA exceeds the pore size of the gel.

In conventional electrophoresis involving a constant electric field, DNA migrates to a distance that is inversely proportional to the logarithm of its length. Thus, for smaller molecules (<5 Kb), relatively small differences in length result in large differences in mobility. Owing to the logarithmic relationship, sensitivity drops with increasing size. Furthermore, all DNA molecules above a size limit that varies with the electrophoretic conditions migrate together, regardless of length; i.e., large DNA molecules migrate abnormally fast. Pulsed-field gel electrophoresis (PFGE) was developed to solve these problems and allow the electrophoretic separation of larger molecules in agarose gels. This first description of PFGE was by Schwartz and Cantor *(2)*. In their method, pulsed, alternating, orthogonal electric fields are applied to a gel. Large DNA molecules in reptation tubes are trapped each time the electric field direction changes and only once again migrate after they have reoriented along the new field axis. The larger the DNA molecule, the longer the time required for reorientation. DNA molecules whose reorientation time is less than the duration of the electric pulse will therefore be fractionated according

From: *Methods in Molecular Medicine, vol. 67: Meningococcal Disease: Methods and Protocols*
Edited by: A. J. Pollard and M. C. J. Maiden © Humana Press Inc., Totowa, NJ

to their size. The limit of resolution of PFGE depends on several factors, including:

1. The uniformity of the two electric fields,
2. The duration of the electric pulses,
3. The ratio of the pulse times for each of the alternating electric fields,
4. The angles of the two electric fields to the gel, and
5. The ratio of the strengths of the two electric fields.

The original method described by Schwartz and Cantor *(2)* could resolve DNA up to 2000 Kb in length. However, improvement to the technique allow current resolution of up to 5000 Kb.

By permitting the separation of large molecules in agarose, PFGE has extended the size range of molecules amenable to molecular analysis and has profoundly altered the study of genes and genomes. For some organisms, intact chromosomes can be separated from each other by PFGE, allowing gene mapping by Southern hybridization and providing a source of purified chromosomal DNA. Application of PFGE can reveal chromosome-length polymorphisms, thus facilitating evolutionary and population studies in a number of species. For chromosomal DNA that is too large to be separated as intact molecules, PFGE extend traditional mapping techniques such as restriction and deletion mapping to regions up to thousands of kilobases in length, thus enabling the constructions of long range maps.

As both a preparative and an analytical tool, PFGE has played a fundamental role for the pathogenic neisseriae in the development of large-fragment cloning *(3)*, detailed physical mapping ***(4,5)***, and as a powerful tool for monitoring bacterial epidemic spread ***(6–10)***.

2. Materials

2.1. Preparation of Meningococcal DNA for PFGE (for 10 Blocks)

1. All nonspecified chemicals were analysis grade and purchased from Merck. Water is autoclaved, glass-distilled water.
2. GC agar plates for growth of Neisseria strains: dissolve 36 g GC medium base (Difco laboratories) per liter H_2O and autoclave at 1 atm at 120°C for 20 min. Allow to cool to 50°C. For each liter of medium, dissolve 100 mg L-glutamine (Sigma-Aldrich) and 300 mg L-cysteine (Calbiochem) in 0.17% 10 mL $Fe(NO_3)_3.9H_2O$. Mix with 12.4 mL 40% glucose (*see* below), 25 mL dialyzed yeast extract (*see* below), 3 mg vancomycin (Sigma-Aldrich), 7.5 mg polymyxin B sulfate (Sigma-Aldrich), and 2 mg nystatin (Sigma-Aldrich) and add the mixture to the GC medium. The 40% glucose consists of 40 g of D(+)glucose-monohydrate in 100 mL H_2O. After autoclaving and sterile dispensing in appropriate lots, it can be stored at room temperature. Glucose contaminates very readily and lots should only be used once. Dialyzed

yeast extract: 125 g Yeast extract (Difco Laboratories) is dissolved with heating in 500 mL H_2O. The solution is poured into 1 m of dialysis tubing (SpectraPor Membrane, diam. 32 mm, MW cutoff 6-8000, Spectrum, Laguna Hills, CA), the ends knotted and the filled tube is placed into a sterile 5-L beaker. Two L H_2O and a magnetic stir bar are added, the beaker is covered, and dialysis is allowed to proceed with magnetic stirring a 4°C overnight. The material outside the dialysis tube is aliquoted, autoclaved, and stored at room temperature.

3. Phosphate-buffered saline (PBS): 140 m*M* NaCl, 1.5 m*M* KH_2PO_4, and 8.1 m*M* $Na_2HPO_4.2H_2O$. 20X PBS solution consists of 160 g NaCl, 28.8 g $Na_2HPO_4.2H_2O$, and 4 g KH_2PO_4, per liter H_2O. The pH should be 7.4. Dispense, autoclave, and store.
4. 1% low-melting agarose (Small DNA Low Melt, Biozym, Hess.Oldendorf, Germany): 100 mg is suspended in 10 mL H_2O and melted in a microwave oven. Cool the melted agarose in a water bath to 42°C.
5. *Escherichia coli* lysis buffer: 6 m*M* Tris-HCl, 1 *M* NaCl, 100 m*M* ethylenediammetetraacetic acid (EDTA), 1% sarkosyl, and 1 µg/mL DNAse-free RNAse. For a 500-mL solution, mix 3 ml of 1 *M* Tris-HCl, pH 8.0 (Trizma Hydrochloride, Sigma-Aldrich), 100 mL of 5 *M* NaCl, 100 mL of 0.5 *M* EDTA, pH 8.0, 5 g sarkosyl (N-lauroyl-sarcosine, Sigma-Aldrich) and 200 mL of H_2O. After dissolving, add 25 µL of DNAse-free RNAse (20 mg/mL, Ribonuclease A, Sigma-Aldrich) and fill to 500 mL with H_2O.
6. ESP (EDTA, sarkosine, Proteinase K): 0.5 *M* EDTA, 1% sarkosyl, and 1 mg/mL of proteinase K. For 25 mL of solution, mix 25 mL of 0.5 *M* EDTA, pH 8.0, 250 mg of sarkosyl, and 25 mg of proteinase K (Boehringer).
7. TE buffer: 10 m*M* Tris-HCl and 0.1 m*M* EDTA, pH 8.0. For 2 L buffer, use 20 mL of 1 *M* Tris-HCl, pH 8.0, and 0.4 mL of 0.5 *M* EDTA, pH 8.0.

2.2. DNA Restriction

To be useful for PFGE, restriction endonucleases should generate large restriction fragment (rare cutting enzymes) and be unaffected by the presence of agarose. These enzymes must be extremely pure because even small amounts of contaminating nucleases will degrade DNA during the long incubations. We generally use *NheI* and *SpeI* but *SmaI*, *SfiI*, and *XhoI* are also suitable.

1. *NheI* and *SpeI* from New England Biolabs.
2. 10X NE Buffer 2: 0.5 *M* NaCl, 100 m*M* Tris-HCl, 100 m*M* $MgCl_2$, 10 m*M* dithiothreitol [DTT], pH 7.9; (New England Biolabs).
3. 100 µg/mL acetylated bovine serum albumin (BSA); New England Biolabs.

2.3. Preparation of the Gel

1. 1% agarose (Sea Kem GTG Agarose, FMC Bioproducts, Rockland, ME). Use 1.1 g agarose in 110 mL running buffer.
2. Running buffer (0.5X TBE): 50 m*M* Tris, 40 m*M* H_3BO_3, 0.5 m*M* EDTA. Per gel chamber dilute 125 mL 10X TBE buffer to 2.5 L with water. For 1 L 10X TBE

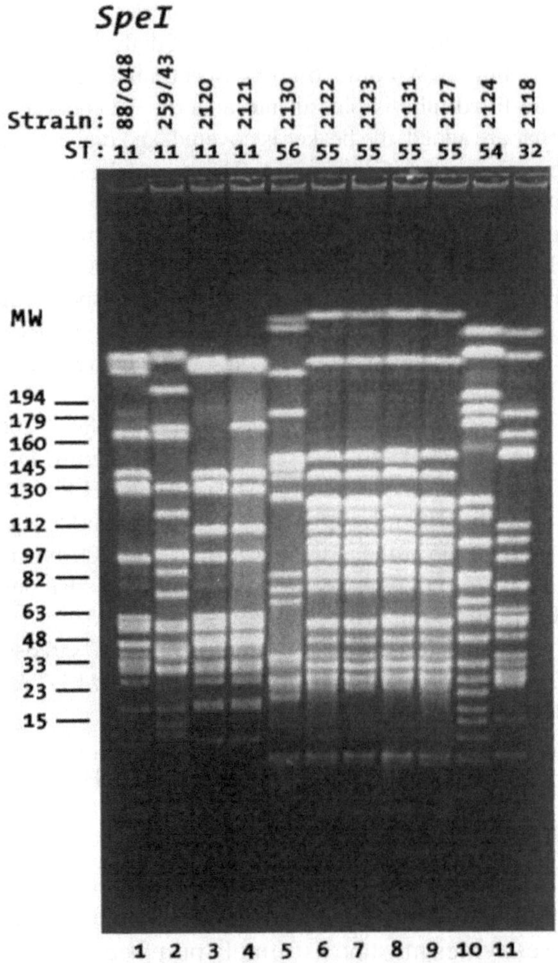

Fig. 1. Pulsed-field gel of 11 meningococcal strains restricted with *SpeI*. The size of the bands ranges between less than 15Kb and more than 194 Kb.

buffer, dissolve 121.1 g Tris-base (Trizma Base, Sigma-Aldrich), 51.35 g H_3BO_3 and 3.72 g EDTA and fill to 1 L with H_2O. Autoclave and store.

2.4. Molecular Weight Markers

A wide variety of molecular-weight markers exist that are suitable for PFGE. We use MidRange I PFG Marker and LowRange PFG Marker (New England Biolabs), which consist of concatemers of lambda DNA mixed with diverse restriction fragments. We always load at least one lane per gel with each marker for increased resolution over using either marker alone.

2.5. Electrophoresis Equipment

1. Gene Navigator™ System (Amersham Pharmacia Biotech).
2. Electrophoresis power supply EPS 500/400 (Amersham Pharmacia Biotech).
3. Multi Temp II™ thermostatic circulator (Amersham Pharmacia Biotech).

2.6. Gel Staining and Photographing

Staining solution: 10 mg/mL ethidium bromide (EtBr; Cal Biochem). Resuspend 1 g EtBr in 100 mL H_2O and store it in a dark bottle. This agent is a mutagen. It should be handled with gloves only and an anti-inhalation mask should be worn while weighing it. Solutions containing EtBr should be decontaminated with a waste reduction unit (bondEX EtBr-50, Macherey-Nagel, Dueren, Germany).

3. Methods

3.1. Preparation of Meningococcal DNA for PFGE

To avoid shearing during extraction of large DNA molecules, cells are lysed *in situ* in an agarose plug *(2)*. Bacterial cells are resuspended in low melting-temperature agarose and solidified in blocks. A variety of substances are infused into the plugs in order to lyse the cells and to remove proteins from the DNA. The DNA obtained by this procedure is both intact and susceptible to restriction *in situ*. After digestion with an appropriate restriction enzyme, the block can be melted and loaded on the gel.

1. Inoculate a supplemented GC agar plate from a frozen stock of *N. meningitidis* and incubate for 16 h at 37°C, 5% CO_2 and 95% humidity.
2. Harvest a small amount of the bacterial culture with a sterile glass rod and resuspend in 10 mL of PBS (*see* **Note 1**).
3. Mix well and adjust the concentration to approx 5×10^8 cells/mL. We use a Klett-Summerson colorimeter for these purposes because they are more reproducible than photometers (*see* **Note 2**).
4. Transfer 10 mL of the bacterial suspension to a 14-mL plastic disposable centrifugation tube (Greiner, Germany) and centrifuge at 1500*g* at room temperature for 5 min. Decant the supernatant and invert the tubes on filter paper for at least 2 min to allow draining.
5. After use, clean blocks formers (insert moulds; Pharmacia) with 70% ethanol and rinse extensively with water. They are stored dry at room temperature. At this point, seal the bottom of the formers with autoclaving tape and label it.
6. Resuspend the cell pellet with 1 mL of 1% low-melting agarose (stored in a water bath at 42°C) with the aid of a pipet. Avoid the formation of air bubbles.
7. Pipet the agar suspension quickly into the block formers (approx 100 µL per well). For each strain, prepare 5–6 blocks. Keep the block former(s) on crushed ice for about 20 min (*see* **Note 3**).

8. Using a small spatula, poke the blocks out of the form into *E. coli* lysis buffer (40–50 mL per 5–6 blocks from one strain in 50 mL plastic [Falcon] centrifuge tubes) and incubate at 30°C overnight.
9. Replace the buffer with 2.5 mL ESP per tube. Incubate at 50°C overnight.
10. Wash the blocks at 37°C in 50 mL of TE buffer four times for 30 min each with shaking at 50–100 rpm. The blocks can then be stored at 4°C for at least 6 mo.

3.2 DNA restriction

1. Cut 1/4 block on a sterile surface such as Parafilm with a sterile scalpel (*see* **Note 4**) and place it in a 1.5-mL Eppendorf tube; equilibrate the 1/4 block with 0.5 mL of digestion buffer at room temperature for at least 20 min. This step dilutes the EDTA inside the block. One such wash is sufficient for *NheI* and *SpeI* but for other enzymes more washes may be required.
2. Remove all the equilibration buffer with a Pasteur pipet. Add 100 µL of the appropriate restriction mix (10 µL 10X restriction buffer, 1 µL of 100 µg/mL acetylated BSA [if recommended by the manufacturer for the particular enzyme], 5–10 U of restriction enzyme plus H_2O to 100 µL volume).
3. Incubate at 37°C overnight.
4. Stop the reaction by removing the restriction mix and adding 0.5 mL of running buffer.

3.3. Preparation of the Gel

1. For a 15 × 15 cm gel, melt 110 mL of 1% agarose in a microwave oven or in a water bath. Allow the agarose to cool at room temperature while stirring with a magnetic bar.
2. Ensure that the conical holes in the plastic tray are free of agarose. These holes prevent the gel from floating due to circulation of the buffer during the run.
3. Place the gel supporting tray on a leveled table such that the slits are on the sides. For proper buffer circulation, the slits must be parallel to the East (right) and West (left) walls.
4. Clean the gel frame with ethanol and make sure that the "ridged" side of the rubber frame is at the bottom and the comb position marks are on top. The ridges seal the frame when slight pressure is applied. The conical holes at the bottom of the tray must be visible within the gel-casting frame. Test the assembly by putting a 0.5 mm comb in the position indicated by the thick red line inside the square on the gel support tray. Adjust the plastic clips such that the teeth of the comb touch the bottom of the tray. With the plastic clips in position, remove the comb for now.
5. Pour the agarose into the frame, making sure that the conical holes are filled. If the gel contains air bubbles, remove them with a Pasteur pipet. Place the comb in the gel and allow the gel to solidify for at least 30 min.
6. To remove the comb, tilt it slowly backwards and forward to break its contact with the agarose and lift it carefully from both ends. Remove the rubber gel-casting frame.

7. Use the gel within 1–2 h or cover it with plastic wrap for later use. If you want to store the gel, flood it with buffer before covering it and store it at 4°C.

3.4. Sample and Marker Loading

1. Remove all equilibration buffer from the tube containing the sample.
2. Incubate the sample for 15–20 min at 65°C (thermo-block) till the agarose is melted.
3. Load 10 μL of melted agarose per well with a 10 μL micropipet. Loading should be very quick to avoid premature solidification. For combs with 25 teeth, leave the first and last wells empty (*see* **Note 5**).
4. The markers are supplied in a GelSyringe dispenser. Using a razor blade, cut a slice on parafilm as above that is slightly narrower than the width of the comb. Transfer the slice to the gel with the help of a fine spatula and let it glide into the well with help of a second spatula. The slice should be placed in close contact with the front of the wells (*see* **Note 6**).

3.5. Electrophoresis Conditions

The conditions will differ with the manufacturer. The instructions here are for a typical PFGE experiment using the Pharmacia Gene Navigator™ System.

1. Start the cooling equipment at least 30 min before the begin of gel electrophoresis to ensure a buffer temperature of 12°C. We need to set the temperature of our cryostat to 10°C to achieve 12°C within the chamber (*see* **Note 7**).
2. Fill the gel chamber with 2.5 L of running buffer and start the external pump that circulates buffer. Always make sure that there is buffer in the tank when the pump is running. After the samples are loaded, place the gel-support tray into the tank. To avoid entrapping air bubbles beneath the gel-support tray, insert one side of the tray first and then lower the remainder carefully into place. If the buffer is insufficient to cover the gel, add more.
3. Adjust the voltage to constant 165 V. The conditions we use for electrophoresis are a 16 h ramp 6–13 s followed by an 8 h ramp from 13–30 s.

3.6. Gel Staining

1. Turn off the power supply before removing the lid. To remove the gel, slide a scalpel under it to cut the agarose in the conical holes and release the gel from the bottom of the tray. Then slide the gel into a plastic dish containing 0.5 μg/mL of EtBr in 0.5X TBE. Be carefully not to break the gel. Incubate at room temperature with shaking (50 rpm) for 30 min, remove the gel, and wash it with tap water. Photograph using UV light (254 nm). Ultraviolet (UV) radiation is dangerous, especially for eyes. Wear protective goggles and a full safety mask that efficiently blocks UV light, and gloves because of EtBr. We use Polaroid 665 film and 15–30 s exposure at f 3.8. Figure 1 from **ref.** ***8*** gives an example of a gel obtained with this method.

4. Notes

1. Plan your time schedule such that you can harvest the cells after 15–16 h growth. Longer incubation periods result in lysis of the meningococci and subsequent smears after electrophoresis. To this end, make sure that all the bacterial strains to be harvested are completed within 1 h after harvesting is begun.
2. The bacterial concentration needs to be adjusted very precisely. Achieving uniform concentrations is critical for the reproducibility, for the resolution of bands of similar size, and for the comparison between different strains.
3. Chilling the agarose adequately is necessary for avoiding later problems with removing the agarose plugs from the formers.
4. Always use clean and sterile tools when handling the blocks to avoid bacterial contamination. Sterile blocks will keep for 6 mo.
5. Correct loading is critical for success. Small air bubbles present while pipetting, or damage to the wells, will result in irregular bands and smears.
6. Positioning the slice very close to the well front is important for obtaining sharp marker bands. Make sure that the slices are not wider than the well.
7. A frequent cause of poor results is inadequate temperature control because the pump stopped or flow was blocked by air bubbles. Proper buffer flow is indicated by fluid moving through the tubing connecting the gel chamber and the cryostat. Check the temperature at the beginning and the end of each run.

References

1. Lerman, L. S. and Frisch, H. L. (1982) Why does the electrophoretic mobility of DNA in gels vary with the length of the molecules? *Biopolymers* **21,** 995.
2. Schwartz, D. C. and Cantor, C. R. (1984) Separation of yeast chromosome-sized DNAs by pulsed field gradient gel electrophoresis. *Cell* **37,** 67–75.
3. Klee, S. R., Nassif, X., Kusecek, B., Merker, P., Beretti, J.-L., Achtman, M., and Tinsley, C. R. (2000) Molecular and biological analysis of eight genetic islands that distinguish *Neisseria meningitidis* from the closely related pathogen *Neisseria gonorrhoeae. Infect. Immun.* **68,** 2082–2095.
4. Dempsey, J. A. F., Litaker, W., Madhure, A., Snodgrass, T. L., and Cannon, J. G. (1991) Physical map of the chromosome of *Neisseria gonorrhoeae* FA1090 with locations of genetic markers, including *opa* and *pil* genes. *J. Bacteriol.* **173,** 5476–5486.
5. Dempsey, J. A. F., Wallace, A. B., and Cannon, J. G. (1995) The physical map of the chromosome of a serogroup A strain of *Neisseria meningitidis* shows complex rearrangements relative to the chromosomes of two mapped strains of the closely related species *N. gonorrhoeae. J. Bacteriol.* **177,** 6390–6400.
6. Bygraves, J. A. and Maiden, M. C. J. (1992) Analysis of the clonal relationships between strains of *Neisseria meningitidis* by pulsed field gel electrophoresis. *J. Gen. Microbiol.* **138,** 523–531.

7. Morelli, G., Malorny, B., Müller, K., Seiler, A., Wang, J., del Valle, J., and Achtman, M. (1997) Clonal descent and microevolution of *Neisseria meningitidis* during 30 years of epidemic spread. *Mol. Microbiol.* **25,** 1047–1064.
8. Vogel, U., Morelli, G., Zurth, K., Claus, H., Kriener, E., Achtman, M., and Frosch, M. (1998) Necessity of molecular techniques to distinguish between *Neisseria meningitidis* isolated from meningococcal disease and from their healthy contacts. *J. Clin. Microbiol.* **36,** 2465–2470.
9. Kwara, A., Adegbola, R. A., Corrah, P. T., Weber, M., Achtman, M., Morelli, G., et al. (1998) Meningitis caused by a serogroup W135 clone of the ET-37 complex of *Neisseria meningitidis* in West Africa. *Trop. Med. Internat. Health* **3,** 742–746.
10. Gagneux, S., Hodgson, A., Erhard, I., Morelli, G., Genton, B., Smith, T., et al. (2000) *Trop. Med. Internat. Health* **5,** 280–287.

11

Nucleotide Sequencing of Antigen Genes of *Neisseria meningitidis*

Rachel Urwin

1. Introduction

The cell-surface structures of *Neisseria meningitidis* play a critical role in the interaction of the bacterium with the human host both as variable antigens that evade immune eradication and by promoting colonization of and adherence to epithelial cells in the nasopharynx. Surface molecules are also implicated in the pathogenicity of some meningococci by facilitating invasion of host cells, survival in the bloodstream, and resistance to phagocytosis. The antigenic diversity among cell-surface components has also been exploited for the development of classification schemes for *N. meningitidis*, which have in turn been used for epidemiological monitoring of meningococcal disease.

Nucleotide-sequence determination and analysis of antigen-encoding genes have been employed to identify the genetic mechanisms used by the meningococcus to modulate the expression (phase variation) of surface structures during the infection process and to generate antigenic diversity in response to host-immune pressure. In this chapter, a number of key surface antigens are described and the impact nucleotide-sequence analyses of the genes encoding these antigens has had on our understanding of meningococcal pathogenesis, epidemiology, and population structure is reviewed. The technical aspects determining the nucleotide sequences of two antigen genes, the porin protein genes *porA* and *porB*, and an iron-limitation protein gene, *fetA* (otherwise known as *frpB*), of *N. meningitidis* are then presented.

1.1. The Polysaccharide Capsule

One of the meningococcal surface antigens that is important both for vaccine development and isolate characterization is the polysaccharide capsule.

From: *Methods in Molecular Medicine, vol. 67: Meningococcal Disease: Methods and Protocols*
Edited by: A. J. Pollard and M. C. J. Maiden © Humana Press Inc., Totowa, NJ

Chemical differences in the capsule allow the classification of meningococci into 13 serogroups ***(1,2)***, only 5 of which (A, B, C, W135,Y) are responsible for most meningococcal disease. The polysaccharide capsule is important for the survival of meningococci in aerosol droplets but also provides a defensive barrier against the host immune system. Indeed, much of the bactericidal effect of human serum has been attributed to the presence of antibodies against the capsular polysaccharides ***(3)***. This observation led first to the development of purified capsular polysaccharide vaccines against serogroups A, C, W135, and Y meningococci and more recently to development of polysaccharide-protein conjugate vaccines for longer-lived protection against serogroup A, C, and W135 meningococcal disease ***(4–7)***. Serogroup B, C, Y, and W135 polysaccharide capsules are all composed of sialic acid, with all genes involved in the biosynthesis and transport of the capsule located within the chromosomal *cps* gene cluster ***(8)***. The meningococcus can switch from expression of one of the sialic acid-containing capsules to another by horizontal genetic exchange of the alpha-2,8 polysialyltransferase gene (*siaD*) ***(9,10)***, a feature that should be considered when designing monovalent vaccination programs ***(11)***.

Phase variation of the polysaccharide capsule is a strategy utilized by the meningococcus to promote colonization and infection: capsule-negative organisms adhere to and invade mucosal epithelial cells most efficiently ***(12)***, whereas capsule expression is essential for survival in the bloodstream. Slipped-strand mispairing resulting from the insertion or deletion of a cytidine residue within a run of seven cytidines in the *siaD* gene has been shown to correlate with the reversible loss of expression of the serogroup B capsule ***(13)***, although in a small proportion of capsule-negative meningococci, capsule expression is reversibly inactivated by the insertion of a naturally occurring insertion element *IS1301* into the sialic acid biosynthesis gene *siaA* ***(14)***.

1.2. Pili

Pili are hypervariable, filamentous lectins that extend considerable distances from the meningococcal cell surface and are involved in adhesion to glycoconjugate structures in the membranes of host epithelial cells ***(15–18)***. They also play a role in the acquisition of exogenous DNA for genetic recombination and transformation ***(19)***. A single pilus is composed of thousands of pilin polypeptide subunits ***(20)***, encoded by the *pilE* gene, which is highly variable as a result of unidirectional DNA exchange with copies of the silent *pilS* gene. These variations in pilin sequence together with post-translational modifications are thought to contribute to the observed variation in epithelial-cell adherence ***(16,21,22)***. Although important for adherence of encapsulated meningococci to endothelial and epithelial cells ***(16)***, mutations in the *pilE* gene are thought to switch off expression of pili following invasion of the mucosal surfaces *(23)*.

1.3. Iron-Limitation Proteins

Meningococci express several iron-regulated surface proteins that are responsible for the acquisition of iron from the human host and its transport into the cell. The transferrin binding proteins, which are encoded by tandomly arranged *tbpA* and *tbpB* genes *(24)*, have been shown to be an essential virulence factor for human infection by the pathogenic *Neisseria (25)* and are therefore considered as potential components for vaccines against serogroup B disease *(26)*. There is no evidence of phase variation in Tbp proteins, with the only signal required for protein expression being iron limitation *(27)*. Nucleotide sequence analysis of *tpbB* shows that this protein is highly variable (J. Bygraves, personal communication) which may limit this protein's eligibility as a vaccine candidate.

An alternative vaccine candidate is the 76-kDa outer-membrane protein (OMP) FetA (previously referred to as FrpB), a protein that is abundantly expressed during iron limitation *(28)*. This protein binds ferric enterobactin and may be involved in the transport of the siderophore into the cell *(29)*. FetA shows sequence homology to the TonB-dependant family of receptors that include the *Escherichia coli* enterobactin receptor, FepA *(30)*. A topology model of the meningococcal FetA protein has been developed from nucleotide-sequence data that predicts 13 surface-exposed loops *(31)*, with bactericidal anti-FetA antibodies targeting the variable epitope that resides in the largest and most variable of these (loop 7) *(32)*. Recent analysis of *fetA* gene sequences among 107 hypervirulent meningococci shows that this protein is highly variable among serogroup B meningococci, with antigenic diversification a result of positive selection from the immune response and abundant genetic recombination (E. M. Thompson, personal communication).

1.4. Major OMPs

Among the surface proteins expressed by *N. meningitidis* are the major OMPs, with five classes (class 1 to class 5) identified *(33,34)*. The heat modifiable class 5 proteins, Opa and Opc, are thought to be important for adhesion and invasion of host epithelial cells *(35–37)*. The Opa proteins are highly heterogeneous and expression of the Opc protein can be varied, so within a single meningococcal strain the antigenic nature and relative amounts of class 5 proteins expressed is hypervariable. The translational phase variation of meningococcal Opa proteins occurs by addition or deletion of CTCTT repeats in the signal sequence-encoding region of *opa* genes *(38)*, whereas the variable number of cytidine residues in the promoter sequence of the *opc* gene are responsible for transcriptional regulation of Opc phase variation ***(39)***.

Almost all meningococcal isolates express the largest of the OMPs—the class 1 (PorA) protein—and all strains possess either a class 2 (PorB2) or a class 3 (PorB3) protein. The PorB2 and PorB3 OMPs are the predominant proteins of the outer membrane, are mutually exclusive, and are expressed by alternate alleles (*porB2* and *porB3*) at the *porB* locus ***(40)***. Modulation of expression of PorA is regulated at the transcriptional level and exhibits three levels of expression depending on the length of the polyguanidine stretch in the promoter region of the *porA* gene ***(41)***. There is no evidence that PorB proteins are subject to phase variation.

Three-dimensional homology models of these porin proteins have been developed from a combination of sequence data and crystal structures of *E. coli* porins. These models predict eight surface-exposed loops interspersed with highly conserved outer membrane-spanning sequences ***(42)***. The antigenically important variable epitopes that are targeted in the host immune response and by serological typing reagents reside in the surface-exposed loops of PorA and PorB ***(43–46)***. Analyses of *porA* and *porB* sequence data indicate that there is positive selection for amino acid change in surface-loop encoding regions of these genes ***(47,48)*** and that the other evolutionary process generating dramatic diversification of these proteins is intra-species genetic recombination. As a consequence of the variability of these proteins, serological typing for long term epidemiological studies of meningococcal disease are problematic. Furthermore, the insensitivity of serosubtyping monoclonal antibodies (MAbs) has been reported ***(49)*** and *porB* sequencing of serologically similar meningococci demonstrated that isolates were not closely related genetically ***(50,51)***. However, the characterization of *porA* and *porB* gene sequences for short-term epidemiological studies has proven successful; for instance, in resolving the relationships among meningococci causing localized outbreaks of disease ***(52)***.

2. Materials

2.1. Polymerase Chain Reaction

Apart from the amplification primers utilized, which were specifically designed for a target antigen gene, in our laboratory the components of the polymerase chain reactions (PCRs) are essentially the same. All PCR components are stored at –20°C. If small volumes are being used, it is advisable to prepare multiple lots of the reaction buffer, $MgCl_2$, dNTP mix and genomic DNA template to minimize the number of freeze-thaw cycles.

1. DNA polymerase: AmpliTaq DNA polymerase (Applied Biosystems, Cat. no. N808-0153, supplied at 5 U/μL). This enzyme is stored at –20°C.
2. Reaction buffer: 10X reaction buffer II (500 m*M* KCl, 100 m*M* Tris-HCl, pH 8.3), lacking Mg^{2+}, is supplied with the enzyme.
3. $MgCl_2$: 25 m*M* $MgCl_2$ is also supplied by Applied Biosystems with the enzyme.
4. dNTPs: A dNTP set is supplied by Applied Biosystems (Cat. no. N808-0260) comprising a single solution containing 2.5 m*M* each of dATP, dCTP, dGTP, and dTTP. Dilution of this stock solution with an equal volume of deionized water gives a 5 m*M* dNTP working solution (1.25 m*M* each of dATP, dCTP, dGTP, and dTTP).
5. Genomic DNA template: Rapid DNA preparations are made using the Isoquick Nucleic Acid Extraction Kit (Orca Research Inc., Cat. no. MXT-020-100), following the manufacturer's instructions. A boiled heavy suspension of *N. meningitidis* cells in water may also be used directly for PCR but this is not a suitable method if long term storage of template DNA is intended.
6. Oligonucleotide primers: All oligonucleotides are synthesized by Oswel Research Products Limited on a 0.2/μmol synthesis scale, without high-performance liquid chromatography (HPLC) purification. Stock solutions are diluted to 10 μ*M* working solutions with deionized water. The primers in **Table 1** are used for *porA*, *porB*, and *fetA* amplification. Primer locations are shown in **Fig. 1**.
7. Plasticware: PCR master mix is prepared in a 1.5-mL Eppendorf tube (Axygen, Cat. no. 311-04-051). Amplification reactions are carried out in 0.2 mL thin-walled tubes (Axygen, Cat. no. 321-02-101).

2.2. Purification of PCR Products

The method used for purification of the PCR amplified DNA prior to sequencing was first described by Embley *(53)*.

1. Polyethyleneglycol $(PEG)_{8000}$/NaCl solution: Mix equal volumes of 40% PEG_{8000} (Sigma, Cat. no. P-4463) and 5 *M* sodium chloride (Sigma, Cat. no. S-7653) for a working solution of 20% PEG_{8000}/2.5 *M* NaCl.
2. 70% (v/v) Ethanol.
3. 1.5-mL Eppendorf tubes.

2.3. Agarose Gel Electrophoresis of PCR Products

PCR reactions are run on an agarose gel, alongside DNA size markers, to confirm that gene amplification has been successful.

1. Agarose: Routine use agarose is suitable (Sigma, Cat. no. A9539).
2. TBE buffer: A 10X (0.89 *M* Tris-borate, pH 8.3, 20 m*M* EDTA) stock solution (National Diagnostics, Cat. no. EC-860) is diluted with deionized water for a 1X TBE working stock.

Table 1
Oligonucleotide Primers Used for *porA, porB,* and *fetA* Amplification

Gene	Forward primer 5′-3′ sequence	Reverse primer 5′-3′ sequence
porA	210, ATGCGAAAAAAACTTACCGCCCTC	211, AATGAAGGCAAGCCGTCAAAAACA
porB	PB-A1, TAAATGCAAAGCTAAGCGGCTTG	PB-A2, TTTGTTGATACCAATCTTTTCAG
fetA	A4, GCAGAAAATAATGCCAAGGTC *(32)*	A5, GGCTGCAGAGGGTATTGGTCCAGCGTTG *(32)*
	A14, ATCCTGCCAAACCTTAACGG *(29)*	

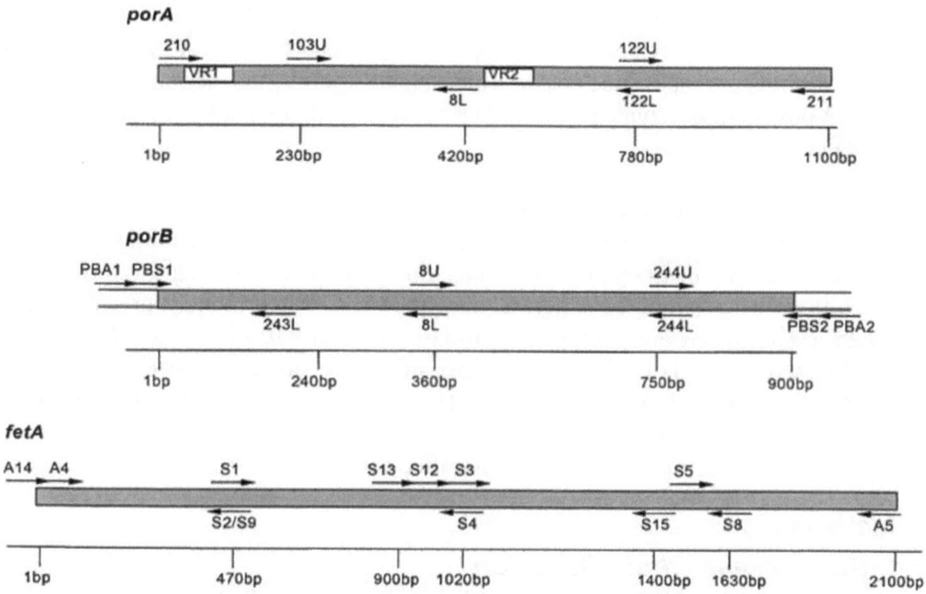

Fig. 1. Location of oligodeoxyribonucleotide primers used for PCR amplification and nucleotide sequencing of *Neisseria meningitidis* porin genes, *porA* (the locations of VR1 and VR2 for *porA* are shown), *porB*, and *fetA*, with arrows to represent the orientation of each primer in relation to gene transcription.

3. Ethidium bromide: To eliminate handling of this mutagen in powder form, we use a pre-mixed 10 mg/mL ethidium bromide solution (Sigma, Cat. no. E-1510) that is stored in the dark at room temperature.
4. Loading buffer: 10X concentration: 67% sucrose, 0.42% bromophenol blue in TE buffer, pH 8.0. Ready-made loading buffer is also produced commercially.
5. DNA molecular weight markers: 100 bp DNA ladder (Promega, Cat. no. G2101).

2.4. Sequencing Reactions

We employ the chain-termination method for automated nucleotide sequencing ***(54)***, in which one of four fluorescently labeled dideoxynucleotides are incorporated during primer extension, resulting in chain termination. Following separation by electrophoresis in an automated sequencer, DNA fragments are detected when the instrument's scanning argon ion laser excites the fluorescent dyes on the 5′ end of the terminated fragments and the fluorescent signal is amplified, interpreted, and assembled with other signals into a DNA sequence. There are several automated sequencing systems commercially available. We follow a protocol that uses the reagents and technology available from Applied Biosystems.

1. Termination mix: BigDye™ Terminator Cycle Sequencing Ready Reaction Kit with AmpliTaq DNA polymerase, FS (Applied Biosystems, Cat. no. 4303152) contains dye terminators, deoxynucleoside triphosphates, buffer, magnesium chloride, and DNA polymerase enzyme premixed in a single tube. Store in 200–500-μL aliquots at –20°C.
2. Oligonucleotide primers: Oligonucleotide sequencing primers are listed in **Table 2**. **Figure 1** shows the location and orientation of each primer. Primers are designed in order that complete sequence will be determined on both forward and reverse strands of the gene. All sequencing primers are diluted to 10-μ*M* stock solutions with deionized water, as described for PCR primers. For sequencing, 625 nM solutions are prepared by dilution of 1 part 10 μ*M* stock with 15 parts deionized water (1:15 dilution). Primer stocks are stored at –20°C.
3. Ethanol: Analytical-grade absolute EtOH is diluted in deionized water to 95% (v/v) and 70% (v/v) solutions.
4. Plasticware: Individual 0.2 mL thin-walled tubes (as for PCR).

3. Methods

3.1. Polymerase Chain Reaction

1. Prepare a master mix containing all of the PCR components except template DNA in a 1.5-mL Eppendorf tube. **Table 3** shows the volumes required for one 50 μL reaction: multiply these volumes according to the number of reactions required, including a negative control, plus one extra (to ensure that there is enough master mix for all reactions). After thorough mixing, dispense 49.5 μL of the master mix into 0.2-mL thin-walled PCR tubes. Inoculate each tube with 0.5 μL of the appropriate genomic DNA.
2. Place the reactions in a thermal cycling machine (we use MJ Research PTC-200 and Applied Biosystems 9700 thermal cyclers) and incubate as follows:
   a. *porA* amplification: 25 cycles consisting 94°C for 1 min, 60°C for 1 min, and 72°C for 2 min. Follow by a further incubation at 72°C for 3 min.
   b. *porB* amplification: Two min at 94°C and then for 30 cycles as follows: 1 min at 94°C; 1 min 60°C; 2 min at 72°C. At the end of the 30 cycles, incubate the reactions for a further 2 min at 72°C. Following incubation, incubate all reactions at 4°C until removed from the thermal cycler.

3.2. Purification of PCR Products

1. Transfer each PCR reaction mix from the PCR tube into an appropriately labeled 1.5-mL Eppendorf tube. If reactions are less than 100 μL, add deionized water to give 100 μL total volume.
2. Add 60 μL 20% (w/v) PEG_{8000}, 2.5 *M* NaCl solution to each tube. Mix the contents of each tube by vortexing and then incubate at 37°C for 15 min or at 4°C overnight.

Table 2
Oligonucleotide Primers Used for *porA, porB*, and *fetA* Nucleotide-Sequence Determination[a]

Gene	Forward primer 5′-3′ sequence	Reverse primer 5′-3′ sequence
porA	210, ATGCGAAAAAAACTTACCGCCCTC	211, AATGAAGGCAAGCCGTCAAAAACA
	103U, GAGCAAGACGTATCCGTT	122L, GGCGAGATTCAAGCCGCC
	122U, GGCGGCTTGAATCTCGCC	8L, GGAGAATCGTAGCGTACGGA
porB	PB-S1, GCAGCCCTTCCTGTTGCAGC	PB-S2, TTGCAGATTAGAATTTGTG
	8U, TCCGTACGCTACGATTCTCC	8L, GGAGAATCGTAGCGTACGGA
	244U, CGCCCCGCGTTTCTTACG	244L, CGTAAGAAACGCGGGGCG
		PB260, AGTGCGTTTGGAGAAGTCGT
fetA	A4, GCAGAAAATAATGCCAAGGTC	A5, GGCTGCAGAGGGTATTGGTCCAGCGTTG
	A14, ATCCTGCCAAACCTTAACGG	S2, CCGAATACGCTTGCGCCG
	S1, CGGCGCAAGCGTATTCGG	S4, GCGGTTTGATTTCCTGATGG
	S3, CCATCAGGAAATCAAACCGC	S8, CGCGCCCAATTCGTAACCGTG
	S5, CCATCAAAGACGCGCTTGCC	S9, CCGAATACGCTGGCACCG
	S12, TTCAACTTCGACAGCCGCCTT	S15, TTGCAGCGCGTCRTACAGGCG
	S13, TACGCAGGCAATGTAAAAGGC	

[a]*See* **Notes 3** and **4** for additional information.

Table 3
The Components in a 50 mL PCR Reaction[a]

Reagent (stock concentration)	Volume (µL)	Final concentration
Deionized H_2O	23.25	—
10X reaction buffer	5.0	1X
PCR primer 1 (10 µ*M*)	5.0	1 µ*M*
PCR primer 2 (10 µ*M*)	5.0	1 µ*M*
$MgCl_2$ (25 m*M*)	3.0	1.5 m*M*
dNTP mix (5 m*M*)	8.0	800 µ*M*
Taq DNA polymerase (5,000 U/mL^{-1})	0.25	1.25 U

[a]Multiply the reagent volumes listed by the number of PCR reactions required + 1 to make up a single master mix, which can then be dispensed in 49.5-µL amounts into reaction tubes (also described in Chapter 12).

3. Pellet the precipitated PCR products by spinning in a microcentrifuge at 13,000*g* for 10 min. Remove the supernatant from each tube using an automatic pipettor, taking care not to disturb the DNA pellet.
4. Wash the DNA pellets by adding 0.5 mL 70% ice-cold ethanol to each tube, and spin again at 13,000*g* for a further 5 min. Remove the supernatant from each tube using an automatic pipettor then dry the DNA pellets using a spinning vacuum desiccator, or allow to air-dry.
5. Resuspend pellets in 10–20 mL deionized water.

3.3. Agarose Gel Electrophoresis of PCR Products

1. Dissolve 1% (w/v) agarose in 1X TBE buffer on a heated plate. When molten, add 0.5 µg mL^{-1} ethidium bromide to the agarose gel mixture, and pour into a gel casting tray and allow to set at room temperature.
2. Mix the DNA samples (5–10 µL of unpurified PCR reactions or 2 µL of purified product made up to 10 µL with deionized water) with 1 µL loading buffer and pipet into the individual preformed wells of the agarose gel, that is submerged in 1X TBE. For size estimation, run DNA markers alongside the DNA samples.
3. Following electrophoresis at a current of 50–100 mA, visualize the EtBr-stained DNA on an ultraviolet (302 nm) transilluminator to confirm the presence of a single band of the correct size in each PCR reaction. The approximate PCR product sizes obtained using the amplification primers listed above are: *porA*, 1100 bp; *porB*, 900–1000 bp; *fetA*, 2000–2100 bp. There should be no product visible in the negative control reaction.

3.4. Sequencing Reactions

1. For each cycle-sequencing reaction, mix the following reagents in a labeled thin-walled tube: 2 µL appropriate sequencing primer; 2 µL BigDye Terminator Cycle Sequencing Ready Reaction mix; 1 µL template DNA.

2. Place the reactions in a thermal cycling machine and incubate as follows: 25 cycles of 96°C for 10 s, 50°C for 5 s, 60°C for 2 min. The reactions are then incubated at 4°C.

Following cycle sequencing, purify the extension products to remove any unincorporated termination mix:

1. Make up the reaction mixes to a total volume of 36 μL with deionized water (for 5 μL reactions add 31 μL water) then transfer into 1.5-mL microcentrifuge tubes containing 64 μL of 95% ethanol. Mix the contents of the tubes by vortexing and incubate at room temperature for 15 min.
2. Pellet the reaction products by spinning tubes in a microcentrifuge at 13,000*g* for 15–30 min. Aspirate the supernatant from the tubes with a micropipettor, taking care not to disturb the pellet, which may or may not be visible at this stage.
3. Wash the pellets by adding 500 μL of 70% ethanol to each tube. Centrifuge the tubes at 13,000*g* for a further 10 min. Carefully aspirate the alcohol solution with an automatic pipet and dry the pellets in a vacuum desiccator.
4. Store the dried pellets at 20°C and resuspend in loading buffer following the manufacturer's protocol prior to loading on an automated sequencer.

3.4.1. Sequence Analysis Software

There are a number of sequence analysis software packages available for the editing of trace files (raw sequence data), and their assembly into contiguous double-stranded gene sequences. These include relatively expensive commercial packages for Macintosh or Windows such as Sequence Navigator (Applied Biosystems), Lasergene99 (DNAstar), and Sequencher (Gene Codes Corporation). We edit and assemble nucleotide sequence data using UNIX-based Staden software *(55)*. Assembled sequences are then reformatted to 'GCG' format and aligned in Seqlab using the Wisconsin package, version 10.1 (Genetics Computer Group, Madison, WI) before being exported for further analysis. Some of the methods used to analyze these sequence data are described in Chapter 23.

Acknowledgments

The oligonucleotide primer sequences and PCR parameters for *porA* and *fetA* amplification were kindly provided by Emily Thompson, Janet Suker, and Joanne Russell.

4. Notes

1. For both amplification reactions and sequencing reactions, the protocols given in this chapter use individual capped tubes for each reaction. If high throughput sequencing of antigen genes is required, please refer to the methods described in Chapter 12, which use 48- or 96-well micotiter plates, for guidance.

2. For *fetA* amplification reactions, primers A4 and A5 are used routinely. PCR failure in a small number of strains may be owing to polymorphisms in the primer A4 binding site, in which case amplification with primers A14 and A5 is recommended.
3. Not all listed *fetA* oligonucleotide sequencing primers need to be used to obtain double-stranded sequence for the *fetA* gene, however, we recommend users try all primers initially and choose those which work best for them.
4. For *fetA* nucleotide sequence determination, primer S9 is very occasionally used when there are polymorphisms in the primer S2 binding site. To determine the nucleotide sequence of the *fetA* variable region only, primers S12 (or S13) and S15 are used.
5. Use primers 210 and 8L to determine the *porA* VR1 sequence, and primers 103U and 122L to sequence the *porA* VR2 sequence.
6. Confirmation of successful amplification reactions by agarose-gel electrophoresis of PCR products can be performed either directly after PCR or following purification of products by PEG precipitation, or on both occasions. The advantage of running the gel after template purification is that successful purification can also be confirmed.
7. The final reaction volume of each sequencing reaction is 5 μL: this is one-quarter of the volume recommended in the manufacturer's protocol. Other users may find it necessary to scale up reactions depending on the gene being sequenced and the primers, chemistries, and automated sequencer being used, although this will increase the cost of each reaction.
8. Please also refer to the **Notes 7** and **8** of Chapter 12 for additional information about ethanol precipitation of sequencing reactions as these are also pertinent to this chapter.

References

1. Eldridge, J., Sutcliffe, E. M., Abbott, J. D., and Jones, D.M. (1978) Serological grouping of meningococci and detection of antigen in cerebrospinal fluid by coagglutination. *Med. Lab. Sci.* **35,** 63–66.
2. Davis, D. M., Dulbecco, R., Eisen, H. N., and Ginsberg, H. S. (1980) The *Neisseriae*, in *Microbiology* (Gotschlich, E. C., ed.), Harper, New York, NY, pp. 635–644.
3. Goldschneider, I., Gotschlich, E. C., and Artenstein, M. S. (1969) Human Immunity to the Meningococcus. II. Development of Natural Immunity. *J. Exp. Med.* **129,** 1327–1348.
4. Jennings, H. J. and Lugowski, C. (1981) Immunochemistry of groups A, B, and C meningococcal polysaccharide-tetanus toxoid conjugates. *J. Immunol.* **127,** 1011–1018.
5. Costantino, P., Viti, S., Podda, A., Velmonte, M. A., Nencioni, L., and Rappuoli, R. (1992) Development and phase 1 clinical testing of a conjugate vaccine against meningococcus A and C. *Vaccine* **10,** 691–698.

6. Richmond, P., Goldblatt, D., Fusco, P. C., Fusco, J. D., Heron, I., Clark, S., Borrow, R., and Michon, F. (1999) Safety and immunogenicity of a new *Neisseria meningitidis* serogroup C-tetanus toxoid conjugate vaccine in healthy adults. *Vaccine* **18,** 641–646.
7. Campagne, G., Garba, A., Fabre, P., Schuchat, A., Ryall, R., Boulanger, D., et al. (2000) Safety and immunogenicity of three doses of a *Neisseria meningitidis* A + C diphtheria conjugate vaccine in infants from Niger. *Pediatr. Infect. Dis. J.* **19,** 144–150.
8. Frosch, M., Weisgerber, C., and Meyer, T. F. (1989) Molecular characterization and expression in Escherichia coli of the gene complex encoding the polysaccharide capsule of *Neisseria meningitidis* group B. *Proc. Natl. Acad. Sci. USA* **86,** 1669–1673.
9. Edwards, U., Muller, A., Hammerschmidt, S., Gerardy-Schahn, R., and Frosch, M. (1994) Molecular analysis of the biosynthesis pathway of the alpha-2,8 polysialic acid capsule by *Neisseria meningitidis* serogroup B. *Mol. Microbiol.* **14,** 141–149.
10. Swartley, J. S., Marfin, A. A., Edupuganti, S., Liu, L. J., Cieslak, P., Perkins, B., et al. (1997) Capsule switching of *Neisseria meningitidis*. *Proc. Natl. Acad. Sci. USA* **94,** 271–276.
11. Maiden, M. C. J. and Spratt, B. G. (1999) Meningococcal conjugate vaccines: new opportunities and new challenges. *Lancet* **354,** 615–616.
12. Stephens, D. S., Spellman, P. A., and Swartley, J. S. (1993) Effect of the (alpha 2→8)-linked polysialic acid capsule on adherence of *Neisseria meningitidis* to human mucosal cells. *J. Infect. Dis.* **167,** 475–479.
13. Hammerschmidt, S., Muller, A., Sillmann, H., Muhlenhoff, M., Borrow, R., Fox, A., et al. (1996) Capsule phase variation in *Neisseria meningitidis* serogroup B by slipped-strand mispairing in the polysialyltransferase gene (*siaD*): correlation with bacterial invasion and the outbreak of meningococcal disease. *Mol. Microbiol.* **20,** 1211–1120.
14. Hammerschmidt, S., Hilse, R., van Putten, J. P., Gerardy-Schahn, R., Unkmeir, A., and Frosch, M. (1996) Modulation of cell surface sialic acid expression in *Neisseria meningitidis* via a transposable genetic element. *EMBO J* **15,** 192–198.
15. Heckels, J. E. (1989) Structure and function of pili of pathogenic *Neisseria* species. *Clin. Microbiol. Rev.* **2S,** S66–S73.
16. Virji, M., Saunders, J. R., Sims, G., Makepeace, K., Maskell, D., and Ferguson, D. J. P. (1993) Pilus-facilitated adherence of *Neisseria meningitidis* to human epithelial and endothelial cells: modulation of adherence phenotype occurrs concurrently with changes in primary amino acid sequence and the glycosylation status of pilin. *Mol. Microbiol.* **10,** 1013–1028.
17. Virji, M., Kayhty, H., Ferguson, D. J., Alexandrescu, C., Heckels, J. E., and Moxon, E. R. (1991) The role of pili in the interactions of pathogenic Neisseria with cultured human endothelial cells. *Mol. Microbiol.* **5,** 1831–1841.
18. McLeod Griffiss, J. (1995) Mechanisms of host immunity, in *Meningococcal Disease* (Cartwright, K. A. V., ed.), John Wiley and Sons, Chichester, UK, pp. 35–70.

19. Poolman, J. T., van der Ley, P. A., and Tommassen, J. (1995) Surface structures and secreted products of meningococci, in *Meningococcal Disease* (Cartwright, K. A. V., ed.), John Wiley and Sons, Chichester, UK, pp. 21–34.
20. Hart, C. A. and Rogers, T. R. F. (1993) Meningococcal disease. *J. Med. Microbiol.* **39,** 3–25.
21. Virji, M., Alexandrescu, C., Ferguson, D. J., Saunders, J. R., and Moxon, E. R. (1992) Variations in the expression of pili: the effect on adherence of Neisseria meningitidis to human epithelial and endothelial cells. *Mol. Microbiol.* **6,** 1271–1279.
22. Nassif, X., Lowy, J., Stenberg, P., O'Gaora, P., Ganji, A., and So, M. (1993) Antigenic variation of pilin regulates adhesion of *Neisseria meningitidis* to human epithelial cells. *Mol. Microbiol.* **8,** 719–725.
23. de Vries, F. P., van der Ende, A., van Putten, J. P., and Dankert, J. (1996) Invasion of primary nasopharyngeal epithelial cells by *Neisseria meningitidis* is controlled by phase variation of multiple surface antigens. *Infect. Immun.* **64,** 2998–3006.
24. Legrain, M., Mazarin, V., Irwin, S. W., Bouchon, B., Quentin Millet, M. J., Jacobs, E., and Schryvers, A. B. (1993) Cloning and characterization of *Neisseria meningitidis* genes encoding the transferrin-binding proteins Tbp1 and Tbp2. *Gene* **130,** 73–80.
25. Cornelissen, C. N., Kelley, M., Hobbs, M. M., Anderson, J. E., Cannon, J. G., Cohen, M. S., and Sparling, P. F. (1998) The transferrin receptor expressed by gonococcal strain FA1090 is required for the experimental infection of human male volunteers. *Mol. Microbiol.* **27,** 611–616.
26. Lissolo, L., Maitre Wilmotte, G., Dumas, P., Mignon, M., Danve, B., and Quentin Millet, M. J. (1995) Evaluation of transferrin-binding protein 2 within the transferrin-binding protein complex as a potential antigen for future meningococcal vaccines. *Infect. Immun.* **63,** 884–890.
27. Schryvers, A. B. and Stojiljkovic, I. (1999) Iron acquisition systems in the pathogenic *Neisseria. Mol. Microbiol.* **32,** 1117–1123.
28. Dyer, D. W., West, E. P., McKenna, W., Thompson, S. A., and Sparling, P. F. (1988) A pleiotropic iron-uptake mutant of *Neisseria meningitidis* lacks a 70-kilodalton iron-regulated protein. *Infect. Immun.* **56,** 977–983.
29. Carson, S. D. B., Klebba, P. E., Newton, S. M. C., and Sparling, P. F. (1999) Ferric enterobactin binding and utilisation by *Neisseria gonorrhoeae. J. Bacteriol.* **181,** 2895–2901.
30. Thulasiraman, P., Newton, S. M. C., Xu, J., Raymond, K. N., Mai, C., Hall, A., et al. (1998) Selectivity of ferric enterobactin binding and cooperativity of transport in Gram-negative bacteria. *J. Bacteriol.* **180,** 6689–6696.
31. Pettersson, A., Maas, A., van Wassenaar, D., van der Ley, P., and Tommassen, J. (1995) Molecular characterization of FrpB, the 70-kilodalton iron-regulated outer membrane protein of *Neisseria meningitidis. Infect. Immun.* **63,** 4181–4184.
32. van der Ley, P., van der Biezen, J., Sutmuller, R., Hoogerhout, P., and Poolman, J. T. (1996) Sequence variability of FrpB, a major iron-regulated outer-membrane protein in the pathogenic neisseriae. *Microbiology* **142,** 3269–3274.

33. Tsai, C.-M., Frasch, C. E., and Mocca, L. F. (1981) Five structural classes of major outer membrane proteins in *Neisseria meningitidis. J. Bacteriol.* **146,** 69–78.
34. Barlow, A. K., Heckels, J. E., and Clarke, I. N. (1989) The class 1 outer membrane protein of *Neisseria meningitidis*: gene sequence and structural and immunological similarities to gonococcal porins. *Mol. Microbiol.* **3,** 131–139.
35. Virji, M. (1996) Meningococcal disease: epidemiology and pathogenesis. *Trends Microbiol.* **4,** 466–469.
36. Virji, M., Makepeace, K., Ferguson, D. J., Achtman, M., and Moxon, E. R. (1993) Meningococcal Opa and Opc proteins: their role in colonization and invasion of human epithelial and endothelial cells. *Mol. Microbiol.* **10,** 499–510.
37. Virji, M., Makepeace, K., Ferguson, D. J. P., Achtman, M., Sarkari, J., and Moxon, E. R. (1992) Expression of the Opc protein correlates with invasion of epithelial and endothelial cells by *Neisseria meningitidis*. *Mol. Microbiol.* **6,** 2785–2795.
38. van der Ley, P., Heckels, J. E., Virji, M., Hoogerhout, P., and Poolman, J. T. (1991) Topology of outer membrane porins in pathogenic *Neisseria* spp. *Infect. Immun.* **59,** 2963–2971.
39. Sarkari, J., Pandit, N., Moxon, E. R., and Achtman, M. (1994) Variable expression of the Opc outer membrane protein in *Neisseria meningitidis* is caused by size variation of a promotor containing poly-cytidine. *Mol. Microbiol.* **13,** 207–217.
40. Hitchcock, P. J. (1989) Unified nomenclature for pathogenic *Neisseria* species. *Clin. Microbiol. Rev.* **2,** S64–S65.
41. van der Ende, A., Hopman, C. T. P., Zaat, S., Oude Essink, B. B., Berkhout, B., and Dankert, J. (1995) Variable expression of class 1 outer membrane protein in *Neisseria meningitidis* is caused by variation in the spacing between the -10 and -35 regions of the promoter. *J. Bacteriol.* **177,** 2475–2480.
42. Derrick, J. P., Urwin, R., Suker, J., Feavers, I. M., and Maiden, M. C. J. (1999) Structural and evolutionary inference from molecular variation in *Neisseria* porins. *Infect. Immun.* **67,** 2406–2413.
43. Frasch, C. E., Zollinger, W. D., and Poolman, J. T. (1985) Serotype antigens of *Neisseria meningitidis* and a proposed scheme for designation of serotypes. *Rev. Infect. Dis.* **7,** 504–510.
44. Saukkonen, K., Leinonen, M., Abdillahi, H., and Poolman, J.T. (1989) Comparative evaluation of potential components for group B meningococcal vaccine by passive protection in the infant rat and *in vitro* bactericidal assay. *Vaccine* **7,** 325–328.
45. Maiden, M. C. J., Suker, J., McKenna, A. J., Bygraves, J. A., and Feavers, I. M. (1991) Comparison of the class 1 outer membrane proteins of eight serological reference strains of *Neisseria meningitidis*. *Mol. Microbiol.* **5,** 727–736.
46. Bash, M. C., Lesiak, K. B., Banks, S. D., and Frasch, C. E. (1995) Analysis of Neisseria meningitidis class 3 outer membrane protein gene variable regions and type identification using genetic techniques. *Infect. Immun.* **63,** 1484–1490.
47. Smith, N. H., Maynard Smith, J., and Spratt, B. G. (1995) Sequence evolution of the *porB* gene of *Neisseria gonorrhoeae* and *Neisseria meningitidis*: evidence of positive Darwinian selection. *Mol. Biol. Evol.* **12,** 363–370.

48. Urwin, R. (1998) PhD Thesis: *Variation in Meningococcal PorB Proteins.* University of Staffordshire, Stoke-on-Trent, UK.
49. Suker, J., Feavers, I. M., and Maiden, M. C. J. (1996) Monoclonal antibody recognition of members of the P1.10 variable region family: implications for serological typing and vaccine design. *Microbiology* **142,** 63–69.
50. Urwin, R., Fox, A. J., Musilek, M., Kriz, P., and Maiden, M. C. J. (1998) Heterogeneity of the PorB protein in serotype 22 *Neisseria meningitidis. J. Clin. Microbiol.* **36,** 3680–3682.
51. Urwin, R., Feavers, I. M., Jones, D. M., Maiden, M. C. J., and Fox, A. J. (1998) Molecular variation of meningococcal serotype 4 antigen genes. *Epidemiol. Infect.* **121,** 95–101.
52. Bygraves, J. A., Urwin, R., Fox, A. J., Gray, S. J., Russell, J. E., Feavers, I. M., and Maiden, M. C. J. (1999) Population genetic and evolutionary approaches to the analysis of *Neisseria meningitidis* isolates belonging to the ET-5 complex. *J. Bacteriol.* **181,** 5551–5556.
53. Embley, T. M. (1991) The linear PCR reaction: a simple and robust method for sequencing amplified rRNA genes. *Lett. Appl. Microbiol.* **13,** 171–174.
54. Sanger, F., Nicklen, S., and Coulson, A. R. (1977) DNA sequencing with chain-terminating inhibitors. *Proc. Nat. Acad. Sci. USA* **74,** 5463–5467.
55. Staden, R. (1996) The Staden sequence analysis package. *Mol. Biotechnol.* **5,** 233–241.

12

Multi-Locus Sequence Typing

Keith A. Jolley

1. Introduction

It has recently become apparent that many bacterial populations undergo extremely high levels of horizontal genetic exchange, such that traditional clonal models of bacterial diversity are now inadequate ***(1–3)***. Such recombination is especially apparent in naturally transformable bacteria such as members of the genus *Neisseria* ***(4)***. This has implications for epidemiology, because it is not possible to assign accurate phylogenies to isolates by looking at variation at a single genetic locus if that locus, or part of it, is randomly exchanged within the population ***(5)***. Further, apparent phylogenies based on data from different loci are likely to be in disagreement with each other ***(6)***. The study of antigen genes, although undoubtedly useful for short-term epidemiology, provides limited information for longer-term analysis of the relatedness of strains as they are under immune selection and hence levels of recombination and mutation proximal to such genes are likely to be significantly higher than around other sites ***(7,8)***.

For these reasons, the indexing of neutral variation of housekeeping genes in a typing system is desirable. The use of multiple genetic markers, distributed around the genome provides both a discriminating and robust means of determining strain diversity. The first major technique to characterize the neutral variation at housekeeping loci was multi-locus enzyme electrophoresis (MLEE) ***(9)***. This approach indexes variations in metabolic enzymes by differences in their electrophoretic mobility in starch gels and has been applied to the population biology of a range of pathogens ***(9–11)***.

Unfortunately, MLEE has a number of disadvantages that has prevented its universal use. On a practical level, the technique requires a relatively high investment

From: *Methods in Molecular Medicine, vol. 67: Meningococcal Disease: Methods and Protocols*
Edited by: A. J. Pollard and M. C. J. Maiden © Humana Press Inc., Totowa, NJ

in training to set up and results are not easily portable among laboratories; for example, in order to compare results, a number of reference standards need to be run alongside the samples. More fundamentally, the electrophoretic profile is an indirect measure of the genetic change and much diversity at the primary sequence level will be missed as small differences may not alter the rate of migration *(12)*.

Multi-locus sequence typing (MLST) *(13)* has all the advantages of MLEE but improves on it in a number of ways. In MLST, fragments of housekeeping genes, approx 430–500 bp in length are sequenced. Nucleotide-sequence data are the most fundamental measure of genetic diversity and require no specialist interpretation and no reference standards. Additionally, the data are truly portable and are easily stored and transmitted. The MLST approach assigns unique numbers to alleles in the order that they are discovered, with no assumptions about relatedness made based on the similarity of individual allele sequences. This is because in bacterial populations with high levels of recombination, alleles with multiple differences may be generated by a single recombination event. Consequently, alleles with a small number of point mutations may have undergone more change than one with a large number of differences.

As nucleotide sequence-determination technology continues to improve, the technique is becoming cheaper and more accessible. Sequence data can be submitted to the MLST web site (http://mlst.zoo.ox.ac.uk) to assign alleles and sequence types (allelic profiles) and to determine whether an isolate belongs to a particular clonal group. The MLST data gathered to date for *Neisseria meningitidis* has provided further evidence of the nonclonal nature of the organism. Phylogenetic trees constructed from individual housekeeping loci are not congruent with each other or with phylogenies determined from allelic profiles, confirming that recombination must be occurring frequently. The use of MLST to study populations not intimately associated with disease should provide insights into the underlying population structure of the organism and will enable inferences on its evolution to be made. Historically, strain collections have largely focused on disease-causing isolates, leading to an overly narrow view on the inter-relationships between strains. Current studies on neisserial carrier populations will begin to address these issues.

In the *N. meningitidis* MLST scheme, internal fragments of the following seven housekeeping genes are amplified and sequenced: *abcZ* (putative ABC transporter), *adk* (adenylate kinase), *aroE* (shikimate dehydrogenase), *fumC* (fumarate hydratase), *gdh* (glucose-6-phosphate dehydrogenase), *pdhC* (pyruvate dehydrogenase subunit), and *pgm* (phosphoglucomutase). Nested sequencing primers are used as they generally produce better sequencing results and nonspecific amplified products are not sequenced. They also allow the use of

Table 1
Primers Used in MLST Amplification Reactions

Gene	Forward primer 5′-3′ sequence	Reverse primer 5′-3′ sequence
abcZ	AATCGTTTATGTACCGCAGG	GTTGATTTCTGCCTGTTCGG
adk	ATGGCAGTTTGTGCAGTTGG	GATTTAAACAGCGATTGCCC
aroE	ACGCATTTGCGCCGACATC	ATCAGGGCTTTTTTCAGGTT
fumC	CACCGAACACGACACGATGG	ACGACCAGTTCGTCAAACTC
gdh	ATCAATACCGATGTGGCGCGT	GGTTTTCATCTGCGTATAGAG
pdhC	GGTTTCCAACGTATCGGCGAC	ATCGGCTTTGATGCCGTATTT
pgm	CTTCAAAGCCTACGACATCCG	CGGATTGCTTTCGATGACGGC

lower-stringency conditions to amplify the gene fragments, which increases sensitivity.

2. Materials

2.1. Polymerase Chain Reaction

1. Oligonucleotide primers: The primers in **Table 1** are used to amplify internal fragments from the seven housekeeping genes. The primers are synthesized commercially on a 0.2 μmol scale and come dissolved in 1 mL of water. Concentrations of these stocks vary but are generally in the range 75–125 μ*M*. Working stocks (10 μ*M*) are prepared by dilution in Milli-Q water and stored at –20°C. Multiple lots should be stored to minimize freeze/thaw cycles.
2. AmpliTaq DNA polymerase (PE Biosystems, Cat no. N808-0153, supplied at 5 U/μL) and 10X reaction buffer II (500 m*M* KCl, 100 m*M* Tris-HCl, pH 8.3), lacking $Mg2^+$, supplied with the enzyme. The enzyme is stored at –20°C.
3. 5 m*M* dNTP solution: 1.25 m*M* dATP, 1.25 m*M* dCTP, 1.25 m*M* dGTP, and 1.25 m*M* dTTP in deionized water. We use a dNTP set supplied by PE Biosystems (Cat. no. N808-0260). The dNTPs are supplied in a single solution at individual concentrations of 2.5 m*M*. This is diluted with an equal volume of Milli-Q water to make the working stock. The stock is stored at –20°C and multiple freeze-thaw cycles are avoided.
4. 25 m*M* $MgCl_2$. Supplied by PE Biosystems with the enzyme.
5. Genomic DNA template: A boiled thick suspension of *N. meningitidis* cells in water may be used directly for PCR. For long-term storage, we prefer to extract total DNA using the Isoquick Nucleic Acid Extraction Kit (Orca Research Inc., Cat. no. MXT-020-100), following the manufacturer's instructions.
6. Individual 0.2-mL thin-walled tubes (Axygen, Cat. no. 321-02-101) or Thermo-fast 48-well plates (ABgene, Cat. no. AB-0648) for carrying out the reaction. The 48-well plates can be sealed with polymerase chain reaction (PCR) adhesive sealing sheets (ABgene, Cat. no. AB-0558).

Table 2
Primers Used in MLST Sequencing Reactions

Gene	Forward primer 5′-3′ sequence	Reverse primer 5′-3′ sequence
abcZ	AATCGTTTATGTACCGCAGG	GAGAACGAGCCGGGATAGGA
adk	AGGCTGGCACGCCCTTGG	CAATACTTCGGCTTTCACGG
aroE	GCGGTCAAYACGCTGATT*	ATGATGTTGCCGTACACATA
fumC	TCCGGCTTGCCGTTTGTCAG	TTGTAGGCGGTTTTGGCGAC
gdh	CCTTGGCAAAGAAAGCCTGC	GCGCACGGATTCATATGG
pdhC	TCTACTACATCACCCTGATG	ATCGGCTTTGATGCCGTATTT
pgm	CGGCGATGCCGACCGCTTGG	GGTGATGATTTCGGTTGCGCC

*Y – C/T degenerate base.

2.2. Agarose Gel Electrophoresis of the PCR Products

1. 6X Loading buffer: 0.25% (w/v) bromophenol blue, 0.25% (w/v) xylene cyanol FF, 40% (w/v) sucrose in deionized water.
2. Agarose (Helena Biosciences, Cat. no. 8201-07).
3. TBE buffer: A 10X stock (0.89 *M* Tris borate, pH 8.3, 20 m*M* EDTA) can be purchased from National Diagnostics (Cat. no. EC-860)
4. 10 mg/mL Ethidium bromide (Sigma, Cat. no. E-1510). This agent is a mutagen and should be handled in a contained area by personnel wearing suitable protective clothing. The chemical is stored at room temperature in the dark.
5. DNA molecular weight markers (Promega 100 bp DNA ladder, Cat. no. G2101).

2.3. Purification of PCR Products

1. Polyethylene glycol (PEG) 8000 (Sigma, Cat. no. P-4463).
2. Sodium chloride (Sigma, Cat. no. S-7653).
3. Ethanol: 70% (analytical grade) in Milli-Q water.
4. 1.5-mL Microcentrifuge tubes (Axygen, Cat. no. 311-04-051).

2.4. Sequencing Reactions

1. Oligonucleotide primers: The primers in **Table 2** are used to sequence the amplified gene fragments. As with the amplification primers, 10 μ*M* stocks are prepared. For sequencing, these stocks are diluted 1:16 with Milli-Q water (625 nM final). All stocks are stored at –20°C and freeze/thaw cycles are minimized.
2. BigDye Terminator Cycle Sequencing Ready Reaction Kit with AmpliTaq DNA polymerase, FS (PE Biosystems, Cat. no. 4303152).
3. Ethanol: 70% and 95% (analytical grade) in Milli-Q water.
4. Individual 0.2-mL thin-walled tubes (as for PCR) or Thermo-fast 96-well plates (ABgene, Cat. no. AB-0600) for carrying out the reaction. The 96-well plates can be sealed with PCR adhesive sealing sheets.

Table 3
PCR Mixture for One 50 mL Reaction[a]

Reagent	Volume (μL)	Final concentration
10X Reaction buffer	5.0	1X
PCR primer 1 (10 μ*M*)	5.0	1 μ*M*
PCR primer 2 (10 μ*M*)	5.0	1 μ*M*
$MgCl_2$ (25 m*M*)	3.0	1.5 m*M*
dNTP mix (5 m*M* total)	8.0	800 μ*M* (total)
Deionized water	23.3	—
Taq DNA polymerase	0.25	1.25 U

[a]A master mix is prepared by multiplying these volumes by the required number of reactions. 49.5 μL of the master mix is pipetted into reaction tubes and 0.5 μL template DNA added.

3. Methods

3.1. Polymerase Chain Reaction

3.1.1. Reactions in Individual Tubes

1. Prepare a master mix based on the volumes in **Table 3** (which shows volumes for a single 50 μL reaction). Prepare enough master mix for the number of reactions required, including a negative control, plus one extra.
2. Dispense 49.5 μL of the mix into each 0.2-mL thin-walled PCR tube.
3. Inoculate with 0.5 μL of genomic DNA, boiled cell suspension or water for the negative control.
4. Subject the reaction tubes to thermocycling in either an MJ Research PTC-200 or a PE Applied Biosystems 9700 thermal cycler as follows: an initial denaturation is carried out at 94°C for 2 min, followed by 30–35 cycles of 94°C for 1 min, 55°C for 1 min and 72°C for 1 min. A final extension step of 72°C for 2 min follows before the tubes are kept at 4°C until the machine is switched off.

3.1.2. Reactions in 48-Well Plates

1. Label the plate using a permanent marker so that its orientation can be determined.
2. Prepare a master mix using the volumes in **Table 4**. This makes enough for 50 reactions of 25 μL each.
3. Pipet 24.5 μL of this mixture into each well of the plate.
4. Inoculate all but one of the wells with 0.5 μL of genomic DNA. The remaining well acts as a negative control to test for contamination.
5. Subject the reaction plate to thermocycling in the same way as for individual tubes.

Table 4
PCR Master Mix for Reactions in 48-Well Plates[a]

Reagent	Volume (μL)	Final concentration
10X Reaction buffer	125	1X
PCR primer 1 (10 μ*M*)	125	1 μ*M*
PCR primer 2 (10 μ*M*)	125	1 μ*M*
$MgCl_2$ (25 m*M*)	75	1.5 m*M*
dNTP mix (5 m*M* total)	200	800 μ*M* (total)
Deionized water	581.3	—
Taq DNA polymerase	6.25	1.25 U

[a]24.5 μL of the master mix is pipetted into each well; 0.5 μL of template DNA is then added.

3.2. Agarose Gel Electrophoresis of the PCR Products

1. Mix one-tenth of the reaction mixture (5 μL for individual tubes or 2.5 μL for 48-well plates) with 1 μL of 6X loading buffer and load onto an agarose gel for electrophoresis. The gel consists of 1% (w/v) agarose in 1X TBE buffer and contains 0.5 μg/mL ethidium bromide. Load an additional lane with DNA molecular weight markers.
2. Perform electrophoresis at ~5 V/cm (measured as the distance between the electrodes) until the dyes in the loading buffer have separated 2–4 cm.
3. Visualize the gel under ultraviolet (UV) light to confirm the presence of a single band in the inoculated reactions. If a band is present in the negative control, there is contamination in the reactions and they must all be discarded.

3.3. Purification of PCR Products

3.3.1. Reactions in Individual Tubes

1. Transfer the contents of each reaction tube to 1.5-mL microcentrifuge tubes and make up the volumes of reactions to 100 μL by the addition of 50 μL Milli-Q water.
2. Add 60 μL of a 20% (w/v) PEG 8000, 2.5 *M* NaCl solution to each tube and mix by vortexing briefly.
3. Incubate the tubes at either 37°C for 15 min, 20°C for 30 min or at 4°C overnight. Longer incubations do not have a detrimental effect on the clean-up procedure.
4. Spin down the precipitated PCR products at maximum speed (~13,000*g*) in a microcentrifuge for 10 min. Remove as much of the supernatants as possible with an automatic pipet and then wash the pellets by the addition of 0.5 mL 70% ice-cold ethanol. Spin the tubes again (with no mixing) at maximum speed for a further 5 min. Remove as much of the ethanol as possible, as before, and then dry the DNA pellet either with a SpeedVac for approx 5 min, or by air-drying.

5. The pellets can be stored dry at –20°C indefinitely. Prior to sequencing, resuspend in 10–15 µL Milli-Q water or equivalent.

3.3.2 Reactions in 48-Well Plates

1. Following thermal cycling, make the reactions up to 50 µL by the addition of 25 µL Milli-Q water.
2. Add 60 µL of a 20% (w/v) PEG_{8000}, 2.5 *M* NaCl solution to each well using a multi-channel, multi-dispensary automatic pipet. Reseal the plate tightly and then mix vigorously using a vortex mixer. Centrifuge the plate briefly at low speed (500*g*) to ensure that all the mixture is at the bottom of the wells.
3. Incubate the plate as for individual tubes –37°C for 15 min, 20°C for 30 min or at 4°C overnight.
4. Spin down the precipitated PCR products by centrifuging at 2750*g* at 4°C for 1 h.
5. For the rest of the clean-up procedure, care must be taken not to agitate the plates in any way as the pellets may become dislodged. Remove the plate seal and discard the supernatant immediately by spinning the plate upside-down on to a piece of cut-to-size Whatman chromatography paper at 500*g* for 1 min.
6. Wash the DNA pellets twice by adding 150 µL of 70% ice-cold ethanol, spinning at 2750*g* at 4°C for a further 10 min and then discarding the supernatants as before.
7. Re-seal the plate. This can be stored dry at –20°C indefinitely. Prior to sequencing, resuspend the DNA pellets in 5 µL Milli-Q water. To aid re-suspension, vortex the plate briefly and spin down at low speed to ensure the solution is at the bottom of the wells.

3.4. Nucleotide-Sequence Determination

We use the PE Applied Biosystems BigDye terminators, which are suitable for use on the ABI Prism 310, ABI Prism 377, and ABI Prism 3700 automated sequencing machines. They may also be used with ABI 373 sequencers with an ABI Prism BigDye filter wheel installed. Sequencing on other systems will require the use of different chemistries and users should refer to the documentation supplied with the machine. For each PCR template, two sequencing reactions are required: one each for the forward and reverse strands. We use 1/4 sized (5 µL) reactions (*see* **Note 5**).

3.4.1. Reactions in Individual Tubes

1. Label 0.2-mL thin-walled PCR reaction tubes appropriately with a permanent marker pen.
2. Add 2 µL of the forward primer (625 nM) into half the tubes. Add 2 µL of the reverse to the other tubes.

3. Add 2 μL of BigDye Ready Reaction Termination Mix to all tubes.
4. Add 1 μL of each PCR product to the appropriate tube, so that each PCR product is present in two separate reactions, one with the forward primer and one with the reverse.
5. Centrifuge the tubes briefly to ensure the mixtures are at the bottom and then place in the thermal cycler.
6. Perform thermal cycling using the following program: 25 cycles of 96°C for 10 s, 50°C for 5 s, and 60°C for 2 min. The thermal cycler should then cool tubes to 4°C until they are removed from the machine.

3.4.2. Reactions in 96-Well Plates

The use of multi-dispensing automatic pipets (multi-channel if appropriate) is highly recommended for 96-well plate set-up.

1. On the left-hand half (48 wells) of the 96-well plate, add 2 μL of the forward primer (625 nM). Add 2 μl (l of the reverse primer to the right-hand half).
2. Add 2 μL of BigDye Ready Reaction Termination Mix to all the wells.
3. Using a multi-channel automatic pipet, transfer 1 μL of each PCR reaction directly from the PCR plate to the sequencing plate, with each PCR template going to the same relative position on both the left- and right-hand sides of the plate.
4. Move the reaction components towards the bottom of the wells by gently tapping the plate on to the workbench. Tightly seal the plate with an adhesive sheet (*see* **Note 6**) and centrifuge briefly to ensure that all the liquid is at the bottom before placing in the thermal cycler.
5. Use the same thermal cycling program as for sequencing in tubes.

3.5. Purification of Sequencing Reactions

There are a number of different protocols suitable for cleaning up sequencing reactions, and which one works best for any particular set-up may need to be determined empirically. Precipitation methods are cheap and fast, but may leave behind some unincorporated dye-labeled terminators. Commercial spin columns cost more and the procedure may take longer, but they should remove more of the terminators. In our hands, ethanol precipitation yields very good results. The procedure detailed below should yield products suitable for loading on all machines.

3.5.1. Reactions in Individual Tubes

1. Make up individual reactions to 36 μL with Milli-Q water, i.e., for 1/4 scale (5 μL) reactions, add 31 μL water. Transfer the mixtures to 1.5-mL microcentrifuge tubes.

2. Add 64 μL of 95% ethanol, vortex the tube briefly and then incubate at 20°C for 15–30 min.
3. Spin the tubes at maximum speed in a microcentrifuge for 30 min. After spinning, aspirate the supernatants immediately with an automatic pipet.
4. Wash the pellets by the addition of 500 μL ice-cold 70% ethanol (no mixing) and spin again at maximum speed for 10 min. Remove as much of the ethanol as possible with an automatic pipet and then vacuum or air-dry the pellets for a few minutes. The dried pellets can be stored at –20°C until ready for loading when they are resuspended in 3–4 μL of the appropriate loading buffer for the sequencing machine to be used.

3.5.2. Reactions in 96-Well Plates

1. Make up reactions to 36 μL with Milli-Q water, preferably using a multi-channel automatic pipet.
2. Add 64 μL of 95% ethanol to each well. Re-seal the plate tightly and vortex briefly to mix. Centrifuge the plate briefly to ensure that all the mixture is at the bottom. Incubate at 20°C for 15–30 min.
3. Centrifuge the plate at 2750*g* at 4°C for 1 h. Remove the adhesive cover immediately after spinning and gently invert the plate onto tissues or blue roll. Spin the plate inverted on to a piece of cut-to-size Whatman chromatography paper at 500*g* for 1 min to remove any residual ethanol from the wells.
4. Add 150 μL of 70% ice-cold ethanol to each well. Re-seal the plate and centrifuge at 2750*g* at 4°C for 10 min. Remove the ethanol by inversion, as before. Remove residual ethanol by spinning on to Whatman paper at 500*g* for 1 min. The plate can be stored at –20°C until ready for loading when the samples are resuspended in an appropriate volume of loading buffer as above.

3.6. Assembly of Sequence Traces and Determination of Allele Numbers and Sequence Types

Sequence assembly can be performed using a variety of computer packages available for different platforms. We recommend the use of Staden ***(14)*** which is available free for noncommercial use on UNIX platforms. Sequences need to be trimmed to the correct size so that they correspond exactly to the region used to define alleles. The sizes and an example allele of each locus are shown in the appendix. Alleles and sequence types can be assigned by interrogating the MLST database (at http://mlst.zoo.ox.ac.uk), where instructions can be found also for submitting new data.

4. Notes

1. To avoid problems of contamination with the PCR, we routinely set up reactions in a class II laminar flow hood, used exclusively for the task. Designated auto-

matic pipets are also used, which never come into contact with amplified DNA. We also recommend the use of filter tips.

2. For high-throughput sequencing, genomic DNA from 47 strains can be added to a 48-well plate, leaving room for the negative control. This enables rapid inoculation of PCR reactions using a multi-channel pipet. This plate can be used to inoculate the reactions for each of the seven housekeeping loci or any other genes required. In our hands, using such a method, it is possible to set up four loci sets of reactions (188 individual reactions) in approx 1 hr.
3. For routine samples, it is not always necessary to run every PCR product on an agarose gel. As long as the negative control is tested for contamination, a few samples (~5) may be run to verify that the reactions have worked, i.e., that there are no omissions to the master mix and that the thermal cycler is performing correctly. Often we only run the gel for about 10 min, which is sufficient to determine whether there is a PCR product or not. The gel can be re-used many times for this purpose.
4. After centrifuging with inverted plates containing the PEG/NaCl solution, care must be taken to wipe the carrier buckets and inner surfaces of the centrifuge to prevent corrosion.
5. For sequencing, we find that using 1/4 sized reactions (i.e., 2 μL of BigDye) produces robust results with our equipment. Better sequence electropherograms may be achieved with 1/2 scale or even full-size reactions, although the cost increases are significant. Use of automated set-up procedures, i.e., robotics, may enable reactions to be scaled down further. Cost savings may also be achieved by the use of BigDye dilution buffers, enabling lower concentrations of the reagent to be used, although we make no recommendation of their use.
6. When sealing the sequencing plate, it is important that the reaction components are not half-way up the sides of the wells. If they are, static on the adhesive sheet may cause the liquid to jump from the wells.
7. Some ethanol precipitation procedures use sodium acetate to help precipitate products. This is fine if the extension products are to be run on slab gel machines such as the 377. If capillary machines, such as the 3700, are used any residual salt left in the reactions will compete with the extension fragments during the electrokinetic injection, resulting in weak signals and eventual damage to the capillary array.
8. In the 95% ethanol precipitation of sequencing reaction-extension products, it is important that the ethanol concentration is accurate. It is recommended that nondenatured ethanol is purchased at a concentration of 95%. Absolute (100%) ethanol gradually absorbs water from the atmosphere, decreasing its concentration, so if this is to be diluted to 95%, it is better to use ethanol from a fresh, recently opened bottle.

5. Appendix

Example alleles from each housekeeping locus:

abcZ-1: 433 bp

TTTGATACTG	TTGCCGAAGG	TTTGGGCGAA	ATTCGCGATT	TATTGCGCCG
TTATCATCAT	GTCAGCCATG	AGTTGGAAAA	TGGTTCGAGT	GAGGCCTTAT
TGAAAGAGCT	CAACGAATTG	CAACTTGAGA	TCGAAGCGAA	GGACGGCTGG
AAGTTGGATG	CGGCGGTGAA	GCAGACTTTG	GGCGAACTCG	GTTTGCCGGA
AAACGAAAAA	ATCGGCAACC	TCTCCGGCGG	TCAGAAAAAG	CGCGTCGCCT
TGGCGCAGGC	TTGGGTGCAG	AAGCCCGACG	TATTGCTGCT	CGATGAACCG
ACCAACCATT	TGGACATCGA	CGCGATTATT	TGGTTGGAAA	ACCTGCTCAA
AGCGTTTGAA	GGCAGCCTGG	TTGTGATTAC	CCACGACCGC	CGTTTTTTGG
ACAATATCGC	CACGCGGATT	GTCGAACTCG	ATC	

adk-1: 465 bp

GAAGCGAAAA	AAATCATTGA	CGAAGGCGGC	TTGGTGCGCG	ACGACATCAT
TATCGGCATG	GTCAAAGAAC	GCATCGCGCA	AGACGACTGC	AAAAACGGTT
TCCTGTTCGA	CGGTTTCCCG	CGCACATTGG	CACAAGCCGA	AGCGATGGTT
GAAGCAGGCG	TGGATTTGGA	TGCAGTCGTT	GAAATCGACG	TGCCTGACAG
CGTGATTGTC	GACCGTATGA	GCGGCCGCCG	CGTGCATTTG	GCTTCCGGCC
GTACTTACCA	CGTTACCTAC	AACCCGCCCA	AAGTTGAAGG	CAAAGACGAC
GTAACCGGCG	AAGATTTGAT	TCAGCGCGAC	GACGACAAAG	AAGAAACCGT
GAAAAAACGC	CTTGCCGTTT	ACCACGAGCA	AACCGAAGTT	TTGGTCGATT
TTTACAGCAA	ACTGGAAGGC	GAACACGCGC	CTAAATATAT	CAAAGTTGAC
GGCACTCAGC	CGGTA			

aroE-1: 490 bp

TATCGGTTTG	GCCAACGACA	TCACGCAGGT	CAAAAACATT	GCCATCGAAG
GCAAAACCAT	CTTGCTTTTG	GGCGCGGGCG	GCGCGGTGCG	CGGCGTGATT
CCTGTTTTGA	AAGAACACCG	TCCTGCCCGT	ATCGTCATTG	CCAACCGCAC
CCACGCCAAA	GCCGAAGAAT	TGGCGCGGCT	TTTCGGCATT	GAAGCCGTCC
CGATGGCGGA	TGTGAACGGC	GGTTTTGATA	TCATCATCAA	CGGCACGTCC
GGCGGCTTGA	GCGGTCAGCT	TCCTGCCGTC	AGTCCTGAAA	TTTTCCTCGG
CTGCCGCCTT	GCCTACGATA	TGGTTTACGG	CGACGCGGCG	CAGGAGTTTT
TGAACTTTGC	CCAAAGCAAC	GGTGCGGCCG	AAGTTTCAGA	CGGACTGGGT
ATGCTGGTCG	GTCAAGCGGC	GGCTTCCTAC	GCCCTCTGGC	GCGGATTTAC
GCCCGATATC	CGCCCTGTTA	TCGAATACAT	GAAAGCCATG	

fumC-1: 465 bp

```
GAAGCCTTGG GCGGACGCGA TGCCGCCGTT GCCGCTTCGG GCGCATTGAA
AACGCTGGCG GCAAGCCTGA ATAAAATCGC CAACGACATC CGCTGGCTGG
CAAGCGGCCC GCGCTGCGGT TTGGGCGAAA TCAAAATCCC CGAAAACGAG
CCGGGTTCGT CCATCATGCC GGGCAAAGTC AACCCGACCC AATGCGAAGC
GATGACCATG GTGTGCTGCC AAGTGTTCGG CAACGACGTT ACCATCGGTA
TGGCGGGCGC GTCGGGCAAT TTCGAGCTGA ACGTCTATAT GCCCGTCATC
GCCTACAACC TCTTGCAATC CATCCGCCTG TTGGGCGACG CGTGCAACAG
CTTCAACGAA CACTGCGCCG TCGGCATTGA ACCCGTACCG GAAAAAATCG
ACTATTTCCT GCACCATTCC CTGATGCTCG TTACCGCGTT AAACCGCAAA
ATCGGTTACG AAAAC
```

gdh-1: 501 bp

```
ATGTTCGAGC CGCTTTGGAA CAATAAATAC ATCGAAAGCG TGCAGCTTAC
CATCGCCGAG CAGTTGGGCG TGGAAGAACG CGGCGAGTTT TACGACATTA
CCGGCGCGTT GCGCGATATG GTGCAAAACC ACTTGATGCA AATGCTGTGC
ATGACTGCGA TGGAAGCCCC CGCCAGCTTG GATGCCGACG CGGTGCGCGA
TGAAAAAGTC AAAGTCATCA AGTCATTGAA GCCGCTGACC GTCGAATCTG
TCAATGAAAA TGTCGTGCGC GGACAATATA CCGCCGCCAA AGGCATGAAC
GGCTATCTTG AAGAAATCAA CGTTCCGCAA GACAGCTTTA CCGAAACCTA
CGTCGCCATT AAAGCCGAAA TCGAAAACGA ACGCTGGAAG GGCGTTCCCT
TCTACCTGCG TACCGGCAAG CGCATGGCGG GCAAAGTGGC GGAAATCGTT
TTGAACTTCA AAGATTTGAA CAGCCATATT TTTGAAGGCA GTCGCACCGC
G
```

pdhC-1: 480 bp

```
ATGCCCGAAG GTGCGGAACA AGACATCTTG AAAGGTATGT ACCTGCTGAA
AGCCGGCGGC AAAGGCGACA AGAAAGTCCA ACTGATGGGT TCCGGTACGA
TTTTGCAAGA AGTGATTGCC GGTGCCGAGC TGCTGAAAGC CGACTTCGGC
GTGGAAGCAG ACATTTGGTC TTGCCCATCT TTCAACCTGT TGCATCGCGA
TGCTATCGAA GCAGAACGTT TCAACCGCCT GAATCCTTTG GAAACTGCAA
AAGTACCGTT TGTTACTTCT CAACTGCAAG GTCATGACGG CCCGGTGATT
GCCGCTACCG ACTATATCCG TAGCTATGCT GACCGCATCC GTGCCTACAT
CCCTAACGAC TACCACGTCT TGGGTACTGA CGGCTTCGGC CGCTCCGACA
GCCGTGCCAA CCTGCGTAGC TTCTTCGAAG TTGACCGCTA CAACGTTGCC
GTTGCTGCAT TGAGCGCATT GGCCGATCAA
```

pgm-1: 450 bp

```
GTGGTTACCA AAGACGGCAA CATTATTTAT CCCGACCGCC AACTGATGCT
GTTCGCCCAA GACGTTTTGA ACCGCAATCC CGGCGCGAAA GTCATTTTCG
ACGTGAAGTC CACCCGCCTG CTTGCGCCTT GGATTAAAGA ACACGGCGGC
AAAGCCATAA TGGAAAAAAC CGGCCACAGC TTTATCAAAT CCGCCATGAA
AGAAACCGGC GCGCCGGTTG CCGGCGAAAT GAGCGGACAC ATCTTCTTCA
AAGAACGCTG GTTCGGCTTC GACGACGGTC TGTACGCCGG CGCACGCCTC
TTGGAAATCC TGTCTGCCTC CGATAATCCG TCCGAAGTGT TAAACAACCT
GCCGCAAAGC ATTTCCACGC CCGAACTCAA CATCGCCCTG CCCGAAGGCA
GCAACGGCCA TCAGGTTATC AACGAACTCG CCGCCAAAGC CGAATTTGAA
```

Acknowledgments

The author would like to thank Martin Maiden and all the members of the Molecular Genetics group at the Wellcome Trust Centre for the Epidemiology of Infectious Disease, University of Oxford, for their support and advice.

References

1. Maynard Smith, J. (1991) The population genetics of bacteria. *Proc. R. Soc. Lond. B Biol. Sci.* **245,** 37–41.
2. Maynard Smith, J., Dowson, C. G., and Spratt, B. G. (1991) Localized sex in bacteria. *Nature* **349,** 29–31.
3. Maynard Smith, J., Smith, N. H., O'Rourke, M., and Spratt, B. G. (1993) How clonal are bacteria? *Proc. Natl. Acad. Sci. USA* **90,** 4384–4388.
4. Maiden, M. C. J. (1993) Population genetics of a transformable bacterium: the influence of horizontal genetical exchange on the biology of *Neisseria meningitidis. FEMS Microbiol. Lett.* **112,** 243–250.
5. Spratt, B. G. and Maiden, M. C. J. (1999) Bacterial population genetics, evolution and epidemiology. *Proc. R. Soc. Lond. B Biol. Sci.* **354,** 701–710.
6. Holmes, E. C., Urwin, R., and Maiden, M. C. J. (1999) The influence of recombination on the population structure and evolution of the human pathogen *Neisseria meningitidis. Mol. Biol. Evol.* **16,** 741–749.
7. Feavers, I. M., Heath, A. B., Bygraves, J. A., and Maiden, M. C. (1992) Role of horizontal genetic exchange in the antigenic variation of the class 1 outer membrane protein of *Neisseria meningitidis. Mol. Microbiol.* **6,** 489–495.
8. Li, J., Nelson, K., McWhorter, A. C., Whittam, T. S., and Selander, R. K. (1994) Recombinant basis of serovar diversity in *Salmonella enterica. Proc. Natl. Acad. Sci. USA* **91,** 2552–2556.
9. Selander, R. K., Caugant, D. A., Ochman, H., Musser, J. M., Gilmour, M. N., and Wittam, T. S. (1986) Methods of multilocus enzyme electrophoresis for bacterial population genetics and systematics. *Appl. Environ. Microbiol.* **51,** 837–884.
10. Ochman, H., Whittam, T. S., Caugant, D. A., and Selander, R. K. (1983) Enzyme polymorphism and genetic population structure in *Escherichia coli* and *Shigella. J. Gen. Microbiol.* **129,** 2715–2726.

11. Ochman, H. and Selander, R. K. (1984) Evidence for clonal population structure in *Escherichia coli*. *Proc. Natl. Acad. Sci. USA* **81,** 198–201.
12. Feil, E., Carpenter, G., and Spratt, B. G. (1996) Electrophoretic variation in adenylate kinase of *Neisseria meningitidis* is due to inter- and intraspecies recombination. *Proc. Natl. Acad. Sci. USA* **92,** 10,535–10,539.
13. Maiden, M. C. J., Bygraves, J. A., Feil, E., Morelli, G., Russell, J. E., Urwin, R., et al. (1998) Mutilocus sequence typing: a portable approach to the identification of clones within populations of pathogenic microorganisms. *Proc. Natl. Acad. Sci. USA* **95,** 3140–3145.
14. Staden, R. (1996) The Staden sequence analysis package. *Mol. Biotechnol.* **5,** 233–241.

13

Capsular Operons

Ulrich Vogel, Heike Claus, and Matthias Frosch

1. Introduction

The major factor determining the different pathogenicities of meningococci and their close relatives, the gonococci, is the polysaccharide capsule. The capsule protects meningococci from complement attack and phagocytosis and is indispensable for systemic spread of the bacteria during sepsis and meningitis *(1–5)*. The influence of the capsule on transmission of the bacteria, colonization of the human host, entry into the bloodstream, and passage of the blood-brain barrier (BBB), respectively, is less well-understood. Colonizing meningococci may be acapsular *(6,7)*, and at least in serogroup B meningococci, there is evidence that transient loss of encapsulation owing to genetic-switching mechanisms facilitates entry into epithelial cells *(8,9)*. Characterization of meningococcal capsules in disease and carrier isolates is important as part of the meningococcal typing scheme of outbreak isolates. Typing is performed to determine the transmission of index strains. Capsular serogrouping is of particular importance in the assessment of the suitability of vaccination in outbreak management (reviewed in **ref.** ***10***). This chapter describes serological and molecular techniques used for the determination of serogroups and capsular genotypes.

1.1. Capsular Polysaccharides

Until now, 12 capsular serogroups have been described (reviewed in **ref.** ***11***). The serogroups differ in the chemical composition of the capsules, and thus in the reactivity with specific antisera. Sialic acid is a component of the polysaccharide in serogroups B, C, W135, and Y *(12–15)*. Meningococcal disease isolates from blood, the cerebrospinal fluid (CSF), or respiratory samples usually express the capsular serogroups A, B, C, W135, and Y, respectively. These serogroups are also found among colonizing nasopharyngeal isolates. However, carrier isolates may

From: *Methods in Molecular Medicine, vol. 67: Meningococcal Disease: Methods and Protocols*
Edited by: A. J. Pollard and M. C. J. Maiden © Humana Press Inc., Totowa, NJ

be acapsular, or express capsules other than A, B, C, W135, or Y *(16)*. Serogroup B and C meningococci, which cause the majority of cases of meningococcal disease in the Northern hemisphere, express homopolymers of sialic acid (α-2,8- and α-2,9-linked polysialic acid, respectively). Because the mammalian neural cell adhesion molecule (N-CAM) carries α-2,8-linked polysialic acid as a post-translational modification *(17)*, the serogroup B capsule, in contrast to the serogroup A, C, W135, and Y capsules, is poorly immunogenic, and no vaccines based on the serogroup B polysaccharide antigen have been designed to date. Serogroup W135 and Y meningococci express heteropolymeric polysialic acid capsules, in which the sialic acid residue is linked to galactose and glucose, respectively *(14)*. Naturally occurring isogenic derivatives of virulent serogroup C meningococci, which express the serogroup W135 and Y capsule, are less serum-resistant than their parent strains (U. Vogel, unpublished). This finding might explain why serogroup W135 and Y meningococci are less frequently associated with systemic disease in Europe than serogroup B and C meningococci *(18)*. The capsular polysaccharide of serogroup A meningococci, which cause large outbreaks of meningococcal disease in Africa (reviewed in **ref.** *19*), does not consist of sialic acid, but of α-1,6-linked N-acetyl-D-mannosamine-1-phosphate *(20)*. This polymer is immunogenic in humans.

1.2. Antibodies to Capsular Polysaccharides

One means to determine the capsular serogroup of meningococci in a microbiological laboratory is the detection by specific antibodies to the bacterial surface. This can be achieved most easily by the use of latex-bead agglutination (*see* Chapter 4) *(21)* or by enzyme-linked immunosorbent assays (ELISA) (*see* Chapter 9) *(6)*. Agglutination is much more rapid than the ELISA technique, but may give rise to nonspecific results, because poly-agglutination with several serogroup-specific antibodies may occur. A variety of antibodies directed to diverse meningococcal capsules has been published *(21–26)*. In this chapter, we will describe the use of the monoclonal antibody (MAb) NmeB 735 in an ELISA format. MAb NmeB 735 is one of few class IgG antibodies directed against α-2,8-linked polysialic acid, which binds with high affinity to the serogroup B capsule as well as to glycosylated N-CAM *(25,27)*. Colony-blot analysis allows the investigation of a large number of colonies in mixed populations, which is used for scientific purposes. Therefore, colony-blot analysis of the serogroup B capsule is described in this chapter as well.

1.3. Molecular Techniques for the Determination of the Capsular Genotype

1.3.1. Organization of Capsular Operons

The genes required for the expression of a capsular polysaccharide in meningococci are clustered in the *cps* locus *(28)*. To our current knowledge, the organization of *cps* is comparable in serogroup A, B, C, W135, and Y meningococci ***(28–32)***. According to the data of the *Neisseria meningitidis* sequencing group at the Sanger Centre, UK ***(32)*** the *cps* of the serogroup A strains comprises 22,877-bp, and 22 open reading frames (orfs). In accordance to previously published data, 7 regions are observed (**Fig. 1**):

1. The *siaA-D* genes ***(31–34)*** (synonymous *synA-D*) of the region A encode enzymes responsible for the synthesis of polysialic acid in serogroup B, C, W135, and Y meningococci. The *mynA-D* genes in serogroup A meningococci are needed for the synthesis of the serogroup A polysaccharide ***(30)***.
2. Region C: this region is composed of four orfs (*ctrA-D*) responsible for capsular transport across the bacterial membranes ***(29,35,36)***. Genes of this regions have been successfully used to establish the detection of meningococcal DNA in clinical samples ***(37)*** (*see* also Chapter 3).
3. Region B: this region comprises the *lip* genes responsible for phospholipid substitution of the polysaccharide ***(35)***. This region is found adjacent to the region D′ in serogroup A meningococci (**Fig. 1**).
4. Region D is not involved in capsular synthesis. In contrast, deletion of the region D will alter the LPS structure ***(38–40)***. The region D is found in gonococci as well ***(41,42)***.
5. Region D′: this region probably resulted from duplication of the region D in meningococci ***(42)***.
6. Region D′ is followed by three orfs, which exhibit homologies to methyltransferase genes.
7. Region E: this region comprises one orf of unknown function ***(28)***, which also occurs in gonococci. The deduced amino acid sequence is more than 50% identical to the regulatory protein Tex of *Bordetella pertussis* (GenBank accession number Q45388) ***(43)***.

1.3.2. Theoretical Basis for the Molecular Analysis of the Capsular Genotype

The region A of the *cps* harbors genes responsible for the synthesis of capsular polysaccharide. Therefore, the determination of the capsular genotype relies on the amplification of serogroup-specific genes within the region A. The *myn* genes of the region A are unique to the serogroup A, and they can be used for the analysis of the serogroup A capsular operon ***(30)***. The *siaA-C* genes of serogroup B, C, W135, and Y meningococci are similar, because they are necessary for the synthesis of the essential component of the polysaccharides, the sialic acid ***(31,34)***. Therefore, distinction of these serogroups has to rely on the serogroup-specific *siaD* genes ***(6,37,44,45)***. The *siaD* genes of serogroup B and C meningococci are 64.4% identical ***(31,34)***. These genes are unrelated to the *siaD* genes of serogroup W135 and Y meningococci, which

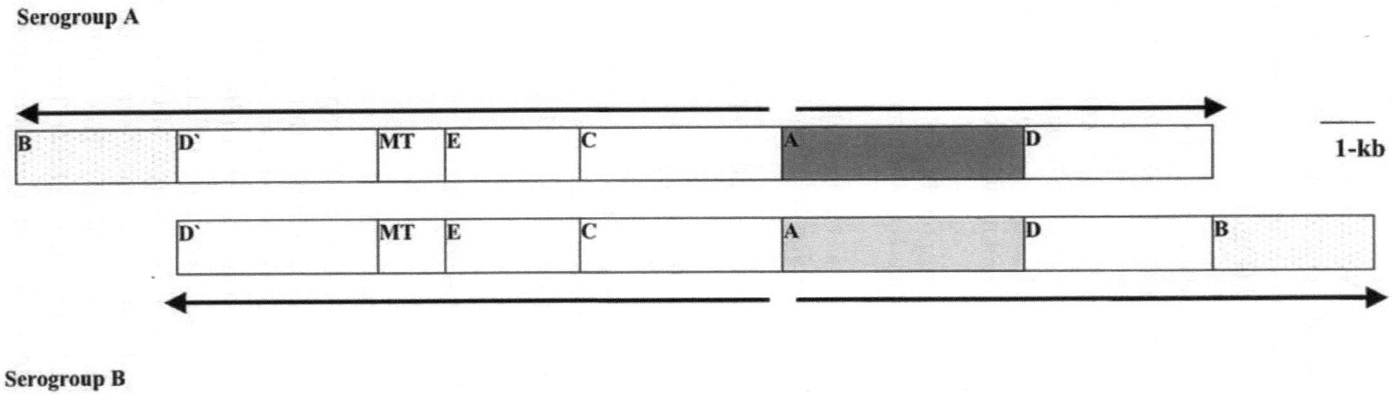

Fig. 1. Comparison of the *cps* loci of the strains Z2491 (serogroup A) and B1940 (serogroup B). The *cps* of strain Z2491 was deduced from data of the *Neisseria meningitidis* sequencing group at the Sanger Centre ***(32)***. The structure of the *cps* of the serogroup B strain B1940 was deduced from several publications ***(28,29,33,35,36,38,42)***. B1940 was selected to illustrate a differing location of the region B obvious in some meningococcal strains. The arrows indicate the direction of transcription of the genes. The letters represent the nomenclature of the regions of *cps*, MT indicates genes with homologies to methyltransferase genes inserted between the regions E and D′. The differences between the regions A of both serogroups are demonstrated by different colors.

share more than 98% identity *(31)*. There is one polymorphic region, between nucleotides 885 and 1,029 of the 3,114-bp *siaD* genes, which distinguishes the serogroup W135 and Y *siaD* genes. By the analysis of serogroup W135 and Y meningococci derived from several genetically diverse sequence types, we could demonstrate that these polymorphisms are serogroup-specific, and that they can be used to distinguish serogroup W135 and Y meningococci (U. Vogel, M. Achtman, H. Claus, unpublished).

1.3.3. Necessity of Capsular Genotyping

Why is the molecular analysis of the capsular genotype mandatory to complete the serological analysis of the serogroup? When we investigated healthy contacts of a patient with meningococcal disease, we observed that 5 of 10 meningococcal carrier isolates were not serogroupable with antibodies directed against the serogroups B, C, W135, and Y, respectively *(6)*. Of the five nongroupable isolates, three possessed the region A either of the serogroup C or of the serogroup Y. This example indicates that a comprehensive serogroup analysis of carrier isolates needs molecular techniques. The acapsular phenotype might be reversible, and two mechanisms of a reversible loss of encapsulation have been described: 1) integration of an insertion element into the region A *(8)*, and 2) slipped-strand mispairing inside the *siaD* gene *(9)*. Therefore, even pathogenic isolates after transmission from the patient to a healthy contact might appear transiently in an acapsular phenotype.

2. Materials

2.1. ELISA

1. Microtiter plates.
2. Phosphate-buffered saline (PBS): 10 m*M* K_2HPO_4/KH_2PO_4, pH 7.4, 0.15 *M* NaCl.
3. Poly-D-lysine: 25 μg/mL in PBS.
4. Glutaraldehyde: 0.05 % in PBS.
5. First antibody: MAb NmeB 735 *(25)* (the antibody can be obtained from Dade Behring Marburg GmbH, P.O. Box 11 49, 35001 Marburg, Germany, if the investigator signs an investigator´s declaration regulating the use of the antibody. At our institute, limited amounts of MAb NmeB 735 ascites fluid prepared years ago is still in use.).
6. Second antibody: peroxidase-conjugated goat anti-mouse IgG+IgM (H+L) (Jackson ImmunoResearch Laboratories, West Grove, PA).
7. Color-development substrate: One ABTS® (2,2′-Azino-di-[3-ethylbenzthiazoline sulfonate (6)] diammonium salt) tablet is dissolved in 5 mL ABTS® buffer (Roche, Mannheim, Germany, Cat. no. 1112422 and 1112597). Safety note: ABTS is an irritant substance.
8. Titertek Multiskan (ICN Biochemicals, Costa Mesa, CA).

2.2. Colony Blot

1. Nitrocellulose-membrane filter (pore size 0.45 μm).
2. Whatman filter paper 3 MM.
3. Denaturing solution: 0.5 *N* NaOH. Safety note: NaOH is a corrosive substance.
4. Neutralizing solution: 0.5 *M* Tris-HCL, pH 7.5, 1.5 *M* NaCl.
5. 20x SSPE: 3.6 *M* NaCl, 0.1 *M* Na_2HPO_4, 0.1 *M* NaH_2PO_4 and 0.02 *M* EDTA.
6. 70% ethanol. Safety note: ethanol is highly flammable.
7. PBS: 10 m*M* K_2HPO_4/KH_2PO_4, pH 7.4, 0.15 *M* NaCl.
8. PBS/1% bovine serum albumin (BSA).
9. PBS/0.2% BSA.
10. First antibody: MAb NmeB 735 ***(25)*** (*see* **Subheading 2.1.**).
11. Second antibody: alkaline phosphatase-conjugated goat anti-mouse IgG + IgM (H + L) (Jackson ImmunoResearch Laboratories, West Grove, PA).
12. 0.1 *M* Tris-HCl, pH 9.6.
13. Color-development substrate: 9 mL 0.1 *M* Tris-HCl, pH 9.6, 20 μL 2 *M* $MgCl_2$, 1 mL 0.1% NBT (4-Nitro blue tetrazolium chloride) dissolved in 0.1 *M* Tris-HCl, pH 9.6, 100 μL 0.5% BCIP (5-bromo-4-chloro-3-indolyl-phosphate) dissolved in 0.1 *M* Tris-HCl, pH 9.6.

2.3. Polymerase Chain Reaction

1. Oligonucleotide primers: Oligonucleotide stocks (100 pmol/μL) are prepared in distilled, deionized water and stored at –20°C for 6 mo. Working dilutions (20 pmol/μL) are stored at –20°C for 1 mo. The primers and their target genes are listed in **Table 1**. The primer combinations used for the serogroup detection are given in **Table 2**.
2. dNTP solution: Lyophilized dNTPs are dissolved in distilled, deionized water to a final concentration of 100 m*M* and stored at –20°. The stock solutions are diluted 1:50 using distilled, deionized water to yield the working solution containing 2 m*M* of each dNTP. Aliquots of the working solution are stored at –20°C.
3. Ampli*Taq*® DNA polymerase (5 U/μL) is supplied with 10X PCR buffer II (100 m*M* Tris-HCl, pH 8.3 [at 25°C], 500 m*M* KCl) and 25 m*M* $MgCl_2$ solution (PE Biosystems, Foster City, CA, Cat. no. N808-0156). All solutions are stored at –20°C.
4. Templates: Suspensions of heat-killed meningococci are used. Bacteria are suspended in PBS ($OD_{600\ nm}$ 1–2) and killed by heating for 10 min at 100°C. Stock solutions are stored at –20°C. Dilutions of 1:10 serve as PCR templates. Safety note: Strictly follow biosafety recommendations when working with *Neisseria meningitidis*.
5. Reaction tubes.
6. Thermal cycler.

2.4. Agarose-Gel Electrophoresis of the PCR Products

1. GEBS: 20% glycerol, 50 m*M* EDTA, 0,05% bromophenol blue, 0,5% N-lauroylsarcosin.

Table 1
Oligonucleotides

Oligonucleotide	Sequence (5′–3′)	Target	Position	Accession no.	Reference
NT2	ATACTTAATAACAGAAAATGGCG	*mynB*	1,605–1,627	GenBank AF019760	*(30)*
NT4	ATGATGGTAATGGGAAAAGAGT	*mynB*	3,222–3,201	GenBank AF019760	*(30)*
UE12	CGCCTTTGCATCTGTCGTAGC	*siaC*	2,861–2,881	EMBL M95053	*(29)*
UE13	GGAGATCAGAAGTCATAGTA	$siaD_B$ downstream	4,641–4,622	EMBL M95053	*(29)*
HC2	AAATCTATAAATTGACTC	$siaD_C$ upstream	94–75 nt upstream of *siaD*	Unpublished	
HC4	GGAGATTTGTTTAGCT	$siaD_C$ downstream	552–537 nt downstream of *siaD*	Unpublished	
HC39	GTGTATGATATTCCAATCGTTG	$siaD_{W135}$	1,103–1,124	EMBL Y13970	*(6,31)*
HC44	GGCTTTGGTTATATATTTCTAG	$siaD_Y$	1,073–1,094	EMBL Y13969	*(6,31)*
HC65	CGAGATTCATTGATGCCTTG	$siaD_{W135/Y}$	3,045–3,026	EMBL Y13969/70	*(31)*

Table 2
PCR Conditions

Serogroup	Primer combination	Annealing temperature (°C)	Fragment length (bp)	Extension time (s)
A	NT2/NT4	56	1,617	90
B	UE12/UE13	52	1,780	120
C	HC2/HC4	40	2,125	120
W	HC39/HC65	54	1,942	120
Y	HC44/HC65	54	1,972	120

2. DNA molecular-weight marker (e.g., 1 kb ladder, Life Technologies, Rockville, MD)
3. Agarose.
4. 1X TBE: 100 m*M* Tris, 100 m*M* boric acid, 2.5 m*M* EDTA. Safety note: boric acid is an irritant substance.
5. Horizontal gel electrophoresis chamber.
6. 50 mg/L ethidium bromide in distilled, deionized water. This agent is stored protected from light at room temperature. Safety note: ethidium bromide is mutagenic and therefore harmful. Carefully follow handling and storage instructions provided by your institution.
7. Transilluminator (λ = 312 nm).

3. Methods

3.1. ELISA

1. Incubate microtiter plates with 50 µL/well poly-D-lysine solution for 1 h at room temperature.
2. Wash three times with PBS and then incubate in a biosafety cabinet with 20 µL of bacterial suspensions in PBS (OD_{600nm}: 0.15) for 2 h. Prepare a positive control (e.g., serogroup B isolate MC58, *see* **Table 3**) and a negative control (e.g., serogroup C isolate 2120, *see* **Table 3**) in the same way. Use PBS/1% BSA for the blank value. Analyze all suspensions in duplicates or triplicates.
3. Cross-link bacteria to poly-D-lysine by adding 100 µL glutaraldehyde solution/well for 10 min.
4. Wash the plates three times with PBS and then block nonspecific binding sites with 150 µL of PBS/1% BSA for 1 h.
5. After washing three times, the plates are incubated with MAb NmeB 735 ascites fluid diluted 1:4,000 in PBS/1% BSA for 1.5 h (20 µL/well).
6. Wash three times with PBS prior to addition for 1 h of 20 µL/well of peroxidase-conjugated goat anti-mouse immunoglobulin diluted 1:2,500 in PBS/1% BSA.
7. Wash three times with PBS. Finally, add 20 µL substrate solution to each well and measure the absorbance at 414 nm after 10 min using a Titertek Multiskan. The absorbance of the positive control should be higher than 1,000 and the absor-

Table 3
Positive Controls for PCR

Serogroup	Reference strain	ET[a]	ST[b]	Reference
A	Z2491	Subgroup IV-1	4	***(46)***
B	MC58	ET-5 complex	Unknown	***(47)***
C	2120	ET-37 complex	11	***(6)***
W135	171	ET-37 complex	11[c]	***(31)***
Y	172	Unknown	166[c]	***(31)***

[a]Electrophoretic type.
[b]Sequence type.
[c]U. Vogel and M. Achtman, unpublished.

bance of the negative control should be lower than 200. A value is regarded as positive, if it exceeds the negative control by more than threefold.

3.2. Colony Blot

1. Transfer bacterial colonies after overnight growth from the nutrient agar to nitrocellulose filters.
2. Dry filters for 1 h in a biosafety cabinet.
3. Meanwhile, soak four Whatman filter papers with denaturing solution, neutralizing solution, 2X SSPE, and 70% ethanol, respectively.
4. Consecutively place dried nitrocellulose filters on each Whatman filter paper for exactly 2 min with the colonies on top. Filters of a positive control (e.g., serogroup B strain MC58, see **Table 3**) and of a negative control (e.g., serogroup C strain 2120; see **Table 3**) are prepared in the same manner.
5. After drying, place the nitrocellulose filters in Petri dishes and block unspecific binding sites by incubation with PBS/1% BSA for 30 min. All incubations are carried out on a shaker (70 rpm) at room temperature.
6. MAb NmeB 735 ascites fluid diluted 1:1,000 in PBS/1% BSA is added for 1 h.
7. Wash the filters three times for 10 min with PBS/0.2% BSA.
8. Detect bound antibody with alkaline phosphatase-conjugated goat anti-mouse Ig (diluted 1:5,000 in PBS/1% BSA), which is incubated for 1 h.
9. Wash the filters twice with PBS/0.2% BSA and once with 0.1 M Tris-HCl, pH 9.6. Then incubate the filters in the color-development solution *without* shaking.
10. Stop the reaction by incubation in distilled, deionized water. The developing time is approx 5–10 min, but depends on the reaction of the controls.

3.3. PCR

1. Prepare the PCR master mix according to **Tables 1**, **2**, and **4**. **Tables 1** and **2** show the oligonucleotides used for the PCR and their combinations for the detection of serogroup specific genes, respectively. **Table 4** demonstrates the compo-

Table 4
PCR Mix

Component		Final concentration
10X PCR buffer II (PE Biosystems)	5 μL[a]	1X
dNTP solution (2 m*M* each dNTP)	5 μL	200 μ*M* each dNTP
25 m*M* $MgCl_2$	3 μL	1.5 m*M*
Primer 1 (20 μ*M*)	0.5 μL	2 nM
Primer 2 (20 μ*M*)	0.5 μL	2 nM
Ampli*Taq*® DNA Polymerase (5 U/μL)	0.1 μL	0.5 U/50 μL
Template	4 μL	4×10^8 CFU/50 μL
Distilled, deionized water	31.9 μL	—

[a]Values are given for one PCR reaction (final volume 50 μL).

sition of the standard 50 μL PCR mix. PCR reactions include at least one negative control without template and one positive control (the strains used for positive controls in our hands are shown in **Table 3**). Add 46 μL of master mix to each reaction tube.

2. Add 4 μL of the bacterial suspensions. For the negative controls use 4 μL distilled, deionized water.
3. The PCR conditions are as follows: initial denaturation is carried out at 94°C for 10 min, followed by 36 cycles of primer annealing for 1 min, extension at 72°C, and denaturation at 94°C for 1 min. The annealing temperatures and the extension times are given in **Table 1**. After a further annealing step, a final extension is carried out at 72°C for 10 min.
4. Mix 10 μL of the PCR products with 5 μL GEBS and load a 1% agarose gel.
5. Electrophoresis is carried out at 200 V until the bromophenol blue dye has migrated approx 8 cm.
6. Place the gel into the ethidium bromide solution for 10 min and then visualize DNA on a transilluminator. The expected sizes of the products are shown in **Table 2**.

4. Notes

1. The determination of the serogroup by ELISA is very robust. It may be worth trying to coat the ELISA plates with heat-killed meningococci in order to avoid the incubation step with live bacteria in a biosafety cabinet. Please note that for reasons unknown to us, the capsule of group A meningococci seems to be very sensitive to heat and ELISAs tend to be falsely negative. Therefore, heat inactivation can only be recommended for group B, C, W135, and Y meningococci.
2. The interpretation of the colony-blot results may be difficult. The following observation can be helpful with unclear results: colonies of encapsulated bacteria are surrounded by capsular polysaccharide shed to the environment. Therefore, positive reactions are not only characterized by dark colonies, but also by a deli-

cate reaction of the surroundings of the colony. This observation facilitates the interpretation. Alternative protocol: treat the dried filters with 70% ethanol only, omitting incubation with NaOH, Tris/NaCl, and SSPE.

3. For the analysis of the serogroup C *siaD* gene by PCR, we use primers, which are derived from the up- and downstream regions, respectively, of the gene (*see* **Table 1**). The PCR works well with serogroup C meningococci derived from different electrophoretic types and geographic origins (e.g., cluster A4, USA; ET-5 complex, Norway; ET-47, Czech Republic; ET-37 complex, Italy; ET-164, The Netherlands). Therefore the primers are very reliable for the detection of the serogroup C. However, alternative primers have been described by Borrow et al. (**ref.** ***44***; *see* also **Chapter 3**).
4. We recently published a PCR amplifying a *cps* fragment comprising the genes *siaA*, *siaB*, and *siaC*. These genes are conserved in the serogroups B, C, W135, and Y (*see* **Subheading 1.3.2.**). The primers SH39 and UE16 used for the *siaA-C* PCR have been published ***(6)***. The *siaA-C* PCR can be used to screen a large number of strains for the presence of the capsular genotypes B, C, W135, and Y, which are all positive in the *siaA-C* PCR.

Acknowledgments

The authors thank Gabriele Heinze for technical assistance and helpful advice.

References

1. Vogel, U. and Frosch, M. (1999) Mechanisms of neisserial serum resistance. *Mol. Microbiol.* **32,** 1133–1139.
2. Mackinnon, F. G., Borrow, R., Gorringe, A. R., Fox, A. J., Jones, D. M., and Robinson, A. (1993) Demonstration of lipooligosaccharide immunotype and capsule as virulence factors for *Neisseria meningitidis* using an infant mouse intranasal infection model. *Microb. Pathog.* **15,** 359–366.
3. Kahler, C. M., Martin, L. E., Shih, G. C., Rahman, M. M., Carlson, R. W., and Stephens, D. S. (1998) The (alpha 2 → 8)-linked polysialic acid capsule and lipooligosaccharide structure both contribute to the ability of serogroup B *Neisseria meningitidis* to resist the bactericidal activity of normal human serum. *Infect. Immun.* **66,** 5939–5947.
4. Vogel, U., Weinberger, A., Frank, R., Müller, A., Kohl, J., Atkinson, J. P., and Frosch, M. (1997) Complement factor C3 deposition and serum resistance in isogenic capsule and LOS sialic acid mutants of serogroup B *Neisseria meningitidis*. *Infect. Immun.* **65,** 4022–4029.
5. Vogel, U., Hammerschmidt, S., and Frosch, M. (1996) Sialic acids of both the capsule and the sialylated lipooligosaccharide of *Neisseria meningitidis* serogroup B are prerequisites for virulence of meningococci in the infant rat. *Med. Microbiol. Immunol. Berl.* **185,** 81–87.
6. Vogel, U., Morelli, G., Zurth, K., Claus, H., Kriener, E., Achtman, M., and Frosch, M. (1998) Necessity of molecular techniques to distinguish between *Neisseria*

meningitidis strains isolated from patients with meningococcal disease and from their healthy contacts. *J. Clin. Microbiol.* **36,** 2465–2470.

7. Block, C., Gdalevich, M., Buber, R., Ashkenazi, I., Ashkenazi, S., and Keller, N. (1999) Factors associated with pharyngeal carriage of *Neisseria meningitidis* among Israel Defense Force personnel at the end of their compulsory service. *Epidemiol. Infect.* **122,** 51–57.
8. Hammerschmidt, S., Hilse, R., van Putten, J. P., Gerardy-Schahn, R., Unkmeir, A., and Frosch, M. (1996) Modulation of cell surface sialic acid expression in *Neisseria meningitidis* via a transposable genetic element. *EMBO J.* **15,** 192–198.
9. Hammerschmidt, S., Müller, A., Sillmann, H., Mühlenhoff, M., Borrow, R., Fox, A., et al. (1996) Capsule phase variation in *Neisseria meningitidis* serogroup B by slipped strand mispairing in the polysialyltransferase gene (*siaD*): correlation with bacterial invasion and the outbreak of meningococcal disease. *Mol. Microbiol.* **20,** 1211–1220.
10. Begg, N. (1995) Outbreak management, in *Meningococcal Disease* (Cartwright, K. A. V., ed.) John Wiley and Sons, Chichester, UK, pp. 285–305.
11. Poolman, J. T., van der Ley, P., and Tommassen, J. (1995) Surface structures and secreted products of meningococci, in *Meningococcal Disease* (Cartwright, K. A. V., ed.), John Wiley and Sons, Chichester, UK, pp. 21–34.
12. Vann, W. F., Liu, T. Y., and Robbins, J. B. (1978) Cell-free biosynthesis of the O-acetylated N-acetylneuraminic acid capsular polysaccharide of group C meningococci. *J. Bacteriol.* **133,** 1300–1306.
13. Liu, T. Y., Gotschlich, E. C., Dunne, F. T., and Jonssen, E. K. (1971) Studies on the meningococcal polysaccharides. II. Composition and chemical properties of the group B and group C polysaccharide. *J. Biol. Chem.* **246,** 4703–4712.
14. Bhattacharjee, A. K., Jennings, H. J., Kenny, C. P., Martin, A., and Smith, I. C. (1976) Structural determination of the polysaccharide antigens of *Neisseria meningitidis* serogroups Y, W-135, and BO1. *Can. J. Biochem.* **54,** 1–8.
15. Bhattacharjee, A. K., Jennings, H. J., Kenny, C. P., Martin, A., and Smith, I. C. P. (1975) Structural determination of the sialic acid polysaccharide antigens of *Neisseria meningitidis* serogroups B and C with carbon 13 nuclear magnetic resonance. *J. Biol. Chem.* **250,** 1926–1932.
16. Gold, R., Goldschneider, I., Lepow, M. L., Draper, T. F., and Randolph, M. (1978) Carriage of *Neisseria meningitidis* and *Neisseria lactamica* in infants and children. *J. Infect. Dis.* **137,** 112–121.
17. Mühlenhoff, M., Eckhardt, M., and Gerardy-Schahn, R. (1998) Polysialic acid: three-dimensional structure, biosynthesis and function. *Curr. Opin. Struct. Biol.* **8,** 558–564.
18. Connolly, M. and Noah, N. (1999) Is group C meningococcal disease increasing in Europe? A report of surveillance of meningococcal infection in Europe 1993–6. European Meningitis Surveillance Group. *Epidemiol. Infect.* **122,** 41–49.
19. Achtman, M. (1995) Global epidemiology of meningococcal disease, in *Meningococcal Disease* (Cartwright, K. A. V., ed.) John Wiley and Sons, Chichester, UK, pp. 159–175.

20. Liu, T. Y., Gotschlich, E. C., Jonssen, E. K., and Wysocki, J. R. (1971) Studies on the meningococcal polysaccharides. I. Composition and chemical properties of the group A polysaccharide. *J. Biol. Chem.* **246,** 2849–2850.
21. Nato, F., Mazie, J. C., Fournier, J. M., Slizewicz, B., Sagot, N., Guibourdenche, M., et al. (1991) Production of polyclonal and monoclonal antibodies against group A, B, and C capsular polysaccharides of *Neisseria meningitidis* and preparation of latex reagents. *J. Clin. Microbiol.* **29,** 1447–1452.
22. Azmi, F. H., Lucas, A. H., Raff, H. V., and Granoff, D. M. (1994) Variable region sequences and idiotypic expression of a protective human immunoglobulin M antibody to capsular polysaccharides of *Neisseria meningitidis* group B and Escherichia coli K1. *Infect. Immun.* **62,** 1776–1786.
23. Hurpin, C. M., Carosella, E. D., and Cazenave, P. A. (1992) Bactericidal activity of two IgG2a murine monoclonal antibodies with distinct fine specificities for group B *Neisseria meningitidis* capsular polysaccharide. *Hybridoma* **11,** 677–687.
24. Raff, H. V., Devereux, D., Shuford, W., Abbott Brown, D., and Maloney, G. (1988) Human monoclonal antibody with protective activity for *Escherichia coli* K1 and *Neisseria meningitidis* group B infections. *J. Infect. Dis.* **157,** 118–126.
25. Frosch, M., Gorgen, I., Boulnois, G. J., Timmis, K. N., and Bitter-Suermann, D. (1985) NZB mouse system for production of monoclonal antibodies to weak bacterial antigens: isolation of an IgG antibody to the polysaccharide capsules of *Escherichia coli* K1 and group B meningococci. *Proc. Natl. Acad. Sci. USA* **82,** 1194–1198.
26. Hutchins, W. A., Adkins, A. R., Kieber Emmons, T., and Westerink, M. A. (1996) Molecular characterization of a monoclonal antibody produced in response to a group C meningococcal polysaccharide peptide mimic. *Mol. Immunol.* **33,** 503–510.
27. Kibbelaar, R. E., Moolenaar, C. E., Michalides, R. J., Bitter-Suermann, D., Addis, B. J., and Mooi, W. J. (1989) Expression of the embryonal neural cell adhesion molecule N-CAM in lung carcinoma. Diagnostic usefulness of monoclonal antibody 735 for the distinction between small cell lung cancer and non-small cell lung cancer. *J. Pathol.* **159,** 23–28.
28. Frosch, M., Weisgerber, C., and Meyer, T. F. (1989) Molecular characterization and expression in *Escherichia coli* of the gene complex encoding the polysaccharide capsule of *Neisseria meningitidis* group B. *Proc. Natl. Acad. Sci. USA* **86,** 1669–1673.
29. Frosch, M., Edwards, U., Bousset, K., Krausse, B., and Weisgerber, C. (1991) Evidence for a common molecular origin of the capsule gene loci in gram-negative bacteria expressing group II capsular polysaccharides. *Mol. Microbiol.* **5,** 1251–1263.
30. Swartley, J. S., Liu, L. J., Miller, Y. K., Martin, L. E., Edupuganti, S., and Stephens, D. S. (1998) Characterization of the gene cassette required for biosynthesis of the (alpha 1→6)-linked N-acetyl-D-mannosamine-1-phosphate capsule of serogroup A *Neisseria meningitidis*. *J. Bacteriol.* **180,** 1533–1539.

31. Claus, H., Vogel, U., Mühlenhoff, M., Gerardy-Schahn, R., and Frosch, M. (1997) Molecular divergence of the sia locus in different serogroups of *Neisseria meningitidis* expressing polysialic acid capsules. *Mol. Gen. Genet.* **257,** 28–34.
32. Parkhill, J., Achtman, M., James, K. D., Bentley, S. D., et al. (2000) Complete DNA sequence of a serogroup A strain of Neisseria menigitidis Z2491. *Nature* **404,** 502–506.
33. Edwards, U., Müller, A., Hammerschmidt, S., Gerardy-Schahn, R., and Frosch, M. (1994) Molecular analysis of the biosynthesis pathway of the alpha-2,8 polysialic acid capsule by *Neisseria meningitidis* serogroup B. *Mol. Microbiol.* **14,** 141–149.
34. Swartley, J. S., Marfin, A. A., Edupuganti, S., Liu, L. J., Cieslak, P., Perkins, B., Wenger, J. D., and Stephens, D. S. (1997) Capsule switching of *Neisseria meningitidis. Proc. Natl. Acad. Sci. USA* **94,** 271–276.
35. Frosch, M. and Müller, A. (1993) Phospholipid substitution of capsular polysaccharides and mechanisms of capsule formation in *Neisseria meningitidis. Mol. Microbiol.* **8,** 483–493.
36. Frosch, M., Müller, D., Bousset, K., and Müller, A. (1992) Conserved outer membrane protein of *Neisseria meningitidis* involved in capsule expression. *Infect. Immun.* **60,** 798–803.
37. Gray, S. J., Sobanski, M. A., Kaczmarski, E. B., Guiver, M., Marsh, W. J., Borrow, R., et al. (1999) Ultrasound-enhanced latex immunoagglutination and PCR as complementary methods for non-culture-based confirmation of meningococcal disease. *J. Clin. Microbiol.* **37,** 1797–1801.
38. Hammerschmidt, S., Birkholz, C., Zähringer, U., Robertson, B. D., van Putten, J., Ebeling, O., and Frosch, M. (1994) Contribution of genes from the capsule gene complex (*cps*) to lipooligosaccharide biosynthesis and serum resistance in *Neisseria meningitidis. Mol. Microbiol.* **11,** 885–896.
39. Lee, F. K., Stephens, D. S., Gibson, B. W., Engstrom, J. J., Zhou, D., and Apicella, M. A. (1995) Microheterogeneity of Neisseria lipooligosaccharide: analysis of a UDP-glucose 4-epimerase mutant of *Neisseria meningitidis* NMB. *Infect. Immun.* **63,** 2508–2515.
40. Jennings, M. P., van der Ley, P., Wilks, K. E., Maskell, D. J., Poolman, J. T., and Moxon, E. R. (1993) Cloning and molecular analysis of the *galE* gene of *Neisseria meningitidis* and its role in lipopolysaccharide biosynthesis. *Mol. Microbiol.* **10,** 361–369.
41. Robertson, B. D., Frosch, M., and van Putten, J. P. (1993) The role of *galE* in the biosynthesis and function of gonococcal lipopolysaccharide. *Mol. Microbiol.* **8,** 891–901.
42. Petering, H., Hammerschmidt, S., Frosch, M., van Putten, J. P., Ison, C. A., and Robertson, B. D. (1996) Genes associated with meningococcal capsule complex are also found in *Neisseria gonorrhoeae. J. Bacteriol.* **178,** 3342–3345.
43. Fuchs, T. M., Deppisch, H., Scarlato, V., and Gross, R. (1996) A new gene locus of *Bordetella pertussis* defines a novel family of prokaryotic transcriptional accessory proteins. *J. Bacteriol.* **178,** 4445–4452.

44. Borrow, R., Claus, H., Guiver, M., Smart, L., Jones, D.M., Kaczmarski, E. B., et al. (1997) Non-culture diagnosis and serogroup determination of meningococcal B and C infection by a sialyltransferase (*siaD*) PCR ELISA. *Epidemiol. Infect.* **118,** 111–117.
45. Borrow, R., Claus, H., Chaudhry, U., Guiver, M., Kaczmarski, E. B., Frosch, M., and Fox, A. J. (1998) *siaD* PCR ELISA for confirmation and identification of serogroup Y and W135 meningococcal infections. *FEMS Microbiol. Lett.* **159,** 209–214.
46. Dempsey, J. A., Wallace, A. B., and Cannon, J. G. (1995) The physical map of the chromosome of a serogroup A strain of *Neisseria meningitidis* shows complex rearrangements relative to the chromosomes of the two mapped strains of the closely related species *N. gonorrhoeae*. *J. Bacteriol.* **177,** 6390–6400.
47. Dunn, K. L., Virji, M., and Moxon, E. R. (1995) Investigations into the molecular basis of meningococcal toxicity for human endothelial and epithelial cells: the synergistic effect of LPS and pili. *Microb. Pathog.* **18,** 81–96.

14

Molecular Analysis of the Meningococcal LPS Expression

Michael P. Jennings, Andrew W. Berrington, and E. Richard Moxon

1. Introduction

Lipopolysaccharide (LPS) is one of the major virulence factors of *Neisseria meningitidis* *(1)*, with proposed roles in bacterial attachment to the host, invasion of host tissues, serum resistance, evasion of the host immune response, and the pathogenesis of sepsis syndrome. Accordingly it has become an important target for research.

Conventionally, the study of LPS has relied on structural investigations and the use of monoclonal antibodies (MAbs), which in the case of meningococcal LPS have revealed marked heterogeneity and complexity *(2)*. The LPS of *N. meningitidis* can be categorized into 12 immunotypes, L1 to L12, which differ in the structure of the oligosaccharide region of the LPS molecule. In most cases these structures have been elucidated *(3)* (for examples, see **Fig. 1**). The type of LPS expressed is a key factor in interactions with the host. For example, the L3 immunotype is more serum resistant than the L8 immunotype *(4)*, while the L8 immunotype may be more invasive *(5)*. Such studies have provided insights into the role of LPS in the pathogenesis of disease.

Crucially, however, many of the oligosaccharide-linked structures that distinguish these immunotypes are subject to phase variation, which is defined as the high-frequency, reversible, on-off switching of gene expression. This may lead to changes in the immunological reactivity of a strain, which indeed may be one means by which the organism succeeds in evading host immunity during disease. For example, switching may occur between the L3 and L8 immunotypes, between L1 and L8, and between L2 and L4. There is evidence from the mouse model that immunotype switching may play a role in the estab-

From: *Methods in Molecular Medicine, vol. 67: Meningococcal Disease: Methods and Protocols*
Edited by: A. J. Pollard and M. C. J. Maiden © Humana Press Inc., Totowa, NJ

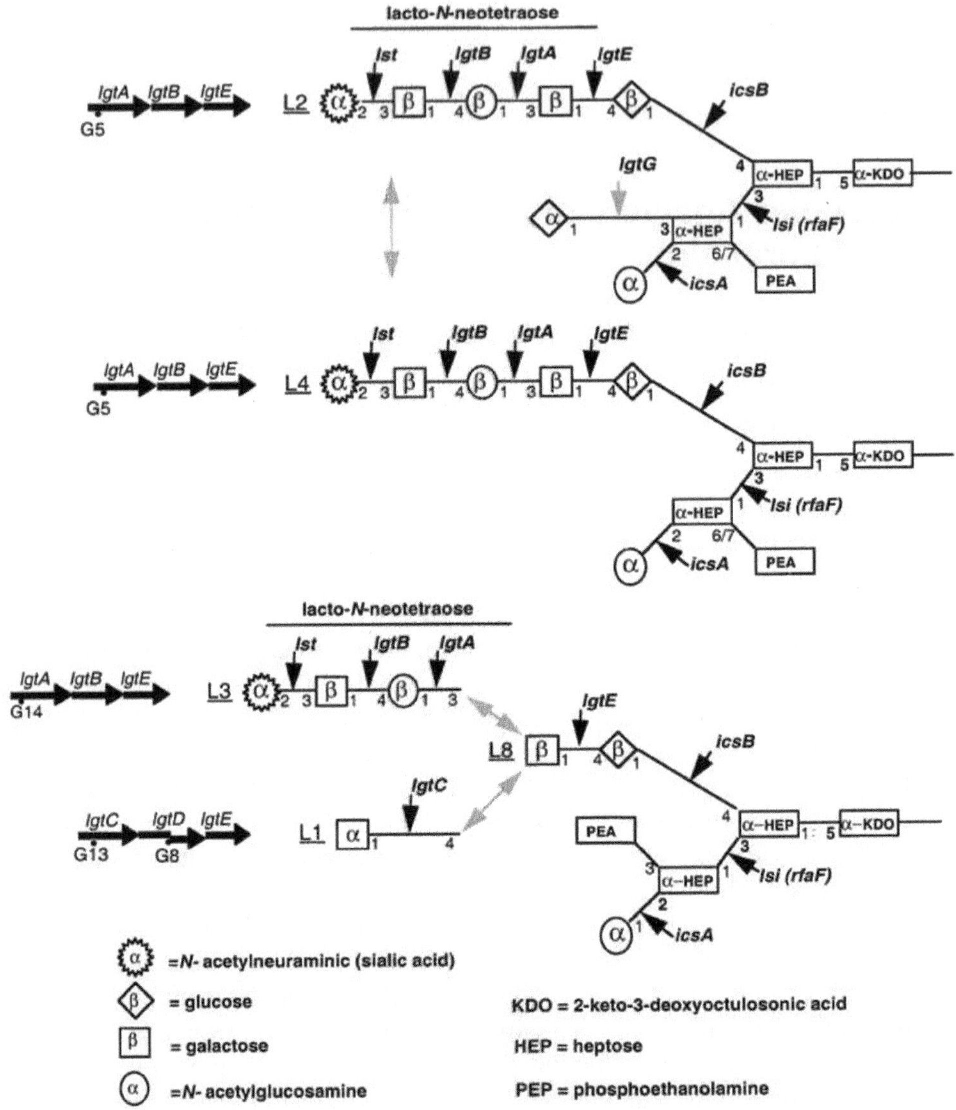

Fig. 1. The primary structure of a selection of meningococcal oligosaccharides of immunotypes L1, L2, L3, L4, and L8. Immunotypes are labeled to the left each structure. Gray arrows show phase variation between structures. Only the terminal structures of L1 and L3 are shown, as they are extensions of the L8 basal structure. The structure of immunotype L6 has the same basal structure as L4, but the terminal two sugars (α-Neu5 Ac-(2-3)-β-D-Gal-) are missing. The enzymatic activities of the *lgtA*, *lgtB*, *lgtC*, *lgtE*, and *lgtG* gene products are indicated with arrows. The *lgt* genes present in each of the type strains are indicated with arrowed lines on the left of the figure. The arabic numbers indicate the position of the binding site; α, β indicate the anomeric configuration. Adapted from **ref. 2**.

lishment of disease *(6)*. However, phase variation means that phenotypic analysis alone may be insufficient to fully document the LPS repertoire of a given strain. This problem may be circumvented by studying the LPS operon at the molecular level *(7)*.

The lgt (lipopolysaccharide glycosyltransferase) operon comprises the closely-linked LPS biosynthetic genes *lgtA*, *lgtB*, *lgtC*, *lgtD*, and *lgtE*. The genes *lgtA*, *lgtB*, and *lgtE* encode the glycosyltransferases required for the biosynthesis of the lacto-N-neotetraose motif of L2, L3 and L4 (**Fig. 1**). The *lgtC* gene encodes a further enzyme for the addition of the N-acetylglucosamine residue found in L1, while *lgtD* catalyses the addition of N-acetylgalactosamine to lacto-N-neotetraose. A sixth gene, *lgtG*, another glycosyltransferase originally discovered in *N. gonorrhoeae* *(8)*, has been observed in *N. meningitidis* but is not closely linked. A given isolate may possess some or all of these genes. In a study of the distribution of the *lgtABCDEG* loci in a global collection of 37 serogroup B strains *(9)*, *lgtA* and *lgtB* were ubiquitous, *lgtC* was present in 14, *lgtE* was present in 36, and *lgtG* in 19. At the time of this writing, *lgtD* has been reported in only one meningococcal strain *(7)*, and is probably more representative of *N. gonorrhoeae*.

Phase variation of these genes is mediated by high-frequency frameshift mutations that occur within homopolymeric tracts situated in the coding regions of *lgtA*, *lgtC*, *lgtD*, and *lgtG* *(7,10)*, and that result in switching between 'on' and 'off' states with respect to expression. This mechanism has been independently confirmed in studies of the *lgt* operon in *N. gonorrhoeae* *(8,11,12)*. For example, the L3 to L8 switching event described earlier occurs via mutation in the poly-G tract within *lgtA*. Tracts of 5, 8, 11, 14, or 17 base pairs in length leave the downstream sequences in frame for transcription (*lgtA* expressed, lacto-N-neotetraose synthesised, L3 immunotype), while tracts of other lengths leave the downstream sequences out of frame (*lgtA* not expressed, L8 immunotype). Similar tracts are found in *lgtC* (poly-G) and *lgtG* (poly-C), and mediate equivalent switching events.

The experimental techniques used to investigate these loci include Southern hybridization to determine the presence or absence of the genes of interest, polymerase chain reaction (PCR) amplification of the regions of those genes that contain homopolymeric tracts, and sequencing of the tracts themselves to determine whether the genes are 'on' or 'off.' This chapter will describe these methodologies. Based on the enzymatic activity of the glycosyltransferases involved, it is possible to predict the LPS structure currently expressed by the strain. For example, **Fig. 1** shows a strain of L3 immunotype with the *lgtA* gene "on" (14 residues in the poly-G tract), which predicts that lacto-N-neotetraose will be made by this strain. Furthermore, this information makes it possible to predict the whole repertoire of immunotypes that a strain might express given

Table 1
Immunotype Control Strains

Immunotype	Strain	Reference
L1	126E	*(2)*
L2	35E	*(2)*
L3	MC58¢3	*(5)*
L4	M891	*(2)*
L5	M981	*(2)*
L6	M992	*(2)*
L8	M978	*(2)*
L10	7880	*(2)*
L11	7889	*(2)*
L12	3200	*(2)*

the appropriate switching events. For example, the L2 strain in **Fig. 1** can be predicted to switch to L4 if *lgtG* is present and switches off.

It is anticipated that studies using techniques such as those described in this chapter will lead to a greater understanding of the mechanisms and functions of LPS immunotype switching.

2. Materials

1. 37°C incubator with 5% CO_2.
2. Centrifuge.
3. Water bath.
4. Thermal cycler.
5. Agarose-gel electrophoresis equipment.
6. Ultraviolet (UV) illuminator and gel-imaging equipment (photographic or digital).
7. Spectrophotometer.

2.2. Cultivation of Meningococci

1. 1% BHI agar (Acumedia) supplemented with 10% Levinthal's base ***(13)***, or equivalent medium capable of supporting the growth of *N. meningitidis*.
2. Control strains for the generation of probes and as controls for Southern blots and PCRs (**Table 1**).

2.3. Probe Preparation

1. PCR reagents: Taq polymerase and buffer, $MgCl_2$, dNTPs, sterile distilled water.
2. Primers (listed in **Table 2**, defined in **Table 5**).
3. Gel-extraction kit, e.g., QiaEx II (Qiagen).
4. DIG High Prime Labeling and Detection Starter Kit 1 (Boehringer Mannheim).

Table 2
Templates and Primers for Generating *lgt* Gene Probes

Probe	Template	Forward primer	Reverse primer	Probe size
lgtA	L3	lic2	lic23	550 bp
lgtB	L3	lic13	lic1	805 bp
lgtC	L1	LgtCF	lgtCR	945 bp
lgtD	L1	F104	xmore37	338 bp
lgtE	L3	x135ext	R110	666 bp
lgtG	L2	LG2	LG3	603 bp

2.4. Extraction of Genomic DNA for Southern Blots

1. Reagents: Phosphate-Buffered Saline (PBS), 10% sodium dodecyl sulphate (SDS), proteinase K, 5 *M* NaCl, 10% CTAB/0.7 *M* NaCl solution, chloroform/isoamyl mixture (24:1), phenol/chloroform/isoamyl mixture (25:24:1), isopropanol, ethanol, TE buffer, RNAse A.

2.5. Restriction Digestion

1. *ClaI* restriction enzyme and buffer, sterile distilled water.

2.6. Southern Blot

1. Equipment: trays, filter paper, paper towels, transfer membrane (e.g., Hybond-N, Amersham International), UV cross linker, hybridisation oven.
2. Denaturing solution: 1.5 *M* NaCl, 0.5 *M* NaOH.
3. Neutralizing solution: 0.5 *M* Tris-HCl, 1.5 *M* NaCl, pH 7.4.
4. 20X SSC stock: 17.5% (w/v) NaCl, 8.82% (w/v) Sodium Citrate, pH 7.0.
5. Transfer buffer: 8X SSC.
6. Standard hybridization buffer: 5X SSC, 0.02% (w/v) SDS, 1X blocking solution (Boehringer Mannheim).
7. Wash buffers: 0.1X SSC, 0.1% SDS; 2X SSC, 0.1% SDS; 0.05X SSC, 0.05% SDS.
8. Maleic acid buffer: 0.1 *M* maleic acid, 0.15 *M* NaCl, pH 7.5.
9. Blocking reagent: 10X blocking solution diluted 1:10 in maleic acid buffer.
10. Anti-digoxigenin-AP, Fab fragments (Boehringer Mannheim).
11. Detection buffer: 0.1 *M* Tris-HCl, 0.1 *M* NaCl, 50 m*M* $MgCl_2$, pH 9.5.
12. NBT: 5% nitro-blue tetrazolium in 70% dimethyl fluoride (DMF).
13. BCIP: 5% 5-bromo-4-chloro-3-indolyphosphate in 100% DMF.

2.7. Amplification of lgt Homopolymeric Tract Regions

1. PCR reagents: Taq polymerase and buffer, $MgCl_2$, dNTPs, sterile distilled water.
2. Primers (listed in **Table 3**, defined in **Table 5**).
3. Gel-extraction kit, e.g., QiaEx II (Qiagen).

Table 3
Primers for Amplifying the Homopolymeric Tract Regions in *lgt* Genes

Gene	Forward primer	Reverse primer
lgtA	lic31ext	lic16ext
lgtC	lgtCF	lgtCR
lgtG	LG1	LG2

Table 4
Primers for Sequencing the Homopolymeric Tract Regions in *lgt* Genes

Gene	Forward primer	Reverse primer
lgtA	lic31ext	lic16ext
lgtC	lgtCF	R99
lgtG	LG6	LG8

2.8. Sequencing of lgt Homopolymeric Tract Regions

1. Primers (listed in **Table 4** and defined in **Table 5**).
2. Ready reaction premix (Big Dye Terminator RR Mix, Applied Biosystems).
3. Ethanol extraction reagents: 3 *M* sodium acetate pH4.6; ethanol.
4. Automated sequencer.

2.9. Sequence Analysis

1. Computer equipment with appropriate software, for example SeqEd (Applied Biosystems).

3. Methods

3.1. General

1. Most methods are as described in Sambrook et al. ***(14)***.
2. A typical sequence of experiments would comprise Southern analysis to determine the *lgt* genes present in the strains of interest, followed by PCR amplification and sequencing of the homopolymeric tracts of the phase-variable genes present.

3.2. Cultivation of Meningococci

1. Streak for single colonies when making PCR template, inoculate plate heavily for extraction of DNA.
2. Incubate at 37°C in 5% CO_2 for 16 h.

Table 5
Sequences, Positions, and References of Primers Used in *lgt* Studies

Primer	Sequence 5′-3′	Position	Reference sequence
F104	ACAACAACACGATGATTATG	2151–2171	U65788
LG1	ATGAAGCTCAAAATAGACATTG	209–230	AF076919
LG2	TTATACGGATGCCAGCATGTC	1244–1264 rc	AF076919
LG3	ATACGGCGTTCCCCCCGAAA	661–680	AF076919
LG6	GATTACGCCGACCTCCTCATCTGC	488–511	AF076919
LG8	GGTAGAGTTCGGGCATATCGGTGC	933–956rc	AF076919
lgtCF	GGAGAAAAGATGGACATCGTATTTTGCGG	652–679	U65788
lgtCR	GTCAATAAATCTTGCGTAAGAATCT	1573–1597 rc	U65788
lic1	GGCACAATGAACTGTTCG	2171–2188 rc	U25839
lic2	ATGCAGACGATATTGCCG	614–631	U25839
lic13	GTTATCAGCTTAGCTTCC	1383–1400	U25839
lic16ext	CGATGATGCTGCGGTCTTTTTCCAT	664–688 rc	U25839
lic23	TTCCGGCAAATGTTTCTCCA	1144–1164 rc	U25839
lic31ext	CCTTTAGTCAGCGTATTGATTTGCG	334–358	U25839
R99	CCCAAATCGGTATCCCATAA	1003–1022	U65788
R110	CCTATCTTTTTCCAAATCGC	3002–3021 rc	U25839
x135ext	CCATGTTATCAGCTTAG	2355–2371	U25839
xmore37	CCTGTCCGGACAAGGCTTTT	2470–2489 rc	U65788

Table 6
Template Strains for Generation of *lgt* Probes

Probe	Template strain	Reference
lgtA	MC58	*(5)*
lgtB	MC58	*(5)*
lgtC	126E	*(2)*
lgtD	126E	*(2)*
lgtE	MC58	*(5)*
lgtG	35E	*(2)*

3.3. Probe Preparation

1. Use lysed whole cells in preference to chromosomal DNA preparations as PCR template: from an overnight plate culture pick 12 isolated colonies to 200 μL sterile distilled water, and boil for 10 min. The strains used to prepare each probe are documented in **Table 6**.
2. Prepare a reaction tube for each specimen containing Taq polymerase buffer and $MgCl_2$ according to the manufacturer's instructions, dNTPs (typically 0.4 μL of a 25 m*M* preparation), 50 pmol of forward and reverse primers, 1 μL of template, and sterilized distilled water to a total volume of 48 μL.
3. After a 5-min hot-start at 94°C, to each tube add 2 μL of a preparation of Taq polymerase diluted in Taq buffer; 0.4 U per reaction is sufficient.
4. Amplify DNA using 35 cycles of 94°C for 1 min, 55°C for 1 min, 72°C for 1 min, followed by final extension at 72°C for 7 min.
5. Purify the PCR product by agarose-gel extraction.
6. Quantitate DNA by comparison with a DNA mass ladder on a 1% agarose gel.
7. Label the probes using the nonradioactive digoxigenin labeling system DIG High Prime Labeling and Detection Starter Kit 1 (Boehringer Mannheim), according to the manufacturer's instructions. Typically, up to 1 μg of PCR product is incubated with 4 μL of labeling reagent and an appropriate volume of sterile distilled water to yield 20 μL of labeled probe.
8. If necessary the yield may be quantified using the DIG Control Teststrips (Boehringer Mannheim), according to the manufacturer's instructions.
9. Denature the probe by boiling for 5 min and cooling rapidly on ice, then add to pre-warmed hybridization buffer. The optimal concentration should be determined by experimentation, but 10 μL of probe diluted in 4 mL of buffer has been used successfully in our laboratory. Following dilution the probe may be kept frozen at –20°C and reused several times.

3.4. Extraction of Genomic DNA for Southern Blots

1. For each strain to be studied, scrape the growth from half a plate into 500 μL PBS. To each tube add 30 μL 10% SDS and 3 μL proteinase K, and heat-kill at 56°C for 1 h.

2. To each tube add 100 µL 5*M* NaCl followed by 80 µL freshly prepared 10% CTAB/0.7 *M* NaCl solution, mix thoroughly, and incubate at 65°C for 10 min in a water bath.
3. To each tube add an equal volume of chloroform/isoamyl (24 : 1), vortex mix, and centrifuge at 14,000 rpm for 5 min.
4. Transfer the aqueous (upper) phase to a fresh tube and add an equal volume of phenol/chloroform/isoamyl (25 : 24 : 1), vortex and centrifuge at 14,000 rpm for 5 min.
5. Transfer the aqueous phase to a fresh tube and add 0.6 volumes of isopropanol, then centrifuge at 14,000 rpm for 5 min to pellet the precipitated DNA.
6. Wash the pellet once with 250 µL 70% ethanol, centrifuge again, remove the supernatant and dry the pellet for 5–10 min.
7. Resuspend the pellet in 80 µL TE buffer containing 10 mg/mL RNAse A.
8. Quantitate the DNA by spectrophotometry at 260 nm.

3.5. Restriction Digestion

1. Digest 5 µg of chromosomal DNA with 5U *ClaI* in enzyme buffer according to the manufacturer's instructions, at 37°C overnight.
2. Separate the fragments on a 0.7% agarose gel, and visualize under UV illumination to ensure complete digestion.

3.6. Hybridization

1. Load control and test digests into a 0.7% agarose gel and run at 100V to maximum separation: store an image for later reference.
2. Agitate the gel in denaturing solution for 30 min.
3. Agitate the gel in neutralizing solution for 30 min.
4. Blot the gel overnight onto transfer membrane using 8X SSC as transfer buffer.
5. Fix DNA to the membrane by UV cross-linking
6. Pre-warm an appropriate volume of hybridisation buffer (20 mL/100 cm^2) and incubate the membrane for 30 min with gentle agitation.
7. Thaw the labeled probe prepared previously and denature by boiling for 5 min and rapidly cooling on ice water.
8. Discard hybridization buffer, add probe (2.5 mL/100 cm^2), and incubate for 16 h in a hybridization oven according to the conditions shown in **Table 7**.
9. Wash the membrane in SSC/SDS solutions as shown in **Table 7**, followed by a final wash with maleic acid solution for 5 min at room temperature. The higher stringency for *lgtD* is necessary to prevent nonspecific binding to homologous *lgtA* sequences.
10. Block the membrane for 30 min in blocking reagent at room temperature.
11. Incubate the membrane at room temperature with a 1 : 5000 solution of labeled antibody (Anti-digoxigenin-AP, Fab fragments, Boehringer Mannheim) in blocking reagent.
12. Wash twice for 15 min at room temperature in maleic acid buffer.
13. Detect bound antibody using a solution of 66 µL NBT and 33 µL BCIP/10 mL of detection buffer. Detection should take place in the dark and without agitation.

Table 7
Hybridization and Washing Conditions

Probe	Conditions	Washes
lgtA	68°C for at least 16 h	Pre-warmed 0.1X SSC, 0.1% SDS 68°C rinse then 2 × 15 min washes
lgtB	68°C for at least 16 h	Pre-warmed 0.1X SSC, 0.1% SDS 68°C rinse then 2 × 15 min washes
lgtC	65°C for at least 16 h	2 × 5 min 2X SSC, 0.1% SDS at room temperature 2 × 15 min 0.1X SSC, 0.1% SDS 65°C
lgtD	68°C for at least 16 h	Pre-warmed 0.05X SSC, 0.05% SDS 68°C rinse then 2 × 15 min washes
lgtE	68°C for at least 16 h	Pre-warmed 0.1X SSC, 0.1% SDS 68°C rinse then 2 × 15 min washes
lgtG	65°C for at least 16 h	2 × 5 min 2X SSC, 0.1% SDS at room temperature 2 × 15 min 0.1X SSC, 0.1% SDS 65°C

3.7. Amplification of lgt *Homopolymeric Tract Regions*

1. Use lysed whole cells in preference to chromosomal DNA preparations as PCR template: from an overnight plate culture pick 12 isolated colonies to 200 μL sterile distilled water, and boil for 10 min.
2. Perform all PCRs in triplicate to reduce the likelihood of introducing lengthening or shortening errors into the homopolymeric tracts.
3. For each specimen prepare three reaction tubes and amplify the DNA as described in **Subheading 3.3.** under probe preparation.
4. Include positive and negative controls. The L1 control strain may be used as a positive control for *lgtC*, while the L2 strain may be used for *lgtA* and *lgtG*.
5. Run 5 μL of product against a molecular weight marker on a 1% gel to confirm amplification.
6. Pool the remainder of the three PCR products for each specimen, and purify by agarose-gel extraction, or alternatively by spin-column elution.
7. Quantitate the product by comparison with a DNA mass ladder on agarose gel; each sequencing reaction will require 60–90 ng of DNA.

3.8. Sequencing of lgt *Homopolymeric Tract Regions*

1. Sequence the homopolymeric tract region of each pooled triplicate PCR product in both forward and reverse directions to ensure accuracy and conformity.
2. Use between 60 and 90 ng of DNA in each sequencing reaction, depending on the concentration of the PCR product. Add an appropriate volume of DNA to each of two tubes and add sterile distilled water to a total of 10.8 μL. Maintain the specimens on ice until sequencing begins.

3. Prepare dilutions of each primer (*see* **Subheading 2.**) to a concentration of 1 pmol/µL. For each specimen add 3.2 µL of the forward primer to one tube, and 3.2 µL of the reverse primer to the other.
4. Add 6 µL of ready reaction premix (Big Dye Terminator RR Mix, Applied Biosystems).
5. Incubate the extension reactions in a thermocycler: 96°C × 10 s, 50°C × 5 s, 60°C × 4 min for 25 cycles.
6. Extract the product by ethanol precipitation: add 2 µL 3 *M* sodium acetate pH 4.6 and the 20 µL aliquot of sequence reaction to a tube containing 200 µL 100% ethanol, and incubate on ice for 30 min.
7. Centrifuge the samples at 14,000 rpm for 30 min to pellet the DNA.
8. Wash the pellet with 500 µL 70% ethanol and centrifuge at 14,000 rpm for 5 min.
9. Remove the supernatant and air-dry the pellet for 5–10 min.
10. Refrigerate before sequencing on an automated sequencer.

3.9. Sequence Analysis

1. Align the homopolymeric tract sequences generated from forward and reverse primers and confirm that upstream and downstream sequence identity is preserved.
2. Count the number of residues within the homopolymeric tract *(7)* to determine whether the open reading frame is complete or truncated.
3. Check the alignment of the sequence both up- and downstream of the tract to detect other mutations.

4. Notes

1. Preliminary experiments should be performed to determine the optimum amount of template for the PCR. A 1:10 or 1:100 dilution of the initial preparation (12 colonies in 200 µL water) is likely to be most fruitful, using 1 µL of this dilution per 50 µL PCR reaction.
2. *lgtG* sometimes has a deletion that prevents amplification using the primers LG1 and LG2. If the test band on the Southern blot has run further than the control band, or if PCR fails without obvious cause, try using primers LG6 and LG8.

References

1. Verheul, A. F. M., Snippe, H., and Poolman, J. T. (1993) Meningococcal lipopolysaccharides: virulence factor and potential vaccine component. *Microbiol. Rev.* **57,** 34–49.
2. Scholten, R. J. P. M., Kuipers, B., Valkenberg, H. A., Dankert, J., Zollinger, W. D., and Poolman, J. T. (1994) Lipo-oligosaccharide immunotyping on *Neisseria meningitidis* by a whole cell ELISA using monoclonal antibodies and association of immunotype with serogroup, serotype and subtype. *J. Med. Microbiol.* **41,** 236–243.
3. Kogan, G., Uhrin, D., Brisson, J. R., and Jennings, H. J. (1997) Stuctural basis of the *Neisseria meningitidis* immunotypes. *Carbohydr. Res.* **298,** 191–199.

4. Moran, E. E., Brandt, B. L., and Zollinger, W. D. (1994) Expression of the L8 lipopolysaccharide determinant increases the sensitivity of *Neisseria meningitidis* to serum bactericidal activity. *Infect. Immun.* **62,** 5290–5295.
5. Virji, M., Peak, I. R. A., Makepeace, K., Jennings, M. P., Ferguson, D. J. P., and Moxon, E. R. (1995) Opc- and pilus-dependent interactions of meningococci with human endothelial cells: molecular mechanisms and modulation by surface polysaccharides. *Mol. Microbiol.* **18,** 741–754.
6. Mackinnon, F. G., Borrow, R., Gorringe, A. R., Fox, A. J., Jones, D. M., and Robinson, A. (1993) Demonstration of lipooligosaccharide immunotype and capsule as virulence factors for *Neisseria meningitidis* using an infant mouse intranasal infection model. *Microb. Pathogen.* **15,** 359–366.
7. Jennings, M. P., Srikhanta, Y. N., Moxon, E. R., Kramer, M., Poolman, J. T., Kuipers, B., and van der Ley, P. (1999) The genetic basis of the phase variation repertoire of lipopolysaccharide immunotypes in *Neisseria meningitidis*. *Microbiol.* **145,** 3013–3021.
8. Banerjee, A., Wang, R., Uljon, S. N., Rice, P. A., Gotschlich, E. C., and Stein, D. C. (1998) Identification of the gene (lgtG) encoding the lipooligosaccharide beta chain synthesizing glucosyl transferase from *Neisseria gonorrhoeae*. *Proc. Natl. Acad. Sci. USA* **95,** 10,872–10,877.
9. Jennings, M. P., unpublished observation.
10. Jennings, M. P., Hood, D., Peak, I. R. A., Virji, M., and Moxon, E. R. (1995) Molecular analysis of a locus which controls the biosynthesis and phase variable expression of the lacto-N-neotetraose terminal LPS structure in *Neisseria meningitidis*. *Mol. Microbiol.* **18,** 724–740.
11. Danaher, R. J., Levin, J. C., Arking, D., Burch, C. L., Sandlin, R., and Stein, D. C. (1995) Genetic basis of *Neisseria gonorrhoeae* lipooligosaccharide antigenic variation. *J. Bacteriol.* **177,** 7275–7279.
12. Yang, Q. L. and Gotschlich, E. C. (1996) Variation of gonococcal lipooligosaccharide structure is due to alterations in poly-G tracts in lgt genes encoding glycosyl transferases. *J. Exp. Med.* **183,** 323–327.
13. Alexander, H. E. (1965) The *Haemophilus* group, in *Bacterial and Mycotic Infections of Man* (Dabos, R. J. and Hirsch, J. G., eds.), London, Pitman Medical Publishing, pp. 724–741.
14. Sambrook, J., Fritsch, E. F., and Maniatis, T. (1989) *Molecular Cloning: A Laboratory Manual*, 2nd ed. Cold Spring Harbor Laboratory Press, Cold Spring Harbor, NY.

15

Genome Sequencing and Annotation

Alex C. Jeffries, Nigel J. Saunders, and Derek W. Hood

1. Introduction

The availability of complete microbial genome sequences enormously facilitates experimental molecular investigations of the respective organisms by providing complete lists of genes, their genetic contexts, and their predicted functions. This can be used in a number of ways to focus studies on bacterial pathogenesis and also vaccine development *(1,2)*. The complete genome sequences from two unrelated strains of *Neisseria meningitidis*, a derivative of isolate MC58 which originally expressed serogroup B capsule and strain Z2491, which is serogroup A, are now available *(3,4)*. The genome sequences of both these strains were determined using the whole genome shotgun approach *(5)*. In this approach, randomly sheared chromosomal DNA is cloned to make a small insert library (1.5–2.0 kb for MC58, 0.5–0.8 kb and 1.0–1.5 kb for Z2491), then each insert is sequenced from both ends using plasmid-specific primers. For the MC58 genome sequence, a large insert lambda library (8–24 kb) was also used. In the initial sequencing phase, 6–8 times coverage of the estimated size of the genome is generally achieved. The DNA sequences are linked together (assembled) into large contigs (a derivative of the word contiguous). Polymerase chain reaction (PCR) and sequencing of large insert libraries are then used to join the contigs, close gaps, and resolve ambiguities (*see* **ref. *6*** for a review).

Because a complete genome sequence contains all of the genetic information of the sequenced isolate, for the first time we have the opportunity to gain a detailed insight into what specifies one organism and its biology, especially in comparison to other organisms. This genetic information includes each determinant influencing host-microbe interaction, every vaccine candidate, and

From: *Methods in Molecular Medicine, vol. 67: Meningococcal Disease: Methods and Protocols*
Edited by: A. J. Pollard and M. C. J. Maiden © Humana Press Inc., Totowa, NJ

all potential therapeutic and diagnostic targets. In addition, the availability of multiple genome sequences from the same species allows strains to be compared in order to gain insights into their shared and divergent phenotypes; to this end, the genome sequencing of the ET-37 complex, serogroup C meningococcal isolate FAM18 is currently underway at the Sanger Centre and should be finished by the time of publication of this book. Common and distinct sequences can be readily identified between strains and are used as the basis of such comparisons. For instance, the genes within the approx 9% of the genome sequence that differs between MC58 and Z2497 may provide clues as to the different ways in which the bacteria spread through human populations. Comparative genome-sequence analyses can also be extended to closely related species. Thus the genome sequence of the related pathogenic species, *Neisseria gonorrhoeae* strain FA1090, which is soon to be completed, will be of great value. Comparison of the sequences of these two human-specific neisserial pathogens, which preferentially colonize different sites and cause different disease syndromes, will allow identification of chromosomal regions that might determine their disease specificities. It is reasonable to propose that DNA segments specific to the meningococcus will be more likely to be involved in aspects of disease related to meningococcal infection, such as septicemia and inflammation of the meninges.

The annotation of genes in a genome sequence is an essential step in obtaining these insights and is a prerequisite for large-scale analyses of gene function at the bench. However, it should be kept in mind that, in the case of many or possibly all bacteria, genomes are labile, or what is often termed "plastic." Genomes in a population of bacteria may be added to and subtracted from through the processes of natural transformation with genomic DNA, plasmid transfer, transfection with bacteriophage, and by the replicative transposition of mobile elements. In addition, rearrangements of portions of the genome, through inversions, duplications, and translocations, may occur. Genome plasticity often affects the phenotype of the organism and is believed to be an important mechanism whereby bacteria adapt to their environments. Therefore, a microbial genome sequence from a particular strain should not be thought of as the one and only genome sequence for that species, but rather as a reference or index sequence.

Complete microbial genome sequencing is rapidly becoming a routine undertaking and already vast quantities of sequence data have been obtained. Currently, the majority of genes in any given genome have not been experimentally investigated to determine the functions of their protein products. An expedient method of determining the function of proteins encoded in a genome, for which experimental evidence has not yet been obtained, is through inference from genes of known or proposed function on the basis of sequence similarity. Public-domain databases contain large numbers of sequences linked to information about the organisms they come from, their assigned function, and literature where the experimental evidence for their function can be found. Using algorithms that identify and assess similarities between sequences, sequence data from the new genome (query sequences) are compared to those from databases and the sequences that show the highest similarities are noted. A judgement is then made about whether the strength and coverage of the matches are sufficient to allow the assignment of a putative function to the query gene sequence. One premise that is being made in this judgement process is that the query sequence and the database sequence have a common ancestor gene (i.e., they are homologous to each other, the standard definition of homology used in evolution). The corollary to this is that although the genes have diverged from each other through speciation, the assignment of homology lets us infer that the gene products have retained the same or very similar tertiary structures and therefore function(s).

Methods for rapid analysis of genome sequence data are still developing and often provide less than desirable, and sometimes incorrect, assignments of function. A detailed analysis of each putative gene sequence, although desirable, is often too time-consuming to be practical, thus a compromise between speed and thoroughness of analysis must be struck and this is one of the aims of the continued improvement in bioinformatics tools. Still, much in this area can be gained through taking advantage of the methods and resources currently available and by taking into account some of their limitations.

2. General Methodologies for Genome Analysis

Genome sequence analysis can be carried out using two broad methodologies; 1) open reading frame (ORF) based, and 2) non-ORF based. In the first methodology ORFs are initially identified in a sequence, whether it is a complete genome sequence or a relatively large segment of a genome sequence. An ORF consists of a stretch of DNA that lies between a start codon (usually ATG but in many bacteria also TTG and GTG) and a stop codon in the reading frame of that particular start codon. For genomes with normal bacterial %GC content and codon usage, ORFs of at least 300 base pairs (bp) can be considered as strong candidates for the coding regions of genes. However, ORFS smaller than this size can code for functional proteins. Deciding which of these small ORFs represent genes can be helped by looking for significant sequence matches, particularly if these matched sequences are of a similar size. However, until more experimental evidence is available for the function of small ORFs in prokaryotic genomes, the particular cut-off that is chosen is largely an arbitrary decision. For instance, the GLIMMER program (*see* below) uses a default cut-off whereby ORFs of less than 90 bp are ignored.

ORFs can be chosen either manually or by using software such as GLIMMER *(7)* (available from The Institute for Genomic Research [TIGR] web site: http://www.tigr.org), which uses an interpolated Markov model to "learn" from real gene sequences what an ORF should "look" like and then proceeds to identify candidate ORFs on this basis. Once ORFs have been identified using any particular method, each one can be used as a query sequence to search for similar sequences from other organisms that are available in databases. As detailed below, the assignment of homology and possibly function is then made depending on the strength of any sequence similarities.

An alternative approach to genome sequence analysis does not pre-define ORFs before doing sequence-similarity searches. Rather, it uses as its query sequence a segment of DNA that is expected to contain many genes, say 100,000 bp, and maps the sequence similarity matches on top of all the possible start and stop codons in the appropriate six reading frames. This can be done using graphical software such as ACEDB or ARTEMIS (*see* **Subheading 2.1., 2.2.**). By looking at all of this information at once, it is relatively easy to identify the start and stop of ORFs and to make the same judgements about homology as are carried out in the ORF-based methods. One of the advantages of using this methodology when looking at bacterial genome sequences is that it more readily allows the identification of frameshift mutations *(8)* and pseudogenes. Frameshifts are sometimes used by bacteria to regulate gene expression in a reversible process called phase variation. This usually occurs in genes, known as contingency genes, which are adaptive to different environmental conditions *(9)*. The identification of such frameshifts was of particular importance in the annotation of the MC58 genome sequence owing to the relatively high number of repeat-associated phase-variable genes in this genome *(3,10)*. A pseudogene is a term used in genetics to describe a gene that is not expressed owing to the presence of stop codons or frameshifts that interrupt the translation of the full protein. They are generated through the normal processes of mutation when a gene no longer provides a selective advantage for the organism. It is important to identify pseudogenes in a genome sequence because they give information about the evolutionary history of the genome and hence the organism. It is also possible that pseudogenes may have arisen after the isolation and during cultivation of the sequenced strain. Therefore, the wild-type organisms and other isolates may posses functional copies of these genes rather than pseudogenes. In addition, pseudogenes may be reactivated by homologous recombination with a functioning copy of the gene.

2.1. Specific Genome Comparisons

Summary tables of genome sequencing projects, both completed and incomplete, can be found at various websites maintained by genome sequencing and/or database facilities or by individual scientists. Examples of the former are the websites maintained by TIGR and The National Center for Biotechnology Information's (NCBI) Entrez facility (http://www.ncbi.nlm.nih.gov/Entrez/); a good example of the latter is the website of Dr. N. Kyrpides (http://wit.integatzdgenomics.com/gold). These summary tables provide links to data on individual genome-sequencing projects, invariably contain some information on the strain or isolate used for sequencing, and may provide literature references for the organism in question. The MC58 genome sequence web page can be found through the TIGR microbial genomes database site (http://www.tigr.org/), whereas the Z2491 genome sequence web page can be found through the Sanger Center site (http://www.sanger.ac.uk/). In addition, websites for incomplete genome sequences usually include one or more suggested wordings for citing the use of the sequence. Often the websites include facilities for searching the genome-sequence annotations for keywords and gene locus numbers and for searching the sequences for similarities to user-provided query sequences. The NCBI Entrez facility also provides further links to taxonomy tables and to some specific analysis data such as Clusters of Orthologous Groups of proteins (COGs) ***(11,12)***, and taxonomic distribution of homologs (TAXTABLE) (both found through links from the respective complete genome sequence pages within the Entrez website).

Most commonly, the analysis facilities on the genome sequencing project web pages are limited to sequence comparisons using the BLAST (basic local alignment search tool) search software ***(13,14)*** (*see* **Subheading 2.1.**). To facilitate complete genome-sequence comparisons and other more detailed analysis on the user's own computer systems, the genome-sequence data can be downloaded by following the instructions on the respective web pages. Typically three sets of data are made available: 1) the complete genome sequence; 2) all ORFs; and 3) the conceptually translated protein sequences of those ORFs. These files are typically provided in FASTA format, the last two being in multi-FASTA format. The FASTA format consists of a plain text file where the first line of the file is the label for the sequence that follows. The form of this label is a "greater-than" character (i.e., >) followed by a title (e.g., >dnaA1). Only one line can be used for this labeling. On the next and subsequent lines the sequence is given, usually with 80 characters per line. In multi-FASTA format, further sequences with their associated labels are appended one after the other in a single file. There is no need for any special indication of the end of a sequence as this is understood if no further text is found or, if a > character is found, a new label and therefore sequence is expected next.

It is important to note that the sequence files obtained from unfinished sequencing projects will carry with them a disclaimer to the effect that the sequences are not only incomplete but will contain a number of errors. In an unfinished sequencing project, the sequence data is in the form of a number of contigs. Sequencing errors are most apparent as ambiguous residues, given as N rather than A, C, G, or T, but may also lay "hidden" in the form of insertions and/or deletions that may result in frameshifts if located within a coding region. In addition, the contigs may have been assembled incorrectly, a situation that may not become apparent until more sequence data is obtained. This is particularly a problem with genomes that contain a large amount of repeated DNA sequences such as a high number of mobile elements of a particular family as was experienced with the meningococcal genomes. Some preliminary annotations or ORF designations may also be provided. Lastly, the ends of contigs should be treated with caution as they often contain relatively large numbers of sequencing errors owing to the inherent limitations of sequencing-gel read lengths. Most errors, particularly contig assembly, will be corrected in the final release of the sequence. However, it should be kept in mind that a few sequence errors will still exist in the final sequence release (for instance, an error rate of one base in 10,000 is generally considered very low) so one should never view a genome sequence as definitive.

Two widely used sequence search software packages are freely available; Standalone BLAST (available from the NCBI's anonymous ftp server; ftp://ncbi.nlm.nih.gov) and FASTA ***(15)*** (available from; ftp://ftp.virginia.edu/pub/fasta/). Both packages contain a number of different programs, often called "flavors," that are used depending on the type of query sequence and database being used (i.e., DNA or protein sequences). The Standalone BLAST programs are generally quicker than the FASTA programs, but the FASTA programs are considered by many as being more sensitive at identifying distant relatives and the statistics (*see* **Subheading 2.2.**) given by the various programs in the two packages are calculated differently. Where possible, protein vs protein sequence searches should be carried out, with "on-the-fly" translated DNA sequence searches being the next most desirable, followed lastly by DNA vs DNA sequence searches. For protein vs protein, or DNA vs DNA, sequence searches the BLASTP and BLASTN programs should be used, respectively. These programs are quicker than the corresponding FASTA program and give results that are comparable in sensitivity. If time is not a constraint, the more sensitive but slower FASTA package program, SSEARCH3, can be used with protein vs protein sequence searches. There is little added advantage in using this program with DNA vs DNA searches. When using translated DNA query sequences to search a protein database, the FASTX3 or FASTY3 programs should be used because they allow for frameshifts in the DNA query sequence, which the equivalent BLASTX program does not. The FASTY3 program is slower than the FASTX3 program but is more sensitive. For protein query sequences searching translated DNA databases, the TFASTX3 or TFASTY3 programs should be used. Again, these two programs allow for frameshifts in the DNA sequences, and the TFASTY3 program is slightly slower but more sensitive than the TFASTX3 program.

Once a genome sequence has been downloaded, each genome sequence must be converted into a BLAST-searchable database before it can be searched using the BLAST programs. This is done by using the FORMATDB program from the Standalone BLAST package. Detailed instructions for setting up Standalone BLAST, creating searchable databases and for running the various flavors of BLAST are found in the README file that is distributed with the package. Similarly, information for setting up and running the FASTA programs will be found in the associated README file. However, because the FASTA package can take FASTA formatted sequences as its databases, there is no need to pre-format the database as with the BLAST package because the genome sequences are usually obtained already in the FASTA format.

The software used for sequence searches are continuously under development and so the best approach is likely to change over time. The guidelines given here will serve most users well and once experience is gained in the use of these methods it will become easier to adapt to new methods as needed.

2.2. The Assignment of Putative Homology and Function to Sequences

The most important pieces of information for deciding the possible homology of a query sequence are the results from database searches. Both BLAST and FASTA outputs include an expectation value for each match, "E" values for BLAST results and "E()" values for FASTA results. These statistics are an estimate of the number of times one would expect to find the observed match purely by chance given the size and sequence composition of the database that has been searched. To be confident that the match is real and not just a result of chance similarity, one will want this number to be as small as possible. As a rule of thumb, expectation values of 10^{-5} to 10^{-6} can be used as a conservative threshold for the assignment of homology. This threshold can be lowered, to say 10^{-10}, in order to increase the specificity of the search. Alternatively, the threshold may be raised, to say 10^{-3}, if one wants to ensure that fewer potential homologs are missed (i.e., to increase the sensitivity of the search). However, a search with a higher threshold will allow more false-positive matches to be made and because closer attention will then need to be given to the analysis of the results, this strategy is not advisable when analyzing large numbers of genes.

There are a number of parameters that can be changed in the BLAST and FASTA programs that will affect the sensitivity of the searches. One of the most important parameters that can be changed are the substitution matrices. Substitution matrices are tables that list the cost of each possible pairwise amino acid or nucleotide substitution and are used by search and alignment programs to calculate the scores for alignments. The individual costs have been calculated from empirical comparisons of clearly aligned sequences. A number of different scoring matrices have been developed using different methods the most popular of which are the BLOSUM matrices *(16)*. By default BLAST uses the BLOSUM62 matrix whereas FASTA uses the BLOSUM50 matrix. For the identification of more distantly related sequences a lower BLOSUM table, for example BLOSUM45, should be tried. An alternative approach to identifying distantly related sequences is to use the PSI-BLAST (position-specific iterative-BLAST) program *(12)*. This program performs a standard BLASTP search of a database and reports the matches. All matches over a certain user-defined threshold (the default is E = 0.001) are then combined into a summary sequence, which is then used as the query sequence for another iteration of the BLASTP search. Successive iterative searches can be made until no new database matches are found.

One source of potential confusion when interpreting search matches occurs when genes have undergone fusion and/or domain rearrangements *(17,18)*. In these cases, good sequence matches to different genes can be made for different regions of the query sequence. If only the best-matched sequence is considered, an erroneous, or at least not a fully detailed, assignment of function can be made. It is therefore informative to look at all of the sequence matches down to the chosen expectation cut-off and note whether matches to genes with significantly different functions are found.

It is also important to note the possibility of circular annotations in database entries *(19)* when searching databases such as GenBank, EMBL, SwissProt, and PIR. This has become a particular problem with the advent of genome sequencing and automated annotation procedures. This problem arises when genes are annotated only on the basis of sequence similarity without any experimental confirmation. Although the initial annotation of a putative gene may be made on the basis of sequence similarity to an experimentally confirmed gene, subsequent annotations based on similarity to this putative gene, then to the newly annotated gene and so on, can occur to such an extent that an annotation can be made where the newly annotated gene has no real similarity to the initial experimentally confirmed gene.

Further information about the possible homology and/or function of specific sequences can be obtained by searching the sequences for conserved sequence signatures and similarities to domains associated with particular families of proteins or functions. Of most use are the Pfam (protein family) *(20)* (http://www.cgr.ki.se/Pfam/), Prosite *(21)* (http://www.expasy.ch/prosite/), and ProDom (protein domain) *(22)* (http://protein.toulouse.inra.fr/prodom.html) databases. All three databases contain groupings of homologous protein domains that have been compiled by different automated methodologies, but are based on the knowledge that most globular proteins larger than about 200 amino acids are composed of a number of discrete structural domains, which often possess discrete functions *(23)*. Furthermore, these domains have evolved from common ancestors and are distributed among different proteins through tandem duplications and/or recombination. The Prosite database also contains signature sequences for particular protein domains or protein families (*see* **Subheading 2.3.**).

Once an enzymatic function has been assigned the relevant pathway and Enzyme Commission (EC) number can often be found by consulting metabolic pathway information such as those contained within the Expasy website (http://www.expasy.ch/). This site shows the location of the enzyme in a biochemical-pathway map. This data helps in understanding the function of the enzyme and thus adds extra information to the annotation. More information on metabolic pathways including genome by genome analyses can be found at the KEGG (Kyoto encyclopedia of genes and genomes) website (http://www.genome.ad.jp/kegg/) *(24)*. Metabolic pathway information may help in suggesting to the investigator what further genes are likely to be present in the genome in order to complete a particular pathway (*see* **refs. *25,26***).

The organization of a genome-sequence annotation and comprehension of the biochemical capacities of the associated organism can be greatly aided by categorizing each gene according to its broad function, for example, DNA metabolism or energy production. A standardized classification system has been developed and provides a framework that has been widely used in genome-sequence annotations *(27)*.

An exemplar of functional genome-sequence analysis based on homology searches is that undertaken to identify potential virulence factors from the MC58 genome sequence *(3)*. By identifying sequences within the MC58 genome sequence that have homology to known virulence-associated genes from other organisms a list of 31 potential virulence factors previously unidentified in meningococci was compiled. The potential roles of these genes in virulence represent hypotheses that may be tested by experimentation.

Two groups of genes within genomes are implicitly hypothetical owing to a lack of experimental evidence for their expression and therefore function. Genes that are identified in more than one genome sequence, but for which no known function can be assigned, are classified as "conserved hypothetical" or "function unknown" (FUN), while ORFs that appear only within one genome and have no sequence similarity to other sequences in the databases are termed simply "hypothetical." Although it is possible that a FUN gene may turn out to be nonexpressed DNA that fortuitously forms an ORF in more than one organism this possibility is vanishingly small if the FUN gene exists in distantly related genomes. Currently around 40% of ORFs from prokaryotic genome sequences are not assigned a function, but this proportion is likely to become smaller as more functional analyses are done. Still it should be kept in mind that some of the hypothetical ORFs, particularly small ones, may turn out not to be genes.

2.3. Analysis of Gene Families and Gene Organization

Because of whole gene duplications, a further distinction needs to be made when considering related genes within and between genomes. When a gene (α) duplicates in a genome and some degree of divergence occurs (say, $\alpha \rightarrow \alpha$ and β), the duplicated gene(s) and the original gene are called paralogues. If the organism in which this duplication has occurred then diverges through speciation the genes belonging to any one gene lineage, say the β lineage, are called orthologues. Orthologues are likely to have the same functions, whereas paralogues are more likely to have diverged in their functions. Paralogous genes in two or more species are, as defined earlier, related to each other through the ancestral gene-duplication event, thus gene α in one species and gene β in another species are also paralogues of each other. Orthology and paralogy is assessed on the basis of sequence similarity where orthologues are expected to have sequences that are very similar to each other because they have similar functions, whereas more sequence divergence is expected to have occurred between paralogues. Duplication events or gene deletions can occur at any and multiple times during the divergence of organismal lineages as can nonorthologous gene displacement *(28)* giving rise to complex groups of orthologues and paralogues in different genomes, which must be considered carefully during genome-sequence analysis. Gene duplication is a fundamental process in the generation of genetic and biochemical diversity. Because duplicated genes often retain similar functions, it is often informative to group them into families and even superfamilies (for a review, *see* **ref.** ***29***). The identity and size of gene families in a genome sequence can be used as indirect evidence for the importance of the associated biochemical functions to the organism. This in turn may provide insights into niche adaptation (*see* **refs.** ***25,26***). For example, the genome sequence of *Helicobacter pylori* contains a relatively large family of outer-membrane proteins (OMPs) that may testify to the need of this organism to adapt to its gastric niche *(30)*.

Sometimes related genes are clustered together *(31)* on the genome or organized into operons. This may add extra evidence for assigning a function or the cellular process with which an ORF is associated. However, many genomes are far less "operonic" than the model organisms *Escherichia coli* and *Bacillus subtilis* and gene orders become less conserved the larger the evolutionary distance between organsisms, so this approach must be used with caution.

2.4. Visualization of Genome-Sequence Information

Of enormous benefit to the comprehension of database search results and genome organization is a graphical interface. A number have been and continue to be developed. The MC58 genome sequencing project relied heavily on the ACEDB program *(32)* (information and program available from the website; http://www.acedb.org/). A graphical interface allows sequences and database matches to be viewed in a relational or contextual manner. In addition, the flexibility of the ACEDB input format allows extra results to be added. In this way, nonhomology-based analyses such as the identification of repetitive sequences can be carried out *(1)*. Another graphical interface for genome sequence analysis is the ARTEMIS program (available from the Sanger Center website), which is a JAVA-based tool for the annotation of and visualization of pre-annotated genome sequences. Sequences to be viewed must be in either the GENBANK or EMBL formats and similarly are saved in either of these formats *(33)*. Detailed information for installing and running ARTEMIS can be found in the users manual located on the ARTEMIS web page. The principal advantage of this approach is that organization and the sequence context of regions or features of interest can be appreciated in a way that is not possible without a graphical interface.

2.5. Other Specialized Analyses and Uses of Complete Genome Sequences

Large-scale inversions, duplications, or translocations that occur within or between closely related genomes can provide information about the evolution and plasticity of the genomes. Identifying such large-scale genomic rearrangements can be difficult without using special methods because the alignment of very large DNA sequences is not possible with normal alignment programs. In order to carry out analyses and visualize the results, the MUMmer program was developed *(34)* (available from the TIGR software web page). Instructions for installing and running this program on a UNIX machine are contained in the README file. This software uses a suffix-tree algorithm to make an alignment of two closely related genome sequences and the output can be displayed as a dotplot. Software to display the rearrangements in more detail is still under development at the time of writing, although the dotplot can be plotted from the ".out" file using the GNUPLOT program (available from the GNU website; http://www.gnu.org). Detailed instructions for installing and running

GNUPLOT can be found in the README file that is distributed with the program.

There are several ways in which a complete (or near complete) genome sequence can facilitate investigations that are not possible with lesser amounts of sequence data. A number of pressures affect the sequence composition of an organism including the metabolic environment and codon usage, which can influence the %GC content of a sequence and other less well-defined processes, such as relative differences in mutations that occur during replication and error correction owing to differences in the DNA metabolism enzymes. Each sequence, in addition to being a string of single bases, can also be considered to be a string of longer components, including, for example, dinucleotides. Thus, a sequence can also be viewed as a string of dinucleotide pairs. It has been noted that each species has a specific dinucleotide signature (DNS), which is based on the proportion of each dinucleotide pair to the total genome. Differences in the %GC content, codon usage within genes, and regions that have an atypical DNS can all be used to identify regions of DNA that are atypical of the whole genome, and these regions are frequently associated with ORFs that might have been acquired by horizontal transfer ***(35)***. This type of approach can provide information useful in the identification of pathogenicity islands and other genes that have been derived from other species backgrounds or bacteriophages, and was used in the analysis of the MC58 genome sequence ***(3)***.

An example of the use of a genome sequence to address a specific problem was the identification of potential OMPs in the MC58 genome sequence for use as vaccine candidates ***(36)***. No vaccine is currently available that is effective against the diverse strains of serogroup B meningococci. The polysaccharide capsule, used as the basis for conjugate vaccines for serogroup A and C strains, for serogroup B bacteria is structurally identical to epitopes expressed on the surface of brain cells. The MC58 genome sequence was systematically searched for potential surface expressed proteins using a combination of homology and pattern searches, including specific screening for protein sorting and localization sites using the PSORT method (http://psort.nibb.ac.jp), and analysis of the hydrophobicity plots generated using the GCG program PEPPLOT ***(37)***. A total of 570 putative OMPs were identified, of which 350 were successfully cloned and expressed in *E. coli*, their products purified and then used to immunize mice. The degree of conservation of the identified surface proteins was then determined using a group of 22 serogroup B and several serogroup A and C pathogenic isolates. Several conserved surface-accessible proteins that elicited an antibacterial response were selected for further development as vaccine candidates ***(36)***.

Another type of analysis that can only be done using complete sequences are those in which it is possible to show that a certain type of sequence of interest is not present. For example, the absence of any short sequences in sufficient abundance to act as an uptake signal sequence in *H. pylori* was used to conclude that this naturally transformable species differs from *Haemophilus influenzae* and *N. meningitidis* in the way in which this process functions ***(38)***.

Complete genome sequences can also directly assist the experimental investigation of organisms. In the most simple sense, they represent an encyclopedia of ORF sequences such that genes of interest can be identified from short stretches of DNA or amino acid sequence. This facilitates approaches such as signature-tagged mutagenesis or proteomics based studies in which small amounts of sequence data can be used to identify the genes of interest that have been selected. It is also possible to assess the methods that are being used. For example, in a study of Tn916 as a tool for mutagenesis in *H. influenzae*, analysis using the complete genome sequence showed that the nature and location of the insertion sites meant that this was not a useful tool for generalized mutagenesis in this species, and facilitated the identification of a new consensus sequence ***(39)***.

The availability of a complete genome sequence greatly helps in facilitating large-scale functional genomics. A catalog of all genes in an organism is essential for the manufacture of microarrays for use in large-scale, parallel, gene-expression studies (e.g., ***40***) and mutant identification (e.g., ***41***). Similarly the efficient use of mass spectrometry for the identification of proteins in proteomic studies also relies on a complete genome sequence (e.g., ***42***).

Acknowledgments

NJS is supported by a Wellcome Trust Fellowship in Medical Microbiology. We wish to thank E. Richard Moxon and John Peden for critical reading of the manuscript.

References

1. Saunders, N. J. and Moxon, E. R. (1998) Implications of sequencing bacterial genomes for pathogenesis and vaccine development. *Curr. Opin. Biotechnol.* **9,** 618–623.
2. Field, D., Hood, D., and Moxon, E. R. (1999) Contribution of genomics to bacterial pathogenesis. *Curr. Opin. Genet. Dev.* **9,** 700–703.
3. Tettelin, H., Saunders, N. J., Heidelberg, J., Jeffries, A. C., Nelson, K. E., Eisen, J. A., et al. (2000) Complete genome sequence of *Neisseria meningitidis* serotype B strain MC58. *Science* **287,** 1809–1815.
4. Parkhill, J., Achtman, M., James, K. D., Bentley, S. D., Churcher, C., Klee, S. R., et al. (2000) Complete DNA sequence of a serogroup A strain of *Neisseria meningitidis* Z2491. *Nature* **404,** 502–506.
5. Fleischmann, R. D., Adams, M. D., White, O., Clayton, R. A., Kirkness, E. F., Kerlavage, A. R., et al. (1995) Whole-genome random sequencing and assembly of *Haemophilus influenzae* Rd. *Science* **269,** 496–512.

6. Frangeul, L., Nelson, K. E., Buchrieser, C., Danchin, A., Glaser, P., and Kunst, F. (1999) Cloning and assembly strategies in microbial genome projects. *Microbiology* **145,** 2625–2634.
7. Salzberg, S., Delcher, A., Kasif, S., and White, O. (1998) Microbial gene identification using interpolated Markov models. *Nucleic Acids Res.* **2,** 544–548.
8. Saunders, N. J., Peden, J. F., Hood, D. W., and Moxon, E. R. (1998) Simple sequence repeats in the *Helicobacter pylori* genome. *Mol. Microbiol.* **27,** 1091–1098.
9. Moxon, E. R., Rainey, P. B., Nowak, M. A., and Lenski, R. E. (1994) Adaptive evolution of highly mutable loci in pathogenic bacteria. *Curr. Biol.* **4,** 24–33.
10. Saunders, N. J., Jeffries, A. C., Peden, J. F., Hood, D. W., Tettelin, H., Rappuoli, R. and Moxon, E. R. (2000) Repeat-associated phase variable genes in the complete genome sequence of *Neisseria meningitidis* strain MC58. *Mol. Micobiol.* **37,** 207–215.
11. Tatusov, R. L., Koonin, E. V., and Lipman, D. J. (1997) A genomic perspective on protein families. *Science* **278,** 631–637.
12. Tatusov, R. L., Galperin, M. Y., Natale, D. A., and Koonin, E. V. (2000) The COG database: a tool for genome-scale analyses of protein functions and evolution. *Nucleic Acids Res.* **28,** 33–36.
13. Altschul, S. F., Gish, W., Miller, W., Myers, E. W., and Lipman, D. J. (1990) Basic local alignment search tool. *J. Mol. Biol.* **215,** 403–410.
14. Altschul, S. F., Madden, T. L., Schaffer, A. A., Zhang, J., Zhang, Z., Miller, W., and Lipman, D. J. (1997) Gapped BLAST and PSI-BLAST: a new generation of protein database search programs. *Nucleic Acids Res.* **25,** 3389–3402.
15. Pearson, W. R. (2000) Flexible sequence similarity searching with the FASTA3 program package. *Methods Mol. Biol.* **132,** 185–219.
16. Henikoff, S. and Henikoff, J. G. (1992) Amino acid substitution matrices from protein blocks. *Proc. Natl. Acad. Sci. USA* **89,** 10,915–10,919.
17. Galperin, M. Y. and Koonin, E. V. (1998) Sources of systematic error in functional annotation of genomes: domain rearrangement, non-orthologous gene displacement and operon disruption. *In Silico Biol.* **1,** 55–67.
18. Enright, A. J., Iliopoulos, I., Kyprides, N. C., and Ouzounis, C. A. (1999) Protein interaction maps for complete genomes based on gene fusion events. *Nature* **402,** 86–90.
19. Kyrpides, N. C. and Ouzounis, C. A. (1999) Whole-genome sequence annotation: 'Going wrong with confidence.' *Mol. Microbiol.* **32,** 881–891.
20. Bateman, A., Birney, E., Durbin, R., Eddy, S. R., Howe, K. L., and Sonnhammer, E. L. L. (2000) The Pfam protein families database. *Nucleic Acids Res.* **28,** 263–266.
21. Bucher, P. and Bairoch, A. (1994) A generalized profile syntax for biomolecular sequences motifs and its function in automatic sequence interpretation, in *ISMB-94 Proceedings 2nd International Conference on Intelligent Systems for Molecu-*

lar Biology (Altman, R., Brutlag, D., Karp, P., Lathrop, R., and Searls, D., eds.), AAAI Press, Menlo Park, OH, pp. 53–61.

22. Corpet, F., Gouzyl, J., and Kahn, D. (1999) Recent improvements of the ProDom database of protein domain families. *Nucleic Acids Res.* **27,** 263–267.
23. Doolittle, R. F. (1995) The multiplicity of domains in proteins. *Ann. Rev. Biochem.* **64,** 287–314.
24. Kanehisa, M. and Goto, S. (2000) KEGG: Kyoto encyclopedia of genes and genomes. *Nucleic Acids Res.* **28,** 27–30.
25. Galperin, M. Y. and Koonin, E. V. (1999) Functional genomics and genome evolution. *Genetica* **106,** 159–170.
26. Galperin, M. Y., Tatusov, R. L., and Koonin, E. V. (1999) Comparing microbial genomes: how the gene set determines the lifestyle, in *Organization of the Prokaryotic Genome* (Charlebois, R. L., ed.), ASM, Washington, DC, pp. 91–108.
27. Riley, M. (1998) Systems for categorizing functions of gene products. *Curr. Opin. Struct. Biol.* **8,** 388–392.
28. Koonin, E. V., Mushegian, A. R., and Boork, P. (1996) Non-orthologous gene displacement. *Trends Genet.* **12,** 334–336.
29. Henikoff, S., Greene, E. A., Pietrokovski, S., Bork, P., Attwood, T. K., and Hood, L. (1997) Gene families: the taxonomy of protein paralogs and chimeras. *Science* **278,** 609–614.
30. Tomb, J. F., White, O., Kerlavage, A. R., Clayton, R. A., Sutton, G. G., Fleischmann, R. D., et al. (1997) The complete genome sequence of the gastric pathogen *Helicobacter pylori. Nature* **388,** 539–547.
31. Overbeek, R., Fonstein, M., D'Souza, M., Pusch, G. D., and Malsev, N. (1999) The use of gene clusters to infer functional coupling. *Proc. Natl. Acad. Sci. USA* **96,** 2896–2901.
32. Durbin, R. and Mieg, J. T. (1991) A C. elegans database. Documentation, code and data available from anonymous ftp servers at lirmm.lirmm.fr, cele.nrc-imb.cam.ac.uk and ncbi.nlm.nih.gov
33. Ouellette, B. F. F. (1998) The GenBank sequence database, in *Bioinformatics: A Practical Guide to the Analysis of Genes and Proteins* Baxevanis, A. D. and Ouellette, B. F. F., eds.), Wiley, New York, pp. 16–45.
34. Delcher, A. L., Kasif, S., Fleischmann, R. D., Peterson, J., White, O., and Salzberg, S. L. (1999) Alignment of whole genomes. *Nucleic Acids Res.* **27,** 2369–2376.
35. Karlin, S., Campbell, A. M., and Mrazek, J. (1998) Comparative DNA analysis across diverse genomes. *Ann. Rev. Genet.* **32,** 185–225.
36. Pizza, M., Scarlato, V., Masignani, V., Giuliani, M. M., Aricô, B., Baldi, L., et al. (2000) Novel proteins for vaccine development from the meningococcus B genome. *Science* **287,** 1816–1820.
37. Wisconsin Package Version 10.0, Genetics Computer Group (GCG), Madison, WI.
38. Saunders, N. J., Peden, J. F., and Moxon, E. R. (1999) The absence of an uptake sequence in *Helicobacter pylori. Microbiology* **145,** 3523–3528.

39. Hosking, S. L., Deadman, M. E., Moxon, E. R., Peden, J. F., Saunders, N. J., and High, N. J. (1998) An *in silico* evaluation of Tn916 as a tool for generalised mutagenesis in *Haemophilus influenzae* Rd. *Microbiology* **144,** 2525–2530.
40. Wilson, M., DeRisi, J., Kristensen, H-H., Imboden, P., Rane, S., Brown, P. O., and Schoolnik, G. K. (1999) Exploring drug-induced alterations in gene expression by microarray hybridization. *Proc. Natl. Acad. Sci. USA* **96,** 12,833–12,838.
41. Behr, M. A., Wilson, M. A., Gill, W. P., Salamon, H., Schoolnik, G. K., Rane, S., and Small, P. M. (1999) Comparative genomics of BCG vaccines by whole-genome DNA microarray. *Science* **284,** 1520–1523.
42. Wasinger, V. C., Pollack, J. D., and Humphery-Smith, I. (2000) The proteome of *Mycoplasma genitalium* chaps-soluble component. *Eur. J. Biochem.* **267,** 1571–1582.

16

Representational Difference Analysis

Lucas D. Bowler, Aldert Bart, and Arie van der Ende

1. Introduction

Successful pathogens have evolved a variety of specific gene products that facilitate their survival and growth within the host, as well as mechanisms to regulate expression of these virulence-associated genes in response to their environment. In comparison with commensals, the pathogenic phenotype can thus be seen as a consequence of both differences in gene content and gene expression. Not surprisingly, identification of these differences is a frequent goal in modern biomedical research, and as a result, a variety of differential screening methods have been developed over the last few years ***(1,2)***.

Representational Difference Analysis (RDA) is a method by which DNA fragments that are present in one DNA population (Tester), but absent or polymorphic in another DNA population (Driver), are preferentially amplified ***(3)***. Accordingly, the approach can be used as a tool for the identification of both differences in gene content and differences in gene expression. Differences in gene content can be identified by comparing the chromosomal DNA of a more virulent strain or species to a closely related avirulent strain or species, whereas variation in gene expression can be identified by comparison of derived cDNA populations. To this end, RDA has recently been used for detection of differences between *Neisseria meningitidis* strains ***(4–6)***, differences between *Neisseria* species ***(7,8)***, and differences between RNAs isolated from *N. meningitidis* grown under different environmental conditions (i.e., the analysis of differential gene expression) ***(9)***.

RDA belongs to the general class of DNA subtractive methodologies, in which one DNA population (known as the "Driver") is hybridized in excess against a second population (the "Tester"), to remove common (hybridizing)

From: *Methods in Molecular Medicine, vol. 67: Meningococcal Disease: Methods and Protocols*
Edited by: A. J. Pollard and M. C. J. Maiden © Humana Press Inc., Totowa, NJ

sequences, thereby enriching for "target" sequences unique to the Tester population. This is achieved by ligation of defined oligonucleotide adaptors to the 5′ end of the Tester molecules. After annealing of the Tester and Driver sequences, DNA polymerase is used to fill in the 3′ ends of the double-stranded molecules. Only tester molecules that have annealed to other tester-originating sequences will yield molecules with double-stranded adaptor sequences at both the 5′ and 3′ ends of the double-stranded sequences. Accordingly, only these molecules will be exponentially amplifiable by polymerase chain reaction (PCR) (using the specific oligonucleotides as primer), thus facilitating enrichment of Tester-specific sequences.

RDA combines this subtractive approach with positive selection of target sequences by what is termed "kinetic enrichment" ***(3)***. Kinetic enrichment takes advantage of the second-order kinetics of DNA reannealing, i.e., the rate of double-stranded DNA formation is higher for DNA species of higher concentration. Thus, the more abundant DNA species in a mixture of fragments can be further partitioned from less-abundant species by reannealing for low C_0t values (the product of initial concentration and time), and subsequent collection of the resulting double-stranded molecules. The molar ratio of abundant to less-abundant sequences in the product will then be in the order of the square of the initial ratio of the concentrations, which eventually leads to purification of the more abundant species. In RDA, this kinetic enrichment is achieved by degradation of single-stranded molecules after the initial amplification by PCR. The target sequences will be enriched exponentially by this PCR, and will therefore finish at a much higher concentration than nontarget Tester sequences (therefore forming relatively more double-stranded molecules). By degrading the single-stranded DNA using Mung Bean Nuclease, only the double-stranded sequences remain (enriched for the target sequences). Subsequently, the target sequences are further enriched for, by another round of PCR.

A modification of RDA, cDNA RDA, has been described ***(10)*** in which the starting material is derived from mRNA rather than DNA, and accordingly targets only genes that are expressed at the time the RNA is isolated. More recently, the cDNA RDA methodology has been further adapted to facilitate the identification of genes whose expression is modified between different bacterial populations ***(9)***. This approach is illustrated schematically in **Fig. 1**. The method is flexible, sensitive, and relatively inexpensive to perform, and in contrast to alternative methods such as differential-display PCR (DD-PCR), and the conceptually similar technique, RNA fingerprinting by arbitrarily primed PCR (AP-PCR), has the major advantage that sequences common to both groups of cells are eliminated. This greatly simplifies the interpretation of results and identification of the differentially expressed genes. In addition, the exponential degree of enrichment achieved by the use of PCR in cDNA RDA enables the detection of very rare transcripts ***(11)***.

Examination of differential gene expression using cDNA RDA requires the sampling of a population (of cells) grown under the condition(s) of interest and a population grown under conditions that differ only by those of interest. For example, in an study to identify iron-regulated genes in *N. meningitidis*, the bacteria would be grown under iron-limitation (to provide the so-called "Tester" material), and another population would be grown under identical conditions, except that iron would be freely available (to provide the "Driver"). To identify genes whose expression is suppressed under iron-limitation, the converse would apply. mRNA is extracted from both populations, and used as a template for cDNA synthesis. The derived cDNAs are restricted and oligonucleotides ligated to the fragments. PCR, using primers specific to these oligonucleotides, is then used to amplify each population of DNA fragments. After amplification, the oligonucleotides are removed with the same enzyme, and the amplified cDNA fragments purified (these preparations are referred to as representations). For the hybridization and amplification stages, new oligonucleotides are ligated to the Tester DNAs only. Tester and Driver DNAs (the latter in excess) are mixed, denatured, and allowed to hybridize. PCR using primers specific to the new oligonucleotide extensions results in enrichment of sequences unique to the Tester DNA population. By repeating these steps, the degree of enrichment is increased. The result is a number of PCR products (difference products) that represent the messages unique to the Tester population. These can then be cloned and characterized. In order to facilitate detection of upregulated messages, rather than just transcripts from genes whose expression is simply switched on or off, experiments can be performed using representations that have been depleted of low-copy sequences by a process known as melt depletion ***(10)***.

As with RDA, cDNA RDA can be divided into three main phases: 1) The generation of PCR amplicons representative of the RNA isolated from given bacterial populations (the purification of genomic DNA restriction fragments in RDA); 2) the PCR-coupled subtractive hybridization of the different representative amplicons (or genomic restriction fragments); and 3) the cloning and screening of the resultant products (which represent the differences between the two populations that were compared). This chapter will describe the procedures involved in carrying out these analyses.

2. Materials

Other than standard molecular biology laboratory equipment, the following items are required:

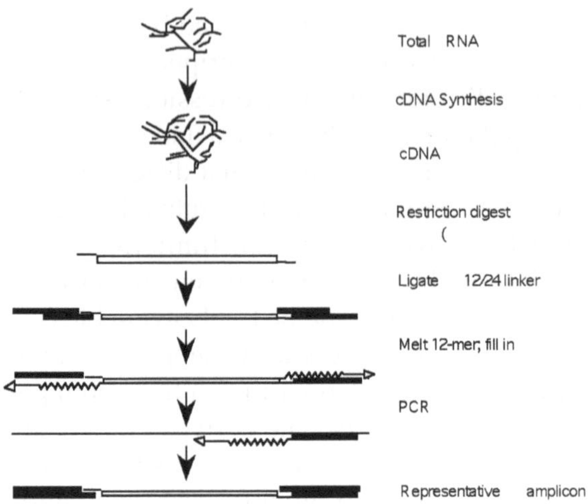
Total RNA
cDNA Synthesis
cDNA
Restriction digest
Ligate 12/24 linker
Melt 12-mer; fill in
PCR
Representative amplicon

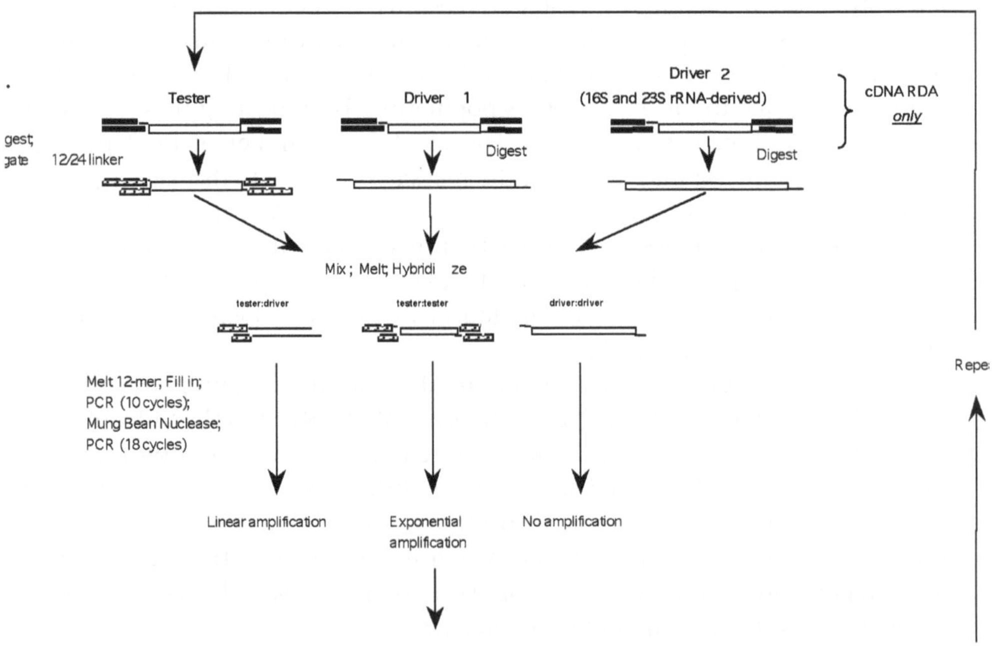
Tester
Driver 1
Driver 2
(16S and 23S rRNA-derived)
cDNA RDA
only
gest;
gate 12/24 linker
Digest
Digest
Mix ; Melt; Hybridi ze
tester:driver
tester:tester
driver:driver
Melt 12-mer; Fill in;
PCR (10 cycles);
Mung Bean Nuclease;
PCR (18 cycles)
Linear amplification
Exponential amplification
No amplification
Repe

1. A high-quality Thermal Cycler.
2. A refrigerated microfuge.

2.1. RDA

2.1.2. Chromosomal DNA Isolation

1. High-quality chromosomal DNA from both bacterial strains to be compared (i.e., Tester and Driver strains). This can be isolated using the protocol in **Subheading 3.1.1.**, using **items 2–11** inclusive, given below. Alternatively, Neisserial chromosomal DNA can be isolated using various commercially available kits, both the Genomic-Tip 100/G system (Qiagen) and the PUREGENE DNA Isolation Kit (Gentra systems) have worked well in our experience.

Fig. 1. *(previous page)* **(A)** Schematic view of the procedure for generation of the initial representations in cDNA RDA. cDNA is produced by random-primed reverse transcription of total RNA. The cDNA is then digested with a restriction enzyme (*e.g. Dpn*II in the cDNA RDA protocol). To the 4 nucleotide-5′ overhang created by the restriction enzyme, 4 nucleotides of the 12-mer oligonucleotide (J-Bgl-12) of the adaptor hybridize. The 24-mer oligonucleotide (J-Bgl-24) of the adaptor hybridizes to the remaining 8 nucleotides of the 12-mer, and can thus be covalently joined to the 5′ phosphate group of the digested starting material. Since the 12-mer is not phosphorylated, it does not become covalently attached, and accordingly dissociates at a higher temperature (72°C in the cDNA RDA protocol). The Taq polymerase is added, and can then "fill in" the sequence complementary to the 24-mer. This creates a binding site for the J-Bgl-24 oligonucleotide that is used as primer in subsequent PCR. Adapted from **ref. *11***. **(B)** Overview of the hybridization/amplification steps in RDA. For cDNA RDA, the adaptors are digested from the representative amplicons of Tester and Driver, and from the 16S and 23S rRNA-derived Driver (Driver 2), which is used in cDNA RDA *only*. For RDA, a digest of genomic DNA is used without generating representative amplicons. A set of adaptors is ligated to the Tester only (in a similar way to that outlined in (A)). The Tester-adaptor DNA is then mixed with excess Driver DNA, melted to obtain single stranded DNA, and allowed to hybridize. Tester sequences present in both the Tester and Driver pools will form heteroduplexes with Driver sequences, whereas unique Tester sequences ("targets") can only hybridize with their complementary Tester-originating sequences. The subsequent "fill in" reaction (*see* (A)) will create molecules with the 24-mer sequence and its complement at both the 5′ and 3′ ends of the molecule for target sequences only. In the following 10 PCR cycles (11 in cDNA RDA), target sequences are amplified exponentially, non-target sequences are linearly amplified or are not amplified at all (Driver-Driver hybrids). Further enrichment is achieved by degradation of single-stranded DNA (including single stranded overhangs of double stranded molecules) with Mung Bean Nuclease, and further PCR amplification. If target sequences are not sufficiently enriched in the first difference product, the procedure can be repeated (in cDNA RDA, generation of DP2 is normal, DP3 can be required in some cases).

2. GTE buffer: 50 m*M* glucose, 50 m*M* Tris-HCl, pH 8.0, 50 m*M* EDTA.
3. Lysozyme (Sigma-Aldrich Co., 30 mg/mL).
4. 20% sodium dodecyl sulphate (SDS).
5. Pronase or Protease K (Calbiochem or Roche Diagnostics, 20 mg/mL).
6. RNAse (Roche Diagnostics, 10 mg/mL).
7. Phenol:chloroform:isoamyl alcohol (25:24:1, [v/v] saturated with 10 m*M* Tris-HCl, 1 m*M* ethylene diamine tetraacetic acid [EDTA], pH 8.0).
8. Chloroform:isoamyl alcohol (24:1, [v/v] saturated with 10 m*M* Tris-HCl, 1 m*M* EDTA, pH 8.0).
9. 3 *M* Sodium acetate, pH 5.3.
10. Ethanol, 100% and 70 %.
11. Sterilized, ultra-high-purity (UHP) water (e.g., from Milli-Q Water System, Millipore).
12. TBE (10X): 1.0 *M* Tris-HCl, 0.9 *M* boric acid, 20 m*M* EDTA, pH 8.3.
13. 1% (w/v) nondenaturing agarose gel in TBE, pH 8.3. The gel should contain 0.1 mg/mL ethidium bromide.
14. Ethidium bromide (10 mg/mL). Store at 4°C in the dark. (**Caution:** Ethidium bromide is highly carcinogenic; handle under appropriate guidelines).
15. DNA molecular size and concentration standards (e.g., 0, 0.5, 1, 2.5, 5, 10 ng/ μL *Hin*dIII digest of lambda phage, New England Biolabs).

2.1.3. Restriction

1. Restriction enzyme *Sau*3A (Boehringer Mannheim GmbH).
2. 10X *Sau*3A buffer (supplied with restriction enzyme).
3. UHP sterilized water.
4. TBE (10X): 0.9 *M* Tris-HCl, 0.9 *M* boric acid, 20 m*M* EDTA, pH 8.3.
5. 1% (w/v) nondenaturing agarose gel in TBE, pH 8.3. The gel should contain 0.1 mg/mL ethidium bromide.
6. Ethidium bromide (10 mg/mL). Store at 4°C in the dark. (**Caution:** Ethidium bromide is highly carcinogenic; handle under appropriate guidelines).
7. DNA molecular size standards (e.g., 100 bp ladder, New England Biolabs, 1 μg/mL).
8. Phenol:chloroform:isoamyl alcohol (25:24:1 [v/v] saturated with 10 m*M* Tris-HCl, 1 m*M* EDTA, pH 8.0).
9. Chloroform:isoamyl alcohol (24:1 [v/v] saturated with 10 m*M* Tris-HCl, 1 m*M* EDTA, pH 8.0).
10. 3 *M* Sodium acetate, pH 5.3.
11. Ethanol, 100% and 70 %.

2.1.4. Ligation of Linkers

1. HPLC-purified linker oligonucleotides, 0.2 mM stocks; *see* **Table 1**.
2. T4 DNA ligase (New England Biolabs, 400 U/μL).
3. 10X T4 DNA ligase buffer (containing ATP, supplied with ligase).

Table 1
HPLC-Purified Linker Oligonucleotides, 0.2 m*M* Stocks

Name	Sequence
R-Bgl-12	5′- GAT CTG CGG TGA -3′
R-Bgl-24	5′- AGC ACT CTC CAG CCT CTC ACC GCA -3′
J-Bgl-12	5′- GAT CTG TTC ATG -3′
J-Bgl-24	5′- ACC GAC GTC GAC TAT CCA TGA ACA -3′
N-Bgl-12	5′- GAT CTT CCC TCG -3′
N-Bgl-24	5′- AGG CAA CTG TGC TAT CCG AGG GAA -3′

2.1.5. Subtractive Hybridization

1. 3X EE buffer: 30 m*M* *N*-(2-hydroxyl) piperazine-*N*''-(3-propanesulfonic acid) (EPPS), 3 m*M* EDTA, pH 8.0.
2. Sterile mineral oil.
3. 5 *M* NaCl.
4. Taq DNA polymerase (Qiagen or Promega, 5 U/μL).
5. 10X PCR buffer (as supplied with *Taq*).
6. 10 m*M* dNTP mix (10 m*M* each dGTP, dATP, dCTP, dTTP, as supplied with Taq).
7. High-performance liquid chromatography (HPLC)-purified linker 24-mer oligonucleotides, 0.2 m*M* stocks (*see* **Subheading 2.1.4.**).
8. Mung Bean Nuclease (New England Biolabs, 10 U/μL).
9. 2X Mung Bean Nuclease buffer (New England Biolabs, as supplied with Mung Bean Nuclease).
10. 50 m*M* Tris-HCl, pH 8.9.
11. TBE (10X): 1.0 *M* Tris-HCl, 90 m*M* Boric acid, 2 m*M* EDTA, pH 8.3.
12. 2% (w/v) non-denaturing agarose gel in TBE, pH 8.3. The gel should contain 0.1 mg/mL ethidium bromide.
13. Ethidium bromide (10 mg/mL). Store at 4°C in the dark. (**Caution:** Ethidium bromide is highly carcinogenic; handle under appropriate guidelines).
14. DNA molecular size standards (e.g., 100 bp ladder, New England Biolabs, 1 μg/mL).
15. Ethanol, 100% and 70 %.

2.1.6. Screening of Difference Products

1. Razor blades or scalpels.
2. Qiaex II DNA purification kit (Qiagen).
3. Cloning system for PCR products (e.g., PCR2.1 TA cloning kit, Invitrogen Co.).

2.2. cDNA RDA

2.2.2. RNA Isolation

RNA is generally very sensitive to the action of ribonucleases. Accordingly, for the successful isolation of high-quality RNA, it is absolutely essential that all solutions and equipment used should be RNase-free. Hands are a major source of nuclease contamination, and powder-free gloves should be worn at all times. (Indeed, it is advisable to change gloves several times during the course of an isolation, because the outsides of the gloves themselves can become contaminated through contact with items in the lab environment.) The use of sterile disposable plasticware is recommended, and where glassware is used, this should be foil-sealed and baked for at least 4 h at 200°C, before use. Because of the potential for residual traces of diethylpyrocarbonate (DEPC) to inhibit some enzymatic processes, we prefer to use untreated ultra high-purity (UHP) water to make up all solutions. These are then filter-sterilized (using nuclease-free filters). UHP water from a good purification system is usually RNase-free, however, it is advisable to check, e.g., using an RNaseAlert kit (Ambion, Inc.).

1. Triisopropylnaphthalene sulphonic acid (TNS, Acros Organics, NJ).
2. *p*-Aminosalicylic acid (PAS, Sigma-Aldrich. Co.).
3. TNS/PAS Lysis solution: 2% TNS, 6% PAS, 1% sodium dodecyl sulfate (SDS), 50 m*M* EDTA, pH 8.0, 250 m*M* NaCl, 200 m*M* MES, pH 6.0, 6% n-butanol, 100 m*M* 2-mercaptoethanol. The TNS/PAS solution should be made up fresh each time in RNase-free water. The 2-mercaptoethanol is added just before use.
4. Acid phenol:chloroform (5:1 [v/v] acid equilibrated to pH 4.7).
5. Chloroform:isoamyl alcohol (49:1 [v/v]).
6. 2.5 *M* LiCl, 25 m*M* EDTA.
7. PRIME RNase inhibitor (5 Prime > 3 Prime, Inc., CO, 0.5–1 U/μL).
8. DNase I buffer: 10 m*M* $CaCl_2$, 10 m*M* $MgCl_2$, 50 m*M* TES, pH 7.5, plus PRIME RNase inhibitor (1 U/30 μL).
9. RNase-free DNase I (e.g., RQ1 RNase-free DNase, Promega Co., 1 U/μL).
10. 10 *M* ammonium acetate.
11. 0.1 m*M* EDTA, plus 1 U/30 μL Prime RNase inhibitor.
12. TBE (10X): 0.9 *M* Tris-HCl, 0.9 *M* boric acid, 20 m*M* EDTA, pH 7.8.
13. 1% (w/v) nondenaturing agarose gel in TBE, pH 7.8. The gel should contain 0.1 mg/mL ethidium bromide.
14. Ethidium bromide (10 mg/mL). Store at 4°C in the dark. (**Caution:** Ethidium bromide is highly carcinogenic; handle under appropriate guidelines).
15. DNA molecular size standards (e.g., 1 Kb plus DNA ladder, Life Technologies, 1 μg/mL).
16. Sterile 50-mL Falcon tubes.
17. Nuclease-free filter tips for micropipets.
18. Nuclease-free microfuge tubes (e.g., from Ambion, Inc.).

2.2.3. cDNA Synthesis

1. TimeSaver cDNA synthesis kit (Amersham Pharmacia Biotech).
2. Superscript II reverse transcriptase (Life Technologies, 200 U/μL).
3. cDNA spun columns (Amersham Pharmacia Biotech).

Table 2
Primer Pairs for Neisserial 16s and 23s Ribosomal RNA Genes

Name	Orientation	Sequence
16Sup	Forward primer	5′-CATAAGAGTTTGATCCTGGCT-3′; 25 pM.
16Sdn	Reverse primer	5′-GTCATGAAGCATACCGTGGT-3′; 25 pM.
23Sup	Forward primer	5′-CAGGT/CGGATGCCTTGGCGA-3′; 25 pM.
23Sdn	Reverse primer	5′-AGAGTCAAGCCTCACGA/GGGCA-3′; 25 pM.

4. *Dpn*II buffer: 100 m*M* NaCl, 50 m*M* Bis Tris-HCl, 10 m*M* $MgCl_2$, pH 6.0. Make up sufficient buffer to equilibrate cDNA spun columns (requires approx 6–7 mL/column).
5. DTT: 0.1 *M* dithiothreitol; store at –20°C.

2.2.4. Isolation of Neisserial 16S and 23S rRNA Genes

1. Neisseria chromosomal DNA (*see* **Subheading 2.1.2.**).
2. PCR primer pairs: *see* **Table 2**.
3. Taq DNA polymerase (e.g., TaKaRa *Ex-Taq*, Takara Shuzo Co., Ltd., 5 U/μL).
4. PCR buffer and dNTPs (as supplied with *Ex-Taq*).
5. 5 *M* Betaine (Sigma-Aldrich Co.).
6. TBE (10X): 1.0 *M* Tris-HCl, 90 m*M* boric acid, 2 m*M* EDTA, pH 8.3.
7. 1% (w/v) nondenaturing agarose gel in TBE, pH 8.3. The gel should contain 0.1 mg/mL ethidium bromide.
8. Ethidium bromide (10 mg/mL). Store at 4°C in the dark. (**Caution:** Ethidium bromide is highly carcinogenic; handle under appropriate guidelines).
9. DNA molecular size standards (e.g., 1 Kb plus DNA ladder, Life Technologies 1 ug/mL).
10. Razor blades or scalpels.
11. QIAquick DNA purification kit (Qiagen).

2.2.5. cDNA RDA

1. Double-stranded cDNA (*see* **Subheading 3.2.2.**).
2. 16S and 23S rRNA amplicons (*see* **Subheading 3.2.3.**).
3. Restriction enzyme: *Dpn*II (New England Biolabs, 50 U/μL).
4. 10X *Dpn*II buffer (as supplied with enzyme).
5. T4 DNA ligase (New England Biolabs, 400 U/μL.
6. 10X T4 DNA ligase buffer (as supplied with enzyme).
7. HPLC (or equivalent)-purified oligonucleotide adaptors/primers: *see* **Table 3**.
8. 10 *M* Ammonium acetate.
9. *Taq* DNA polymerase: *Amplitaq* DNA polymerase (Perkin-Elmer Co., 5 U/μL).
10. PCR buffer (5X): 335 m*M* Tris-HCl, pH 8.9, 20 m*M* $MgCl_2$, 80 m*M* $(NH_4)_2SO_4$, 166 μg/mL BSA.
11. 4 m*M* dNTP mix (4 m*M* each dGTP, dATP, dCTP, dTTP).

Table 3
Oligonucleotide adaptor pairs

Name	Sequence
R-Bgl-12	5′- GAT CTG CGG TGA -3′; 0.25 m*M*
R-Bgl-24	5′- AGC ACT CTC CAG CCT CTC ACC GCA -3′; 0.5 m*M*
J-Bgl-12	5′- GAT CTG TTC ATG -3′; 0.25 m*M*
J-Bgl-24	5′- ACC GAC GTC GAC TAT CCA TGA ACA -3′; 0.5 m*M*
N-Bgl-12	5′- GAT CTT CCC TCG -3′; 0.25 m*M*
N-Bgl-24	5′- AGG CAA CTG TGC TAT CCG AGG GAA -3′; 0.5 m*M*

12. Phenol:chloroform:isoamyl alcohol (25:24:1 [v/v] saturated with 10 m*M* Tris-HCl, 1 m*M* EDTA, pH 8.0).
13. Chloroform:isoamyl alcohol (49:1 [v/v]).
14. 3 *M* Sodium acetate, pH 5.3.
15. TE: 10 m*M* Tris-HCl, 1 m*M* EDTA, pH 7.5.
16.. MicroSpin S-300 HR columns (Amersham Pharmacia Biotech).
17. EE buffer (3X): 30 m*M* EPPS, 3 m*M* EDTA, pH 8.0.
18. 5 *M* NaCl.
19. Mung Bean Nuclease (New England Biolabs, 10 U/μL).
20. Mung Bean Nuclease buffer (as supplied with enzyme).
21. 50 m*M* Tris-HCl, pH 8.9.
22. Yeast tRNA (Life Technologies, 10 mg/mL).
23. Glycogen, (e.g., GlycoBlue, Ambion, Inc., 15 μg/mL).
27. 1.5% (w/v) nondenaturing agarose gel in TBE, pH 8.3. The gel should contain 0.1 mg/mL ethidium bromide.
28. Ethidium bromide (10 mg/mL). Store at 4°C in the dark. (**Caution:** Ethidium bromide is highly carcinogenic; handle under appropriate guidelines).
29. DNA molecular size standards (e.g., 1 Kb plus DNA ladder, Life Technologies 1 ug/mL).
30. Suitable concentration standards (*see* **Note 1**).

2.2.6. Cloning of Difference Products

1. Razor blades or scalpels.
2. QIAquick DNA purification kit (Qiagen).
3. Cloning system for PCR products (e.g., PCR2.1 TA cloning kit or TOPO TA cloning kit, Invitrogen Co.).

3. Methods

3.1. RDA

3.1.1. Isolation of Chromosomal DNA

1. Harvest the growth of one 7-cm plate using a sterile cotton swab, suspend in 1 mL of GTE buffer in a 2-mL Eppendorf tube, pellet by centrifugation for 1 min at 16,000*g* in a microcentrifuge.

2. Resuspend in 500 µL GTE buffer, add 25 µL lysozyme and 25 µL 20% SDS, mix, incubate at 37°C for 1 h or until suspension becomes clear.
3. Add 5 µL Pronase or Protease K, incubate for 4 h at 50°C.
4. Add 5 µL RNAse, incubate 30 min at 50°C.
5. Extract with an equal volume of phenol : chloroform : isoamyl alcohol, then with an equal volume of chloroform : isoamyl alcohol.
6. Precipitate the DNA by adding 0.1 volume of 3 *M* sodium acetate, and 2.5 volumes of 100% ethanol, invert to mix.
7. Centrifuge at 16,000*g* in a microcentrifuge for 15 min, decant the supernatant, and wash the pellet with 1 mL 70% EtOH.
8. Carefully aspirate the ethanol, air-dry the pellet for 15 min at room temperature.
9. Dissolve the DNA in 100 µL sterile UHP water. Store at –20°C.
10. Determine concentration and quality of preparations by comparison of serial dilutions of 2 µL of the DNA on a 1% nondenaturing agarose gel in TBE, pH 8.3, alongside DNA concentration standards.

3.1.2. DNA Restriction

1. Digest 100 µg each of both Tester and Driver chromosomal DNA to completion by adding 2 µL *Sau*3A (10U/µL), 10 µL *Sau*3A buffer (10X), and sterile UHP water to a final volume of 100 µL. Incubate 16 h at 37°C.
2. Test 2 µL for complete digestion by agarose-gel electrophoresis on a 1% gel in TBE, pH 8.3.
3. Extract remaining restrictions with an equal volume of phenol : chloroform : isoamyl alcohol, then with an equal volume of chloroform : isoamyl alcohol.
4. Add 0.1 volume of 3 *M* sodium acetate, pH 5.3, and 2.5 volumes of 100% ethanol, and precipitate on ice for 30 min. Centrifuge for 15 min at 16,000*g*, wash pellet with 70% ethanol, and air-dry.
5. Resuspend Driver DNA in 30 µL sterile UHP water (final concentration approx 2.5 ng/µL), resuspend Tester DNA in 30 µL sterile UHP water, dilute 10 µL of this with 40 µL sterile UHP water (final concentration approx 500 ng/µL). The 20 µL of the undiluted material can be used in a Tester-Tester control (*see* **Note 2**).

3.1.3. Ligation of J-Bgl-Adaptors

1. Ligate J-Bgl-adaptors to the Tester chromosomal DNA by taking 2 µL (approx 1 µg) diluted Tester digest, add 2.5 µL 0.2 m*M* J-Bgl-12, 2.5 µL 0.2 m*M* J-Bgl-24, 3 µL 10X ligase buffer, and 14 µL sterile UHP water.
2. Anneal oligonucleotide adaptors in a PCR thermocycler, by heating the reaction to 50°C for 2 min, then cool to 10°C at no more than 1°C/min.
3. Add 6 µL T4 DNA ligase, mix well, and incubate for 18 h at 16°C.

3.1.4. Subtractive Hybridization

1. Combine 4 µL J-ligated Tester (±0.133 ng) and 4 µL Driver (±10 µg), and 25 µL 100% ethanol. Mix well to precipitate the DNA, centrifuge at 16,000*g*, for 30 min. Carefully wash with 70% ethanol.

2. Air-dry pellet, resuspend thoroughly in 4 μL 3X EE buffer.
3. Overlay with sterile mineral oil, denature DNA at 96°C for 5 min.
4. Add 1 μL 5 *M* NaCl (prewarmed).
5. Hybridize for 20 h at 67°C.
6. To 0.5 μL of the above hybridization mixture, add 40 μL 10X PCR buffer, 12 μL 10 m*M* dNTP, 3 μL *Taq* polymerase, and 343.5 μL sterile UHP water.
7. Incubate in PCR thermocycler for 5 min at 72°C.
8. Add 2 μL 0.2 m*M* J-Bgl-24 primer.
9. Perform 10 cycles of 1 min at 95°C, 3 min at 70°C.
10. Precipitate PCR mix with 2.5 volumes 100% ethanol, centrifuge at 16,000*g* for 30 min. Wash with 70% ethanol.
11. Resuspend pellet in 18 μL sterile UHP water, add 20 μL 2X Mung Bean Nuclease reaction buffer, add 2 μL (10U/μL) Mung Bean Nuclease, mix, incubate for 1 h at 30°C.
12. Inactivate Mung Bean Nuclease by adding 160 μL 50 m*M* Tris-HCl, pH 8.9, incubate for 5 min at 98°C.
13. Use 40 μL of the above mixture as template in a PCR reaction with 40 μL 10X PCR buffer, 12 μL 10 m*M* dNTP, 3 μL *Taq* polymerase (15 U), 2 μL 0.2 m*M* J-Bgl-24 primer, 303 μL sterile UHP water (final volume is 400 μL). Perform 20 cycles of 1 min at 95°C, 3 min at 70°C, followed by a final extension for 10 min at 72°C.
14. Precipitate DNA by adding 0.1 volume 3 *M* sodium acetate, pH 5.3, and 2.5 volumes 100% ethanol, centrifuge at 16,000*g*, for 30 min. Wash with 70% EtOH, resuspend in 50 μL sterile UHP water.
15. Run out a 5 μL sample on a 2% nondenaturing agarose gel. If Tester and Driver contain relatively few differences, discrete amplicons will be visible (*see* **Note 3**).

3.1.5. Cloning of Difference Products

1. Run remainder of each sample on a 2% nondenaturing agarose gel in TBE, pH 8.3, carefully excise each band from the agarose gel, using a sharp razor blade.
2. Purify amplicons using Qiaex II, according to manufacturers instructions.
3. Optional (*see* **Note 4**): re-amplify the amplicon. Use 1 μL of the purified amplicon as template in a PCR reaction with 5 μL 10X PCR buffer, 1 μL 10 m*M* dNTP, 1 μL *Taq* polymerase (5 U), 0.5 μL 0.2 m*M* J-Bgl-24 primer, 42.5 μL sterile UHP water to a final volume of 50 μL. Perform 30 cycles of 1 min at 95°C, 3 min at 70°C, followed by a final extension for 10 min at 72°C.
4. Clone the amplicon in the PCR2.1 vector, according to manufacturers instructions. Recombinant plasmid DNA can then be isolated (using standard methods) and used for sequencing, for identification of the amplicons (*see* **Notes 5** and **6**).

3.2. cDNA RDA

Successful application of the cDNA RDA technique requires the reproducible isolation of high-quality representative RNA preparations from the bacteria. Accordingly, the utmost care should be taken during the RNA isolation procedure. Bacterial RNA is very unstable, and accordingly isolation should carried out quickly and efficiently. A rapid-lysis technique optimized for use with Neisseria is described. (Other methods that result in the production of high quality RNA could be employed.)

Because bacterial mRNA is poorly polyadenylated, it is not possible to purify it efficiently using polyT-affinity methodologies. As a consequence, the protocol for cDNA RDA of bacteria differs from the original cDNA RDA methodology in that it uses total RNA rather than purified message as its starting point. Accordingly, given the abundance of rRNA in total RNA preparations, it is necessary to supplement the derived Driver component with additional rRNA-derived material to increase selection against these common sequences.

3.2.1. RNA Isolation

Total RNA can be isolated by a procedure adapted from the TNS/PAS method of Felipe et. al. *(7)*.

1. Harvest bacterial cultures by centrifugation of 10–20 mL aliquots in Falcon tubes at 7,500*g* for 5 min at 4°C.
2. Quickly and carefully remove supernatant and keeping cells cool, resuspend by vigorously vortexing (approx 3 × 15 s; *see* **Note 7**) cell pellet in 1.5 mL cold, fresh TNS/PAS lysis solution, 1.5 mL acid phenol:chloroform and 300 μL chloroform : isoamyl alcohol.
3. Spin samples at 16,000*g* for 5 min at 4°C and carefully transfer the aqueous phase to new tubes.
4. Re-extract aqueous phase with 1 volume of acid phenol:chloroform and 0.2 volume of chloroform : isoamyl alcohol, and precipitate RNA, following incubation with 2.5 *M* LiCl, 25 m*M* EDTA, for at least 2 h at –20°C, by centrifugation at 16,000*g* for 30 min at 4°C.
5. Wash pellet(s) twice with 70% ethanol, and resuspend to approx 1 μg/μL in DNase I buffer. Add RNase-free DNase I to a final concentration of 30/μg nucleic acid, and incubate for 45 min at 37°C. Terminate reaction by extraction with 1 volume of acid phenol:chloro-form followed by a further extraction with 1 volume of chloroform.
6. Precipitate RNA with 0.2 volume of 10 *M* ammonium acetate and 1 volume of 2-propanol for at least 2 h at –20°C. Collect the precipitate by centrifugation at 16,000*g* for 30 min at 4°C.
7. Wash pellets twice with 70% ethanol, air-dry (do NOT over-dry, RNA can difficult to resuspend. It is easier if pellets are still slightly moist), and resuspend in RNase free H_2O containing 0.1 m*M* EDTA, PRIME RNase inhibitor (1 U/30 μL).
8. Aliquots of the total RNA preparations can be stored at –80°C.
9. Quantitation and crude quality assessment can be carried out by measuring optical density (OD) of the preparation at 260 nm and 280 nm, and by examination on a 1% nondenaturing agarose gel. **Figure 2** shows a typical result obtained with a good-quality RNA preparation.

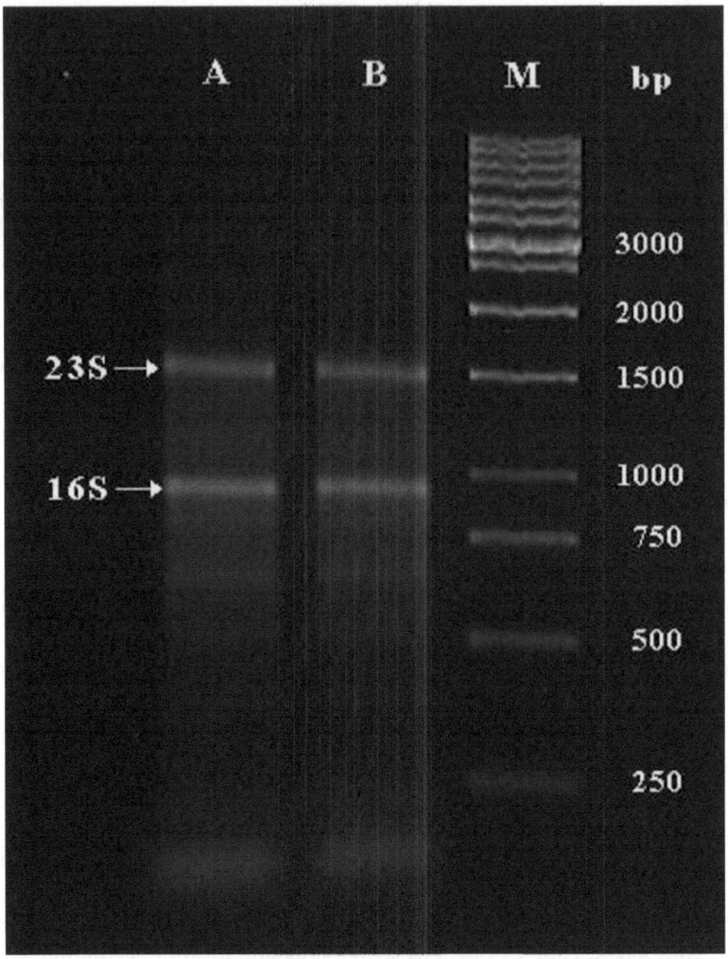

Fig. 2. Total RNA from *N. meningitidis* isolated using the TNS/PAS method. **A**, Total RNA isolated from *N. meningitidis* CE1402 grown under iron-sufficient conditions. **B**, Total RNA isolated from *N. meningitidis* M986 grown under iron-limited conditions. **M**, molecular weight markers, sizes are given in bp. Positions of the dominant 16S and 23S rRNA bands are indicated.

3.2.2. cDNA Synthesis

The synthesis of cDNA is performed by random-priming of total RNA using the Pharmacia TimeSaver cDNA synthesis kit (*see* **Note 8**) The protocol is according to the manufacturer's instructions using 5 μg total RNA (*see* **Subheading 3.2.1.**) as the template, and the random hexamers (as supplied with kit) at 1:200 dilution (0.037 μg/reaction), with the following modifications:

1. After 20 min incubation of the first-strand reaction at 37°C, add 1 μL of Superscript II reverse transcriptase to the reaction mix and continue incubation for a further 1 h.
2. Carry out the second-strand incubation at 12°C for 1 h, then 22°C for a further 2 h.
3. Purify the cDNA using a cDNA spun column, according to manufacturers instructions.
4. Make up volume to 148 μL with *Dpn*II buffer.

3.2.3. Isolation of N. meningitidis *16S and 23S rRNA Genes*

1. Use 0.1–0.5 μg of chromosomal DNA (*see* **Subheading 3.1.1.**) as template in 12X 100 μL reactions for each of the rRNA genes to be isolated.
2. To each template in PCR tube add 10 μL 10X buffer, 8 μL dNTP mixture and 20 μL 5 *M* betaine solution (*see* **Note 9**). Add 1 μL each of the two relevant primers, and make up total volume to 100 μL with sterile UHP water. Denature template DNA in a thermal cycler by heating to 96°C for 5 min. Add 0.5 μL (2.5 U) *Taq* polymerase, cycle reactions: 96°C for 1 min, 58°C for 1 min, and 72°C for 3 min, for 25–30 cycles, with a final extension at 72°C for 10 min.
3. Examine reactions for specificity and yield by running out a 5 μL sample of each on a 1.0% nondenaturing agarose gel. The primer pairs used; 16Sup and 16Sdn, and 23Sup and 23Sdn, should give rise to products of approx 1450 bp and 2850 bp, respectively.
4. Run out remainder (approx 95 μL) of each reaction on a 1% nondenaturing agarose gel. Excise these bands, and purify, e.g., using a QIAquick DNA purification kit (Qiagen), according to manufacturer's instructions. Dilute products to approx 0.5 mg/mL. These purified products constitute the starting material for the generation of the rRNA gene-derived representations.

3.2.4. PCR-Coupled Subtractive Hybridization

The following methodology is adapted from Hubank and Schatz ***(11)***.

The technique of cDNA RDA is very sensitive, and it is important that all possible precautions are taken to prevent cross-contamination of materials. All reagents (including enzymes) should be subdivided before use. Micropipet tips with integral filters should be used throughout and it is recommended that all PCR reactions be set up in an airflow cabinet.

Because the complexity of the derived cDNA populations is considerably less than that of genomic DNA, the simplification of the starting material required for RDA (the generation of a sub-population of amplified restriction fragments) is not essential. However, to be able to utilize PCR to enrich for differences, it is necessary to generate amplified populations of cDNA restriction fragments, although because of the reduced complexity, four-cutter restriction enzymes can be used, thus increasing the proportion of amplifiable fragments generated. For the generation of rRNA-derived Driver, the PCR products from **Subheading 3.2.3.**, are substituted for cDNA.

3.2.4.1. Ligation of R-Bgl-Adaptors

1. Add 1.5 μL DTT (100 m*M*) to 148 μL cDNA preparation (*see* **Subheading 3.2.2.**) in *Dpn*II buffer. Add 1 μL *Dpn*II. Incubate for 3 h at 37°C.
2. To ligate R-Bgl-adaptors to the rRNA-derived amplicons (*see* **Subheading 3.2.3.**), Digest 1–2 μg of each purified PCR product by adding 1 μL of *Dpn*II, 10 μL 10X *Dpn*II buffer, and sterile UHP water to a total volume of 100 μL. Incubate for 3 h at 37°C.
3. Extract the reactions with an equal volume of phenol:chloroform:isoamyl alcohol, then with an equal volume of chloroform:isoamyl alcohol. Add 1 μL (15 μg) glycogen carrier, 30 μL ammonium acetate, 600 μL of cold 100% ethanol, and precipitate on ice for 30 min.
4. Spin down the precipitate at 16,000*g* for 30 min at 4°C. Wash the pellet with 70% ethanol.
5. Air-dry and resuspend the pellet in 20 μL TE, transfer the suspension to a 0.5-mL PCR tube.
6. Add 24 μL sterile UHP water, 6 μL ligase buffer (as supplied with T4 DNA ligase) and 4 μL each of 0.25 m*M* R-Bgl-12 and 0.5 m*M* R-Bgl-24 adaptor/primers.
7. Anneal oligonucleotide adaptors in a PCR machine, by heating the reaction to 50°C for 2 min, followed by cooling to 10°C at no more than 1°C/min.
8. Add 2 μL T4 DNA ligase, mix well, and incubate for 18 h at 14°C.

3.2.4.2. Generation of Representations

Pilot reactions should be carried out for each representation to be generated to establish optimum amplification conditions (*see* **Note 11**). This is to determine the number of PCR cycles required to generate suitable ('good') representations. The criteria are that a 10 μL sample run out on a 1.5% agarose gel should give a smear ranging in size from approx 0.2–1.5 kb and contain approx 0.5 μg DNA. Too few cycles will not provide sufficient material for the subsequent subtraction step, over-amplification will bias the populations and reduce average fragment size (*see* **Note 12**). For the generation of the rRNA-derived representation however, no pilot is required, instead use the same number of cycles determined as optimum for the other Tester and Driver components.

1. Dilute the ligation (*see* **Subheading 3.2.4.1.**) 1:3, by adding 120 μL TE.
2. For each pilot reaction, add 3 μL diluted ligation, 139 μL sterile UHP water, 40 μL PCR buffer, 16 μL 4 m*M* dNTP mix, and 1 μL 0.5 m*M* R-Bgl-24 adaptor/primer to a 0.5-mL PCR tube.
3. Incubate at 72°C for 3 min in a Thermal Cycler. Add 1 μL (5 U) *Amplitaq* DNA polymerase, and continue incubation for a further 5 min.
4. Cycle reactions at 95°C for 1 min and then 72°C for 3 min for 25 cycles. Remove 10-μL aliquots at intervals from about cycle 16 onwards (the optimum number for generation of representations usually lies in the range of 17–24 cycles).

5. Run out the 10 μL samples along with size and concentration standards on a 1.5% nondenaturing agarose gel.
6. From examination of this gel, select the number of cycles that generates suitable representations, and set up 9X 200 μL PCR reactions for each sample intended for use as Driver, and 3X 200 μL reactions for each sample intended for use only as Tester (if reciprocal subtractions are to be carried out, set up 12X 200 μL reactions of each).
7. Cycle reactions for the determined number of cycles, finishing with a 10 min extension at 72°C.
8. Extract reactions with an equal volume of phenol : chloroform : isoamyl alcohol, then with an equal volume of chloroform : isoamyl alcohol. Add 0.1 volume of 3 *M* sodium acetate, pH 5.3, an equal volume of 2-propanol, and precipitate the DNA on ice for 30 min.
9. Pellet the DNA by centrifugation at 16,000*g* for 30 min at 4°C. Wash the pellet with 70% ethanol, air dry, and resuspend in TE to give a concentration of approx 0.5 mg/mL (a rough guideline is to use about 25 μL of TE per reaction).
10. Check quality and concentration of DNAs by running 1 μL samples on a 1.5% nondenaturing agarose gel, alongside standards.

3.2.4.3. Preparation of Driver and Tester Components

1. Digest 100 μg (200 μL) each of Driver and rRNA-derived representations by adding 5 μL *Dpn*II, 60 μL 10X *Dpn*II buffer, and sterile UHP water to final volumes of 600 μL. Incubate 3 h at 37°C.
2. Extract digests with equal volumes of phenol : chloroform : isoamyl alcohol, then chloroform:isoamyl alcohol.
3. Add 0.1 volume of 3 *M* sodium acetate, pH 5.3, and an equal volume of 2-propanol to each digest, and precipitate on ice for 30 min.
4. Collect precipitates at 16,000*g* for 30 min at 4°C. Wash the pellets with 70% ethanol, air-dry, and resuspend in 150 μL TE. Combine 16S and 23S representations.
5. Determine concentration of cut Driver and rRNA-derived representation by running 1 μL samples on a 1.5% nondenaturing gel with standards. Adjust to approx 0.5 mg/mL with TE as necessary. These represent the Driver components (Driver 1 and 2, respectively) shown in **Fig. 1B**.
6. If a representation is to be used as a Tester, digest 10 μg (20 μL) with 0.5 μL *Dpn*II, 6 μL 10X *Dpn*II buffer in a final volume of 60 μL. Incubate 3 h at 37°C.
7. Extract digests with equal volumes of phenol : chloroform : isoamyl alcohol, then chloroform : isoamyl alcohol.
8. Add 0.1 volume of 3 *M* sodium acetate, pH 5.3, and 3 volumes of cold ethanol to each digest, and precipitate at –20°C for 30 min.
9. Collect precipitates at 16,000*g* for 30 min at 4°C. Wash the pellets with 70% ethanol, air-dry, and resuspend in 20 μL TE.
10. Remove digested R-Bgl- adaptors using a spin-column purification system such as MicroSpin S-300 HR columns, according to manufacturer's protocol.

11. Estimate DNA concentration by running a 1 μL sample on a 1.5% nondenaturing gel with standards.
12. Combine 1 μg of spin-column purified DNA, 3 μL 10X T4 DNA ligase buffer, 2 μL 0.5 m*M* J-Bgl-24 adaptor, 2 μL 0.25 m*M* J-Bgl-12 adaptor, and sterile UHP water to a final volume of 29 μL.
13. Anneal oligonucleotide adaptors in a PCR machine, by heating the reaction to 50°C for 2 min, then cool to 10°C at no more than 1°C/min.
14. Add 1 μL T4 DNA ligase, mix well, and incubate for 18 h at 14°C.
15. Dilute the ligation to approx. 10 ng/μL by the addition of 70 μL TE. This preparation is the J-ligated Tester.

3.2.4.4. Subtractive Hybridization

See **Fig. 1B** for schematic representation of proceedure.

1. Combine 5 μg (10 μL) of digested Driver (Driver 1), 5 μg (10 μL) digested rRNA-derived representation (Driver 2) and 0.1 μg (10 μL) of J-ligated Tester in a 0.5-mL microcentrifuge tube. Make up to 100 μL with sterile UHP water. This gives a Driver:Tester ratio of 100:1 (50:50:1).
2. Extract digests with equal volumes of phenol:chloroform:isoamyl alcohol, then chloroform:isoamyl alcohol.
3. Add 0.2 volumes of 10 *M* Ammonium acetate, pH 5.3, and 3 volumes of cold ethanol to each digest, and precipitate at –70°C for 10 min.
4. Incubate the tube containing precipitate at 37°C for 1 min, then sediment at 16,000*g* for 20 min at 4°C to collect DNA. Very carefully wash the pellet with 70% ethanol.
5. Air-dry pellet, and resuspend very thoroughly in 4 μL 3X EE buffer by pipetting up and down for at least 3 min.
6. Incubate at 37°C for 5 min, vortex vigorously, and spin solution to the bottom of the tube.
7. Overlay solution with a few drops of mineral oil (even if PCR machine has heated lid), and denature DNA for 5 min at 98°C. Cool block to 67°C.
8. Incubate hybridization mix at 67°C for 24 h (to allow complete annealing).
9. Remove hybridization mix to a fresh tube, and dilute stepwise in 200 μL TE: add 10 μL TE and mix by pipetting, add a further 25 μL TE and mix, and then make up to 200 μL, and vortex thoroughly. This diluted, hybridized DNA is then used to generate the first difference product (*see* **Note 13**).
10. For each subtraction set up two PCR reactions, comprising: 122 μL sterile UHP water, 40 μL 5X PCR buffer, and 16 μL of 4 m*M* dNTP mix, and 20 μL diluted hybridization mix.
11. In a PCR machine, incubate reactions at 72°C for 3 min, add 1 μL (5 U) *Amplitaq* DNA polymerase, and continue incubation at 72°C for a further 5 min.
12. Add 1 μL of 0.5 m*M* J-Bgl-24 primer, cycle at 95°C for 1 min and 70°C for 3 min for 11 cycles (*see* **Note 14**), with a final extension at 72°C for 10 min.

13. Combine the two reactions in a single microfuge tube. Extract with equal volumes of phenol : chloroform : isoamyl alcohol, then chloroform : isoamyl alcohol. Add 100 μg (10 μL) tRNA, 0.1 volume 3 *M* sodium acetate, pH 5.3, and an equal volume of 2-propanol. Precipitate on ice for 30 min.
14. Sediment the precipitate at 16,000*g* for 20 min at 4°C. Very carefully wash the pellet with 70% ethanol. Resuspend in 20 μL TE.
15. Add 4 μL Mung Bean Nuclease (MBN) buffer, 2 μL Mung Bean Nuclease (MBN), and make up volume to 40 μL with sterile UHP water. Incubate at 30°C for 45 min (*see* **Note 15**).
16. Terminate reaction by the addition of 160 μL of 50 m*M* Tris-HCl, pH 8.9, and heating to 98°C for 5 min. Cool the reaction to 4°C on ice.
17. On ice set up one PCR reaction comprising: 122 μL sterile UHP water, 40 μL 5X PCR buffer, 16 μL dNTP mix, and 1 μL 0.5 m*M* J-Bgl-24 oligo.
18. Add 20 μL of the MBN-treated DNA. Incubate the reactions in a PCR machine at 95°C for 1 min, add 1 μL (5 U) *Amplitaq* DNA polymerase, cycle 95°C for 1 min and 70°C for 3 min, for 18 cycles, with a final extension at 72°C for 10 min.
19. Estimate the DNA concentration by running a 10 μL sample on a 1.5% nondenaturing agarose gel, with standards.
20. Extract the reactions with equal volumes of phenol : chloroform : isoamyl alcohol followed by chloroform : isoamyl alcohol. Add 0.1 volume 3 *M* sodium acetate, pH 5.3, 1 volume 2-propanol, and precipitate on ice for 30 min.
21. Collect precipitates at 16,000*g* for 30 min at 4°C. Wash the pellets with 70% ethanol, air-dry, and resuspend in TE to 0.5 μg/μL (volume necessary is yield dependant, but is typically approx 20–30 μL).
22. This is the first difference product (DP1).

3.2.4.5. Generation of a Second Difference Product

See **Note 16**, and **Fig. 3**.

1. Mix 2 μg (4 μL) of DP1 (*see* **Subheading 3.2.4.4.**) with 84 μL sterile UHP water, add 10 μL 10X *Dpn*II buffer and 2 μL of *Dpn*II. Incubate 3 h at 37°C.
2. Extract the reactions with an equal volume of phenol : chloroform : isoamyl alcohol, then with an equal volume of chloroform : isoamyl alcohol. Add 1 μL (15 μg) glycogen carrier, 0.1 volume sodium acetate, pH 5.3, and 3 volumes cold ethanol. Precipitate at –20° for 30 min.
3. Collect precipitates at 16,000*g* for 30 min at 4°C. Wash the pellets with 70% ethanol, air-dry, and resuspend in 20 μL TE (this gives approx 100 ng/μL).
4. Take 2 μL of the restricted DP1, and add 3 μL 10X ligase buffer, 2 μL each of 0.25 m*M* N-Bgl-12 and 0.5 m*M* N-Bgl-24 adaptors, and make up to a final volume of 29 μL with sterile UHP water.
5. Anneal oligonucleotide adaptors in a PCR machine, by heating the reaction to 50°C for 2 min, then cool to 10°C at no more than 1°C/min.
6. Add 1 μL T4 DNA ligase, mix well, and incubate for 18 h at 14°C.

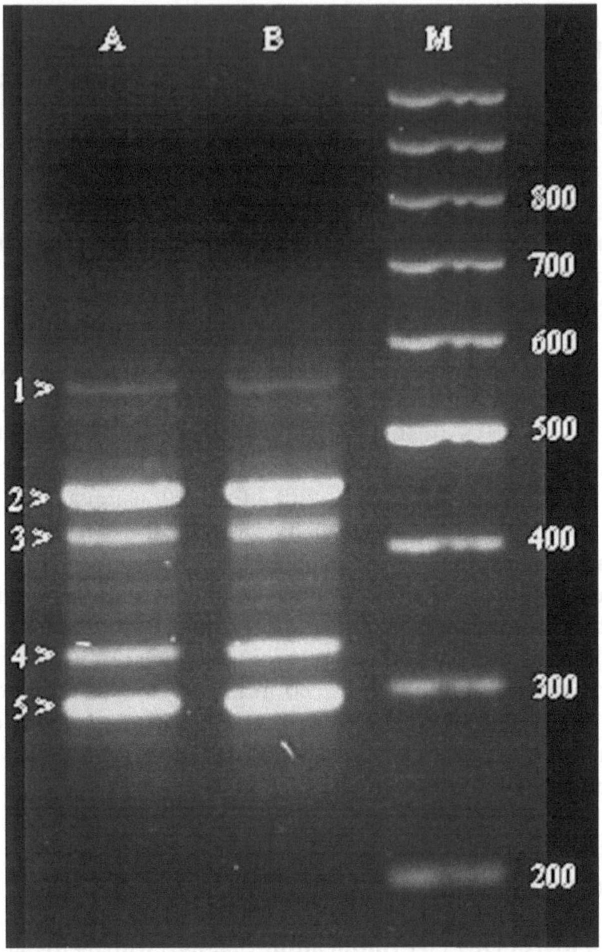

Fig. 3. Difference products generated during an analysis of iron-regulated gene expression in *N. meningitidis* by cDNA RDA. **A** and **B**, show DNA fragments amplified in two independent experiments initiated from separate aliquots of same total RNA preparation (showing reproducibility). **M**, molecular mass markers. Arrows indicate bands selected for isolation, cloning and sequencing. Adapted from **ref. *9***.

7. Dilute ligation mix to approx. 1.25 ng/μL by the addition of 130 μL TE.
8. Combine 5 μg (10 μL) of digested Driver (Driver 1), 5 μg (10 μL) digested rRNA-derived representation (Driver 2) (*see* **Subheading 3.2.4.3.**) Mix 10 μL (approx 10 μg) of Driver with 10 μL (approx 12.5 ng) of N-Bgl-ligated DP1 (*see* **Subheading 3.2.4.4.**). This gives a Driver-Tester ratio of 800:1 (400:400:1).
9. Extract the digests with equal volumes of phenol:chloroform:isoamyl alcohol, then chloroform:isoamyl alcohol.

10. Add 0.2 volumes of 10 *M* Ammonium acetate, pH 5.3, and 3 volumes of cold ethanol to each digest, and precipitate at -70°C for 10 min.
11. Incubate the tube containing precipitate at 37°C for 1 min, then centrifuge at 16,000*g* for 20 min at 4°C to collect DNA. Very carefully wash the pellet with 70% ethanol.
12. Air-dry pellet, and resuspend very thoroughly in 4 μL 3X EE buffer by pipetting up and down for at least 3 min.
13. Incubate at 37°C for 5 min, vortex vigorously, and spin solution to the bottom of the tube.
14. Overlay the solution with a few drops of mineral oil (even if PCR machine has heated lid), and denature DNA for 5 min at 98°C. Cool block to 67°C.
15. Incubate the hybridization mix at 67°C for 24 h (to allow complete annealing).
16. Remove the hybridization mix to a fresh tube, and dilute stepwise in 200 μL TE: add 10 μL TE and mix by pipetting, add a further 25 μL TE and mix, and then make up to 200 μL, and vortex thoroughly. This diluted, hybridized DNA is then used to generate the first difference product.
17. For each subtraction set up two PCR reactions, comprising: 122 μL sterile UHP water, 40 μL 5X PCR buffer, and 16 μL of 4 m*M* dNTP mix, and 20 μL diluted hybridization mix.
18. In a PCR machine, incubate reactions at 72°C for 3 min, then add 1 μL (5 U) *Amplitaq* DNA polymerase, and continue incubation at 72°C for a further 5 min.
19. Add 1 μL of 0.5 m*M* N-Bgl-24 primer, cycle at 95°C for 1 min and 72°C for 3 min for 11 cycles, with a final extension at 72°C for 10 min.
20. Combine the two reactions in a single microfuge tube. Extract with equal volumes of phenol:chloroform:isoamyl alcohol, then chloroform:isoamyl alcohol. Add 100 μg (10 μL) tRNA, 0.1 volume 3 *M* sodium acetate, pH 5.3, and an equal volume of 2-propanol. Precipitate on ice for 30 min.
21. Sediment the precipitate at 16,000*g* for 20 min at 4°C. Very carefully wash the pellet with 70% ethanol. Resuspend in 20 μL TE.
22. Add 4 μL MBN buffer, 2 μL MBN, and make up volume to 40 μL with sterile UHP water. Incubate at 30°C for 45 min.
23. Terminate the reaction by the addition of 160 μL of 50 m*M* Tris-HCl, pH 8.9, and heating to 98°C for 5 min. Cool the reaction to 4°C on ice.
24. On ice, set up two PCR reactions for each subtraction, each comprising: 122 μL sterile UHP water, 40 μL 5X PCR buffer, 16 μL dNTP mix, and 1 μL 0.5 m*M* N-Bgl-24 oligo.
25. Add 20 μL of the MBN-treated DNA to each. Incubate reactions in a PCR machine at 95°C for 1 min, add 1 μL (5 U) *Amplitaq* DNA polymerase, cycle 95°C for 1 min and 72°C for 3 min, for 18 cycles, with a final extension at 72°C for 10 min. Combine each pair of reactions.
26. Estimate DNA concentration by running a 10-μL sample on a 1.5% nondenaturing agarose gel, with standards.

27. Extract the reactions with equal volumes of phenol:chloroform : isoamyl alcohol, then chloroform : isoamyl alcohol. Add 0.1 volume 3 *M* sodium acetate, pH 5.3, 1 volume 2-propanol, and precipitate on ice for 30 min.
28. Collect precipitates at 16,000*g* for 30 min at 4°C. Wash the pellets with 70% ethanol, air-dry, and resuspend in TE to 0.5 μg/μL (volume is yield dependant, but is typically approx 40–50 μL). This is the second difference product (DP2).

3.2.4.6. Generation of Further Difference Products

There are advantages and disadvantages in proceeding to a third difference product (DP3). It can be useful if DP2 contains many poorly defined and/or weak bands. However, a third round of PCR-coupled subtractive hybridization can result in the loss of some difference products, particularly those derived from transcripts expressed at low levels.

For the generation of DP3, the procedure is essentially as in **Subheading 3.2.4.5.**, except:

1. Digest DP2 (*see* **Subheading 3.2.4.5.**) with *Dpn*II to remove the N-Bgl-adaptors, and replace with J-Bgl-adaptors.
2. Dilute the J-Bgl-ligated DP2 to 1 ng/μL with TE. Set up hybridizations (*see* **Subheading 3.2.4.5., steps 8–15**) using driver to tester ratios of between 5,000–20,000 : 1 (2,500 : 2,500 : 1–10,000 : 10,000 : 1). To achieve this, vary quantity of J-Bgl-ligated Tester and keep the combined Driver concentration at 10 μg/mL (i.e., 5 μg/mL each of Driver 1 and 2; *see* **Subheading 3.2.4.3.**).
3. Generate DP3 according to protocol given in **Subheading 3.2.4.5., steps 16–28**, setting up four PCR reactions for each subtraction.
4. Resuspend pellet from the four combined reactions (from each subtraction) to a final concentration of approx 0.5 μg/mL in TE. This is DP3.

3.2.4.7. Cloning of Difference Products

1. Run out each difference product on a 1.5% nondenaturing gel in TBE, pH 8.3. **Figure 3** shows a typical result.
2. Carefully excise each band from the agarose gel, using a sharp razor blade. Purify amplicons using Qiaex II, according to manufacturer's instructions.
3. Clone the amplicon in the PCR2.1 vector, according to manufacturer's instructions. Recombinant plasmid DNA can then be isolated (using standard methods) and inserts sequenced for identification of the differentially expressed genes (*see* **Note 17**).

4. Notes

1. It is vital concentrations are accurately determined. Suitable standards can be prepared by digesting genomic DNA of known concentration (sheared to an average length of about 20 kb), with *Dpn*II. Dilutions of this standard (say between 0.1–1.0 μg) should be loaded on the agarose gels, alongside the PCR product to be quantified.

2. It is extremely useful to include both positive and negative controls in the experiments. As a positive control, original Tester DNA supplemented with an appropriate target (e.g., Bacteriophage lambda DNA or a known plasmid) should be used as a +ve Control-Tester, with Tester DNA without supplement as +Control-Driver. As a negative control, original Tester DNA can be used as both –Control-Tester and –Control-Driver. The positive control should give rise to target-derived amplicons, the negative control should not yield any amplicon.
3. The number of discrete amplicons depends on the number of differences between Tester and Driver DNA populations. A relatively low number of differences yields discrete amplicons after one round of subtractive hybridization. If a smear appears, this indicates more differences and/or relatively inefficient subtractive hybridization. In this case, a second round of subtractive hybridization can be performed, using a second different adaptor pair of oligonucleotides.
4. Re-amplification can be of use if bands observed at end of **Subheading 3.1.4.** are weak.
5. Multiple transformants should be tested for each amplicon, as amplicons are heterogenous, i.e., different DNA species can have the same electrophoretic mobility. This is particularly important if differences in intensity of the amplicon bands are seen after gel electrophoresis.
6. Identification of the amplicons can be carried out by sequencing of the insert of the resultant recombinant plasmids. Because the identified differences should either be absent in the driver, or have a restriction-site polymorphism, each putative difference should be checked for validity by Southern hybridization against the original genomic restrictions.
7. Amount of vortexing, depends on how well the cells have pelleted. It is important that the bacteria are well-suspended in the lysis mixture. More mixing may be required.
8. The modified Amersham-Pharmacia cDNA synthesis kit and protocol were found to give very good results in our hands, although other methodologies could be used.
9. The addition of betaine to the PCR reaction mix aids amplification of the rRNA sequences.
10. During generation of the representations, the resulting products are limited in their complexity by the ability for each product to be amplified within the mixture, under the conditions used. In general, templates (cDNA) restriction fragments that are either too large (in excess of approx 1 kb), or too small (under approx 0.2 kb) do not amplify efficiently. The product (representation) therefore only "represents" the amplifiable proportion of the digest. Accordingly, to ensure the greatest proportion of differentially expressed genes are identified, it is advisable to repeat the cDNA RDA analyses with a variety of different restriction enzymes (and relevant oligonucleotide adaptor/primers). The choice of alternative restriction enzymes to be used can be facilitated by examination of available sequence data.

11. Pilot reactions should also be carried out on a negative reverse transcription (RT) control (i.e., on total RNA preparations to which attempts to ligate the J-Bgl-adaptors have been made). This is to check for contamination with genomic DNA.
12. It is important that the PCR amplification to produce representations is kept within the linear range if the relative proportions of individual species are to be maintained with respect to the starting RNA populations. Accordingly, it is vital that care is taken over this "titration" (*see* **Subheading 3.2.4.2.**). This is particularly important for the detection of relative (rather than absolute) differences in expression.
13. During reannealing, three types of hybrid molecules can be formed (*see* also **Fig. 1B**): Given the abundance of material, Driver-Driver hybrids are most common, but lacking adaptors, cannot generate primer-binding sites during the T4 DNA polymerase "fill-in" reaction and are therefore not amplified. Driver-Tester hybrids are the next most common products, but because the Driver strand cannot generate a primer-binding site, these molecules can only be amplified linearly (i.e., DNA synthesis can only be primed from one strand (the tester). Tester-Tester hybrids on the other hand (representing the differentially expressed genes) will possess primer-binding sites at both ends, and will thus be amplified exponentially.
14. The initial 11-cycle PCR helps prevent loss of genuine, but less-abundant difference products during the precipitation steps prior to the MBN treatment.
15. The MBN treatment removes all single-stranded nucleic acids, including linear products of Driver-Tester hybrids, tRNA carrier, etc. It is also advisable to check efficiency of the MBN digestion. This can be done by comparison of treated and untreated aliquots on a 1.5% nondenaturing gel in TBE, pH 8.3. In our experience it is important to have fresh enzyme (it seems to perform poorly if old).
16. Because of random annealing events, many amplified molecules present at the DP1 stage will not represent genuine differences. A second round of PCR-coupled subtractive hybridization is therefore required. However because of the partial enrichment that has occurred, this can be carried out at higher stringencies (Driver-Tester ratios). A high degree of background smearing at this stage can indicate failure of the MBN treatment or incomplete denaturation of Tester and driver components prior to hybridization.
17. Identification/characterization of the difference products is initiated by sequencing of the insert of the resultant recombinant plasmids. Multiple clones arising from the same amplicon should be examined as although bands appear discrete, the amplicons are heterogenous, i.e., can comprise multiple different products. Similarity searches can then be carried out on genuine differences in DNA and Protein databases. Because the identified differences should only be present or upregulated in the Tester, each putative difference should be checked for validity by Southern hybridization against the original representations, and ideally also by RT-PCR, using different independently isolated RNA preparations as template (cloning of high numbers of false-positives usually indicates that the Driver-

Tester ratio used was too low). Gene libraries can be constructed and/or screened by standard techniques to obtain full-length genes.

18. Low yield of any product often means insufficient template was used. In generation of the initial cDNA RDA representations, poor quality RNA and/or cDNA can also be the culprit. During generation of difference products, however, it should be noted that simple failures during preliminary steps, e.g. loss of pellets during resuspension, incomplete/failed digestions, ligations, and so on, can also result in a lack of amplifiable template in the various PCR reactions.

References

1. Sagerström, C. G., Sun, B. I., and Sive, H. L. (1997) Subtractive cloning: past, present, future. *Ann. Rev. Biochem.* **66,** 751–783.
2. Handfield, M. and Levesque, R. C. (1999) Strategies for isolation of in vivo expressed genes from bacteria. *FEMS Microbiol. Rev.* **23,** 69–91.
3. Lisitsyn, N., Lisitsyn, N., and Wigler, M. (1993) Cloning the differences between two complex genomes. *Science* **259,** 946–951.
4. Bart, A., Dankert, J., and Van der Ende, A. (2000) Representational difference analysis of *Neisseria meningitidis* identifies sequences that are specific for the hyper-virulent lineage III clone. *FEMS Microbiol. Lett.* **188,** 111–114.
5. Strathdee, C. A. and Johnson, W. M. (1995) Identification of epidemiologic markers for *Neisseria meningitidis* using difference analysis. *Gene* **166,** 105–110.
6. Claus, H., Friedrich, A., Frosch, M., and Vogel, U. (2000) Differential distribution of novel restriction-modification systems in clonal lineages of *Neisseria meningitidis*. *J. Bacteriol.* **182,** 1296–1303.
7. Tinsley, C. R. and Nassif, X. (1996) Analysis of the genetic differences between *Neisseria meningitidis* and *Neisseria gonorrhoeae*: two closely related bacteria expressing two different pathogenicities. *Proc. Natl. Acad. Sci. USA* **93,** 11, 109–11,114.
8. Perrin, A., Nassif, X., and Tinsley, C. (1999) Identification of regions of the chromosome of *Neisseria meningitidis* and *Neisseria gonorrhoeae* which are specific to the pathogenic *Neisseria* species. *Infect. Immun.* **67,** 6119–6129.
9. Bowler, L. D., Hubank, H., and Spratt, B. G. (1999) Representational difference analysis of cDNA for the detection of differential gene expression in bacteria: development using a model of iron-regulated gene expression in *Neisseria meningitidis*. *Microbiology* **145,** 3529–3537.
10. Hubank, M. and Schatz, D.G. (1994) Identifying differences in mRNA expression by representational difference analysis of cDNA. *Nucleic Acids Res.* **22,** 5640–5648.
11. Hubank, M. and Schatz, D. G. (1999) cDNA representational difference analysis: a sensitive and flexible method for the identification of differentially expressed genes. *Methods Enzymol.* **303,** 325–349.

17

Managing Outbreaks

The Public Health Response

James M. Stuart

1. Introduction

1.1. Chapter Content

Comprehensive practical guidelines for the control of large-scale epidemic meningococcal disease were updated in 1998 by the World Health Organization (WHO) *(1)*. The guidance in this chapter is designed to assist in the management of the smaller-scale outbreaks or clusters, particularly in the educational setting (*see* **Note 1**). It focuses on countries, especially in Europe or North America, that are less prone to major epidemics and will normally have an adequately resourced public-health capacity.

1.2. The Public-Health Response

Outbreaks of meningococcal disease, from the small cluster in a school to the massive epidemic of sub-Saharan Africa, generate high levels of public alarm *(1,2)*. Contributing to this alarm are the high case-fatality rates (usually 5–10%) *(1)*, the rapid progression of severe septicemia, and the susceptibility of the young and healthy. In addition, the lack of predictability and speed of development of outbreaks can confound the efforts of public-health authorities to manage the outbreak. The impression that the authorities are not doing enough to prevent further cases and deaths can develop quickly, and the authority's credibility is on the line. Consequently, the speed of public health response is vital both to implement preventive measures and to manage the understandable public anxiety.

From: *Methods in Molecular Medicine, vol. 67: Meningococcal Disease: Methods and Protocols*
Edited by: A. J. Pollard and M. C. J. Maiden © Humana Press Inc., Totowa, NJ

The nature of the response is usually guided by national policy on management of clusters or outbreaks ***(3–8)***. There is considerable variation in these policies, reflecting the lack of hard evidence to inform best practice ***(3)***.

1.3. Assessing the Risk

Studies of household contacts have consistently shown a raised relative risk in the months following an index case, ranging from 500—1200 in the first month ***(9–12)***.

The risk to contacts in educational settings is lower ***(9–11,13)*** (Rushdy A., unpublished data). Studies show a consistent pattern of highest risk in the first 24 h falling over the next 7 d, but remaining higher than the expected background rate for 2–3 wk. In a 3-yr survey of clusters in England and Wales, relative risks of a second case within 4 wk of an index case in the same educational setting were 4.4, 12.3, and 27.5 for secondary schools, primary schools, and pre-school groups, respectively (Rushdy A., unpublished data). Because background disease rates are very low, usually around 1–7/100,000 per annum in Europe and North America ***(14)***, absolute risk of a second case in such settings is low. Once a second case has occurred, the risk of a third case in that institution may be as high as 30–50% ***(13)*** (Rushdy A., unpublished data).

Relative risk of further cases outside the educational setting has not been formally assessed, but outbreaks in definable social groups, civilian communities, and military recruits are well-described ***(2,15–19)***.

1.4 Managing Clusters in Educational Settings: Benefits and Costs of Interventions

1.4.1. Information

Communicating information about the outbreak to pupils, staff, parents, and local physicians is a low-cost intervention that should help in early identification and treatment of any further cases. The cost-effectiveness of this intervention is not known, but parents usually wish to be informed of cases and the raised relative risk in this setting suggests that heightened awareness is a logical public-health objective.

1.4.2. Chemoprophylaxis

The main intervention that may reduce risk in the short term is chemoprophylaxis. The usual aim of chemoprophylaxis in outbreaks is to eliminate meningococcal carriage in a defined population that is considered to be at higher risk of carriage of the outbreak strain. This population may be children and carers in a nursery, groups of friends, students in the same educational year, or all students in the school. Carriage studies during clusters sometimes but not invariably identify high carriage rates. In two outbreaks in school settings in England between 1995–1996, carriage rates of 25% (5/20 friends of cases) and 16% (8/50 classmates of cases) were found in which all carriers were found to have the outbreak strain (J. M. Stuart, unpublished data). In four other school outbreaks during the same period, carriage rates of the outbreak strain in pupils varied between undetectable and 1%. In one university outbreak, no carriers of the outbreak strain were found among 587 students swabbed *(20)*.

The recommended antibiotics for chemoprophylaxis are usually rifampicin or ciprofloxacin. Ceftriaxone is an alternative for use in pregnancy but is less popular for routine use as it is given by injection and is painful. These antibiotics have all been shown to have a high degree of effectiveness in eradicating carriage *(21–23)*, but their effectiveness in protection against disease is less clear. In household settings, chemoprophylaxis after one case may reduce the risk of further cases by 50% *(10)*, but no controlled trials have been done. In educational settings, effectiveness is not known, thus benefit is possible but uncertain. Costs include possibility of antibiotic resistance *(24)*, side effects, and eradication of commensal organisms that normally assist in generating immunity against meningococcal disease *(25)*.

1.4.3. Selective Carriage Eradication

An alternative to mass chemoprophylaxis is the "hunt and kill" strategy. This involves throat swabbing to identify carriers of the outbreak strain followed by selective carriage eradication *(26)*. This will restrict unnecessary antibiotic use. Disadvantages include the added costs of swabbing and isolation of the organism, the time taken to identify carriers, and the insensitivity of a single throat swab in identification of carriers *(27)*. Nonetheless, this approach has clear attractions for outbreaks evolving over weeks or months rather than days, and could find increasing use when more rapid and sensitive molecular methods for meningococcal identification become available.

1.4.4. Vaccination

If an outbreak is caused by strains of a serogroup for which an effective vaccine exists, vaccination should be considered. Recent data from England and Wales showed that if the serogroup of one case had been identified and another case was diagnosed within 4 wk in the same school, the second case was likely to be of the same strain as the first case (A. Rushdy, personal communication). This may help in decision-making.

Polysaccharide vaccines are safe and relatively inexpensive. They offer short-term protection (not in young children), but will not induce a good antibody response for 10 d after vaccination *(28)*. Giving vaccine without antibiotics would not therefore be expected to prevent cases during the period of highest risk in school outbreaks *(29)*. Vaccination can be used in combination with chemoprophylaxis, or without antibiotics in outbreaks that develop over longer time scales. Because it is anticipated that the newer conjugated vaccines will be more effective, it is likely that they will replace polysaccharide vaccines depending on their cost and availability.

1.4.5. Risk Benefit Analysis

Assessment of risk, benefits, and costs of interventions must then lead to a decision on public-health action. External factors such as availability of staff, antibiotics, vaccine, and feasibility of action (such as holidays just started) may well influence the decision-makers *(30)*. Demand for action from parents and politicians may be intense.

1.5. Managing Community Outbreaks

The same interventions are available for use in community outbreaks. Whether mass chemoprophylaxis works in open civilian communities is not known. It is not often used *(17,18)* and may not even lower attack rates *(31)*, though one trial in military barracks showed a significant effect on disease reduction *(19)*. The larger the population to whom antibiotics are administered, the higher the risk of potential harm from resistance, side effects, and eradication of protective Neisserial strains.

Vaccination in serogroup C outbreaks is recommended for consideration in the US when a defined threshold is reached *(8)*. Vaccination in conjunction with selective eradication of carriage has been proposed in Norway *(32)*.

2. Materials *(1,33; see* Note 2)

1. Letters to parents/students (*see* Appendix A,B).
2. Consent forms (*see* Appendix C).
3. Information on meningococcal disease (*see* Appendix D).
   a. Antibiotics (*see* Appendix E,F).
   b. Vaccine (*see* Appendix G).
4. Supplies of antibiotics, vaccines, syringes, needles.
5. Resuscitation equipment containing adrenaline, antihistamine for injection.
6. Communication facility: telephone, fax.
7. Contact numbers of expert advisers, information line.

3. Method

3.1. Surveillance

- Maintain good relationships with clinicians and microbiologists so that suspected cases are reported and microbiological investigation undertaken promptly. *See* **Table 1**.

Table 1
Suggested Microbiological Investigations[a]

Microscopy and culture of cerebrospinal fluid (CSF) or other deep sites
Culture of blood, throat swab, rash aspirate
Polymerase chain reaction (PCR) testing (where available)
Latex agglutination
Serology

[a]For confirmation of meningococcal infection, and referral to reference laboratory for identification of serogroup/type/subtype and/or genotype.

Table 2
Suggested Case Definitions

Confirmed case: Clinical diagnosis of invasive meningococcal disease confirmed by microbiological tests of high specificity, e.g., organism identified from blood, CSF, or other deep site.
Probable case: Clinical diagnosis where invasive meningococcal disease is the most likely diagnosis. This may or may not be supported by laboratory tests of lower specificity, e.g., culture from throat swab.
Possible case: Clinical diagnosis where invasive meningococcal disease is possible but where other diagnoses are at least as likely.

- Use agreed-upon case definitions and record cases on a database. *See* **Table 2**.
- Manage single cases according to standard protocol, with antibiotics +/– vaccine and information to close contact group. If a single case occurs in an educational setting, consider letter to parents if confirmed or probable case (*see* **Appendix A**).

3.2. Managing Clusters in Educational Settings (*see* Table 3)

3.2.1. Assess the Information

When two or more cases are reported from a school or college, careful and rapid assessment should be made. This should include a review of:

- All available clinical and microbiological data on the cases. If available, serogrouping of strains together with serotype/serosubtype or genotype will help in assessing relatedness of strains;
- Dates of onset of illness and of last attendance at school;
- Evidence of links between cases by age, school year, home address, social activities, friends; and
- The number of students in the school and in each school year.

Table 3
Steps in Cluster Management

Assess the information.
Consider the options.
Make a decision.
Communicate the decision.
Implement the decision.

3.2.2. Consider the Options

A decision must now be reached on public-health action. Rumors are probably already spreading round the school. Parents may be thinking of keeping their children away from school, especially if there has been a death (*see* **Notes 3** and **4**). The media may already have been informed.

Options will include:

- Waiting for more information, e.g., because of uncertain diagnoses;
- Informing parents but no prophylaxis apart from household contacts, e.g., because cases a few weeks apart, large school, big age difference in the cases, no social links, cases due to different serogroups, school has closed for holidays;
- Offering antibiotics with or without vaccine to a defined group of students, e.g., if two cases same school year, short interval between them, both confirmed cases; and
- Vaccination without antibiotics.

3.2.3. Make a Decision

The data on risk suggest a need to act urgently. If uncertain, the following may assist in decision-making:

- Seek expert advice from the national, regional epidemiology center.
- Check with the reference laboratory about interpretation of results and fast-tracking any specimens.
- Talk to the head of the school, assess feasibility of proposed interventions.
- If planning large-scale intervention, call an outbreak-control team meeting. This team may include: public-health physician, microbiologist, pharmacist, school health doctor/nurse, head teacher/education department representative, and press officer.

3.2.4. Communicate the Decision

- Communicate your decision promptly to pupils, teachers, parents, public-health department staff, primary and secondary care staff.

- Prepare a press statement and agree on a single press spokesperson. It is most likely that the press will find out about the outbreak if they have not done so already. The assistance and advice of a communications expert is strongly advised. The level of public interest is likely to depend on factors such as the number of cases, the size of the population at risk, and whether deaths have occurred.
- If high levels of interest are anticipated or already evident, prepare to set up telephone helplines, to allow controlled media access to vaccination sites, to release regular coordinated press briefings, and to hold press conferences *(33)*.

3.2.5. Implement the Decision

If antibiotics +/– vaccine are to be offered to pupils, make urgent arrangement with:

- Community medical/nursing staff to deliver medicines/vaccine to children (*see* **Note 5**);
- Head teacher to inform parents, seek consent, and discuss need for parents' meeting (*see* Appendices B, C, D); and
- Pharmacists to supply antibiotics (in correct formulation, dosage, and information sheets) and vaccines (**Table 4**) (*see* Appendices E, F, G).

3.3. Managing Community Outbreaks

Although school outbreaks must be handled quickly in order control alarm and reduce immediate risk of further cases, wider community outbreaks usually build up more slowly and by their nature are more diffuse. The same management steps apply.

- Assess carefully all the epidemiology at your disposal: confirmed and probable cases, serotyping and/or molecular typing data, dates of onset, population containing the cases. Calculate the attack rates. Although a precise threshold for action is necessarily arbitrary, in the US it is suggested that vaccination be considered if **at least 3** confirmed cases due to vaccine preventable disease have occurred in different households within 3 mo and the overall attack rate is **more than 10/100,000** *(8)*.
- If you are seriously considering an intervention, an outbreak-control team meeting is strongly recommended. Involve an expert adviser from outside the outbreak district.
- Consider all the alternatives for action (*see* **Subheading 1.4.**): information campaign, chemoprophylaxis, vaccination, selective carriage eradication.

One of the major difficulties in targeting a community for vaccination is deciding on the population boundaries, often defined by age group and geography. Such boundaries will of necessity be arbitrary. As far as possible, use existing administrative boundaries that make sense to the people who live within and without them. In any case, there are likely to be people living on the

Table 4
Chemoprophylaxis and Vaccination Recommendations[a]

Age	Dosage
Suggested dosage of rifampicin[b]	
Adults and children over 12 yr	600 mg[c]
Children 1–12 yr	10 mg/kg[c]
Children <1 yr	5 mg/kg[c]
Suggested dosage of ciprofloxacin	
Adults and children over 12 yr	500 mg (single dose)

Notes on chemoprophylaxis and vaccination sessions

- Chemoprophylaxis and vaccination sessions *(33)* need to be planned carefully, preferably using one large open room, e.g., the school hall, with screens to prevent waiting pupils from seeing the vaccinations.
- Clerical staff (usually 1–2 per session) are needed at point of entry to check off names and consent forms.
- A qualified physician should be available to deal with medical queries, reactions, etc.
- More than one antibiotic and vaccine station can be used, depending on numbers to be immunized, numbers of staff, and the space available, allowing at least 40 pupils per hour to go through each antibiotic and vaccine station (up to 60–80 per hour in university settings).
- For antibiotic stations, one nurse is needed to give and observe taking of antibiotics. Pupils then move to vaccine stations staffed by two nurses (one to draw up vaccine and the other to immunize).
- Vaccine batch numbers should be recorded.
- After vaccination, pupils should be seated in a waiting area for 15–30 min.
- Sessions of 2–2.5 h are normally feasible.

[a]*See* **Note 6**.
[b]Adapted from **ref.** ***4***.
[c]Twice daily for 2 d.

other side of the boundary who may feel unjustifiably excluded, who may be worried or angry, and whose anger will be increased if and when cases occur in the nontargeted population! The extent of public concern and press interest should not be underestimated ***(17)*** (*see* **Subheading 3.2.4.**).

4. Notes

1. A cluster may be considered as a grouping of cases and an outbreak as a grouping of cases in excess of expectancy, but an argument about whether two or three cases in a school constitute a cluster or an outbreak should not be allowed to delay pubic-health action.

2. Communication skills and cool judgement are an advantage.
3. A death in a pupil at a school will naturally raise anxiety levels among staff and parents. If you are hesitating between two options and in the absence of strong scientific evidence to inform decision-making, external factors that do not of themselves alter the risk of further cases may reasonably influence your decision making. It is a matter of judgement.
4. Good judgement comes from experience. Experience comes from bad judgement (A. Jaffe, personal communication).
5. If vaccination is to be offered but vaccine supplies are not immediately sufficient, the priority should be to reduce the immediate risk by giving antibiotics. Additional sessions can be organized when vaccine supplies become available.
6. Check if these antibiotics are licensed in your country for chemoprophlyaxis of meningococcal disease. If not, a statement to this effect should be included with the proviso (if true) that it is recommended in national policy.

Appendices

Example of information letter to parents after one or two cases A

Dear Parent or Guardian,

We are writing to inform you that one/two pupil(s) from the school has/have been admitted to hospital with meningitis/septicemia, probably/possibly caused by the meningococcal bacteria. The child/children is/are (status—responding well to treatment, etc.). We have been in contact with doctors at the Health Authority, who have advised that no further action is necessary at the present time. There is no reason to make any change in the school routine and no reason for children to be kept at home.

Meningococcal bacteria are carried in the back of the throat of about 1 in 10 people at any one time but only very rarely cause illness. Most people who carry the bacteria become immune to them. The bacteria do *not* spread easily and those who have had prolonged, close contact with the person are at a slightly greater risk of getting ill. These people have been identified and given antibiotics to stop the bacteria spreading.

Although the risk to your child is very small, it is sensible to be aware of the signs and symptoms, which are detailed in the attached leaflet. If you suspect that a member of your family is suffering from these symptoms, you should contact your doctor immediately. If you have individual worries about this case, you can speak to a member of the Communicable Disease Control Team at .... during normal working hours.

Yours sincerely,

Head Teacher/Public Health Physician

Example of parent letter if antibiotics and/or vaccine program **B**

Dear Parent or Guardian,

Following the recent letter from the head teacher on. . . I am writing to inform you that two/three pupils from the school have been admitted to hospital with meningitis/septicemia, probably/definitely caused by the meningococcal bacteria. The children are (status—responding well to treatment, etc.).

In accordance with national policy, we will be offering preventive antibiotics (and vaccination) to all pupils in the school. A special session for this will be held on .... from ..... to ..... in .... the school hall.

Your child should attend this session and bring with them the enclosed consent form, signed by you. I also enclose an information sheet on meningitis/ciprofloxacin/rifampicin/vaccine for your information.

For further information about this illness, a telephone helpline is available at ....

Yours sincerely,

Public Health Physician

Example of consent form **C**

.... Health Authority ....School

Name of pupil .... Date of birth....../....../......
Address ....
School year ....

I consent to my child receiving meningococcal vaccine*
I consent to my child receiving: Ciprofloxacin (those aged 12 or over)*
Rifampicin (those aged less than 12)*
*Please delete as applicable

Relationship to child: (Mother, Father, Legal Guardian) ....
NAME (Capitals, please) ....

Date: Signed:

Please read the information leaflet attached

Example of information sheet **D**

Extracted and modified from "About Meningitis" leaflet, Meningitis Trust.

Meningitis and septicemia are not easy to spot at first because the symptoms are similar to those of flu. Recognizing the symptoms early could mean the difference between life and death. Someone with meningitis or septicemia will become very ill. The illness may take one or two days to develop, but it can develop very quickly over a few hours. Here are some of the symptoms.

- Vomiting
- Very high temperature
- Violent or severe headache
- Stiff neck
- Disliking bright lights
- Drowsiness or lack of energy
- Painful joints
- Rash. This type of rash may start as tiny blood spots, which look like pin pricks. The spots can be anywhere on the body, even behind the ears or on the soles of the feet. If left untreated, the spots can spread around the body and get bigger so that they look like bruises. The spots or bruises do not turn white when pressed with a glass.

Call a doctor immediately if someone has this rash or if they are ill with these symptoms.

Example of information leaflet on rifampicin E

The drug that you have been prescribed is to prevent you from carrying the bacteria that causes meningitis with which you may have been in contact. It also prevents you passing on the disease. This is a short-term measure only and it is important that everyone offered this medicine takes it at around the same time.

There is a small chance that you may still become ill **and continued vigilance is necessary for everyone**. If you develop a fever, headache, or vomiting, please contact your doctor and show him this letter.

The medicine should be taken TWICE a day for TWO days, i.e., four doses.

It is important that you take your capsules or syrup exactly as directed.

A child's dose depends on the age and weight of the child and will be decided by your doctor. Most children will be given the drug in syrup. The syrup should also be taken for two days.

These doses should be taken at 12-hour intervals, and ONE HOUR BEFORE MEALS (e.g., breakfast and supper) to obtain the best effect.

CHECK WITH THE DOCTOR AVAILABLE AT THE SCHOOL BEFORE TAKING THE TABLETS IF:

1. You have had a previous allergic reaction to rifampicin.
2. You are taking oral contraceptives (extra precautions should be taken during the rest of the month).
3. You are taking any other medication.
4. You have jaundice, liver problems, or porphyria.

PLEASE REMEMBER

1. Rifampicin is colored red, and this may stain your urine, spit, and tears. It can also permanently stain soft contact lenses.
2. Do not drink alcohol during the two days that you are taking Rifampicin.

.... Health authority, telephone....

Example of information leaflet on ciprofloxacin F

The drug (Ciprofloxacin) that you have been prescribed is to prevent you from carrying the bacteria that causes meningitis with which you may have been in contact. It also prevents you passing on the disease. This is a short-term measure only and it is important that everyone offered ciprofloxacin takes the tablets at around the same time.

There is a small chance that you may still become ill and continued vigilance is necessary for everyone. If you develop a fever, headache, vomiting, or any other relevant symptoms, please seek medical advice and show this letter.

The adult dose is ONE 500 mg dose (two tablets, 250 mg each)

It is important that you take your tablets now and exactly as directed

1. The tablets should be swallowed whole with a full glass of water.
2. DO NOT take the tablets if you have taken antacid/indigestion medicines or preparations containing iron or mineral supplements within the last four hours. Please see the doctor available here if this is the case.
3. Do not take alcohol with this medicine because it may make you drowsy, affecting your ability to drive or operate machinery.
4. One possible side effect of the antibiotic is facial swelling. This normally subsides over a period of about half an hour. If you experience this, please see the doctor or nurse here. You may also feel tired or have stomach-ache, but these usually settle quickly and are not a cause for concern.

CHECK WITH THE DOCTOR AVAILABLE AT THE SCHOOL BEFORE TAKING THE TABLETS IF:

5. You have had a previous allergic reaction to ciprofloxacin.
6. You are taking any other medication, particularly for diabetes or epilepsy.
7. You are pregnant or breast-feeding.
8. You have G6PD deficiency.
9. You have any other queries.

.... Health authority, telephone....

Example of information leaflet on A & C meningococcal vaccine G

You are being offered immunization against a particular type of meningitis caused by a germ called the group C meningococcus. This vaccine will help to protect you against this type of meningitis, which has affected other pupils at the school.

This is not a live vaccine and you cannot catch meningitis from receiving the vaccine. The likely side effect of the vaccine is that you may develop a sore arm. You may also develop a mild temperature. The temperature is only likely to last for 24 hours.

The vaccine provides increased protection against group A and C disease for about three years but does not protect you against group B and other forms of meningitis. Therefore it is very important that you should still remain vigilant for the symptoms and signs of meningitis and seek medical help as early as possible if you are concerned.

.... Health Authority, telephone....

Acknowledgments

I am most grateful to Jeanette Spence, Neena Stewart, and Mike Barker for providing practical details and information used in their health districts, and to Mike Barker for his helpful comments.

References

1. World Health Organization (1998) *Control of Epidemic Meningococcal Disease: WHO Practical Guidelines.* World Health Organization, Geneva.
2. Begg, N. (1995) Outbreak management, in *Meningococcal Disease* (Cartwright, K. A. V., ed.), John Wiley and Sons, Chichester, UK, pp. 285–305.
3. Thalanany, M. (1997) The management of clusters of meningococcal disease: survey of 35 European countries, in *Surveillance of Bacterial Meningitis in Europe 1996* (Connolly, M. and Noah, N., eds.). Kings College, London, pp. 34–40.
4. PHLS Meningococcal Infections Working Party and Public Health Medicine Environmental Group (1995) Control of meningococcal disease: guidance for consultants in communicable disease control. *Commun. Dis. Rep. Rev.* **5,** R189–R194.
5. Stuart, J. M., Monk, P. N., Lewis, D. A., Constantine, C., Kaczmarski, E. B., and Cartwright, K. A. V. on behalf of the PHLS Meningococcus Working Group and Public Health Medicine Environmental Group (1997) Management of clusters of meningococcal disease. *Commun. Dis. Rep. Rev.* **7,** R3–R5.
6. Canadian Consensus Conference on Meningococcal Disease (1994) Guidelines for control of meningococcal disease (February 1993). *Can. Comm. Dis. Rep.* **20,** 17–27.

7. Patel, M. S., Collignon, P. J., Watson, C. R., Condon, R. J., Doherty, R. R., Merianos, A., and Stewart, G. J. (1997) New guidelines for management and prevention of meningococcal disease in Australia. *Med. J. Aust.* **166,** 598–601.
8. Centers for Disease Control and Prevention (1997) Control and prevention of meningococcal disease and control and prevention of serogroup C meningococcal disease: evaluation and management of suspected outbreaks. *MMWR* **46,** 1–21.
9. Olivares, R. and Hubert, B. (1992) Clusters of meningococcal disease in France (1987–1988). *Eur. J. Epidemiol.* **8,** 737–742.
10. Hastings, L., Stuart, J., Andrews, N., and Begg, N. (1997) A retrospective survey of clusters of meningococcal disease in England and Wales, 1993–1995: estimated risks of further cases in household and educational settings. *Commun. Dis. Rep. Rev.* **7,** R195–R200.
11. De Wals, P., Hertoghe, L., Borlee-Grimee, I., De Maeyer-Cleempoel, S., Reginster-Haneuse, G., Dachy, A., Bouckaert, A., and Lechat, M. F. (1981) Meningococcal disease in Belgium. Secondary attack rate among household, day-care nursery and pre-elementary school contacts. *J. Infect.* **3,** 53–61.
12. Meningococcal Disease Surveillance Group (1976) Analysis of endemic meningococcal disease by serogroup and evaluation of chemoprophylaxis. *J. Infect. Dis.* **134,** 201–204.
13. Zangwill, K. M., Schuchat A., Riedo, F. X., Pinner, R. W., Koo, D. T., Reeves, M. W., and Wenger, J. D. (1997) School-based clusters of meningococcal disease in the United States. Descriptive epidemiology and a case-control analysis. *JAMA* **277,** 389–395.
14. Noah, N. and Henderson, B. (1999) Surveillance of bacterial meningitis in Europe 1997/8. Public Health Laboratory Service, London.
15. Imrey, P. B., Jackson, L. A., Ludwinski, P. H., England, A. C. I., Fella, G. A., Fox, B. C., Isdale, L. B., Reeves, M. W., and Wenger, J. D. (1996) Outbreak of serogroup C meningococcal disease associated with campus bar patronage. *Am. J. Epidemiol.* **143,** 624–630.
16. Koh, Y. M., Barnes, G. H., Kaczmarski, E., and Stuart, J. M. (1998) Outbreak of meningococcal disease linked to a sports club. *Lancet* **352,** 706–707.
17. Irwin, D. J., Miller, J. M., Milner, P. C., Patterson, T., Richards, R. G., Williams, D. A., Insley, C. A., and Stuart, J. M. (1997) Community immunization programme in response to an outbreak of invasive Neisseria meningitidis serogroup C infection in the Trent region of England 1995–1996. *J. Public Health Med.* **19,** 162–170.
18. Jacobson, J. A., Chester, T. J., and Fraser, D. W. (1977) An epidemic of disease due to serogroup B *Neisseria meningitidis* in Alabama: report of an investigation and community-wide prophylaxis with a sulfonamide. *J. Infect. Dis.* **136,** 104–108.
19. Kuhns, D. M., Nelson, C. T., Feldman, H. A., and Kuhn, L. R. (1943) The prophylactic value of sulfadiazine in the control of Meningococcic meningitis. *JAMA* **123,** 335–339.
20. Gilmore, A., Jones, G., Barker, R. M., Soltanpoor, N., and Stuart, J. (1999) Meningococcal disease at the University of Southampton. *Epidemiol. Infect.* **123,** 185–192.

21. Deal, W. B. and Sanders, E. (1969) Efficacy of rifampicin in treatment of meningococcal carriers. *N. Engl. J. Med.* **281,** 641–645.
22. Cuevas, L. E., Kazembe, P., and Mughogho, G. K. (1995) Eradication of nasopharyngeal carriage of *Neisseria meningitidis* in children and adults in rural Africa: a comparison of Ciprofloxacin and Rifampicin. *J. Infect. Dis.* **171,** 728–731.
23. Schwartz, B., Al-Ruwais, A., A'Ashi, J., Broome, C. V., Al-Tobaiqi, A., Fontaine, R. E., et al. (1988) Comparative efficacy of ceftriaxone and rifampicin in eradicating pharyngeal carriage of group A *Neisseria meningitidis*. *Lancet* 1239–1242.
24. Jackson, L. A., Alexander, E. R., Debolt, C. A., Swenson, P. D. B. J., McDowell, M. G., Reeves, M. W., and Wenger, J. D. (1996) Evaluation of the use of mass chemoprophylaxis during a school outbreak of enzyme type 5 serogroup B meningococcal disease. *Pediatr. Infect. Dis. J.* **15,** 992–998.
25. Gold, R., Goldschneider, I., Lepow, M. L., Draper, T. F., and Randolph, M. (1978) Carriage of *Neisseria meningitidis* and *Neisseria lactamica* in infants and children. *J. Infect. Dis.* **137,** 112–121.
26. Kristiansen, B.-E. and Knapp, A.-B. (1996) Secondary prevention of meningococcal disease:high risk contacts should be given chemoprophylaxis and preventive treatment with penicillin. *BMJ* **312,** 591–592.
27. Jones, D. M. (1996) Secondary prevention of meningococcal disease. *BMJ* **312,** 1537.
28. Jones, D. M. (1987) Meningococcal vaccines. *PHLS Microbiol. Dig.* **4,** 23–24.
29. Round, A. and Palmer, S. (1999) Should we be doing more to prevent Group C meningococcal infection in school age children? How can we decide? *J. Public Health Med.* **21,** 8–13.
30. Ardern, K., Bowler, S., Hussey, R. M., and Regan, C. M. (1999) Managing meningococcal disease case clusters: art or science? *J. Epidemiol. Com. Health* **53,** 565–571.
31. Shehab, S., Keller, N., Barkay, A., Leitner, L., Leventhal, A., and Block, C. (1998) Failure of mass antibiotic prophylaxis to control a prolonged outbreak of meningococcal disease in an Israeli village. *Eur. J. Clin. Microbiol. Infect. Dis.* **17,** 749–753.
32. Smith, I., Lehmann, A. K., Hoiby, E. A., and Halstensen, A. I. (1999) Follow up of meningococcal disease cases in Western Norway. European Monitoring Group on Meningococci. Abstracts of 5th Meeting, **123** (Abstract National Meningococcal Reference Laboratory, Athens, Greece).
33. Barker, R. M., Shakespeare, R. M., Mortimore, A. J., Allen, N. A., Solomon, C. L., and Stuart, J. M. (1999) Practical guidelines for responding to an outbreak of meningococcal disease among university students based on experience in Southampton. *Commun. Dis. Public Health* **2,** 168.

18

Global Trends in Meningococcal Disease

Dominique A. Caugant

1. Introduction

The unambiguous identification of epidemic *Neisseria meningitidis* strains and their clear distinction from other less pathogenic meningococci is required for the global epidemiology of meningococcal disease. Until the recent development of multi-locus sequence typing *(1)*, multi-locus enzyme electrophoresis (abbreviated MEE or MLEE) was the only method to permit large-scale analysis of *N. meningitidis* strains causing disease in various parts of the world and to document the intercontinental spread of particularly pathogenic organisms *(2–8)*.

The MLEE approach has been used extensively in studies of population biology and phylogenetics of both eukaryotes and prokaryotes, and has proven itself to be the gold standard for population genetics of bacteria *(9)*. The technique is based on the analysis of electrophoretic variation in a support, usually starch gel, of a set of chromosomally encoded cytoplasmic enzymes that are detected with specific staining methods. Distinct mobility variants of each enzyme (electromorphs) are equated with alleles at the corresponding gene. Although the allelic variation is measured indirectly at the protein level instead of the nucleotide sequence of the genes, it is a fully validated genotyping method, which indexes the variation present in the whole bacterial genome and gives a representative measure of overall genetic relatedness among isolates *(10)*. The enzymes analyzed in MLEE are essential for the bacterial metabolism and are encoded by housekeeping genes. In such genes, allelic variation is neutral or nearly so, which means that possession of anyone of the alleles does not affect the fitness of the strains. Thus, convergence to the same allele through adaptative evolution is unlikely and differences between strains in a set of

From: *Methods in Molecular Medicine, vol. 67: Meningococcal Disease: Methods and Protocols*
Edited by: A. J. Pollard and M. C. J. Maiden © Humana Press Inc., Totowa, NJ

housekeeping genes reflect the genetic events that have occurred overall in their genome since their divergence from a common ancestor.

The allele profiles obtained by MLEE, designated as electrophoretic types (ETs), correspond to the multi-locus enzyme genotypes of the organisms. Bacterial strains with identical ETs are assumed to be members of the same clone. The allelic profiles can be submitted to computer analyses in order to establish the genetic similarity of any number of strains and to represent it graphically ***(10)***.

In application to *N. mengitidis*, MLEE has proved very effective for analysis of sporadic cases ***(11)***, local outbreaks of disease ***(12–14)***, and for identifying the relationships among epidemics occurring in different parts of the world ***(2–8)***. Although probably all clones of *N. meningitidis* can cause disease when encountering a particularly susceptible individual, important variations in the virulence potential of different meningococcal clones has been demonstrated by comparing the genotypes of strains causing disease with those colonizing the throat of asymptomatic carriers ***(15)***. Significant temporal changes in the clonal composition of the meningococcal population causing disease in a geographic area have been documented ***(16)***, sometimes even during the course of an epidemic ***(17)***.

Hundreds of distinct ETs or clones have been identified among the many thousands of individual strains subjected to MLEE analyses in the past 15 years. Most ETs have been identified once in a single individual, either a healthy carrier or a patient, but dozen or so clones have been isolated from patients repeatedly over several decades and in various parts of the world ***(18)***. These predominant clones have been usually associated with an increased incidence of disease, showing that epidemics and hyperendemic waves of disease are associated with the spread of an especially virulent bacterium in a susceptible population ***(6,7)***.

A number of other clones, represented by a limited number of strains and usually recovered in a single geographic location, differed from the epidemic meningococcal clones at only one or two of the enzyme loci as shown by MLEE analyses. These closely related variants are assumed to result essentially from recent recombinational events between the epidemic strains and other strains of *Neisseria* species circulating in the human population ***(19,20)***. These genetic groups of clones that are different from one another, but still sufficiently closely related for a common origin to be recognized, have been designated as subgroups for serogroup A strains ***(21)*** and clone-complexes, clusters, or lineages for strains of other serogroups ***(2,16,18)***. The patterns of epidemic spread of the genetic groups that have reached an intercontinental distribution are presented here, followed by the protocol for MLEE analyses of *N. meningitidis* that is used by most laboratories presently performing the technique.

1.1. Global Trends Associated with the Spread of Epidemic Clones

MLEE analysis of *N. meningitidis* strains expressing the serogroup A capsular polysaccharide has shown that they represent a distinct phylogenetic subpopulation of the species *(18)*. Serogroup A strains are unusual in that they may provoke large epidemics, with incidence rates of over 500/100,000, which sometimes encompass several countries or even continents in a short period of time. Since the Second World War, these epidemics have been restricted to China and the Sahel region of sub-Saharan Africa, called the meningitis belt. Achtman and co-workers have characterized serogroup A isolates representing the organisms responsible for most epidemics or outbreaks in the world since the 1960s *(3,21)* and demonstrated the existence of 8 genetic subgroups among serogroup A strains. Two of these, subgroups I and III, have undergone pandemic spread. The other subgroups of serogroup A strains, although associated with serious epidemics, have shown a more limited geographical distribution. Subgroup IV-1 was responsible for both endemic disease and epidemics in West Africa from the early 1960s to the early 1980s; subgroup IV-2 has been associated with epidemics in the United States and Great Britain during the two World Wars; subgroups V, VII, and VIII were exclusively found in China; and subgroup VI has been identified solely in Russia and Eastern Europe *(21)*.

1.1.1. Subgroup I

The first recognized subgroup I strain was isolated in the UK in 1941 *(6)*. At the beginning of the 1960s, subgroup I was identified in North Africa and in countries of the African meningitis belt. In the early 1970s, subgroup I clones caused outbreaks of disease in Brazil, the US, and Canada. Subgroup I clones were also found at that time in Europe and were in the late 1970s responsible for epidemics in Nigeria and Rwanda *(6)*. Subgroup I has been identified in South Africa since 1968 and led in 1991 to an outbreak among refugees from Mozambique *(7)*; it was still the predominant serogroup A clone in South Africa in 1996 *(22)*. Outbreaks among Maoris in New Zealand and the aboriginal population in Australia in the 1980s and 1990s were also traced to subgroup I clones *(6,21)*. A world map illustrating the places of identification of subgroup I up to the 1980s is presented in **ref.** *5*.

1.1.2. Subgroup III

Strains of subgroup III have been responsible for two pandemics that both had their origin in China, some 15 years apart. The first one, starting in China in the 1960s, spread to Romania, Russia, and Scandinavia in 1969. It resulted in a severe epidemic in Finland, starting in 1973. Subsequently, subgroup III led a major epidemic in Brazil in the mid-1970s *(3)*.

Subgroup III strains started a new epidemic in China in the early 1980s, and thereafter spread to Nepal and most likely India. Subgroup III bacteria, probably carried by pilgrims from South Asia, caused 7,000 cases of meningococcal disease during the annual Haj pilgrimage to Mecca, Saudi Arabia, in 1987 *(4)*. The clone was then spread to all continents by returning pilgrims. Cases were reported among the travellers and their close-contacts, in the US, England, and France, but the strain was not further transmitted in these countries and no epidemics developed *(6)*. In the African continent, however, where subgroup III strains had not been identified previously, the situation was quite different. Major epidemics occurred in Ethiopia, Sudan, Chad, and Kenya in 1988 and 1989. In the following years, the other countries of the meningitis belt, as well as African countries outside that traditional meningitis region, such as Burundi, Zambia, Cameroon, Uganda, and Rwanda, were reached by outbreaks caused by subgroup III strains *(23)*. In 1996, the sub-Saharan region of Africa was reached by a new subgroup III epidemic of unprecedented scale with over 150,000 reported cases and 16,000 deaths, affecting principally Burkina Faso and Nigeria. South Africa was reached by subgroup III strains for the first time also in 1996 *(22)*. Major international efforts were set up to prevent further epidemics in West Africa *(24)*, but epidemics are still occurring. In 1997, meningitis outbreaks caused by clones of subgroup III were seen again in Burkina Faso, Ghana, Togo, and Benin, and in 1998 in Guinea-Bissau *(8,25)*. In 1999, Sudan experienced its third subgroup III epidemic in 10 years *(25)*, while Senegal was reached for the first time by a subgroup III epidemic *(26,27)*. Thus, the introduction of subgroup III strains in Africa, after the Haj pilgrimage of 1987, led to epidemics and outbreaks encompassing essentially the whole continent.

1.1.3. The ET-5 Complex

In the mid 1970s, an increased incidence of serogroup B meningococcal disease was noted both in Norway and in Spain. Analysis of patient isolates by MLEE demonstrated that both epidemics were caused by the same group of closely related clones, the ET-5 complex *(2)*. The same clone represented the predominant genotype of the isolates in both countries, although the strains differed in their two major serotyping antigens: the ET-5 complex strains from Norway were nearly all serotype 15:P1.7,16, while the strains from Spain usually had another serotype: serosubtype combination, 4:P1.19,15. In the following years, the ET-5 complex spread from these two foci to much of Western Europe, where it caused increases in disease incidence and localized outbreaks. In the mid 1990s, after periods of low incidence of disease, Iceland and Finland were also reached by severe outbreaks caused by ET-5 *(7)*.

Strains of the ET-5 complex, that were B:4:P1.19,15 as in Spain, were also responsible for the severe epidemic that started in Cuba in the beginning of the 1980s *(2)*, and produced an elevated disease incidence in Brazil, especially in the

Sao Paulo region, in the late 1980s. Bacteria of the ET-5 complex, expressing a new serotype:serosubtype combination, B : 15 : P1.7b,3 were also responsible for a severe epidemic in Chile that started in the town of Iquique in 1985 and then spread throughout the country. In the early 1990s, the ET-5 complex was also identified in Argentina, but represented less than 20% of the patient strains *(7)*. Members of the ET-5 complex were sporadically identified in the US and Canada from the late 1970s, but until the 1990s it did not seem to establish itself as an important source of disease in North America. In 1994, substantial increases in incidence of serogroup B meningococcal disease were noted in parts of Washington State and in Oregon, associated with ET-5 complex strains presenting the same serological characteristics as the Norwegian ones, B:15:P1.7,16 *(28,29)*.

Organisms of the ET-5 complex have been present in South Africa since the late 1970s, representing about 25% of the cases in the Cape Province. Elsewhere in the African continent they have been detected solely in Morocco and Algeria, where they were the predominant clonal group in the 1990s among serogroup B isolates *(7,30)*. Clones of the ET-5 complex caused disease in Australia, where they were first recognized among patients immigrating from East Asia, and among the few serogroup B patient strains analyzed from China, Japan, and Thailand, demonstrating a global distribution. A world map showing the distribution of outbreaks caused by clones of the ET-5 complex is shown in **ref.** *7*.

Retrospective analyses have shown that bacteria of the ET-5 complex were not a common source of disease before the 1970s. Although comprehensive epidemiological data from many countries are available from that period on, the exact routes of spread of the ET-5 complex have been difficult to establish accurately, because of the relatively low transmissibility of the clone. In contrast to the nearly immediate occurrence of the first wave of epidemics after introduction of subgroup III strains in the African continent, a delay of several years has been noticed in several countries between the introduction of clones of the ET-5 complex and the onset of the epidemic. Epidemics caused by the ET-5 complex, although giving only a moderate increase in disease incidence, may last for several decades. In Norway, only in 1999, 25 years after the onset of the epidemic, is the incidence back to the endemic level of disease.

Individual clones of serogroup A meningococci present essentially the same antigenic characteristics and only limited variation in the housekeeping genes used in MLEE analyses in the course of a pandemic *(31)*. In contrast, numerous genetic changes have been evidenced during the global spread of strains of the ET-5 complex. In practice, all genes that have been studied in ET-5 complex isolates have showed allelic variation, which often could be traced as a consequence of recombinational events. Some of this microvariation seems to be selected for as an escape mechanism for meningococci to avoid the immune pressure of the human host.

1.1.4. The ET-37 Complex

The oldest identified bacterium of the ET-37 complex was a serogroup B strain isolated in the US in 1917. Outbreaks and epidemics traced to the ET-37 complex (also designated as cluster B2 in **ref. *18*** and as lineage IX in **ref. *16***) have been documented since the 1960s, when it was responsible for numerous cases of meningococcal disease in the U.S. Army ***(32)***. The ET-37 complex was probably the origin of the large serogroup C outbreak in Brazil in the early 1970s (which was followed by a subgroup III epidemic) and was the dominant clone of the serogroup B epidemic in South Africa in the late 1970s ***(18)***. Serogroup C strains of the ET-37 complex have been regularly isolated from cases of sporadic disease and local outbreaks in the 1980s in the US, Europe, and Africa. In Africa, strains of the ET-37 complex recovered from patients may belong to serogroup C, Y, or W135.

In the 1990s, the appearance of a variant within the ET-37 complex resulted in increased incidence of serogroup C disease in various regions of the world. This new ET, designated ET-15, was first identified in Canada in 1986. ET-15 differed from ET-37 by having an allele at the fumarase locus that is otherwise infrequent in meningococcal strains ***(33)***. In the following years, ET-15 was responsible for large outbreaks of the serogroup C disease in Canada, leading to several mass-immunization campaigns between 1992 and 1994 ***(34)***. Then, increases in serogroup C disease were reported in different regions of the US, and ET-15 was associated with several of these outbreaks ***(35)***. ET-15 strains reached Iceland in 1991, causing most of the serogroup C disease from 1993; and Finland was reached in 1992 ***(7)***. In 1993, outbreaks of serogroup C disease in Israel ***(36)*** and the Czech Republic ***(37)*** were traced to the ET-15 clone, and the increase in serogroup C disease that occurred in England since 1995 ***(38)*** was also mainly associated with the same clone. ET-15 was identified in Norway first in 1994, but its introduction did not result in an increase in serogroup C disease. In Australia, however, its importation in 1994 led to many cases, especially in New South Wales ***(13)***. In 1998, an outbreak in Germany during a carnival was also owing to this new variant ***(39)***.

With ET-15 we experienced the emergence and rapid intercontinental spread of a new variant within a group of clones that already had a world-wide distribution. ET-15 organisms had a significantly higher case-fatality ratio than other invasive meningococcal disease isolates, which may result from lower herd immunity to the newly emerged clone ***(40)***. Additional molecular techniques have been employed in an attempt to identify determinants that may be associated with the increased virulence of ET-15 compared to other ET-37 complex strains ***(41,42)***, but no clear answer has yet been provided.

1.1.5. Cluster A4

Another clone-complex that has been associated with epidemics and hyperendemic waves of disease has been named cluster A4 ***(18)***, also called Lineage II in **ref. *16***. The earliest identification of cluster A4 was in the Netherlands in 1961. Starting in the mid 1960s, an hyperendemic wave of disease caused by cluster A4 was noted in the Netherlands, followed a few years later by another wave owing to a closely related clone of the same complex ***(16)***.

Cluster A4 has been a common cause of disease in the 1970s in the US, Canada, the UK, Iceland, and many other European countries, and was responsible for a severe serogroup B epidemic in Cape Town, South Africa from 1979, which followed the ET-37 complex epidemic ***(17,18)***. In the last few years, cluster A4 clones have been associated with a high incidence of serogroup B disease in children in Greece ***(7)*** and an increase in serogroup C disease in Brazil ***(43)***. Isolates of cluster A4 were identified as the cause of outbreaks in Australia in the early 1990s and are the major cause of serogroup B meningococcal disease in Argentina ***(25)***.

1.1.6. Lineage III

A retrospective survey of serogroup B cases strains in the Netherlands since 1958 identified a new clone-complex, designated as lineage III that started to give disease in 1980 ***(16)***. Lineage III became the most prevalent clone-complex in the Netherlands in 1990, representing about 20% of the disease isolates ***(44)***, and resulted in a moderate increase in the incidence of disease. It was then also recognized at a low frequency in several other European countries, including Iceland, Finland, Norway, the UK, Greece, and Austria. In Belgium, however, lineage III strains, spreading from the Netherlands, led to an increase in the incidence of serogroup B disease in 1997 ***(45)***. Lineage III was associated with the ongoing epidemic of meningococcal disease in New Zealand that started in the early 1990s and is affecting especially the Maori and Pacific Islander populations ***(46,47)***.

MLEE analyses have demonstrated the huge spreading ability of a few virulent clones of *N. meningitidis*. A new disease-causing clone in one area may reach a global distribution in the course of a few years, with a complete replacement of the strains associated with disease in the human population. Although the introduction of a clone with an epidemic potential in a region does not necessarily mean that an epidemic will ensue, the clone-complexes responsible for an increased incidence of disease in one country have often been associated with outbreaks and epidemics elsewhere. In spite of the improved understanding of the epidemiology of meningococcal disease that has been provided by clonal analyses, it is still impossible to predict reliably the occurrence of epidemics. Epidemiological surveillance on a global scale, including clonal analyses of the disease-causing organisms, needs to be pursued to be able to establish appropriate preventive measures.

2. Materials

2.1. Preparation of Bacterial Extracts

1. Safety cabinet with vertical airflow.
2. 100 mL overnight Tryptic Soy Broth (TSB) cultures.
3. Refrigerated centrifuge with appropriate rotors.
4. 300-mL centrifuge bottles and 10-mL centrifuge tubes.
5. Lysis buffer: 10 m*M* Tris-HCl, 1 m*M* ethylene diamine tetraacetic acid (EDTA), pH adjusted to 6.8 with concentrated HCl. All buffers and solutions should be prepared with deionized water.
6. Vortex mixer.
7. Disposable membrane filters with 0.45-μm pore size.
8. Freezer (–70°C).

2.2. Electrophoresis

1. One-L Erlenmeyer flasks with thick walls.
2. Starch, hydrolyzed for gel electrophoresis (Connaught, Toronto, Canada).
3. Gel and electrode buffers (*see* **Table 1**).
4. Acrylic gel molds (18 × 20 × 1 cm).
5. Plastic foil.
6. Horizontal electrophoresis apparatus consisting of 2 acrylic tanks (20 × 6 × 6 cm) with platinum electrodes (*see* **Note 1**).
7. Power supplies with a minimum capacity of 100 mA at 300 V.
8. Whatman filter paper no. 3, cut into pieces of 6 × 9 mm.
9. Amaranth dye solution (100 mg amaranth dissolved in 1 mL ethanol, plus 19 mL water).
10. Sponge wicks (18 × 14 cm).
11. Glass plates (20 × 30 × 0.3 cm).
12. Metal pans (20 × 30 × 5 cm).

2.3. Staining of Enzymatic Activities

1. Acrylic slicing plate (17 × 28 cm) with a 4 mm wide × 1 mm thick edge on each side of the length of the plate.
2. Slicer (thin metal wire stretched on an acrylic handle).
3. Clear plastic boxes for staining of the enzymes.
4. Chemicals and staining solutions (*see* **Table 2**).
5. Incubator (37°C).
6. Light box.
7. Fixing solution: 1:5:5 mixture of acetic acid, methanol, and water.

Table 1
Three Buffers Systems Used for MLEE Analysis of *N. meningitidis*

System	Electrode buffer	Gel buffer	Voltage (V)	Enzymes
A	Tris-citrate, pH 8.0 83.20 g Tris, 33.09 g citric acid monohydrate, water to 1 L	Tris-citrate, pH 8.0 Electrode buffer diluted 1:29	130	ME, malic enzyme; G6P, glucose 6-phosphate dehydrogenase; PEP, peptidase; IDH, isocitrate dehydrogenase; ACO, aconitase; GD1 and GD2, two glutatmate dehydrogenases; ADK, adenylate kinase
C	Borate, pH 8.2 18.50 g boric acid, 2.40 g NaOH, water to 1 L	Tris-citrate, pH 8.7 9.21 g Tris, 1.05 g citric acid monohydrate, water to 1 L	250	ADH, alcohol dehydrogenase
D	Lithium hydroxide, pH 8.1 1.20 g LiOH monohydrate, 11.89 g boric acid, water to 1 L	Lithium hydroxide, pH 8.3 Electrode buffer diluted 1:9 in 6.20g Tris, 1.60 g citric acid monohydrate, water to 1L	325	FUM, fumarase; ALK, alkaline phosphatase; IP1 and IP2, two indophenol oxidases

Table 2
Staining Solution for Enzymes Used in MLEE Analysis of *N. meningitidis*

Enzyme	EC no.	Agar overlay[a]	Staining solution
Aconitase (ACO)	4.2.1.3	Yes	15 mL Tris-HCl,[b] 10 mL $MgCl_2$,[c] 25 mg cis-aconitic acid, 10 U isocitrate dehydrogenase, 1 mL NADP,[d] 0.5 mL PMS,[e] 1 mL MTT[f]
Adenylate kinase (ADK)	2.7.4.3	Yes	25 mL Tris- HCl,[b] 100 mg glucose, 25 mg ADP, 1 mg hexokinase, 1 mL $MgCl_2$,[c] 15 U glucose 6-phosphate dehydrogenase, 1 mL NADP,[d] 0.5 mL PMS,[e] 0.5 mL MTT[f]
Alcohol dehydrogenase (ADH)	1.1.1.1	No	3 mL 96% ethanol, 2 mL isopropanol, 2 mL NAD,[g] 0.5 mL PMS,[e] 1 mL MTT[f]
Alkaline phosphatase (ALP)	3.1.3.1	No	50 mL 0.05 *M* Tris-HCl, pH 8.5, 1 g NaCl, 2 mL $MgCl_2$,[c] 2 mL 0.25 *M* $MnCl_2$, 50 mg β-naphthyl acid phosphate, 100 mg polyvinylpyrrolidone, 50 mg fast blue BB salt
Fumarase (FUM)	4.2.1.2	No	50 mL Tris-HCl,[a] 50 mg fumaric acid, 50 U malic dehydrogenase, 2 mL NAD,[g] 0.5 mL PMS,[e] 1 mL MTT[f]
Glutamate dehydrogenase (NAD-dependent) (GD1)	1.4.1.2	No	50 mL Tris-HCl,[b] 2.1 g glutamic acid, 2 mL NAD,[g] 0.5 mL PMS,[e] 1 mL MTT[f]
Glutamate dehydrogenase (NADP-dependent) (GD2)	1.4.1.4	No	50 mL Tris-HCl,[b] 2.1 g glutamic acid, 1 mL NADP,[d] 0.5 mL PMS,[e] 1 mL MTT[f]
Glucose 6-phosphate dehydrogenase (G6P)	1.1.1.49	No	50 mL Tris-HCl,[b] 100 mg glucose 6-phosphate, 1 mL $MgCl_2$,[c] 1 mL NADP,[d] 0.5 mL PMS,[e] 1 mL MTT[f]
Indophenol oxidase (IPO)	1.15.1.1	No	40 mL Tris-HCl,[b] 1 mL $MgCl_2$,[c] 0.5 mL PMS,[e] 1 mL MTT[f]; expose to light

Isocitrate dehydrogenase (IDH)	1.1.1.42	No	50 mL Tris-HCl,b 2 mL 0.1 *M* isocitric acid, 2 mL $MgCl_2$,c 1 mL NADP,[d] 0.5 mL PMS,[e] 1 mL MTT[f]
Malic enzyme (ME)	1.1.1.40	No	40 mL Tris-HCl,[a] 6 mL 2 *M* malic acid, 2 mL $MgCl_2$,[b] 1 mLNADP,[c] 0.5 mL PMS,[d] 1 mL MTT[e]
Peptidases (PEP)	3.4.–.–	Yes	25 mL Tris-HCl,[b] 2 mL 0.25 *M* $MnCl_2$,[h] 10 mg peroxidase, 10 mg o-dianisidine di-HCl, 10 mg venom from Crotalus atrox, 20 mg phenyl-alanyl-leucine

[a]Boil 0.5 g agar in 25 mL of Tris-HCl[b] in a microwave oven until dissolved and cool to 60°C before mixing with the other ingredients.
[b]0.2 *M* Tris-HCl, pH 8.0: 24.2 g Tris in 1 L water; adjust pH with concentrated HCl.
[c]0.1 *M* $MgCl_2$: 2.03 g $MgCl_2 . 6H_2O$ in 100 mL water.
[d]NADP solution: 1% (w/v) in water. Keep the solution refrigerated.
[e]PMS (phenazine methosulfate) solution: 1% (w/v) in water. Keep the solution refrigerated and in the dark.
[f]MTT (dimethylthiazol tetrazolium) solution: 0.8% (w/v) in water. Keep the solution refrigerated and in the dark.
[g]NAD solution: 1% (w/v) in water. Keep the solution refrigerated.
[h]0.25 *M* $MnCl_2$: 4.90 g $MnCl_2 . 4H_2O$ in 100 mL water.

3. Methods

3.1. Lysate Preparation

1. An overnight 100 mL pure culture of each isolate is transferred to a 300-mL centrifuge bottle within the safety cabinet (*see* **Note 2**).
2. The cells are harvested by centrifugation (10 min at 15,000*g*).
3. After discarding the supernatant, the cells are suspended in 1 mL of lysis buffer, transferred to a 10-mL centrifuge tube, vortexed a few seconds, and frozen at –20°C overnight (*see* **Note 3**).
4. After thawing, the cellular debris are pelleted by centrifugation at 20,000*g* for 20 min at 4°C. The bacterial suspension must be kept cool at all time under the lysis process, and thereafter.
5. The supernatant is filtrated through a 0.45-μm membrane, before storage of the lysate in a glass tube at –70°C until electrophoresis.

3.2. Gel Preparation

1. In a 1-L Erlenmeyer flask, mix thoroughly 48 g starch in 420 mL of gel buffer. Three different buffer systems are used depending on the enzymes to be stained (*see* **Table 2**).
2. The mixture is heated over a Bunsen burner with continuous and vigorous hand swirling until the suspension starts to boil and develop large air bubbles (*see* **Notes 4** and **5**).
3. The gel is degassed for 1 min and immediately poured into a gel mold. If air bubbles are visible in the gel after pouring, they should be quickly removed by aspiration with a Pasteur pipet.
4. After solidification, either at room temperature for 2 h or at room temperature for 30 min followed by 30 min at 4°C, the gel is wrapped in a plastic film to prevent desiccation. Care should be taken that no air bubbles are trapped between the surface of the gel and the plastic film. Normally, gels are stored overnight at room temperature before electrophoresis. For optimal results, a gel must be used within 24 h of its preparation.

3.3. Electrophoresis

1. The protein extracts are thawed and immediately put on ice.
2. The gel is unwrapped and cut through with a scalpel, at 5 cm from the shorter end of the gel mould.
3. Using forceps, a piece of Whatman filter paper is dipped in the cell lysate, blotted on a filter paper to eliminate the excess of liquid, then inserted into the slit in the gel, leaving a 1-cm space from the left end of the gel. Repeat the procedure with the next lysate, leaving a 2–3-mm space between the papers. Up to 20 samples can be loaded on an 18-cm wide gel. Pieces of filter paper, dipped in amaranth dye, are placed in the spaces remaining at each end of the slit to mark the migration of the buffer front.

4. The two pieces of the gel are carefully pressed together, to eliminate the air between the filter papers and avoid protein denaturation.
5. The slit of the gel with the filter papers is covered with the plastic film, which is then folded back at 2.5 cm from the end of the gel.
6. The electrophoresis tanks are filled with about 250 mL of electrode buffer (*see* **Table 1**).
7. Place the gel mold on top of the electrode trays.
8. Contact between gel and buffer is provided by the sponge wicks: one is aligned with the row of samples over the plastic film, the other one is placed 10 cm apart directly on the gel. The plastic film is folded back to cover both sponge wicks.
9. A glass plate is centered on top of the gel.
10. During electrophoresis, the gel is cooled by ice in the metal tray supported by the glass plate (*see* **Note 6**).
11. Connect the electrodes, with the cathode nearest the samples as the proteins will migrate towards the anode in these buffer systems. A constant voltage is maintained during electrophoresis (*see* **Table 1**).
12. The duration of electrophoresis varies from 4–6 h depending on the buffer system. Standardization of the migration between gels is assured by measuring the migration of the amaranth dye (10 cm).

3.4. Slicing and Staining of the Gel

1. After electrophoresis, the ice pan, the glass plate, the plastic film, and the sponge wicks are removed from the gel.
2. With a scalpel, a slit is cut at 2–3 mm on each side of the length of the gel and at the level of the migration of the amaranth dye. All but the central part of the gel (10 × 17 cm piece) is discarded. Cut a corner of the central piece of gel to mark its orientation.
3. Carefully remove the filter papers that were used to load the protein extracts and place the gel piece, bottom down, on the slicing plate.
4. Press the wire through the gel, supported on the 1 mm edge of the slicing plate.
5. Turn the whole gel bottom up and carefully lift the 1-mm-thick slice into a staining box, labeled with the gel number and the name of the enzyme to be stained.
6. Turn the remainder of the gel bottom down and cut additional slices in a same way (up to 4 slices can be cut from a gel).
7. Staining methods for the 14 enzyme loci used in meningococci are given in **Table 2** (*see* **Note 7**). The dry ingredients can be weighted in advance, but the solutions must be added immediately before staining (*see* **Note 8**). All the components must be mixed thoroughly before adding the agar solution, cooled down to 60°C, as indicated (*see* **Table 2**).
8. Pour the solution onto the gel.
9. The gels are incubated at 37°C in the dark, until appearance of the enzyme reaction (colored bands), except for indophenol oxidase that is stained on the light box, at room temperature. Enzyme activity for this enzyme shows as white bands

on a dark background. Depending on the enzyme, the staining reaction may take from a few minutes to several hours (*see* **Note 9**).

10. After staining, the solution is poured off and the gel slice rinsed in water, if no agar overlay was used. The gels are fixed except for those stained for indophenol oxidase, which should be kept in water.

3.5. Interpretation of the Gels

1. The bands of enzyme activity should be narrow and clearly visible to assure good resolution. Relative mobilities of each enzyme from the different isolates must be compared visually against one another on the same gel. Distinctive electromorphs are numbered in order of decreasing anodal mobility, i.e., the electromorph that has migrated the farthest is assigned no. 1.
2. On gels stained for the glutamate dehydrogenases (*see* **Note 10**) and sometimes on gels stained for other dehydrogenases, an additional band of activity that has migrated further away from the origin appears. This unknown dehydrogenase is polymorphic and has been included as one of the enzymes routinely scored for epidemiological analysis of the meningococcus.
3. One or a few strains may occasionally lack activity for an enzyme. Although the stained enzymes are encoded by housekeeping genes, they are not always needed for survival, especially when the strain has been passed in the laboratory for a long time. Null alleles are recorded as such. It is essential, however, to assess that they do not result from a poor preparation or storage of the protein lysate (*see* **Note 11**).
4. Electromorphs are identified by side-by-side comparison on the same gel slice. In practice, this means that the protein extract from an isolate will be electrophoresed and stained for the same enzyme many times before its electromorph can be unambiguously identified. When analyzing a new set of meningococcal strains, it is recommended to include on the gel the extracts from at least two reference strains, presenting distinct electromorphs at most enzymes assayed (for example an ET-5 and an ET-37 strain; *see* **Table 3**). The first electrophoresis permits a rough evaluation of the electromorphs of the unknown strains in comparison with the two standards. Accurate electromorph assignment for each individual enzyme will be obtained by rerunning the strains side by side with different reference electromorphs, until identity is ascertained.

3.6. Analysis of the Data

For each isolate, an electromorph is assigned to each of the 14 enzyme loci. This combination of electromorphs represents the allelic profile (ET) of the meningococcus. The allele profiles of the epidemic clones presented earlier are given in **Table 3**. The strains can then be grouped according to their ET.

Further analyses of the data are performed using computers. Programs for analysis of MLEE data for bacterial strains have been developed by Dr. T. S. Whittam ***(10)***. A statistical package including five programs—ETDIV,

Table 3
Allele Profiles of the Dominant Epidemic Clones of *N. meningitidis* Described.[a]

Clonal group	Serogroup	Main serotypes	Electromorph at indicated enzyme locus													
			ME	G6P	PEP	IDH	ACO	GD1	GD2	ADH	FUM	ALK	IP1	IP2	ADK	UDH
Subgroup I	A	4,21:P1.10	1	3	2	3	4	1	3	3	1	8	2	5	2	3
Subgroup III	A	4,21:P1.20,9	1	4	5	6	4	1	3	2	1	8	2	3	2	2
ET-5 complex	B, (C)	15:P1.7,16; 15:P1.7b,3; 4:P1.19,15	1	1	7	8	4	2	3	2	1	1	2	3	2	3
ET-37 complex	C, B, (W135,Y)	2a:P1.5,2; 2a:P1.5,y	4	3	4	5	2	1	4	1	1	8	2	3	2	3
Cluster A4	B and C	2b:P1.2; 2b:P1.3	3	3	4	9	2	1	3	2	1	8	2	3	2	3
Lineage III	B	4:P1.4	5	3	5	12	4	1	3	2	1	3	2	3	2	3

[a]Enzyme abbreviations are as indicated in **Table 2**.

ETCLUS, ETMEGA, ETLINK, and ETBOOT—is now available through the internet at Dr. Whittam's laboratory home page: (http://www.bio.psu.edu/People/Faculty/Whittam/Lab/programs).

ETDIV provides a list of the distinct allelic profiles, indicates the number of isolates of each ET, and lists the name of isolates belonging to each ET that is represented by more than one strain. For each enzyme locus, the alleles identified are indicated together with their frequency, and from the allele frequencies the genetic diversity is calculated as $h = (1 - \sum xi^2)\ [n/(n-1)]$, where xi is the frequency of the ith allele and n is the number of ETs ***(48)***. Mean diversity per locus (H) is the arithmetic average of h values over the loci studied.

The strains to be analyzed can be grouped before analysis into defined populations, according to specific parameters, such as their geographical origin, clinical source, serogroup, serotype, and so on. ETDIV will analyze the allele frequencies and genetic diversity concomitantly for isolates in each population and for the whole sample. A table will be generated indicating the ET diversity within the populations and in the whole sample, together with the coefficient of genetic differentiation (Gst) for each locus and in average over loci ***(49)***.

ETDIV also generates a file named ETLIST.DAT that is used as the input of the ETCLUS program. ETCLUS provides a dendrogram of genetic relationships between ETs based on the average-linkage algorithm (UPGMA), as described by Sneath and Sokal ***(50)***. Distances are measured as the proportion of loci at which mismatches occur between pairs of ETs. The program generates the distances between the ETs and their nearest relative and provides a simple drawing of the dendrogram.

The other programmes are for more advanced population genetics analyses.

4. Notes

1. The electrophoresis equipment presented here is easy to produce and is a cheap alternative to commercial horizontal electrophoresis apparatus.
2. Cells can be grown on 3–4 agar plates instead of the 100-mL broth culture. In that case, the cells scraped from plates are directly suspended in the lysis buffer.
3. The cells can be kept in the lysis buffer at –20°C for a few days, if necessary.
4. Starch from Connaught Laboratories shows little batch-to-batch variation and produces gel slices of regular good quality. Altering of the boiling time may be necessary when changing starch batch.
5. Cautions should be taken when boiling the gels. Even Erlenmeyer flasks that tolerate heat and vacuum can break during gel preparation. Heat-insulating gloves and protective eyeglasses must be worn.
6. During electrophoresis, the ice needs to be changed after 2–3 h. Make sure that the ice tray is well-centered on the top of the gel.

7. Some authors have used other enzymes for clonal analyses of *N. meningitidis*. Staining methods for these additional enzymes may be found in **refs. *10*** and ***51***. The principles of the staining reactions are described in **ref. *51***.
8. Many of the chemicals used for staining the enzymes represent a health hazard and must be handled with great care, following the manufacturer's instructions. Wearing gloves and a mask when handling the stain is recommended.
9. The two glutamate dehydrogenases can be stained on the same slice of gel. First, incubate with the staining solution for the NAD-dependent glutamate dehydrogenase (GD1). When the enzyme activity is visible for all strains, add 1 mL of NADP into the staining box and incubate again a for a few minutes.
10. Caution should be taken when staining for glucose 6-phosphate dehydrogenase (G6P) and isocitrate dehydrogenase (IDH) as the staining reaction may develop in just a few minutes.
11. Although the lysates can be thawed and frozen several times, the stability of the enzymes differed. Aconitase is rather unstable and should be one of the first ones to be studied.

References

1. Maiden, M. C., Bygraves, J. A., Feil, E., Morelli, G., Russell, J. E., Urwin, R., et al. (1998) Multilocus sequence typing: a portable approach to the identification of clones within populations of pathogenic microorganisms. *Proc. Natl. Acad. Sci. USA* **95,** 3140–3145.
2. Caugant, D. A., Frøholm, L. O., Bøvre, K., Holten, E., Frasch, C. E., Mocca, L. F., et al. (1986) Intercontinental spread of a genetically distinctive complex of clones of *Neisseria meningitidis* causing epidemic disease. *Proc. Natl. Acad. Sci. USA* **83,** 4927–4931.
3. Olyhoek, T., Crowe, B. A., and Achtman, M. (1987) Clonal population structure of *Neisseria meningitidis* serogroup A isolated from epidemics and pandemics between 1915 and 1983. *Rev. Infect. Dis.* **9,** 665–692.
4. Moore, P. S., Reeves, M. W., Schwartz, B., Gellin, B. G., and Broome, C. V. (1989) Intercontinental spread of an epidemic group A *Neisseria meningitidis* strain. *Lancet* **ii,** 260–263.
5. Achtman, M. (1990) Molecular epidemiology of epidemic bacterial meningitis. *Rev. Med. Microbiol.* **1,** 29–38.
6. Achtman, M. (1995) Global epidemiology of meningococcal disease, in *Meningococcal Disease* (Cartwright, K.A.V., ed.), John Wiley and Sons, Chichester, UK, pp. 159–175.
7. Caugant, D. A. (1998) Population genetics and molecular epidemiology of *Neisseria meningitidis*. *APMIS* **106,** 505–525.
8. Wenger, J. D. and Perkins, B. A. (1998) Patterns in the emergence of epidemic meningococcal disease, in *Emerging Infections* (Scheel, W. M., Armstrong, D., and Hughes, J. M., eds.), American Society for Microbiology Press, Washington, DC, pp. 125–136.

9. Boerlin, P. (1997) Applications of multilocus enzyme electrophoresis in medical microbiology. *J. Microbiol. Methods* **28,** 221–231.
10. Selander, R. K., Caugant, D. A., Ochman, H., Musser, J. M., Gilmour, M. N., and Whittam, T. S. (1986) Methods of multilocus enzyme electrophoresis for bacterial population genetics and systematics. *Appl. Environ. Microbiol.* **51,** 873–884.
11. Raymond, N. J., Reeves, M., Ajello, G., Baughman, W., Gheesling, L. L., Carlone, G. M., et al. (1997) Molecular epidemiology of sporadic (endemic) serogroup C meningococcal disease. *J. Infect. Dis.* **176,** 1277–1284.
12. Wedege, E., Kolberg, J., Delvig, A., Høiby, E. A., Holten, E., Rosenqvist, E., and Caugant, D. A. (1995) Emergence of a new virulent clone within the ET-5 complex of serogroup B meningococci in Norway. *Clin. Diagn. Lab. Immunol.* **2,** 314–321.
13. Imrey, P. B., Jackson, L. A., Ludwinski, P. H., England III, A. C., Fella, G. A., Fox, B. C., et al. (1996) Outbreak of serogroup C meningococcal disease associated with campus bar patronage. *Am. J. Epidemiol.* **143,** 624–630.
14. Jelfs, J., Jalaludin, B., Munro, R., Patel, M., Kerr, M., Daley, D., et al. (1998) A cluster of meningococcal disease in western Sydney, Australia initially associated with a nightclub. *Epidemiol. Infect.* **120,** 263–270.
15. Caugant, D. A., Kristiansen, B.-E., Frøholm, L. O., Bøvre, K., and Selander, R. K. (1988) Clonal diversity of *Neisseria meningitidis* strains isolated from a population of aymptomatic carriers. *Infect. Immun.* **56,** 2060–2068.
16. Caugant, D. A., Bol, P., Høiby, E. A., Zanen, H. C., and Frøholm, L. O. (1990) Clones of serogroup B *Neisseria meningitidis* causing systemic disease in the Netherlands, 1958–1986. *J. Infect. Dis.* **162,** 867–874.
17. Caugant, D. A., Zollinger, W. D., Mocca, L. F., Frasch, C. E., Whittam, T. S., Frøholm, L. O., and Selander, R. K. (1987) Genetic relationships and clonal population structure of serotype 2 strains of *Neisseria meningitidis*. *Infect.Immun.* **55,** 1503–1513.
18. Caugant, D. A., Mocca, L. F., Frasch, C. E., Frøholm, L. O., Zollinger, W. D., and Selander, R. K. (1987) Genetic structure of *Neisseria meningitidis* populations in relation to serogroup, serotype, and outer membrane protein pattern. *J. Bacteriol.* **169,** 2781–2792.
19. Maynard Smith, J., Smith, N. H., O'Rourke, M., and Spratt, B. G. (1993). How clonal are bacteria? *Proc. Natl. Acad. Sci. USA* **90,** 4384–4388.
20. Maiden, M. C. J., Malorny, B., and Achtman, M. (1996) A global gene pool in the neisseriae. *Mol. Microbiol.* **21,** 1297–1298.
21. Wang, J.-F., Caugant, D. A., Li, X., Hu, X., Poolman, J. T., Crowe, B. A., and Achtman, M. (1992). Clonal and antigenic analysis of serogroup A *Neisseria meningitidis* with particular reference to epidemiological features of epidemic meningitis in China. *Infect. Immun.* **60,** 5267–5282.
22. McGee, L., Koornhoof, H. J., and Caugant, D. A. (1998) Epidemic spread of subgroup III of *Neisseria meningitidis* serogroup A to South Africa in 1996. *J. Infect. Dis.* **27,** 1214–1220.

23. Guibourdenche, M., Høiby, E. A., Riou, J.-Y., Varaine, F., Joguet, C., and Caugant, D. A. (1996) Epidemics of serogroup A *Neisseria meningitidis* of subgroup III in Africa, 1989–94. *Epidemiol. Infect.* **116,** 115–120.
24. Tikhomirov, E., Santamaria, M., and Esteves, K. (1997) Meningococcal disease: public health burden and control. *Rapp. Trimest. Statist. Sanit. Mond.* **50,** 170–177.
25. Caugant, D. A., unpublished data.
26. Nicolas, P., Raphenon, G., Guibourdenche, M., Decousset, L., Stor, R., and Gaye, A. B. (2000) The 1998 Senegal epidemic of meningitis was due to clonal expansion of A:4:P1.9, clone III-1, sequence type 5 *Neisseria meningitidis* strains. *J. Clin. Microbiol.* **38,** 198–200.
27. Sow, A. I., Caugant, D. A., Cisse, M. F., Høiby, E. A., and Samb, A. (2000) Molecular characteristics and susceptibility to antibiotics of serogroup A *Neisseria meningitidis* strains isolated in Senegal in 1999. *Scand. J. Infect. Dis.* **32,** 185–187.
28. Reeves, M. W., Perkins, B. A., Diermayer, M., and Wenger, J. D. (1995) Epidemic-associated *Neisseria meningitidis* detected by multilocus enzyme electrophoresis. *Emerg. Infect. Dis.* **1,** 53–54.
29. Diermayer, M., Hedberg, K., Hoesly, F., Fischer, M., Perkins, B., Reeves, M., and Fleming D. (1999) Epidemic serogroup B meningococcal disease in Oregon: the evolving epidemiology of the ET-5 strain. *JAMA* **281,** 1493–1497.
30. Tali-Maamar, H. and Caugant, D. A., unpublished data.
31. Achtman, M. (1997) Microevolution and epidemic spread of serogroup A *Neisseria meningitidis*: a review. *Gene* **192,** 135–140.
32. Wang, J.-F., Caugant, D. A., Morelli, G., Koumaré, B., and Achtman, M. (1993) Antigenic and epidemiological properties of the ET-37 complex of *Neisseria meningitidis*. *J. Infect. Dis.* **167,** 1320–1329.
33. Ashton, F. E., Ryan, J. A., Borczyk, A., Caugant, D. A., Mancino, L., and Huang, D. (1991) Emergence of a virulent clone of *Neisseria meningitidis* serotype 2a that is associated with meningococcal group C disease in Canada. *J. Clin. Microbiol.* **29,** 2489–2493.
34. Kertesz, D. A., Coulthart, M. B., Ryan, J. A., Johnson, W. M., and Ashton, F. E. (1998) Serogroup B electrophoretic type 15 *Neisseria meningitidis* in Canada. *J. Infect. Dis.* **177,** 1754–1757.
35. Jackson, L. A., Schuchat, A., Reeves, M. W., and Wenger, J. D. (1995) Serogroup C meningococcal outbreaks in the United States. *JAMA* **273,** 390–394.
36. Block, C., Keller, N., and Caugant, D. A. (1998) The epidemiology of meningococcal disease in Israel. The activity of familiar and less familiar clone-complexes, in *Eleventh International Pathogenic Neisseria Conference* (Nassif, X., Quentin-Millet, M.-J., and Taha, M.-K., eds.), Editions EDK, Paris, p. 256.
37. Kriz, P., Giorgini, D., Musilek, M., Larribe, M., and Taha, M. K. (1999) Microevolution through DNA exchange among strains of *Neisseria meningitidis* isolated during an outbreak in the Czech Republic. *Res. Microbiol.* **150,** 273–280.

38. Kaczmarski, E. B. (1997) Meningococcal disease in England and Wales: 1995. *Commun. Dis. Rep. Rev.* **7,** R55–R59.
39. Ehrhard, I., Hauri, A. M., Caugant, D. A., Kriz, P., Frank, U., Ammer, J., et al. (1999) Outbreak of serogroup C meningococcal disease in Bavaria during carnaval period 1998. 5th meeting of the European Monitoring Group on Meningococci, Crete, Greece, p. 24.
40. Whalen, C. M., Hockin, J. C., Ryan, A., and Ashton, F. (1995) The changing epidemiology of invasive meningococcal disease in Canada, 1985 through 1992. Emergence of a virulent clone of *Neisseria meningitidis*. *JAMA* **273,** 390–394.
41. Strathdee, C. A. and Johnson, W. M. (1995) Identification of epidemiological markers for *Neisseria meningitidis* using difference analysis. *Gene* **166,** 105–110.
42. Jelfs, J., Munroe, R., Ashton, F., Rawlinson, W., and Caugant, D. A. (1998) Global study of variation in a new variant of the ET-37 complex of *Neisseria meningitidis*, in *Eleventh International Pathogenic Neisseria Conference* (Nassif, X., Quentin-Millet, M.-J., and Taha, M.-K., eds.), Editions EDK, Paris, p. 5.
43. Sacchi, C. T., Zanella, R. C., Caugant, D. A., Frasch, C. E., Hidalgo, N. T., Milagres, L. G., et al. (1992) Emergence of a new clone of serogroup C *Neisseria meningitidis* in Sao Paulo, Brazil. *J. Clin. Microbiol.* **30,** 1282–1286.
44. Scholten, R. J. P. M., Poolman, J. T., Valkenburg, H. A., Bijlmer, H. A., Dankert, J., and Caugant, D. A. (1994). Phenotypic and genotypic changes in a new clone complex of *Neisseria meningitidis* causing disease in the Netherlands, 1958–1990. *J. Infect. Dis.* **169,** 673–676.
45. Looveren, M., Vandamme, P., Hauchecorne, M., Wijdooghe, M., Carion, F., Caugant, D. A., and Goossens, H. (1998) Molecular epidemiology of recent Belgian isolates of *Neisseria meningitidis* serogroup B. *J. Clin. Microbiol.* **36,** 2828–2834.
46. Martin, D. R., Walker, S. J., Baker, M. G., and Lennon, D. R. (1998). New Zealand epidemic of meningococcal disease identified by a strain with phenotype B:4:P1.4. *J. Infect. Dis.* **177,** 497–500.
47. Martin, D. R., Walker, S. J., Glennie, A. C., Baker, M. G., Eyles, R. F., Lennon, D. R., and Roberts, A. P. (1998). Continuation of meningococcal disease epidemic in New Zealand, in *Eleventh International Pathogenic Neisseria Conference* (Nassif, X., Quentin-Millet, M.-J., and Taha, M.-K., eds.), Editions EDK, Paris, p. 8.
48. Nei, M. (1978) Estimation of average heterozygosity and genetic distance from a small sample of individuals. *Genetics* **89,** 583–590.
49. Nei, M. (1977) F-statistics and analysis of gene diversity in subdivided populations. *Ann. Hum. Genet.* **41,** 225–233.
50. Sneath, P. H. A. and Sokal, R. R. (1978) *Numerical taxonomy*. W. H. Freeman and Company, San Francisco.
51. Harris, H. and Hopkinson, D. A. (1976). *Handbook of Enzyme Electrophoresis in Human Genetics*. North-Holland Publishing Company, Amsterdam.

19

Epidemiology, Surveillance, and Population Biology

Carriage Studies

Keith Cartwright

1. Introduction

Seven years after meningococci were first grown from patients with meningitis *(1)*, Kiefer reported the isolation of the organisms from the nasopharynx of cases of meningococcal disease, and from their contacts *(2)*. The importance of nasopharyngeal acquisition and carriage as a key step in the development of invasive meningococcal infection was rapidly appreciated, as was the far greater frequency of the carrier state when compared with the relatively small numbers of individuals developing invasive disease. Attempts to interpret the significance of variations in the bacteria themselves as a factor influencing the outcome of the interaction between humans and meningococcus had to await the development of the first typing systems based on serological reagents *(3)*. It became clear rapidly that meningococcal strains isolated from the blood or cerebrospinal fluid (CSF) of patients with invasive disease were more likely to be typable than strains from the nasopharynx of individuals who were asymptomatic carriers.

These early forays into meningococcal typing, carried out by British army doctors during World War I, were driven by the substantial outbreaks of meningococcal disease that affected new recruits. The first, classical epidemiological studies of meningococcal acquisition and carriage were undertaken by Capt. J. A. Glover of the Royal Army Medical Corps, working at the Guards Depot, Caterham, in South London, over the period 1915–1919. Glover showed that rates of meningococcal carriage rose in recruits during periods of severe

From: *Methods in Molecular Medicine, vol. 67: Meningococcal Disease: Methods and Protocols*
Edited by: A. J. Pollard and M. C. J. Maiden © Humana Press Inc., Totowa, NJ

overcrowding, and that cases of disease started to occur when threshold carriage rates of 20% were breached. In the first demonstration of the application of the results of carriage studies to disease control, Glover showed that by maintaining meningococcal carriage rates below the "danger level" of 20% (mainly by means of reducing overcrowding), cases of meningococcal disease could be prevented ***(4)***. Though later workers cast doubt on the validity of an association between carriage rates and risk of disease ***(5,6)***, Glover's findings, and his successful intervention, are a landmark in the epidemiology of meningococcal infection.

Other milestones in the elucidation of the dynamics of meningococcal carriage and disease include:

- Careful longitudinal studies of meningococcal carriage ***(7)***, identifying short- and long-term carriers and the phenomenon of "intermittent" carriage;
- In 1950, the reconciliation of the two principal typing systems that had developed in France and England, with agreement to base the nomenclature of serogrouping on the designations A, B, C, and so on ***(8)***;
- The isolation, identification, and characterization of *Neisseria lactamica* ***(9,10)***, a human nasopharyngeal commensal very closely related to the meningococcus, permitting the differentiation of the two species;
- The application of selective media (first Thayer-Martin ***[11]***, and then New York City medium ***[12]***), to the isolation of meningococci from nasopharyngeal cultures, simplifying laboratory isolation dramatically;
- The use of multi-locus enzyme electrophoresis (MLEE) in meningococcal typing ***(13)***, permitting the unequivocal identification of clones, and marking the beginning of the end for phenotypic characterization of meningococci for epidemiological purposes;
- Demonstration of the dependence of the meningococcus on acquisition of iron from human transferrin ***(14)***, providing an explanation for the selective colonization of humans by the meningococcus; and
- The development of automated DNA sequencing, facilitating the application of multi-locus sequence typing to meningococci ***(15)*** and the potential to understand the genetic basis for phenotypic variation among meningococcal strains.

1.1. Interpreting the Literature

The voluminous literature on meningococci and meningococcal disease that has accumulated over the last hundred years is liberally adorned with accounts of studies of meningococcal nasopharyngeal carriage. Most older carriage studies are now of limited value. In all studies carried out before the 1960s, meningococci were not distinguished from *Neisseria lactamica*, yet in infants and toddlers *N. lactamica* is found far more frequently than *N. meningitidis*. The importance of methodological differences in carriage studies has long been appreciated and was summarized concisely by Broome in her 1986 review ***(16)***.

Some of the methodological variables that now need to be taken into account in designing new studies are considered further.

Today, we enjoy a better understanding of the limitations of "snapshot" studies of meningococcal carriage. They provide a cross-section of meningococcal carriage in the targeted study population at a single moment in time, but in any individual carrier it cannot be determined whether colonization occurred a day, a week, a month, or a year before the positive swab was obtained. Similarly, without follow-up swabbing, it cannot be established how long colonization persists after documenting a positive swab. The same limitations apply to individuals found to be free of carriage on a single occasion. In addition to the known insensitivity of a single swab in confirming freedom from carriage of meningococci, a single negative swab cannot exclude the possibility that the subject sampled was colonized only days, or even hours before the swab was taken.

1.2. Carriage vs Acquisition

Meningococcal carriage rates in a population at any moment in time are determined both by the acquisition rate (numbers of new subjects in the population becoming colonized within any specified time period) and by the duration of carriage. Acquisition rates (particularly of virulent meningococci) are believed to be far more important than carriage rates in determining the risk of invasive infection. Most meningococci isolated from the nasopharynx have little or no invasive potential, and on the contrary, probably help to reinforce local and systemic immunity.

Military recruits and first-year undergraduates at universities with halls of residence (communal living and sleeping accommodation) are known to have very high acquisition rates ***(17,18)***. Thus, data on meningococcal acquisition and carriage that are derived from such "special" populations cannot be applied meaningfully to general populations.

1.3. Duration of Carriage

There are few good studies on duration of meningococcal carriage. The question of whether duration of carriage varies between meningococcal strains or between human populations cannot be answered with any degree of confidence. However, there is some suggestion that duration of carriage of serogroup A strains in sub-Saharan Africa (half life of 3 mo ***[19]***) may be shorter than that of serogroup B strains in Europe (half life of 9 mo or more (***20***; Cartwright and Stuart unpublished data).

1.4. Molecular Characterization

The recent widespread availability of automated DNA sequencing, polymerase chain reaction (PCR) testing, and other molecular techniques has driven a rapid expansion in our understanding of the genetic basis for phenotypic variation in carried meningococci. This, allied to a rapidly increasing knowledge of the sophisticated control systems for meningococcal gene expression, has gone a long way towards explaining some of the apparent paradoxes that were thrown up by past studies of carriage and disease that were dependent on classical phenotyping (grouping, typing and subtyping) to explain the epidemiology *(21)*.

2. Why Are Carriage Studies Undertaken? What Do They Tell Us?

2.1. Populations Sampled

Most published studies are point prevalence ("snapshot in time") carriage studies undertaken in response to clusters or outbreaks of disease. A bias towards carriage studies during or after outbreaks (as opposed to studies in normal, healthy populations) is easy to understand. Though swabbing the posterior pharynx via the mouth (or for infants, via the nose) is relatively noninvasive, it is nevertheless an unpleasant procedure. It may be difficult to persuade healthy individuals to participate in such studies unless they can see a perceived health benefit to themselves or to others as a result of their participation. Nowadays, ethical committees may have greater reservations about the balance between intrusion and benefit associated with such studies.

Despite these difficulties, many such studies have been carried out, either in healthy general populations ***(19,22,23)***, or in more selected populations such as infants and young children ***(24)***, schoolchildren ***(20)***, university students ***(18)***, military recruits ***(17,25,26)***, jail inmates ***(27)***, contacts of meningococcal disease cases ***(28–30)***, or in populations experiencing high rates of meningococcal disease ***(31—33)***. In a number of studies, serial swabbing over weeks, months, or years has enabled estimates to be made of acquisition rates, and/or the duration of carriage, with varying degrees of accuracy ***(17,19,20,22, 24,26,34,35)***.

2.2. Risk Factors for Carriage

Attempts have been made (more frequently in recent years) to unravel some of the risk factors for carriage, in addition to the known influences of age and gender ***(17,18,23,27,36–39)***. Other than having close contact with a case of meningococcal disease, or with another known carrier, smoking (both active and passive) is perhaps the best-documented factor affecting carriage rates ***(40)***. Strangely, despite the very strong seasonality of meningococcal disease, both in temperate and tropical countries, most evidence to date from longitudinal carriage studies suggests that there is little seasonal variation in rates of meningococcal carriage.

2.3. Effect of Carriage on Expression of Class 1 Outer-Membrane Protein

In one recent longitudinal study, the effect of carriage on the stability of expression of the class 1 outer-membrane protein (OMP), currently an important vaccine candidate for serogroup B meningococcal disease, was investigated *(41)*.

2.4. Effect of Conjugated Vaccines on Meningococcal Carriage

Administration of conjugated Hib vaccines results in a great reduction in the nasopharyngeal carriage rate of Hib bacteria *(42)*, associated with high levels of serum antibody against the capsular polysaccharide. In the UK, there is now evidence of lower rates of Hib disease in unimmunized older people *(43)*, presumably through a reduction of carriage in children, and the consequent reduction in exposure to carriers.

In the UK, most serogroup C meningococcal disease is caused by strains of the ET-37 complex. Following the recent introduction of conjugated meningococcal serogroup C vaccines into the childhood immunization schedule in the UK in November 1999, large studies of meningococcal carriage are now in progress. The aim is to determine the effect on carriage of meningococci in the vaccinated population, and in particular, the prevalence of carriage of strains expressing the serogroup C polysaccharide, and the prevalence of carriage of ET-37 strains expressing other capsular polysaccharides. Recently it has become clear that capsule switching within meningococcal clones can and does occur *(44)*. This has heightened concern that by increasing selectively the prevalence of immunity to a single meningococcal antigen (the serogroup C capsular polysaccharide) within a large population, there may be an expansion of virulent ET-37 clone strains expressing other capsular polysaccharides *(45)*, with potential compromise of the new immunization program.

2.5. Carriage Studies to Inform Interventions During Outbreaks

Since the early part of the last century, it has been appreciated that most cases of meningococcal disease were sporadic, i.e., they followed transmission of a pathogenic meningococcus from an asymptomatic to a susceptible individual. When sulphonamides (and later, other powerful antibiotics) became available, and the possibility of eliminating meningococci from the nasopharynx of colonized individuals became a reality, the concept of "hunt and kill the meningococcus" offered attractions to public-health medicine specialists. Indeed, a driver for the development of the first meningococcal polysaccharide vaccines in the 1960s was the emergence of sulphonamide-resistant meningococci in US army recruit camps, and the consequent failure of control of clusters of cases by use of sulphonamide chemoprophylaxis. Meningococcal carriage studies in response to outbreaks have also seemed attractive because of the perplexing nature of such outbreaks. It has proven almost irresistible to attempt to explain outbreaks on the basis of particular patterns of meningococcal carriage in the affected community. More recently, with the ever-increasing interest of the media in meningococcal disease clusters and outbreaks, allied to our inability to control outbreaks, particularly of serogroup B disease, carriage studies may be undertaken for reasons that are at least in part political (better to be seen to be doing something rather than nothing. . .).

The reality is that few, if any, community-wide carriage studies that have been undertaken in response to outbreaks over the last 20 years, have shed sufficient light on the dynamics of transmission to support a clear intervention strategy. Most have found a low carriage rate of the disease-producing (or "epidemic") strain. This is true for both serogroup B and C outbreaks. The value of swabbing studies in serogroup A epidemics in the meningitis belt of Africa is equally unclear. Recommended determinants for vaccine interventions have been set out clearly by the World Health Organization (WHO), based on changes in the weekly disease incidence, and not on rates of carriage of serogroup A strains. Recently, the validity of this strategy has been challenged ***(46)***.

2.6. Carriage Studies to Enhance Understanding of Meningococcal Disease Epidemiology

A pessimistic view of the value of carriage studies based solely on their utility in informing cluster or outbreak management, is perhaps an oversimplification and overly retrospective. With the improved genetic typing tools now at our command ***(47)***, carriage studies may now be undertaken to improve our understanding of the epidemiology of meningococcal carriage, and thereby, albeit indirectly, of meningococcal disease as well. It is no exaggeration to say that the capacity to extract useful information from carriage studies and to understand better the dynamics of meningococcal transmission between humans, and its relationship to invasive disease, will be revolutionized by the deployment of molecular methods of meningococcal characterization.

2.7. Sources of Variability in Carriage Studies

There are numerous reasons why the interpretation (and comparison) of data from published meningococcal carriage studies is fraught with difficulty. The most obvious variable is the population studied. Patterns of meningococcal acquisition and carriage in different age groups, in different ethnic groups, and in different countries (e.g., temperate and tropical) cannot be compared meaningfully. As well as these obvious population variables, some technical sources of variability and error are listed below.

2.7.1. Swabbing

1. Route of access to the posterior pharyngeal wall. Olcén et al. have shown that the per-oral route is modestly superior to the per-nasal route ***(48)***.
2. Site of sampling in the throat. The posterior pharyngeal wall behind the uvula should be sampled, but some recommend sampling the tonsils in addition. Touching the posterior pharyngeal wall often induces a gag reflex and may make further attempts to swab difficult. A decisive (though not aggressive) sweep of the posterior pharyngeal wall is recommended.
3. Anogenital carriage. Swabbing the anogenital region for meningococcal carriage is only practical (and probably ethical) in special settings such as clinics for sexually transmitted diseases.
4. Use of pernasal swabs. Infants and young children (and many cases of meningococcal disease) cannot cooperate with per-oral swabbing but may still be sampled via the per-nasal route. The technique is not too intrusive, but two assistants may be required, one to steady the patient's or subject's head, and one to hold the child's hands away from the swab.
5. Variability of efficiency of swabbing. Variability of technique and success between swabbers is inevitable. In large studies, where a number of different swabbers will be employed, a standardized technique should be agreed upon, and training given. For studies where swabbing is planned to take place over several days or over longer periods, a supervisor should check regularly that swabbing is being conducted in line with the agreed technique. Individual swabbers can verify the reproducibility of their own technique if they sample a proportion of individuals twice (with swabs separated by a few minutes) and demonstrate that culture results are similar.

   Two swabs collected from the same individual within a short space of time but by two different swabbers and yielding similar results on culture will help to give confidence in the reproducibility of technique between swabbers. Comparisons of percentages of positive swabs collected by different swabbers will provide further reassurance.

   Failure to isolate a meningococcus on a selective medium does not exclude the possibility that the swab used to inoculate the plate failed to make contact with the posterior pharyngeal wall, a site richly endowed with a variety of upper respiratory commensal bacteria. Confirming that the posterior pharyngeal wall was sampled can be achieved by inoculating a proportion of swabs on to a nonselective medium, e.g., chocolate agar (Oxoid Ltd., Wade Road, Basingstoke, Hants., UK, RG24 8PW, Columbia agar enriched with 5% sterile defibrinated, chocolated horse blood) and checking for the growth of other commensals (after the swabs have been used for meningococcal isolation). Noncapsulated haemophili are suitable "control" organisms for this purpose, or pneumococci if the population consists of young children.
6. Type of swab used: charcoal or plain. Dr. Dennis Jones, past Director of the Public Health Laboratory Service (PHLS) Meningococcal Reference Unit (MRU), used to attest to the superiority of charcoal-impregnated swabs. This

may be important if swabs are to spend many hours in transit, but is probably less important if swabs are plated directly. Plain cotton-tipped swabs (Medical Wire & Equipment Co. [Bath] Ltd., Corsham, Wilts., UK, SN13 9RT) are satisfactory for direct plating.

7. Direct or delayed plating. Direct plating and early incubation at 37°C in 5% CO_2 is optimal. If plating will be delayed a good quality semi-solid transport medium such as Stuart's medium (Oxoid Ltd.) should be used.

2.7.2. Selective Culture Medium

Because of the abundant and diverse normal flora of the human nasopharynx, the use of selective culture media, e.g., modified New York City agar (Oxoid Ltd.) has revolutionized swabbing surveys. There is a price to pay for this increased ease of isolation of meningococci. Meningococci vary somewhat in their sensitivity to antibiotics, e.g., the trimethoprim concentration used in a selective agar is a trade-off between suppression of commensal flora and suppression of meningococci: 3 mg/L is the normal concentration used, but it will inhibit a few meningococci.

2.7.3. Inherent Insensitivity of Swabbing

Numbers of meningococci isolated on swabbing seem to fluctuate enormously from day to day (and perhaps from hour to hour). Colonized individuals may yield positive cultures only intermittently ***(7,35)***, and therefore any figure for the rate of carriage will be at best an underestimate.

2.7.4. Carriage of Multiple Strains: How Many Colonies to Pick?

Simultaneous carriage of multiple meningococcal strains is infrequent but well-documented. The likelihood of detecting simultaneous carriage of more than one strain of meningococcus, or of simultaneous carriage of meningococci and *N. lactamica*, is increased by the number of suspected neisserial colonies picked from the primary plate for further characterization. In most large studies, only a single colony is picked for detailed characterization, unless colonial variants are easily detectable by naked-eye examination of the primary plates. If this question is of particular importance, multiple picks (up to five) may be required.

2.7.5. Strain Characterization Methods: Phenotypes vs Genotypes

Carried meningococci form a diverse, nonclonal, or weakly clonal, population. Lineages of meningococci (such as the ET-37 complex) may contain meningococcal strains that express more than one capsular polysaccharide. For example, the ET-37 complex that is normally associated with expression of the serogroup C capsular polysaccharide, also includes meningococci that express the serogroup B and W-135 capsular polysaccharides, and possibly other capsular polysaccharides as well. In order to understand the relationship between carried strains and disease-producing isolates, it is necessary to go beyond traditional phenotypic methods of characterization.

A further complication is the fact that the majority of meningococci isolated from the nasopharynx do not agglutinate (or only agglutinate weakly) with grouping sera. This is thought to be owing to downregulation of expression of capsular polysaccharide as a response to the carrier state. A greater proportion of carried than invasive strains may also fail to express type and/or subtype antigens (class 2/3 and class 1 OMPs, respectively). At its worst, meningococci may be isolated from the nasopharynx that can only be described phenotypically as "nongroupable, nontypable, nonsubtypable" (NG; nt; nst). This unsatisfactory state of affairs can be remedied by the application of molecular techniques to detect the presence of the respective underlying genes (*siaD*, *porB*, and *porA*), that may be found to be present.

3. Methods: Design and Planning of Carriage Studies

Many issues need to be considered in the design, planning, and execution of meningococcal carriage studies.

3.1. Establishing and Setting Out the Aims of the Study

Of fundamental importance is a clear statement of the purpose of the study and/or of the hypothesis or hypotheses to be tested. Studies can no longer be justified simply on grounds such as "to investigate patterns of meningococcal nasopharyngeal carriage." There should be good reasons to undertake carriage studies. They should yield new information, or if planned as part of the management of an outbreak of disease, they should offer the potential to alter the management of the outbreak.

3.2. Meningococcal Strain Characterization Methods

Classical phenotypic methods of strain characterization have been used in the past. Increasingly, they are likely to be supplanted by molecular methods of strain differentiation. The particular methods chosen ***(47)*** will be shaped by the aims of the study and by the resources available.

MLEE is capable of assigning meningococci unambiguously to specific clones ***(13)***, but is time- and labor-intensive.

Genotyping methods are now so far superior to classical phenotypic characterization and are so well-suited to characterization of meningococci isolated from the nasopharynx, that serious consideration should be given to their use in future carriage studies.

3.3. Incorporation of, or Collaboration with, Other Studies

An early issue to decide is the desirability of "piggy-backing" any other studies on to the original carriage study, e.g., a serological study or a risk-factor questionnaire, or the identification of a cohort of subjects for a subsequent longitudinal study of acquisition and duration of carriage.

3.4. What Population to Study? What Size of Population?

Establishing clearly the hypothesis to be tested will lead naturally to the choice of a suitable population or populations to be sampled. It will also lead to estimates of the size of the population to be studied. For example, longitudinal studies to investigate acquisition rates and duration of carriage are best carried out in small, easily accessible populations with known high acquisition rates. Such groups include military recruits and undergraduates (recruits may have the edge in terms of accessibility!). In contrast, studies of the effect of the introduction of conjugated serogroup C vaccines on carriage require thousands of subjects to give sufficient power to detect significant differences in carriage rates between vaccinated and unvaccinated groups (owing to the very low natural carriage rate of serogroup C meningococci). It is of critical importance to involve a statistician (ideally one with experience in the field) at the earliest stages of planning a carriage study.

If a large study is planned, multiple collaborators may be needed to cope with the logistics of the exercise. Sampling 5,000+ individuals in the village of Stonehouse in 1986 took two weeks of daily swabbing and required the resources of three local Public Health Laboratories and the local Department of Public Health Medicine to cope with the swabbing itself and with initial processing of inoculated plates. It also required extra teams of staff at the MRU to handle the resulting meningococcal cultures. Stuart et al. ***(49)*** have described many of the practical measures to be considered in the design, planning, and execution of such large studies.

3.5. Population Biases: Actual and Potential

Depending on the purpose(s) of the proposed study, consideration will need to be given to the representativeness of the population to be sampled. Examples of populations that may not be generally representative include:

1. High carriage rate to be expected:
   a. Cases of meningococcal infection,
   b. Families and close contacts of cases,
   c. Families and close contacts of carriers,
   d. Young adults,
   e. Smokers or those exposed to passive smoking, and
   f. Military recruits, university students in the first 8 wk of term.

2. High carriage rate of an outbreak strain possible:
   a. Outbreak populations may have high carriage rates of the outbreak strain (but not of all meningococci).
3. Low carriage rate to be expected:
   a. Recipients of conjugated meningococcal vaccines,
   b. Those who have had recent antibiotic treatment.
4. Carriage rate comparisons of dubious validity:
   a. Different countries, e.g., Africa vs Europe and North America,
   b. Different age groups (young adults have the highest carriage rates),
   c. Different gender mixes (males generally carry more often than females),
   d. Different socio-economic classes (owing to differences in exposure to smoking),
   e. (Possibly) studies carried out in different seasons or different years (especially in Africa), and
   f. Studies in "normal" and "outbreak" populations.

3.6. Recruitment of Subjects

Estimates will need to be made of the likely recruitment rate into the proposed study. It is worth bearing in mind that though young adult males have the highest meningococcal acquisition and carriage rates, they are also the age and gender group least accessible to medical interventions, and the group least likely to participate in a voluntary study. It is better to make pessimistic assumptions about recruitment rates and to be pleasantly surprised than to carry out a study that demonstrates a trend towards the tested hypothesis, but lacks the power to confirm the significance of the findings.

Recruitment can be improved by providing good information to the subjects well before the start of the study, by means of good publicity (*see* below).

3.7. Risk and Benefit

Swabbing the nasopharynx is a very low-risk procedure. However, the author has encountered faints, tonic-clonic seizures, and a variety of other complications (fortunately, none as yet fatal). Swabbing may cause psychological, as well as physical distress. Fainting can be infectious, as can uncontrollable crying, particularly in adolescent girls. Swabbing should never be carried out in an open room (e.g., a school hall), with subjects waiting their turn being given powerful aural and visual stimuli. If a school population is to be sampled, swabbing of individuals should always be carried out in a separate room, ideally with swabbed subjects not returning immediately to mix with those yet to be swabbed.

Early on, consideration must be given to the management of:

1. Carriers of outbreak strains: will any or all be offered antibiotics or vaccines?
2. Carriers of nonoutbreak strains: how will they be reassured?

3. Noncarriers: will they be falsely reassured by apparent freedom from meningococcal carriage?
4. The possibility of rare, serious adverse events (e.g., a true convulsion or even a death) occurring during swabbing (whether or not related to swabbing): first aid should be at hand; and
5. A patient and his/her relatives who develops meningococcal disease just after swabbing, and before the swab result is available.

3.8. Ethical Approval

Ethical approval for the study should be obtained at the earliest possible opportunity. As well as approving the overall design of the study, practical aspects will be scrutinized in detail. Once satisfied about the design, power, and overall validity of a study, ethics committees will often focus on the quality and accessibility of patient information, underpinning, as it does, the granting of informed consent. Ethics committees may also be expected to focus on ensuring adequate protection of the very young and of groups with whom communications may require special consideration, e.g., non-English language speakers. Participation in studies should be open to all members of the eligible population.

3.9. Data

Key decisions are made at an early stage in the design of carriage studies regarding the amount and nature of data to be recorded. Points to consider include:

1. Data ownership issues: who will act as custodian and guarantor of the data?
2. The amount of demographic data to be requested and recorded; only that required for the purposes of the study should be collected;
3. Whether individuals will be invited to complete a "registration card" to be handed over at the time of swabbing for later entry on to computer, or whether this information will be obtained by a clerical officer at the time of swabbing;
4. Data entry to computer: will any (or all) data be entered twice to check accuracy of entry?
5. Data security against loss through hardware or software failure, fire or theft; databases should be anonymized (if appropriate), duplicated (at least twice), password-protected, kept locked and in secure physical environments, and with copies kept in different buildings (to guard against hard disk failure, theft, and fire)
6. Data manipulation and analysis: what software is to be used?
7. Duration of storage: are there legal, ethical, or scientific obligations regarding the period for which the dataset must be retained?
8. "Future proofing:" consideration should be given to the value of carriage datasets to others, e.g., modellers.

4. Practical Issues

4.1. Publicity

If a large study is planned, the local news media can be used to ensure that the study has a high profile. Such is the newsworthiness of meningococcal disease, there is little to fear that the media will not respond wholeheartedly to requests for publicity. Information can be disseminated via posters, leaflets, mailshots, through the local press, radio and television, and through press conferences. Having a principal (or a single) spokesperson ensures that a single, clear message is transmitted. In the UK, the national meningitis charities (the Meningitis Trust, Fern House, Bath Road, Stroud, Gloucestershire GL5 3TJ, tel. 01453 768000, email: support@meningitis-trust.org.uk, and the Meningitis Research Foundation, 13 High Street, Thornbury, Bristol BS12 2AE, tel. 01454 281811, email: info@meningitis.org) can also be relied upon for practical help.

Providing plenty of information about the proposed study and its objectives encourages the targeted population to "buy into" the study. It allows questions to be asked (and answered), and it promotes ownership of the study by the study population. Pointing out the high rate of meningococcal infection in teenagers and young adults may help to enlist the participation of these otherwise potentially inaccessible age groups.

Seeking support for the study from local medical practitioners and other health professionals is critical. Doctors, nurses, and health visitors are highly influential opinion-makers, as are local politicians. Politicians are (perhaps rightly) exquisitely sensitive about any hint of exclusion from events that affect their constituents. For large studies, it may be advisable to provide the local police with the proposed sampling plan.

Expectations of all groups must be managed. For example, it is important to give clear messages about the expected outcomes of the study, and the timeframe within which those outcomes can be expected.

4.2. Human Resources: Getting the Team Involved

The target population is not the only group that needs to be involved in the planning process. Those involved in carrying out the swabbing and processing of plates and cultures must also be involved at an early stage in the planning process. In a large study, these will include at least:

1. Reception and secretarial staff:
   a. patient reception and management in clinics,
   b. recording of demographic information,
   c. administration of any planned questionnaire,
   d. data entry on to a computer, and
   e. data validation.

2. Swabbers (nurses, doctors, health visitors).
3. "Platers:" if different from swabbers.
4. First aiders (or other medical support).
5. Drivers.
6. Laboratory and reference laboratory staff.
7. Administrators.
8. Collaborators in other centers.

4.3. Other Resources

Consumables must be costed accurately, based on the anticipated response rates. A good laboratory manager is essential for this exercise. Additional capital items such as incubators and computers may be required. The collaborating reference laboratory will need to prepare its budget, based on the anticipated meningococcal isolation rate and on the proportion of strains that are to be characterized. A small contingency fund is strongly advisable.

4.4. Funding

There are many potential sources of funding for carriage studies. An important point is that money will need to be committed in large amounts prior to the collection of the first swab. This needs to be understood by any funding organization.

4.5. Timing of Clinics

Especially in large studies, swabbing sessions or clinics need to be arranged at locations and at times convenient for the study population. Walk-in clinics may be an attractive option, but an alternative is to invite attendance of specified portions of the target population on specific days and at specific times. This helps to reduce waiting times and makes life easier for swabbing and laboratory staff.

4.6. Pilot Studies

There is much to be said for carrying out a small pilot study in advance of any larger community-based carriage study. A pilot may not always be feasible, but if it can be undertaken, it helps to identify at an early stage many wrinkles and unforeseen difficulties.

4.7. Contingency Planning

In large studies, especially those with multiple collaborators, it is inevitable that some things will go wrong. It may not be possible or reasonable to plan for every eventuality, but the following are worthy of consideration:

1. Intercurrent staff illness;
2. Bad weather—effects on turnout rates and on logistics;

3. Road traffic accidents involving vehicles carrying inoculated plates;
4. Accidental loss of inoculated plates;
5. Late arrival of plates in a laboratory;
6. Failure of incubators, gas supplies, batches of media, etc.;
7. Inability of laboratories to cope with workload (in the middle of the 2-wk Stonehouse survey, an outbreak of legionnaires' disease occurred locally, diverting resources away from the carriage study).

4.8. Audit Trails

Careful records should be kept of all stages of the swabbing and culture process, including the names of the individuals who collected the swabs, those who carried out the plating and those who isolated and characterised the resulting meningococci. This will enable identification of variability between swabbers, as well as any failure in processing particular batches of swabs.

4.9. Learning from Experience

Especially if a large study is planned, there is much to be said for consulting with other people who have done one before!

4.10. Dissemination of Results

A single lead person for the study is required, who will take responsibility for the coordination of the whole project, including bringing it to completion. Research studies are pointless (and unethical) if the results are not made available to others. For large-scale carriage studies, this will normally involve submission of at least the principal findings for peer-reviewed publication, but also timely and accessible dissemination of results to individual participants. Because of the emotive nature of meningococcal disease, it is worth considering having available further counseling for individual participants who need help in understanding the significance of results, especially in personal terms.

5. The Future: DNA Amplification Rather Than Culture?

The availability of molecular methods of detection of meningococcal DNA in clinical specimens by PCR amplification raises the question of whether such methods could or should be applied to studies of nasopharyngeal carriage. Possible advantages include improved sensitivity: it is very likely that PCR amplification of meningococcal DNA in nasopharyngeal swabs would result in a much-increased yield of positives. Amplification of relevant genes would permit detailed characterization (multi-locus sequence type, serogroup, type, and subtype). An additional advantage is that the logistics of carriage studies would be made simpler. There would be no need to process swabs in the minutes or hours after collection. Swabs could be stored at low temperature and processed by automated methods at leisure.

To balance these undoubted advantages must be set the current relatively high cost of the PCR test and gene sequencing. Further, nasopharyngeal secretions are frequently inhibitory to PCR DNA amplification. Though this nonspecific inhibition can be overcome by further technical development of the methodology, such development has yet to take place. Before any such molecular methods could be applied to large carriage studies, sensitivity and specificity and positive and negative predictive values would have to be determined and validated carefully, not a small task.

Finally, the interpretation of a positive PCR result in this setting requires some consideration. A positive meningococcal PCR result could be owing to the presence of dead bacteria, with consequent unknown significance.

Despite these caveats, it seems very likely that molecular diagnosis of meningococcal carriage in large-scale carriage studies will be attempted in the coming years.

Acknowledgment

I am grateful to many colleagues who have provided advice over the years addressing practical issues that arise in the design and implementation of swabbing studies, but particular thanks are due to Dr. James Stuart and Dr. Dennis Jones.

References

1. Weichselbaum, A. (1887) Ueber die aetiologie der akuten meningitis cerebrospinalis. *Fortschr. Med.* **5,** 573–583, 620–626.
2. Kiefer, F. (1896) Zur differential diagnose des erregers der epidemischen cerebrospinal meningitis und der gonorrhoe. *Berl. Klin. Woch.* **33,** 628–630.
3. Gordon, M. H. and Murray, E. G. (1915) Identification of the meningococcus. *J. R. Army Med. Corps.* **25,** 411–423.
4. Glover, J. A. (1920) Observations on the meningococcus carrier rate and their application to the prevention of cerebro-spinal fever. Special Report series of the Medical Research Council (London).
5. Laybourn, R. L. (1931) A study of epidemic meningitis in Missouri: epidemiological and administrative considerations. *South. Med. J.* **24,** 678–686.
6. Dudley, S. F. and Brennan, J. R. (1934) High and persistent carrier rates of *Neisseria meningitidis*, unaccompanied by cases of meningitis. *J. Hyg. (Camb.)* **34,** 525–541.
7. Rake, G. (1934) Studies on meningococcus infection. VI. The carrier problem. *J. Exp. Med.* **59,** 553–576.
8. Branham, S. E. (1956) Milestones in the history of the meningococcus. *Can. J. Microbiol.* **2,** 175–188.
9. Mitchell, M. S., Rhoden, D. L., and King, E. O. (1965) Lactose-fermenting organisms resembling *N. meningitidis*. *J. Bacteriol.* **90,** 560.

10. Hollis, D. G., Wiggins, D. L., and Weaver, R. E. (1969) *Neisseria lactamicus* sp. n., a lactose fermenting species resembling *Neisseria meningitidis*. *Appl. Microbiol.* **17,** 71–77.
11. van Peenen, P. F. D., Suiter, L. E., Mandel, A. D., and Mitchell, M. S. (1965) Field evaluation of Thayer-Martin medium for identification of meningococcus carriers. *Am. J. Epidemiol.* **82,** 329–333.
12. Faur, Y. C., Weisburd, M. H., and Wilson, M. E. (1973) A new medium for the isolation of pathogenic *Neisseria* (NYC Medium). II. Effect of amphotericin B and trimethoprim lactate on selectivity. *Health Lab. Sci.* **10,** 55–60.
13. Olyhoek, T., Crowe, B. A., and Achtman, M. (1987) Clonal population structure of *Neisseria meningitidis* serogroup A isolated from epidemics and pandemics between 1915 and 1983. *Rev. Infect. Dis.* **9,** 665–692.
14. Schryvers, A. B. and Gonzalez, G. C. (1990) Receptors for transferrin in pathogenic bacteria are specific for the host's protein. *Can. J. Microbiol.* **36,** 145–147.
15. Maiden, M. C. J., Bygraves, J. A., Feil, E., Morelli, G., Russell, J. E., Urwin, R., et al. (1998) Multilocus sequence typing: a portable approach to the identification of clones within populations of pathogenic organisms. *Proc. Natl. Acad. Sci. USA* **95,** 3140–3145.
16. Broome, C. V. (1986) The carrier state: *Neisseria meningitidis*. *J. Antimicrob. Chemother.* **18(Suppl. A),** 25–34.
17. Riordan, T., Cartwright, K., Andrews, N., Stuart, J., Burris, A., Fox, A., et al. (1998) Acquisition and carriage of meningococci in marine commando recruits. *Epidemiol. Infect.* **121,** 495–505.
18. Neal, K. R., Nguyen-Van-Tam, J., Jeffrey, N., Slack, R. C. B., Madeley, R. J., Ait-Tahar, K., et al. (2000) Changing carriage rate of *Neisseria meningitidis* among university students during the first week of term: cross sectional study. *BMJ* **320,** 846–849.
19. Blakebrough, I. S., Greenwood, B. M., Whittle, H. C., Bradley, A. K., and Gilles, H. M. (1982) The epidemiology of infections due to *Neisseria meningitidis* and *Neisseria lactamica* in a northern Nigerian community. *J. Infect. Dis.* **146,** 626–637.
20. De Wals, P., Gilquin, C., De Maeyer, S., Bouckaert, A., Noel, A., Lechat, M. F., and Lafontaine, A. (1983) Longitudinal study of asymptomatic carriage in two Belgian populations of schoolchildren. *J. Infect.* **6,** 147–156.
21. Vogel, U., Morelli, G., Zurth, K., Claus, H., Kriener, E., Achtman, M., and Frosch, M. (1998) Necessity of molecular techniques to distinguish between *Neisseria meningitidis* strains isolated from patients with meningococcal disease and from their healthy contacts. *J. Clin. Microbiol.* **36,** 2465–2470.
22. Greenfield, S., Sheehe, P. R., and Feldman, H. A. (1971) Meningococcal carriage in a population of "normal" families. *J. Infect. Dis.* **123,** 67–73.
23. Caugant, D. A., Hoiby, E. A., and Magnus, P., et al. (1994) Asymptomatic carriage of *Neisseria meningitidis* in a randomly sampled population. *J. Clin. Microbiol.* **32,** 323–330.

24. Gold, R., Goldschneider, I., Lepow, M. L., Draper, T. F., and Randolph, M. (1978) Carriage of *Neisseria meningitidis* and *Neisseria lactamica* in infants and children. *J. Infect. Dis.* **137,** 112–121.
25. Caugant, D. A., Hoiby, E. A., Rosenqvist, E., Froholm, L. O., and Selander, R. K. (1992) Transmission of *Neisseria meningitidis* among asymptomatic military recruits and antibody analysis. *Epidemiol. Infect.* **109,** 241–253.
26. Andersen, J., Berthelsen, L., Bech Jensen, B., and Lind, I. (1998) Dynamics of the meningococcal carrier state and characteristics of the carrier strains: a longitudinal study within three cohorts of military recruits. *Epidemiol. Infect.* **121,** 85–94.
27. Tappero, J. W., Reporter, R., Wenger, J. D., Ward, B. A., Reeves, M. W., Missbach, T. S., et al. (1996) Meningococcal disease in Los Angeles County, California, and among men in the county jails. *N. Engl. J. Med.* **335,** 833–840.
28. Marks, M. I., Frasch, C. E., and Shapera, R. M. (1979) Meningococcal colonization and infection in children and their household contacts. *Am. J. Epidemiol.* **109,** 563–571.
29. Cartwright, K. A. V., Stuart, J. M., and Robinson, P. M. (1991) Meningococcal carriage in close contacts of cases. *Epidemiol. Infect.* **106,** 133–141.
30. Kristiansen, B.-E., Tveten, Y., and Jenkins, A. (1998) Which contact of patients with meningococcal disease carry the pathogenic strain of *Neisseria meningitidis*? A population-based study. *BMJ* **317,** 621–625.
31. Cartwright, K. A. V., Stuart, J. M., Jones, D. M., and Noah, N. D. (1987) The Stonehouse survey: nasopharyngeal carriage of meningococci and *Neisseria lactamica*. *Epidemiol. Infect.* **99,** 591–601.
32. Olsen, S. F., Djurhuus, B., Rasmussen, K., Joensen, H. D., Larsen, S. O., Zoffman, H., and Lind, I. (1991) Pharyngeal carriage of *Neisseria meningitidis* and *Neisseria lactamica* in households with infants within areas with high and low incidences of meningococcal disease. *Epidemiol. Infect.* **106,** 445–457.
33. Fernandez, S., Arreaza, L., Santiago, I., Malvar, A., Berron, S., Vazquez, J. A., et al. (1999) Carriage of a new epidemic strain of *Neisseria meningitidis* and its relationship with the incidence of meningococcal disease in Galicia, Spain. *Epidemiol. Infect.* **123,** 349–357.
34. Artenstein, M. S., Rust, J. H., Hunter, D. H., Lamson, T. C., and Buescher, E. L. (1967) Acute respiratory disease and meningococcal infection in army recruits. *JAMA* **201,** 1004–1008.
35. Pether, J. V. S., Lightfoot, N. F., Scott, R. J. D., Morgan, J., Steele-Perkins, A. P., and Sheard, S. C. (1988) Carriage of *Neisseria meningitidis*: investigations in a military establishment. *Epidemiol. Infect.* **101,** 21–42.
36. Conley Thomas, J., Bendana, N. S., Waterman, S. H., Rathburn, M., Arakere, G., Frasch, C. E., et al. (1991) Risk factors for carriage of meningococcus in the Los Angeles County men's jail system. *Am. J. Epidemiol.* **133,** 286–295.
37. Imrey, P. B., Jackson, L. A., Ludwinski, P. H., England III, A. C., Fella, G. A., Fox, B. C., et al. (1995) Meningococcal carriage, alcohol consumption, and campus bar patronage in a serogroup C meningococcal disease outbreak. *J. Clin. Microbiol.* **33,** 3133–3137.

38. Tayal, S. C., Rashid, S., Muttu, K. M. S., and Hildreth, A. J. (1997) Meningococcal carriage: prevalence and sex-related risk factors. *J. Infect.* **34,** 101–105.
39. Block, C., Gdalevich, M., Buber, R., Ashkenazi, I., Ashkenazi, S., and Keller, N. (1999) Factors associated with pharyngeal carriage of *Neisseria meningitidis* among Israel Defense Force personnel at the end of their compulsory service. *Epidemiol. Infect.* **122,** 51–57.
40. Stuart, J. M., Cartwright, K. A. V., Robinson, P. M., and Noah, N. D. (1989) Effect of smoking on meningococcal carriage. *Lancet* **ii,** 723–725.
41. Jones, G. R., Christodoulides, M., Brooks, J. L., Miller, A. R. O., Cartwright, K. A. V., and Heckels, J. E. (1998) Dynamics of carriage of *Neisseria meningitidis* in a group of military recruits: subtype stability and specificity of the immune response following colonization. *J. Infect. Dis.* **178,** 451–459.
42. Murphy, T. V., Pastor, P., Medley, F., Osterholm, M. T., and Granoff, D. M. (1993) Decreased *Haemophilus* colonization in children vaccinated with *Haemophilus influenzae* type b conjugate vaccine. *J. Pediatr.* **122,** 517–523.
43. Sarangi, J., Cartwright, K., Stuart, J., Brookes, S., Morris, R., and Slack, M. (2000) Invasive *Haemophilus influenzae* disease in adults. *Epidemiol. Infect.* **124,** 441–447.
44. Swartley, J. S., Marfin, A. A., and Edupuganti, S., et al. (1997) Capsule switching of *Neisseria meningitidis*. *Proc. Natl. Acad. Sci. USA* **94,** 271–276.
45. Maiden, M. C. J. and Spratt, B. G. (1999) Meningococcal conjugate vaccines: new opportunities and new challenges. *Lancet* **354,** 615–616.
46. Bovier, P. A., Wyss, K., and Au, H. J. (1999) A cost-effectiveness analysis of vaccination strategies against *N. meningitidis* meningitis in sub-Saharan African countries. *Soc. Sci. Med.* **48,** 1205–1220.
47. Yakubu, D. E., Abadi, F. J. R., and Pennington, T. H. (1999) Molecular typing methods for *Neisseria meningitidis*. *J. Med. Microbiol.* **48,** 1–10.
48. Olcén, P., Kjellander, J., Danielsson, D., and Lingquist, B. L. (1979) Culture diagnosis of meningococcal carriers: yield from different sites and influence of storage in transport medium. *J. Clin. Pathol.* **32,** 1222–1225.
49. Stuart, J. M., Cartwright, K. A. V., Jones, D. M., Noah, N. D., Wall, R. J., Blackwell, C. C., et al. (1987) An outbreak of meningococcal disease in Stonehouse: planning and execution of a large-scale survey. *Epidemiol. Infect.* **99,** 579–589.

20

Surveillance of Meningococcal Disease in Europe

Norman Noah

1. Introduction

For a technique often now referred to as "the backbone of public health," it is curious how only recently surveillance has come to be recognized as important. As soon as recording of disease events began, so of course did surveillance, but the first application of the term to "the ongoing scrutiny of disease" is thought to have been by Langmuir *(1)* in the 1950s. The use of the term has helped to focus attention on it as a technique and a discipline in its own right, and there are now books devoted to the subject *(2,3)*. The technique is also being applied increasingly to chronic disease *(2)*.

For meningococcal infection, it can be argued that any laboratory investigation any more sophisticated than making that diagnosis is "academic" unless it is being used for surveillance and epidemic management. The management and treatment of individual cases of meningococcal infection is not dependent on the results of grouping, subtyping, or serotyping, nor indeed is chemoprophylaxis. The availability of a vaccine against groups C, A, W135, and Y strains but not group B does now mean that grouping of strains is helpful in local epidemic situations in which the use of the vaccine is being considered.

Nevertheless, it has to be said that the surveillance of meningococcal infection, although undoubtedly useful, is at present somewhat limited in being able to tell us what we would like—and need—to know. The reasons for this will become apparent later in this chapter. This chapter will outline the general principles of surveillance, and at the same time apply them to the specific example of meningococcal infection at national and European level. A more detailed textbook account of the general principles and practice of surveillance is available *(4)*.

From: *Methods in Molecular Medicine, vol. 67: Meningococcal Disease: Methods and Protocols*
Edited by: A. J. Pollard and M. C. J. Maiden © Humana Press Inc., Totowa, NJ

2. Definition of Surveillance

The definition of surveillance is continuous analysis, interpretation, and feedback of systematically collected data, generally using methods distinguished by their practicality, uniformity, and rapidity rather than by accuracy or completeness. By observing trends in time, place, and persons, changes can be observed or anticipated and appropriate action, including investigative or control measures, can be taken *(5)*.

This definition is useful because it illustrates the rough and ready approach that can still work in surveillance. Useful information can often emerge from the intelligent use of what may appear to be unpromising data. Nevertheless constant efforts must be made to improve scope, accuracy and detail as the surveillance develops.

3. Methods

The "traditional" four main steps in surveillance are: collection, analysis, interpretation, and feedback. To these may be added the preliminary assessment before surveillance begins and the action that may need to be taken at the end.

3.1. Preliminary Assessment

It is difficult to be dogmatic about the several factors that may have to be taken into account in assessing whether surveillance should be conducted for a disease like meningococcal infection. Obviously the infrastructure has to be present: this will include a reliable death certification system; doctors to notify and/or laboratories with the necessary competence and facilities; local (district) public health or microbiological personnel to collect information for local action before passing it on centrally; and a central organization with the facilities and expertise to collect and analyze, and the ability to make something of the data before providing feedback.

Other factors to consider before setting up a surveillance program, and that will affect the design of the system, includes the political structure of country, the organization and financing of its health system, the use of health care outside this system, the communications systems and level of computerization, as well as the level of training of personnel.

The cost and priorities—which will depend not only on the incidence of the disease but also on its relative importance compared with other conditions—clearly matter. One cannot always take the motivation of reporting sources for granted, and persuasion may be needed. The quality and relevance of feedback are important here.

3.2. Collection

This has to be systematic and accurate, timely, consistent, and representative.

Table 1
Case Definition of Meningococcal Infection and Sources of Information

Death certification	Primary cause of death Underlying cause of death
Notifications/clinical diagnosis	Meningitis Septicemia Septicemia and meningitis Other invasive
Laboratory diagnosis	Light microscopy Culture: CSF, blood, skin rash, other Throat only Nonculture methods, e.g., PCR, Ig antibody

3.3. Systematic and Accurate Reporting

Reporting has to be systematic and accurate to make sense. Part of the systematic process is to have a case definition that is clearly understood by all participants. Meningococcal infection provides a particularly good example of how difficult this can be, especially in an European or international context.

3.3.1. Case Definition and Sources of Data

There are difficulties and dilemmas with the definition of meningococcal infection (*see* **Table 1**).

3.3.1.1. Death Certifications

Death certification reporting for meningococcal disease may be the most complete, but may lack accuracy. Death certifications often have to be accepted at face value, but there are uncertainties in the accuracy of diagnosis, especially with clinical diagnoses. Group and serotype data may be difficult to obtain. Moreover, deaths may not necessarily reflect incidence, especially for comparisons between European countries, as case fatality ratios often vary considerably between countries. Missing data are also a problem: some cases can be missed altogether; deaths can be certified as acute bacterial meningitis, or even acute meningitis, and it is usually difficult, if not impossible, to know how many of these were meningococcal in origin. The problems with septicemia are similar, only worse, because of the large number of deaths attributed to "acute septicemia" without further qualification. Undoubtedly a proportion of these will have been caused by meningococcal infection.

In England and Wales, the primary and underlying causes of death on the death certificate are separated, and meningococcal disease can appear in either section.

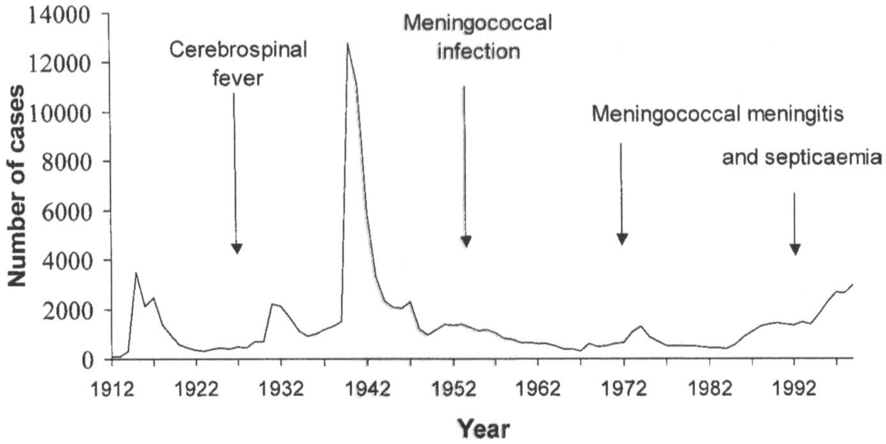

Fig. 1: Notifications of cerebrospinal fever, meningococcal meningitis/septicemia, England and Wales, 1912–1999.

A surveillance system based on death certification alone is unlikely to provide much useful information about meningococcal disease, but is something to start with if nothing else is available. If available for many years it may give an indication of trends, and of the age and sex distribution of meningococcal disease. Death certification can be helpful as an adjunct to surveillance that is based on morbidity data.

3.3.1.2. Notification

Notification systems are generally based on clinical diagnoses, although grouping and typing information may also be available. Completeness and accuracy are certainly problems, but are generally overrated ones. Timeliness, on the other hand, and completeness, are often better than with laboratory data. Much useful information on trends, seasonality, and age and sex distribution are provided by notifications. These trends are shown vividly in **Fig. 1**, which is based on the number of notifications of various notifiable forms of meningococcal disease since 1912 in England and Wales, including a long period when it was notifiable as cerobrospinal fever. The remarkable increase in notified cases during World War II is clearly shown, and occurred in many other Westernized countries.

Completeness and accuracy become important goals of surveillance when a vaccine is introduced and the incidence of the infection approaches low levels.

A case definition is certainly possible for notified cases but it would have to be known and accepted by every doctor in the country, with every case notified having to be checked by the office of the local Director of Public Health. Clinicians do not always take the opportunity of correcting a notification if it turns out subsequently to be wrong. Strict case definition for notification is usually best reserved for the last stages of elimination, when accuracy is essential (as is happening with measles now in the UK and other European countries). Nevertheless, the accuracy of notification of meningococcal disease in most Westernized countries is fairly good, and the value of notification should not be underestimated.

In Europe, for meningococcal disease, a surveillance system based on notifications alone would probably have not been worthwhile, unless it was used to build a network that would eventually report laboratory data. This is mainly because group and serotype data are essential to the goals of European surveillance for meningococcal disease. Also, with the wide variations in accuracy, timeliness, and completeness that are likely to be found between countries in Europe, the information gathered would be difficult to interpret. Some useful information on age distributions could emerge. In the event many countries did start reporting notifications, although most now report laboratory data also.

3.4.3. Laboratory Reporting

Surveillance systems based on laboratory diagnoses are more accurate, but generally are even less complete than notifications, so the two systems can often run in parallel. In some countries, it is possible to correlate notified cases with the laboratory reported cases, so that duplication is avoided, and one "comprehensive" list is compiled (although this may still be incomplete). The amount of work involved in this, especially in larger countries, should not be underestimated. Case definitions are also difficult with laboratory data. The isolation of a meningococcus from cerbrospinal fluid (CSF), blood, or other normally sterile site is generally indisputable. It is "a gold standard" for diagnosis, and for definition of a "case." If however differentiation is being made between meningitis and septicemia, cases may be difficult to classify. In the European Meningococcal Surveillance Unit, we classify isolates in one patient from CSF or both CSF and blood as "meningitis," and from blood only as "septicemia," but some patients have clinical septicemia or clinical meningitis which will be at variance with the diagnosis based on laboratory findings. There is also an increasing tendency to attribute cases clinically to septicemia if they have severe disease or die, which makes case fatality rates based on meningitis or septicemia difficult to interpret.

Decisions have to be made about isolates of meningococci from throat in patients with meningitis or septicemia. In our European surveillance, throat isolates from asymptomatic persons are not included in the routine statistics for analysis, but we accept throat isolates from clinical cases if there is no isolate from a sterile site. However some spurious meningococcal infections undoubtedly slip through the net and are reported; the more complex the case definitions, the greater the scope for inaccuracy.

Nonculture methods of diagnosis should ideally be assessed for sensitivity and specificity before acceptance into the surveillance scheme. Light microscopy showing Gram-positive diplococci in CSF with compatible clinical features are accepted. Polymerase chain reaction (PCR) diagnoses are also accepted. Serotyping data are usually not available when nonculture methods are used. CSF isolates in particular may become more scarce in the future, because of the dangers of lumbar puncture in patients with raised intracranial pressure. Isolation rates may also be affected if patients are treated immediately on clinical suspicion, before blood or CSF can be taken for culture.

The usefulness of pan-European surveillance depends greatly on the grouping, typing, and sub-typing of isolates, and the trend towards nonculture methods may make it less useful in the future.

Although in theory, the iceberg phenomenon is particularly strong with laboratory reporting, and laboratory-confirmed cases may be small in number and possibly unrepresentative, this type of reporting is important. Without it, the usefulness of surveillance in many infections could be questioned. Thus, for meningitis, identification and reporting of the causal organism increases its usefulness many-fold, as does the grouping of meningococci for meningococcal disease. Similarly, the laboratory input to surveillance of food poisoning, influenza, and respiratory infections can be said to "put the color into a black-and-white outline drawing." In general, and arguably, laboratory data may be more important qualitatively than quantitatively.

3.4. Timeliness

Timeliness is important in all forms of infectious disease surveillance. In some surveillance systems, the main objective is outbreak control. This applies particularly to infections in which point- or continuing-source infections are common. Thus with salmonellas and Enternet *(6)* (an EU–wide system for surveillance of enteric infections) early detection of Europe-wide food-borne outbreaks is important and timeliness to within a few days is essential. The objectives for Legionnaires' disease (LD) are similar *(7)*, and the existing surveillance systems for salmonellas and LD are highly successful. For infections such as meningococcal disease, the epidemiology in Europe is fairly stable and Europe-wide outbreaks are less common. The main objectives of meningococcal surveillance are more "descriptive." They would include: to inform vaccine use, to examine the burden of disease, and to detect changes in the distribution of important groups and serotypes. Nevertheless, timeliness is still important in meningococcal surveillance but has been difficult to achieve with all countries in the European Surveillance. Inevitably some can report with little delay, others need longer. The timing of the routine quarterly and annual reports theoretically depends on when the very last report comes in to the Surveillance Unit.

The reasons for this delay are predominantly administrative, in that laboratories may need time in putting the data together in a form suitable for our use. In some countries, laboratory and notification data are correlated and duplicates removed, which takes time. Moreover although we receive most of our reports as single cases, some reporting centers provide a summary form with the data aggregated. This adds to delay and makes analysis less flexible. In our European Meningococcal Surveillance, timeliness of reporting and feedback has room for improvement.

Timeliness is particularly important for outbreaks crossing country borders, as happened in April 2000, and again in February and March 2001, when several cases of meningitis were associated with the Haj in Saudi Arabia *(8)*. Nearly all these cases were caused by one strain, W135:2a:P1.2; P1.5, which was thought to belong to the ET-37 complex. Cases were reported from France, England, the Netherlands, and Germany, and occurred in travellers to the Haj, and in their contacts when they got back home. Much of this type of surveillance is best conducted on the telephone or electronically, and is best coordinated by one center.

3.5. Consistency

It is very difficult to run a surveillance system if reporting is not regular and reliable. Unfortunately, political upheavals and other changes in Europe have often caused these two essentials to a successful surveillance system to be lacking. At various times we have had 38 countries reporting to us, but many of our recent reports have been based on 28–32 countries in Europe, and 3–4 elsewhere. Interpretation of statistics becomes difficult when reporting is irregular. This becomes especially problematic when large countries with patterns well outside "the norm" report irregularly. Thus those with high or low incidence, or with a high proportion of, say, group C strains, will affect the results overall if they are intermittent reporters.

In our European surveillance we have attempted to work on this problem by developing a list of "core reporters," and by undertaking some separate analyses of their data. These countries have reported without a break for a number of years, and by pooling their data we achieved some consistency, albeit at the expense of diminishing coverage.

3.6. Representativeness

There are really two questions here: how representative are the reporting centers of meningococcal infection in their own countries, and how representative are all the reporting countries together of meningococcal disease in Europe?

Data sent from national reference laboratories are likely to be, but are not necessarily, fairly representative. Some of these laboratories may not be acceptable to, or used by, other diagnostic laboratories. This may be especially so with some centers that have developed an interest in grouping and typing meningococci, but have not been designated officially as "reference laboratories."

For European surveillance as a whole, we have high coverage in Western Europe, somewhat lower in Eastern Europe. This is partly owing to there being fewer resources for reagents and typing in Eastern European countries, and fewer reference or "representative" laboratories. Nevertheless, those that do report are willing and enthusiastic, and we are always attempting to increase coverage. In some Eastern European countries, surveillance reports are not national, and we then match cases reported to the base population.

Meningococcal disease is in general too uncommon a disease for sentinel surveillance to be successful.

In general, the consistency of our surveillance results, as judged by age and sex distributions for meningococcal groups, case fatality ratios, and meningitis/septicemia, is good. However with an infection which seems to be fairly stable overall, but is known to cause localized intense outbreaks (such as happened in Stroud in England in the 1980s and in northeastern Czech republic in 1993–1994), there is always concern that some important occurrences are being missed.

3.6.1. Quality Control

A surveillance system, such as the system in Europe in which all participating laboratories are part of a network, provides a natural group for quality control. One or more of the participating laboratories acts as a reference laboratory.

3.7. Enhanced Surveillance

In England and Wales, an enhanced surveillance system for meningococcal disease has been introduced in some regions of the country. In countries in which many of the attributes of a successful surveillance system referred to earlier may be difficult to achieve, concentrating intensive surveillance in a few areas or regions may be more efficient than trying to achieve perfection across the whole country. One disadvantage is that care needs to be taken if the disease under surveillance varies widely geographically. Another problem is that costs will increase, especially if, as is usually necessary, one person—a facilitator—is needed to ensure completeness, timeliness, and accuracy. The main advantages, however, are that completeness is almost assured, cases tend to be investigated more thoroughly, accuracy is improved, and further detail can be obtained if necessary: diagnosis and case-fatality rates are more reliable, for example. Moreover, the data can often be extrapolated to the rest of the country.

3.8. Analysis

This is the process of organizing the raw data so that they can be interpreted, and will include calculating rates, ratios, and proportions and preparing tables, graphs, and charts. When using rates or ratios, it is important to be aware that some of these indices are based on very small numbers, and to take care not to misinterpret when comparing rates.

3.8.1. Rates and Proportions

Rates (usually per 100,000 for meningococcal infection) should be used wherever possible. For incidence, rates should be standardized for age to ensure that comparisons between countries are not biased by their different age structures. For an infection such as meningococcal, in which the age distribution is heavily skewed to infants and children, this is especially important. The differences in crude and standardized incidences are not very different in most countries in Western Europe that have similar population age structures (*see* **Table 2**), and the differences are greater in smaller countries.

For some of the analyses, percentages are used instead of rates. This is a useful technique if, say, it is wished to compare age distributions of meningococcal cases between countries. We then need to "standardize" for different incidence rates, to make comparisons of age distributions somewhat easier. In our annual reports for European meningococcal surveillance, we tend to use percentages for comparing age distributions between countries and also between meningococcal groups and types. It must be remembered that percentages by themselves are of little value, and so must be used mainly for comparisons, as noted earlier.

Examples of using incidence rates and percentages are shown in **Fig. 2A–D**. The incidence rates for groups B and C (**Fig. 2A**) show clearly that the highest incidence for each group is in infants aged 1–11 mo, but also that the incidence of group B infection in those aged 1–4 yr is still higher than that for the peak age of 1–11 mo for group C. They also show that the incidence in teenagers, especially the older teenagers, is about the same in both groups. This indicates that group C has a greater tendency to affect teenagers than group B. This is shown clearly when the ages are shown as proportions (percentages) as in **Fig. 2B**, in which the older age shift of group C compared with group B infection is apparent. Indeed, although the age distributions of infections caused by either group has a bifid pattern, with peaks at 1–4 yr and 15–19 yr, this pattern is more marked in group C infections (**Fig. 2B**). **Fig. 2C** and **D** show similar differences in interpreting incidences and proportions in graphical form, with the age distribution of group C : 2a clearly shifted towards the older age groups. Moreover, although the incidence rates are very different, the age distribution,

Table 2
Meningococcal Disease by Country, Europe 1997–1998: Number of Cases and Incidence

Country	Notifications			Laboratory cases		
	Number	Crude incidence	Age-standardized incidence	Number	Crude incidence	Age-standardized incidence
Austria				94	1.2	1.2
Belgium				238	2.3	2.3
Croatia[a]	27	0.8	n/a			
Czech Republic				123	1.2	1.3
Denmark	199	3.8	n/a	147	2.8	n/a
England and Wales				2045	3.9	2.3[c]
Estonia	2	0.1	0.1	6	0.4	0.0
Finland[b]				29	0.6	n/a
France				338	0.6	0.6
Germany				361	0.4	0.5
Greece	166	1.6	1.5	107	1.0	1.0
Iceland				21	7.8	6.0
Israel				45	0.8	0.5
Latvia	19	0.8	0.7	24	1.0	1.1
Lithuania[b]	34	1.8	n/a			
Malta				25	6.8	6.1
Netherlands	505	3.3	3.1	526	3.4	3.3
Northern Ireland[b]				30	3.6	3.1
Norway				100	2.3	2.4
Portugal[b]	67	1.4	1.4			
Republic of Ireland				328	9.3	7.1
Romania[b]				10	0.1	n/a
Russia (Moscow)				90	1.0	1.2
Scotland				301	5.9	5.5
Slovak Republic	43	0.8	0.8	104	1.9	1.7
Slovenia	5	0.3	0.3	3	0.2	0.2
Spain				644	1.6	1.4
Sweden	53	0.6	n/a			
Switzerland[b]				67	1.9	n/a
Ukraine[d]	33	1.7	n/a			
Europe[e]				**5523**	**1.8**	**1.5**
USA				*3246*	*1.2*	*1.0*
Australia				*323*	*1.8*	*n/a*

[a]Number of cases for 3rd and 4th quarters of 1997 and 1st quarter of 1998 only.
[b]Number of cases for 1st and 2nd quarter of 1998 only.
[c]The age standardized incidence rate for England and Wales appears to be very low compared to the crude incidence because many cases (40%) had no age information. This figure should be treated with caution. (Adjusting for the 40% the figure would be 3.2.)
[d]Number of cases for 3rd and 4th quarters of 1997 only.
[e]20 Countries.
Note: All incidence rates have been adjusted to Annual Rates.

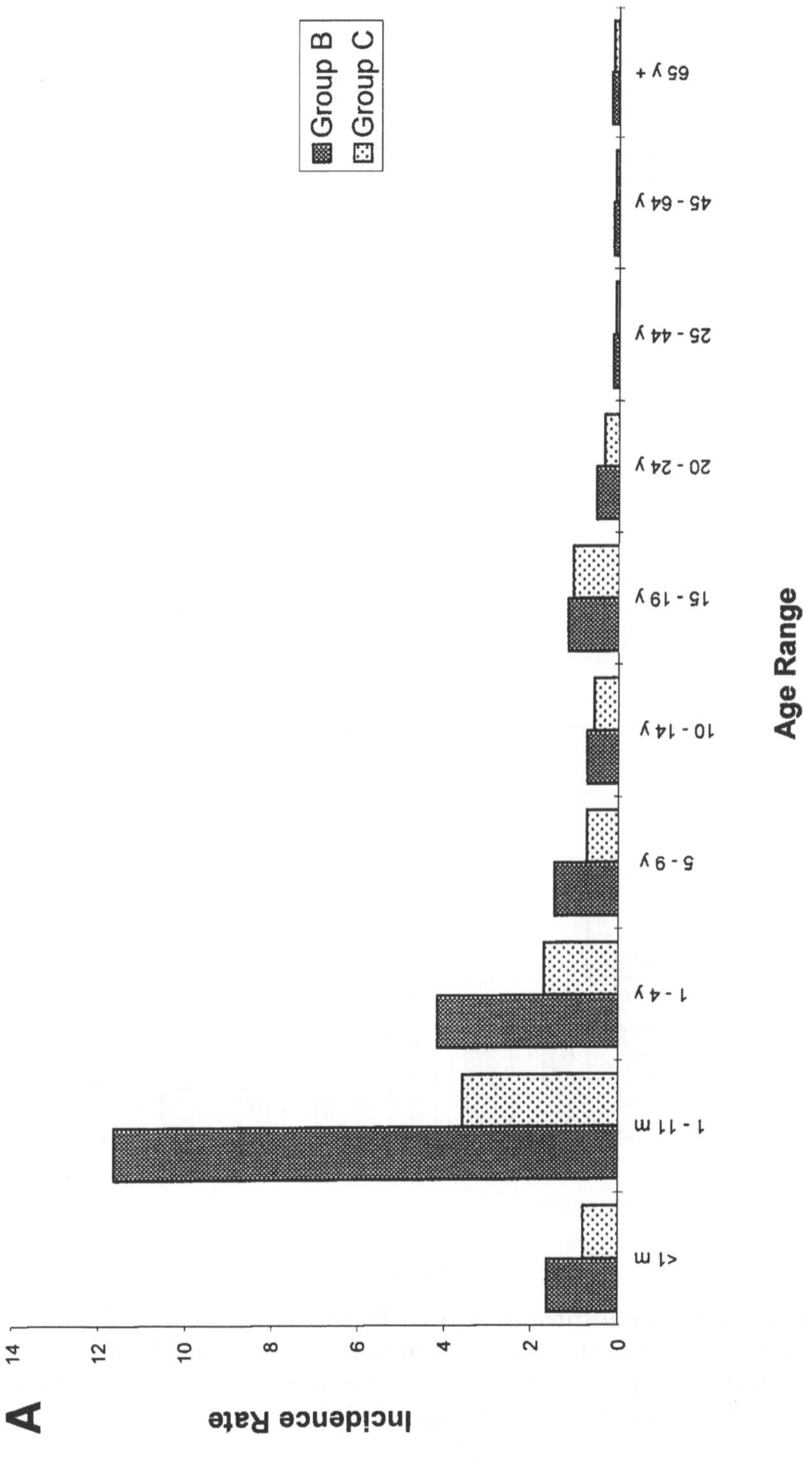

Fig. 2. (A) Age distribution of group B and C meningococcal disease by incidence rate per 100,000, Europe 1997–1998.

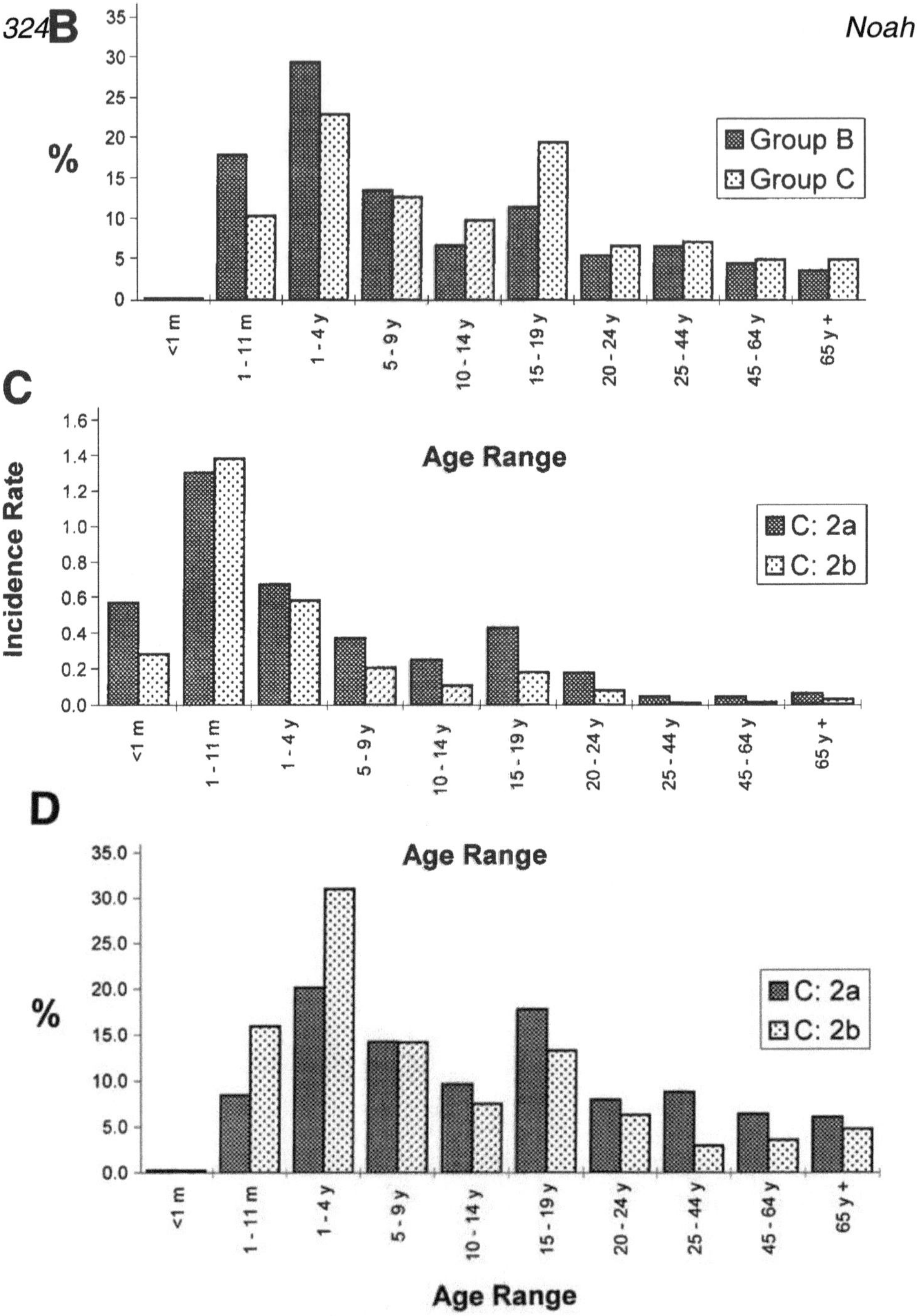

Fig. 2 *(continued)* (**B**) Age distribution of group B and C meningococcal disease by proportion, Europe 1997–1998. (**C**) Age distribution of Type C: 2a and C: 2b by incidence rate per 100,000, Europe 1997–1998. (**D**) Age Distribution of Type C: 2a and C: 2b meningococcal disease by proportion, Europe 1997–1998

as opposed to incidence, of group C:2b is closer to that of group B than to group C:2a.

3.8.2. Case Fatality

Case-fatality rates vary widely between participating countries in our European surveillance (in 1997–1998, between 1% and 33%), but we suspect this is something of a reporting artefact rather than a real reflection of differences in treatment and management. Reasons for countries with apparently too high or too low case-fatality rates include:

1. Low numbers. A country with a high case-fatality rate of 33% had only 9 reported cases, with 3 deaths, during that year.
2. Outcome not reported. If the outcome is not reported in many cases, case-fatality rates will tend to be low. We allow for this by using as a denominator only those cases which have been reported as survived/died. Nevertheless, some countries still have very low rates and the most likely explanation is that they are reported to the reference laboratory as survived before the outcome is truly known. An unlikely alternative possibility is that cases that die are less likely to be investigated microbiologically, and hence not referred to the reference laboratory.
3. Fatal cases more likely to be reported or investigated. Some countries report very high case-fatality rates. In many instances this is unlikely to be real and suggests that patients who die are more likely to have been investigated or reported than those who survive. This is to some extent supported by our data, in that countries with high case-fatality rates tend to have low outcome-reporting rates.

3.8.2.1. Case-Fatality Rates and Ratios

There is an important difference here which is worth discussion. A case-fatality rate strictly should apply to a series of cases followed up for a sufficient period so that the outcome is known in all cases. With meningococcal disease this is rarely possible on a national basis, although there are some smaller countries that do provide high-quality data with reliable case-fatality rates. Usually the so-called case-fatality rate is a ratio of cases ascertained by some means (notification or laboratory) to deaths certified through the official death-registration scheme. The sources of data are not the same. The term case-fatality ratio is much to be preferred for this, as it is not a rate. Case-fatality ratio is useful for looking at trends in "survival" in each country, especially if the sources of deaths and cases have remained the same over the period, and the rates for reporting each have not changed. They may be misleading if the absolute values are accepted uncritically.

The three standard epidemiological analyses are: time, place, person.

3.8.3. Time

Analyses by time include examining annual incidence data within countries over some years, as well as over the whole of Europe. Within countries, total numbers can be used, although rates are preferred. When comparisons between countries are being made, rates should be used. Seasonal trends can be scrutinized weekly, calendar monthly, four-weekly, or quarterly. In pan-European surveillance, weekly analyses are not often helpful: they can be difficult to interpret, and there may be too much "noise." Quarterly distributions are easiest, as most countries report quarterly, but they tend to lack sufficient detail. Four-weekly or monthly analyses are probably the best compromise if it is possible with the data-reporting system. Four-weekly is scientifically the most correct, because each period has the same number of days. Moreover 52 wk of the year can be neatly sub-divided into four equal periods of 13 wk. The disadvantages of four-weekly analyses are that they may be slightly more difficult to interpret in terms of "months" numbered as 13 rather than 12, and the occasional occurrence of years with 53 weeks!

3.8.3.1. Epidemiological Years

It makes sense to use epidemiological years rather than calendar years with an infection that has such a strong winter seasonal pattern as meningococcal disease. It is important to analyze by "epidemic" rather than create an artificial break in the middle of a seasonal outbreak. We have now changed to epidemiological year in our European surveillance.

Temporal patterns in the distribution of the different groups, especially in the proportions of group B to C disease, and of the major serotypes (C:2a, C:2b, B:4, B:15, etc.), are important components of our analyses.

3.8.4. Person

In general, much the most important source of information in surveillance is that relating to person. Analysis of "age" is the most basic and useful of all person characteristics, and for meningococcal infection in particular, surveillance would be much less worthwhile without this information.

In any epidemiological analysis, the age groupings chosen will depend on the age distribution of the disease. As far as it is possible to generalize, no one cell should contain a considerably larger number than the other cells; certainly not more than about 50% (unless there are only about three or four cells). In our reports, the largest cell, of children aged 1–4 yr, contains about 27% of cases, although the incidence is highest in those aged 1–11 mo.

Analyses by age for meningococcal surveillance in Europe include age-specific incidence, fatality rates, analyses by groups and by sero/subtypes. Standard age distributions for meningococcal disease are those shown in **Fig. 3A–D**. It is important however to be flexible in analyzing age, and it is much easier to do this when cases are reported as line lists rather than as aggregated data.

For the use of group C vaccine in teenagers, for example, the distribution within the critical 15–19 yr age group is important in knowing whether to target university entrants or high school pupils.

Sex distribution of meningococcal infection in Europe has always tended to show a clear male predominance, which is as expected. However, some countries show a preponderance of females and the significance of these differences from the "norm" is unclear.

Sometimes information is provided on occupational groups or travel history, but the surveillance is not suitable for routine reporting of information of this nature, and is usually best asked for in outbreaks.

3.8.5. Place

The only information gathered on place is country of origin. More detailed analyses of geographical variations in infection are best done within countries, by their own surveillance schemes. There are considerable variations within countries both in incidence and in serotype distribution, as well as variations between countries.

3.8.6. Other Analyses

Data are also analyzed for antibiotic resistance patterns to sulphonamide, penicillin, and rifampicin. These vary widely between countries.

3.9 Evaluation

Every surveillance system needs to be evaluated, so that the data are not misinterpreted. This can be as a continuous process, or by regular surveys, or a mixture of both. With the widely disparate reporting systems found in Europe, evaluation is difficult but important.

Some of the attributes of a surveillance system that should be evaluated include completeness, representativeness, accuracy, timeliness, and consistency. Laboratory aspects of accuracy are part of quality control. We tend to favor continuous evaluation of our sources, complemented with the occasional questionnaire survey. Countries have been asked to estimate their levels of completeness for example, and this needs perhaps to be undertaken more regularly. Examples of continuous evaluation have been included in various sections of this chapter.

3.10. Interpretation and Feedback

It is possible to be drowning in statistics and yet thirsting for information. Interpretation is the process of turning statistics into information. Together with feedback it is a vital process in surveillance. Many of the pitfalls in interpreting data on meningococcal disease have been described previously. Avoiding these pitfalls will aid in interpreting the analyses correctly, but will not by itself turn statistics into information. The quality of interpretation and feedback affects reporting: reporters will quickly lose motivation if feedback is nonexistent or meaningless.

When interpreting data, their completeness, timeliness, representativeness, and significance (in its literal rather than its statistical sense) need to be taken into account. Care must be taken when comparing incidences between countries because completeness of reporting of meningococcal disease cases will vary. First, not all cases will necessarily be diagnosed correctly clinically. Even when they are, not all will be notified or reported. Second, not all cases will be investigated by the laboratory, and not all true cases of meningococcal disease will be correctly diagnosed. This may be for reasons of poor or inadequate specimens or specimen transport, or limited expertise or availability of reagents. Third, not all those diagnosed will necessarily find their way into a national or trans-continental surveillance system; moreover, reporting laboratories may not represent the entire country. There are also problems of case definition, which were discussed earlier. Analyses using percentages from countries with very small numbers of cases, even if completeness is nearly 100%, can be misleading and have to be interpreted with care. If the completeness of reporting varies considerably between countries with different epidemiological patterns, great care has to be taken in interpreting data. For example, if countries with predominantly group B disease had virtually 100% coverage rates for reporting, whereas those with predominantly group C or A disease had very low rates of reporting, the importance of group B disease will be exaggerated with respect to groups C and A disease.

There may be problems with timeliness, especially if laboratories do sero- and subtyping in batches, and cases may be attributed to the wrong month, quarter, or year.

Case-fatality rates especially need to be interpreted with caution. The reasons for this have already been discussed in **Subheading 3.8.2.** above.

The process of turning statistics into "meaningful information" can be described as setting the findings into context. Trends and patterns, and why they could be important, have to be described. Key changes on which to act to prevent or control disease, e.g., the detection of an increase in incidence of a serotype, should be highlighted. High risk groups should be identified in terms of time, place, and person. The age distribution of meningococcal disease and the distribution of serogroups within those ages are particularly important in assessing the schedule for a vaccine.

When interpreting statistics for feedback, it is probably as well to determine what the most useful items of information are likely to be. With European surveillance of meningococcal disease, the prevalence and incidence of groups and serosubtypes, together with their distribution by age and place, and any changes in them that occur with time, are probably at its heart. The arrival of a new clone, with knowledge of its age distribution and some indication of how virulent it is, should be detected early. The main problem with surveillance of meningococcal disease as it stands is the plethora of sero- and sub-types. This makes it difficult to interpret changes that occur, especially those beyond the serotype level. There is little knowledge with the present typing systems about how close the various strains are, especially as the ET system is at present too limited in scope and too difficult to perform to be applied universally. Without a universally available and coherent typing system, there is inadequate insight into the patterns of spread of meningococcal infection across the continent. Sero- and sub-typing are useful for localized outbreaks, but less good for the broad picture.

We provide regular feedback quarterly and annually. The information is provided in the commentary and tables in the main part of the reports, the "statistics" in the appendices. These appendices consist of detailed tables for those who wish to do further analyses.

An essential adjunct to regular reports is the flexibility to report outbreaks and other acute changes on an *ad hoc* basis. Recent examples of this are a widespread international outbreaks of cases of W135 infection imported into Europe (as well as other parts of the world) following the years 2000 and 2001 Haj *(8)*, as well as the more localized problems confined to one country, as occurred with acute outbreaks of meningococcal disease in Malta (group B) in 1996–1999, Spain (Galicia, Cantabria and Rioja, mainly group C2b:P1.2. P1.5) in 1996 *(9)*, and the Czech republic (C2a:P1.2, P1.5) in 1993–1994 ***(10,11)***. Successful reporting of acute incidents depends on efficient surveillance systems within the reporting countries as well as a network of organizations across Europe with the ability to investigate these incidents epidemiologically. The EPI-ET system has proved itself useful for gathering in this type of information.

Another important function for a successful surveillance system is the ability to respond to individual inquiry. This is as important as the regular reporting system. The data need to be organized and easily accessible to provide information for *ad hoc* inquiries. Assistance or guidance in interpretation is also important.

4. Action

Action depends on the objectives of the surveillance, which in turn is dependent on the type of infection concerned, particularly its mode of propagation. European surveillance of meningococcal infection is quite different from the surveillance of salmonellas or LD. With salmonellas *(6)* and LD *(7)*, the prime objective of surveillance is the early detection of outbreaks. Salmonella outbreaks may be caused by a foodstuff distributed across many countries, and the early detection of an abnormal pattern triggers an intensive and urgent investigation to pinpoint the source and remove it. With LD the source is not a foodstuff but the principles are the same: both these infections are commonly associated with point-source outbreaks. With meningococcal disease, on the other hand, infection is propagated, i.e., spreads directly from case-to-case (albeit with many chains of asymptomatic infection in between). The objectives of surveillance for meningococcal disease are thus quite different. The surveillance of meningococcal disease in Europe as it stands provides a good information basis for action. As judged against the main purposes of surveillance, it can detect changes in groups, sero- and subtypes, quantify morbidity and mortality, and provide information on vulnerable age groups in the population. Antibiotic-resistance patterns are also available. It is possible to use the information for planning for vaccine use. The availability of a conjugated group C vaccine will ensure that the data will be used by manufacturers and planners for implementation. The need for a group B vaccine throughout probably the whole of Europe is already apparent from the surveillance. Continued surveillance after implementation of group C (or indeed any vaccine) is important because of any changes that may occur in serogroup distribution after mass vaccination.

Nevertheless, the network exists for the investigation of (rare) outbreaks of meningococcal disease, as occurred in April and May 2000 following the Haj *(8)*. This is an example of the meningococcal equivalent of a "point source" outbreak, although "control" in the sense of removing a continuing source of infection does not apply. Nevertheless the outbreak can be coordinated epidemiologically and microbiologically through the network, the cases and strains characterized, and the impact of the outbreak evaluated. The need for the inclusion of W135 in a vaccine for pilgrims to the Haj is already apparent.

Further benefits of meningococcal disease surveillance include the use of the network for research and quality control, the standardization of protocols for management, and the comparison of the effects of different protocols. The European meningococcal disease network has been used for all these purposes on several occasions.

5. Dissemination and Communication

Finally, the elegant differentiation, made by Goodman et al. *(12)* between dissemination and communication of information, is fundamental and must be an important goal for any surveillance system. Dissemination is "a one-way process through which information is conveyed from one point to another." Communication, on the other hand, "is a loop," and "a collaborative process." It "facilitates their consequent use for public health actions." It is essentially the process already referred to of turning statistics into information. It is the most difficult and frustrating part of any surveillance network. The European meningococcal surveillance has had moderate success in this transformation, and there always remains room for improvement, as in any surveillance system.

Acknowledgment

European Surveillance for meningococcal infection is run by the author and Brian Henderson B.S.C. They are grateful to all their collaborators in many countries, both in Europe and further afield, and to Wyeth for funding.

References

1. Langmuir, A.D. (1963) The surveillance of communicable diseases of national importance. N. Eng. J. Med. 268, 182–192.
2. Eylenbosch, W. J. and Noah, N. D. (eds.) (1988) *Surveillance in Health and Disease*. Oxford University Press, Oxford, UK.
3. Teutsch, S. M. and Churchill, R. E (1994) *Principles and Practice of Public Health Surveillance*. Oxford University Press, Oxford, UK.
4. Noah, N. D. (1997) Methods—Microbiology in Oxford Textbook of Public Health, 3rd ed., vol. 2 (Detels, R., Holland, W. W., McEwen, J., and Omenn, G. S., eds.) Oxford University Press, Oxford, UK, pp. 929–949.
5. Last, J. M. (ed.) (1995) *A Dictionary of Epidemiology, 3rd ed.* Oxford University Press, New York.
6. Communicable Disease Surveillance Center, de Mateo, S. (1998) *Salmonella enteritidis* PTI outbreak in a hotel in Mallorca. *Eurosurveill. Wkly.* **2,** 9807–9809.
7. Slaymaker, E., Joseph, C. A., Bartlett, C. L. R. on behalf of the European Working Group for Legionella Infections (1999) Travel associated legionnaires' disease in Europe: 1997 and 1998. *Eurosurveillance* **4(11),** 120–124.
8. Ramsay, M. and Handysides, S., et al. (2000) Meningococcal infection in pilgrims returning from the Haj. (and updates) *Eurosurveill. Wkly.* **4,** 407, 413, 427.
9. Fernandez, S., Arreaza, L., Santiago, I., Malvar, A., Berron, S., Vazquez, J. A., Hervada, X., and Gestal, J. J. (1999) Carriage of a new epidemic strain of *Neisseria meningitidis* and its relationship with the incidence of meningococcal disease in Galicia, Spain. *Epidemiol. Infect.* **123,** 349–357.
10. Krizova, P. and Musilek, M. (1995) Changing epidemiology of meningococcal invasive disease in the Czech Republic caused by new clone *Neisseria meningitidis* C:2a: P1.2(P1.5), ET-15/37. *Cent. Eur. J. Public Health* **3,** 189–194.

11. Krizova, P., Musilek, M., and Kalmusova, J. (1997) Development of the epidemiological situation in invasive meningoccal disease in the Czech Republic caused by emerging *Neisseria meningitidis* clone ET-15/37. *Cent. Eur. J. Public Health* **5,** 214–218.
12. Goodman, R. A., Remington, P. L., and Howard, R. J. (1999) Communicating information for action, in *Principles and Practice of Public Health Surveillance.* Oxford University Press (www.euroserve.org/update/).

21

Global Surveillance for Meningococcal Disease

Nancy E. Rosenstein

1. Introduction

The word "surveillance" probably first referred to close supervision of individuals exposed to an infectious disease and their close contacts *(1)*. Currently, though, surveillance refers more frequently to the ongoing accumulation of data so that it can be used for decision-making. A surveillance system includes collection, analysis, and dissemination of data. Surveillance can be used to evaluate trends in disease, to identify outbreaks, to test hypotheses, to evaluate existing programs, and to plan for new programs. Surveillance is the single most important tool for identifying infectious diseases that are emerging, are causing serious public health problems, or are diminishing in importance *(2)*.

Meningococcal disease surveillance often has more than one goal. Because single cases trigger a public-health response in many countries, specifically identification of close contact and administration of chemoprophylaxis to prevent secondary disease, cases must be detected quickly. Timely reporting is also important to promptly identify outbreaks, and surveillance must establish the causative serogroup because vaccines used to control outbreaks are serogroup-specific. Surveillance is used to evaluate trends in the epidemiology over time, which is crucial to facilitate decision-making. For example, the detection of an increased proportion of US meningococcal disease attributed to serogroup Y has prompted greater interest in inclusion of a serogroup Y conjugate component in new meningococcal-conjugate vaccines. Finally, surveillance is essential to estimate the burden of meningococcal disease; surveillance is especially important as many countries prepare for implementation of routine childhood vaccination with new meningococcal vaccines.

From: *Methods in Molecular Medicine, vol. 67: Meningococcal Disease: Methods and Protocols*
Edited by: A. J. Pollard and M. C. J. Maiden © Humana Press Inc., Totowa, NJ

Although multiple countries conduct surveillance for meningococcal disease, methodologies vary dramatically and systematic surveillance is not conducted in many countries. Therefore, evaluating the global burden of meningococcal disease is exceedingly difficult. A recent study estimated that there were 117,000 cases of meningococcal disease in the world in 1990, with the majority of those cases in India (n = 22,000) and China (n = 22,000) *(3)*. Evaluation of the global burden of meningococcal disease can be useful to put meningococcal disease in the context of other diseases, but estimates of the number of cases may not adequately convey the public health importance of this disease. In most developed countries, meningococcal disease affects a relatively small number of people but the high case-fatality and morbidity rates, despite appropriate medical treatment, increase its importance, as does the public concern after even a single case. When a cluster of cases occur, public concern heightens, and when an outbreak is declared, additional intervention is required, including in some cases costly vaccination campaigns.

Although outbreaks of serogroup A meningococcal disease were common in industrialized countries early in the 20th century, they have been rare in these countries since World War II. In contrast, in the developing world, major serogroup A outbreaks occur more frequently, especially in the African "meningitis belt," a broad savannah region in Africa that extends from Ethiopia in the east to Senegal in the west *(4)*. In this region, sporadic infections occur in annual cycles with large-scale outbreaks superimposed every 8–12 yr. These epidemics frequently result in attack rates of 500 to 1,000 cases per 100,000 population, but rates can reach as high as 2000 cases per 100,000 population or 2%. In 1990, the African meningitis belt did not experience a major epidemic; therefore, the study of the global burden of meningococcal disease estimated the cases of meningococcal disease from sub-Saharan Africa as only 17,000 *(3)*. In 1996, the largest epidemic ever recorded occurred in the meningitis belt with the total number of cases was estimated by the World Health Organization (WHO) as 152,813, probably a substantial underestimate *(5)*. Rapid detection and early response to epidemics can reduce illness and deaths through prompt vaccination campaigns; however, the region was not adequately prepared to implement comprehensive control efforts. Essential services and personnel were diverted and limited health budgets strained to cope with the epidemic. Evaluation of the importance of meningococcal disease must therefore not only include surveillance for cases and deaths, but also evaluation of the substantial medical and economic impact of disease.

2. Methods

2.1. Selection of a Population

The surveillance population should be well-defined geographically and age-specific population data should be available so that age-specific rates can be calculated. A stable population (without many people moving in and out) is preferable because accurate surveillance and determination of rates in a highly mobile population is difficult. The residents of the surveillance area should have good access to, and a high utilization of, one or more health facilities that are able to diagnosis meningococcal disease. All health facilities (including all hospitals, public and private) that diagnose and treat meningococcal disease in the surveillance population should be included in the surveillance system. Optimally, surveillance would be conducted throughout the entire population but, especially in developing countries, limited resources may make this difficult. In this setting, the most practical population for surveillance is probably an urban population that is geographically distinct from other population centers and that is served by one or more major health centers.

2.2. Definition of a Case

An appropriate case definition is essential to a surveillance system. A case definition typically includes criteria for person, place, time, clinical or laboratory diagnosis, and epidemiologic features; cases are frequently categorized by the degree of certainty regarding diagnosis as possible, probable, or confirmed. For meningococcal disease, case definitions vary among countries. A patient with clinically compatible illness and laboratory confirmation is generally considered a confirmed case, whereas a patient with clinically compatible illness and no laboratory confirmation is a possible or suspected case *(6)*. In the US, laboratory confirmation includes only isolation of *Neisseria meningitidis* from a normally sterile site (e.g., blood or cerebrospinal fluid [CSF]), and a patient with a positive antigen test in CSF or clinical purpura fulminans is considered a probable case *(6)*. As our understanding of meningococcal disease and its associated laboratory testing improves, case definitions may change. In the UK, a positive polymerase chain reaction (PCR) of blood or CSF is considered laboratory confirmation.

Case definitions evolve over time and may differ by situation. For example, in Africa, surveillance of meningococcal disease is essentially targeted at meningitis, because septicemia is much less frequent and more difficult to recognize and confirm, especially in poorly equipped health facilities. In this region, meningitis surveillance is based on a very simple case definition that can be implemented in any health-care setting. The WHO therefore recommends that while the definition of a confirmed and suspected case is similar to that listed earlier, a probable case is defined as a patient with clinically compatible illness with turbid CSF or an ongoing epidemic *(7)*.

2.3. Collection and Recording of Information

Information on diseases can be obtained in many ways and each mechanism has characteristics that must be balanced against the purpose of the system. In many countries, notification of all meningococcal cases is required, an appropriate strategy for a disease that is potentially catastrophic and has high and urgent preventability constraints. However, laboratory-based systems for meningococcal disease can also provide essential, detailed information on meningococcal serogroups. Existing data sets can provide surveillance data, often more economically or efficiently than a newly initiated system. For example, because most patients with meningococcal disease are hospitalized, hospital discharge records could provide basic data on meningococcal cases.

Surveillance data are collected from multiple sources including physicians, laboratorians, hospitals, and schools. Data-collection instruments should be standardized to facilitate analysis and comparison with data collected in other systems. Data elements should be generally recognized and optimally use computerized formats. Typically, after assurances of privacy and confidentiality, identifying information is kept at a local site (i.e., state health department). Identifying information is often removed before data are transmitted to a agency (i.e., federal health department) to assure the anonymity of the patients.

Surveillance systems are generally characterized as either passive or active. Most routine notifiable disease surveillance relies on passive systems. In many countries, reporting of meningococcal cases is required and health-care providers report disease on a case-by-case basis to the local health department. Passive reporting is simple and not burdensome to the health department, but it has important limitations. Because of the high profile of meningococcal disease, cases are frequently reported but compliance with the case definition cannot be confirmed, reporting can be late, and information is often incomplete. Because of the importance of meningococcal disease, active systems are often used. These systems involve regular outreach to potential reporters to stimulate reporting. Active surveillance can validate the representativeness of passive reporting and assure more complete reporting; it can also include collection of strains of *N. meningitidis* and allow population-based estimates of the burden of disease owing to particular molecular subtypes. Active surveillance can also be used in conjunction with specific epidemiologic investigations. For example, active surveillance will be invaluable to assess the impact of integration of conjugate meningococcal vaccines into routine childhood immunization programs. Active surveillance is, of course, more expensive and because resources are often limited, active systems might be used for brief periods for discrete purposes, such as for early recognition of epidemics in the African meningitis belt.

Optimally, surveillance should utilize modern computing and communication technologies to collect data and transform it into usable information rapidly and effectively. Accurate, efficient data transfer with rapid notification of key partners and constituents is critical and can be enhanced by new technology. In the US, most disease reports received by state health departments originate from clinical laboratories and are received via mail, facsimile, or telephone *(8)*. Automated reporting from clinical laboratories has been proposed as a means to improve the quality and timeliness of disease notification. In one recent study, electronic reporting more than doubled the total number of laboratory-based reports that were received and reports were more timely and more complete *(8)*.

2.4. Data Analysis and Dissemination

Data should be analyzed periodically to provide feedback to reporting sites on their performance, to identify potential problems with surveillance, and to provide information to policy-makers and physicians. Analysis of the data needed to address the salient questions must be assessed to assure that the data source or collection process is adequate. In general, simple analysis should include an assessment both of overall rates and age- and serogroup-specific attack rates. Analysis should also include rates by geographic areas, either at a country, state, or county level.

Data should be analyzed and presented in a compelling manner so that decision-makers at all levels can readily see and understand the implications of the information *(6)*. Although the primary users of surveillance information are public health professionals and health-care providers, providing access to the public and the media may facilitate communication of important public-health messages.

2.5. Evaluation of Surveillance

Evaluation of surveillance systems is essential to developing effective and efficient systems. Evaluation includes assessing the public-health importance of the problem under surveillance, whether the system is meeting its objectives, and what resources are used to operate the system. The surveillance process should also be evaluated to assess the following characteristics: simplicity, flexibility, acceptability, sensitivity, timeliness, and positive predictive value (PPV) *(9)*. While a simple system is preferable, the need to conduct confirmatory laboratory tests often complicates meningococcal disease surveillance. Flexibility entails the ability of a system to accommodate changes in case definitions or the additional of new variables. Because of the severity of illness owing to *N. meningitidis* and the availability of preventive interventions, acceptability is high, and individuals and organizations are generally willing to participate in surveillance. Sensitivity can be defined as the proportion of all true cases detected by the surveillance system. In developed countries, most patients with meningococcal disease seek medical care, but diagnostic tests are imperfect and not all diagnosed cases are reported; therefore, sensitivity is less than 100%. The sensitivity of a system can also be defined as the ability of the system to detect epidemics. In the African meningitis belt, WHO recommends using of 15 cases per 100,000 population over 2 wk as indicative of an epidemic and therefore a useful threshold to initiate a mass vaccination campaign *(7)*. Optimization of this approach requires sensitive and timely surveillance, which is difficult to achieve, but clearly a high priority for not only meningococcal disease but also for other diseases with epidemic potential. PVP is the proportion of patients identified as having cases who actually do have the condition under surveillance, and PVP should be assessed along with its effect on the use of resources. A surveillance system with low PVP and therefore frequent false-positive case reports would lead to wasted resources. For example, because detection of an outbreak of serogroup C meningococcal disease typically prompts mass vaccination, a high PVP is essential ***(10)***. On the other hand, in the context of a meningococcal disease epidemic in the African meningitis belt, once a serogroup A meningococcal disease epidemic is confirmed, diagnostic testing of additional clinical cases may less important *(7)*.

3. Notes

In many countries, surveillance for meningococcal disease is a priority because of the high public awareness of disease and the occurrence of epidemics. Meningococcal disease, however, is only one of a number of communicable diseases causing morbidity and mortality, especially in Africa. Development of surveillance for meningococcal disease should be integrated into a comprehensive integrated surveillance system. An integrated approach does diminish simplicity, but it can markedly improve flexibility and acceptability as well as coordination, efficiency, and sustainability. A strong disease surveillance system is the foundation of an effective disease prevention and control program.

References

1. Thacker, S. B. and Berkelman, R. L. (1988) Public health surveillance in the United States. *Epidemiol. Rev.* **10,** 164–190.
2. Centers for Disease Control and Prevention (1994) Addressing emerging infectious disease threats: a prevention strategy for the United States. U.S. Department of Health and Human Services, Atlanta, GA.
3. Murray C. J. L. and Lopez, A. D. (1996) Anonymous Global Health Statistics: a compendium of incidence, prevalence, and mortality estimates for over 200 conditions. The Harvard School of Public Health on behalf of The World Health Organization and the World Bank, Boston, 283–309.

4. World Health Organization (1996) Cerebrospinal meningitis in Africa. *Wkly. Epidemiol. Rep.* **42,** 318–319.
5. World Health Organization (1997) Epidemic meningitis in Africa, 1997. *Wkly. Epidemiol. Rep.* **42,** 314–318.
6. Centers for Disease Control and Prevention (1997) Case definitions for infectious conditions under public health surveillance. *MMWR* **46(RR-10),** 1–55.
7. World Health Organization Working Group (1995) Control of epidemic meningococcal diseases. WHO Practical Guidelines. Edition Fondation Marcel Merieux, Lyon, France.
8. Effler, P., Ching-Lee, M., Bogard, A., et al. (1999) Statewide system of electronic notifiable disease reporting from clinical laboratories. *JAMA* **282,** 1845–1850.
9. Centers for Disease Control and Prevention (1998) Guidelines for evaluating surveillance systems. *MMWR* **37,** 1–18.
10. Centers for Disease Control and Prevention (1997) Control and prevention of meningococcal disease and Control and prevention of serogroup C meningococcal disease: evaluation and management of suspected outbreaks. Recommendations of the Advisory Committee on Immunization Practices (ACIP). *MMWR* **46(RR-5),** 1–21.

22

Epidemiology of Meningococcal Disease in North America

Andrew J. Pollard, David Scheifele, and Nancy Rosenstein

1. Introduction: *Neisseria meningitidis*

Invasive disease caused by *Neisseria meningitidis* is one of the leading infectious causes of death in childhood in North America *(1)*, but its prevention has not received the same priority on the health agenda as in Europe, Australia, and New Zealand. There are several likely explanations, but the principal one is that disease incidence appears to be lower in both Canada *(2)* and the United States *(3)* than in some of these other countries *(4,5)*. Here, we describe recent epidemiological data concerning meningococcal infection in Canada and the United States and comment on the possible future introduction of vaccination to prevent meningococcal disease across the continent.

1.1. The Organism

N. meningitidis is a Gram-negative diplococcus that normally colonizes the nasopharynx of 10–30% of healthy adults *(6)*. The organism has a wide array of mechanisms that enable it to resist mucosal and tissue defenses. Only rarely do meningococci invade through the mucosal barrier into the bloodstream to cause invasive disease. During invasive disease and transmission, meningococci are surrounded by a polysaccharide capsule, the immunological reactivity of which defines the serogroup *(7)*. The capsule is important in pathogenesis because it is a major factor in enabling the organism to resist phagocytosis and complement deposition. Meningococci expressing capsules of serogroups B, C, Y, and W135 are responsible for a majority of cases of invasive disease in North America and Europe *(8)*. Serogroup A meningococci cause endemic and epidemic disease in Africa and Asia but rarely affect individuals in industrialized nations *(8)*. Beneath

From: *Methods in Molecular Medicine, vol. 67: Meningococcal Disease: Methods and Protocols*
Edited by: A. J. Pollard and M. C. J. Maiden © Humana Press Inc., Totowa, NJ

the polysaccharide capsule is an outer membrane that contains lipopolysaccharide (endotoxin) and a number of outer-membrane proteins (OMPs). Antigenic variation in one of these proteins, PorB, confers the serotype of the organisms, and PorA epitopes determine the serosubtype. The immunotype is determined by the type of lipopolysaccharide present in the outer membrane.

1.2. Surveillance

In the US, meningococcal disease reporting is mandatory with reports collected from clinicians, laboratories, and public-health officials through passive surveillance. In addition the Centers for Disease Control and Prevention (CDC, Atlanta, GA), operate active population-based surveillance for several pathogens, including *N. meningitidis* as part of Active Bacterial Core Surveillance (ABCs) ***(9)***. The population under surveillance includes some 30 million Americans and data is extrapolated from this cohort to the national population (270 million). Currently ABC collects only information about culture-positive cases, but the introduction of polymerase chain reaction (PCR) diagnostics for identifying cases of meningococcal disease is currently being evaluated.

In Canada, data are collected at the federal level through mandated but passive clinical and laboratory reporting; there is no population under active surveillance. PCS diagnosis became available in several provinces in 2001.

1.3. Case Definitions

Slightly different case definitions are used in Canada ***(10)*** and the US ***(11)***. In the US a probable case is defined as a case with a positive antigen test in cerebrospinal fluid (CSF) or clinical purpura fulminans in the absence of a positive blood culture (but positive antigen test results from urine or serum samples are considered unreliable for diagnosis). A confirmed case in the US consists of a compatible clinical presentation that is confirmed in the laboratory through isolation of *N. meningitidis* from a normally sterile site (e.g., blood or CSF or, less commonly, joint, pleural, or pericardial fluid) ***(11)***.

In Canada, a confirmed case is defined similarly, i.e., compatible illness with laboratory confirmation of infection through isolation of *N. meningitidis* from a normally sterile site (blood; CSF, joint, pleural or pericardial fluid) ***(10)***. However, demonstration of *N. meningitidis* antigen in CSF is also compatible with the confirmed case definition. A clinical case is defined as invasive disease with purpura fulminans, even if there is failure to identify any organism in the blood or CSF by either isolation or antigen detection.

2.0. Incidence of Disease

Invasive meningococcal disease affects approx 1 individual per 100,000 population per year in both Canada ***(2)*** and the US ***(3)***. Over time, fluctuations

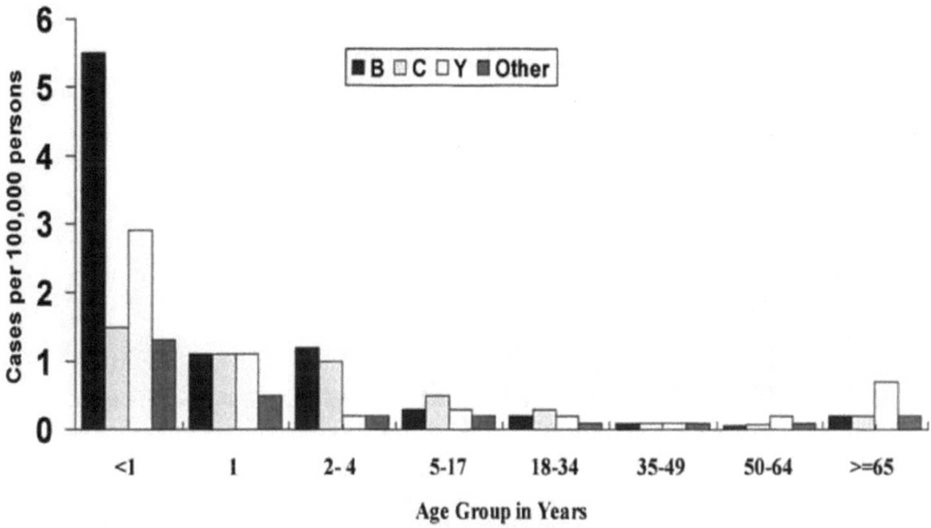

Fig. 1. Serogroup-specific incidence of meningococcal disease by age group, USA, 1997–1999. Adapted with permission from **ref.** ***9***.

in the rate of disease also occur but the reported national rates have remained below 2/100,000 for the last 45 years ***(2,12–14)***.

2.1. Risk Factors for Meningococcal Disease

More than 50% of cases of meningococcal disease involve children with most disease occurring in children under 5 yr of age, with a peak incidence at 6–24 mo old (*see* **Fig. 1** and **2**) ***(2,3)***. Disease is most common in late winter and early spring ***(2,3)*** although sporadic cases occur year round. The attack rate for household contacts exposed to patients who have sporadic meningococcal disease has been estimated to be 4 cases per 1,000 persons exposed, which is 500–800 times greater than the total population ***(15)***. Treatment of close contacts (i.e., household or day-care center contacts) with antimicrobial chemoprophylaxis is very effective for prevention of meningococcal disease and is the primary means for secondary prevention of meningococcal disease in the US. Preceding viral infection, especially with influenza A, has been suggested as a risk factor ***(16,17)***, and active and passive smoking have been clearly linked to an increased risk of disease ***(18–21)***. Overcrowding is an important risk factor as is bar and nightclub patronage during some outbreaks, probably for similar reasons ***(22–24)***. A number of immunodeficiencies are linked with an increased risk of disease, including complement deficiencies ***(25,26)***, hypogammaglobulinaemia ***(27,28)***, asplenia ***(29)***, and a recent study

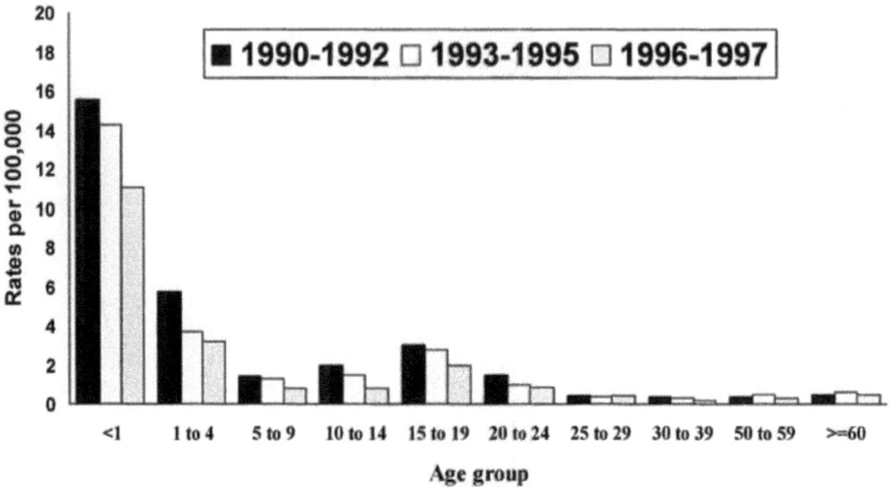

Fig. 2. Incidence of meningococcal disease by year and age group, Canada, 1990–1997. Adapted with permission from **ref. *75***.

suggested a possible link with corticosteroid therapy ***(30,31)***. Individuals with human immunodeficiency virus are probably also at increased risk for sporadic meningococcal disease, but not nearly to the degree associated with their risk of infection with other encapsulated organisms such as *Streptococcus pneumoniae* ***(32)***. In the US, Blacks and those of low-socioeconomic status have been consistently found to be at higher risk for meningococcal disease ***(3,33)***. Race and low socio-economic status are likely to be markers for disease that may reflect differences in fac-tors such as household crowding, urban residence, and exposure to tobacco smoke ***(30)***.

2.2. Mortality and Morbidity

Mortality from meningococcal disease in Canada was most recently reported in 1996 as 6.5% *(2)* and in the US as 10.3% for 1992–1996 *(3)*. The highest case-fatality rate reported in the US followed disease with serogroup W135 (21%) followed by C (14%), Y (9%), and B (6%) *(3)*. Similarly, in Canada, the case-fatality rate was 12% for serogroup C, and 5% for B *(2)*. The serogroup differences in these rates probably represent both differences in virulence of the organism and variation in host susceptibility. Various studies have examined morbidity from meningococcal disease, which is believed to affect 11–19% of survivors ***(34,35)*** and include limb loss, hearing deficit, and neurologic deficits.

2.3. Outbreaks

The US has reported an increase in the number of outbreaks in the past decade ***(36–38)***. Outbreaks of meningococcal disease occur each year and attract much public and media attention. However, these account for less than 3% of all cases in North America ***(39)***. Serogroup C meningococci are responsible for a majority of outbreaks, although some group Y outbreaks have been reported recently ***(3)***.

In the US, meningococcal outbreaks are defined as either “organization-based,” in which there are common affiliations between cases but no close contact (e.g., schools, universities, and prisons) or “community-based,” in which the cases live in the same geographical area but have no common affiliation (e.g., towns, cities, or counties) ***(38)***. In both scenarios an outbreak is declared if there are more than 3 cases within a 3-mo period resulting in an attack rate of greater than 10/100,000.

In addition to these brief outbreaks, hyperendemic meningococal disease (also known as prolonged outbreaks) owing to serogroup B organisms can occur. Hyperendemic group B disease has caused an increased incidence in the Pacific northwest region of the US in recent years, with rates four times higher than in other states ***(40)***; this was caused by meningococci belonging to the ET-5 complex which have caused this epidemiology in a number of countries over the last 20 years. A recent decline in serogroup B disease in this region suggests that this outbreak may be ending ***(41)***.

In Canada, almost all outbreaks of meningococcal disease since 1986 have been caused by a single clone of serogroup C meningococci known as ET-15 ***(42)***, a member of the ET37 complex, leading to several mass-immunization programs in the early 1990s ***(43)***. Five provinces in Canada reported serogroup C outbreaks in early 2001, leading to mass immunization campaigns in each case. Similar large immunization campaigns have been undertaken in the US ***(36)***, where 90% of group C isolates belong to the ET37 complex ***(3)***. In 1999–2000, an outbreak of serogroup C disease occurred in Alberta involving 22 cases, mostly aged 15–19 yr and not apparently linked ***(44)***. In response, the Provincial Government administered some 297,000 immunizations to persons 2–19 yr old ***(44)***. In the US from 1994–1997, 102,000 doses were given in response to 13 outbreaks ***(45)***.

3.0. Serogroup and Disease

The serogroup distribution of meningococcal disease in Canada and the US is outlined in **Figs. 3** and **4**. There has been an increase in the proportion of cases owing to serogroup Y meningococci in the US over the past decade. The prevalent serogroup Y clone is similar but not identical to previous clones as

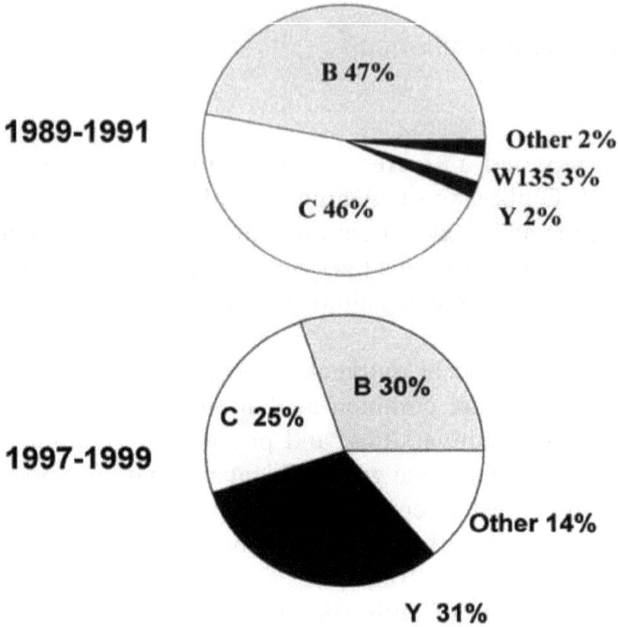

Fig. 3. Meningococcal serogroup distribution in the USA. Adapted with permission from **refs.** ***9*****,*****33*****,** and ***76***.

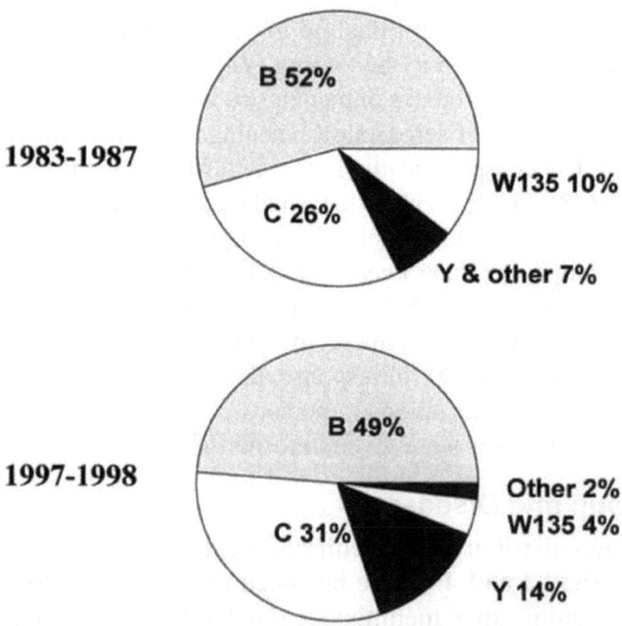

Fig. 4. Meningococcal serogroup distribution in Canada. Adapted with permission from **refs.** ***48*** and ***77***.

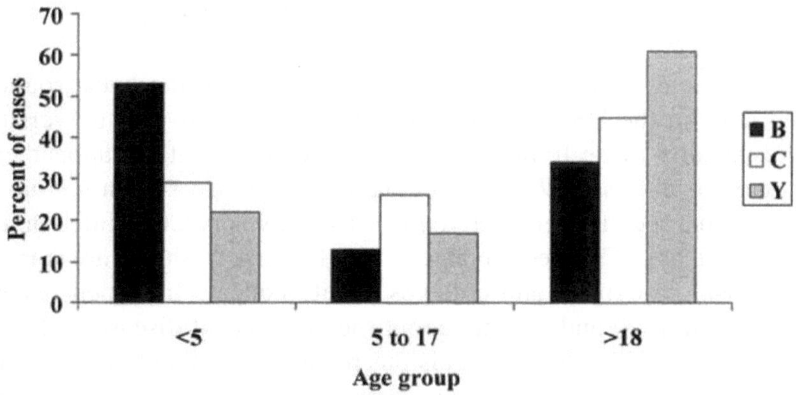

Fig. 5. Age and percentage of cases of meningococcal disease, USA, 1992–1996. Adapted with permission from **ref. *3***.

identified by multi-locus enzyme electrophoresis (MLEE) ***(46)***. Waning population immunity as well as introduction of a new clone may have caused this rise in disease caused by serogroup Y meningococci ***(3)***. Of importance, age appears to alter prevalence of serogroup-specific disease (**Fig. 1** and **Fig. 5**), with a majority of serogroup B cases in early childhood and more then 60% of serogroup Y cases in adults ***(3)***. Changes in serogroup distribution in Canada are presented in **Fig. 4** and suggest a decrease in the proportion of disease caused by W135 and an increase in the proportion of cases with serogroup Y-associated disease ***(2,12,46,47)***. In 2000, the first large international outbreak of serogroup W135 meningococcal disease was reported among Hajj pilgrims returning from Saudi Arabia ***(48)***.

4. Currently Available Vaccines and Their Uses in North America

In the US, the quadrivalent A, C, Y, W135 plain polysaccharide vaccine is the only available vaccine; in Canada, both the quadrivalent and the bivalent plain polysaccharide A, C vaccines are available. Both vaccines are poorly immunogenic in children less than 2 yr of age and the immunity that they generate is of limited duration, especially in young children. However, vaccine efficacy is 85–90% in older children and adults, with a duration of protection of 5–10 yr ***(50)***. There is also evidence that hyporesponsiveness to the polysaccharide vaccine may occur after repeated doses, although the clinical significance of this phenomenon is unknown ***(51)***. In both Canada and the US, therefore, these vaccines are used only for high-risk groups, including those with asplenia, with complement deficiency, high-risk laboratory personnel, and military personnel, and in the control of outbreaks ***(38,39,52–54)***. Meningococcal vaccine is also recommended for travelers to areas where epidemic meningococcal disease activity might be anticipated (i.e. the African "meningitis belt" *(49,55–57)*.

Disease among college students is not higher than the background age-adjusted rates in the US *(58)*. However, freshmen (first-year university students), especially those living in dormitory accommodation, appear to have higher rates of disease *(39,58)*. Vaccination of college students is not cost-effective from a societal perspective *(59)*. The Advisory Committee on Immunization Practices (ACIP) recommended that, because freshmen are at modestly increased risk, caregivers and colleges should educate freshmen (especially those in dormitories) and parents about meningococcal disease and vaccination so that they make informed decisions regarding vaccination *(39)*. No such national policy exists in Canada and there are no studies of disease burden among college students, although there is a documented rise in disease incidence among adolescents as described in the US and elsewhere.

4.1. Polysaccharide-Protein Conjugate Vaccines

Polysaccharide-protein conjugate vaccines, similar in design to those in widespread use against *Haemophilus influenzae* type b (Hib), offer the advantages of infant immunization, immunologic memory, and potentially herd immunity that could not be achieved with plain polysaccharide vaccines. Clinical trials are now underway for A, C, Y, and W-135 polysaccharides-protein conjugate vaccines, but published data are available only from studies of A and C conjugate vaccines and a serogroup C immunization program has been implemented in the UK *(61)*. None of these vaccines has been licensed in Canada or the US. In Canada, a C polysaccharide-protein conjugate vaccine was licensed in 2001.

4.2. Immunization Priorities in North America

Streptococcus pneumoniae is the most common cause of community-acquired invasive bacterial disease in North America, causing significantly more disease than *N. meningitidis* (*see* **Fig. 6**). Furthermore, increasing rates of penicillin and cephalosporin resistance in the US *(62)* and Canada *(63)* impact on clinical decisions in the management of pneumococcal infections, making control of this organism of importance. In 2000, a 7-valent pneumococcal polysaccharide-protein conjugate vaccine was shown to be efficacious *(64)* and was introduced in the US for infant immunization *(65)*. Similarly, in Canada, licensure of the 7-valent pneumococcal vaccine is expected imminently and implementation may precede consideration of meningococcal vaccines.

In Canada, infant immunization against the five usual pathogens (polio, diphtheria, tetanus, pertussis, and Hib) requires a single injection per visit, making introduction of new antigens into the schedule quite straightforward. Addition of further antigens into the crowded US schedule is likely to be par-

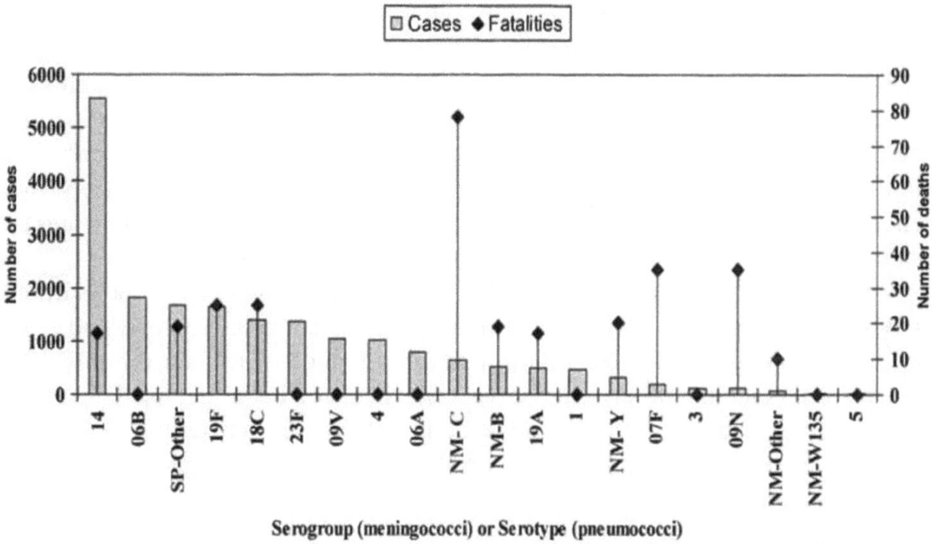

Fig. 6. Distribution of number of invasive bacterial isolates by year, based on ABCs surveillance data, USA (approx 30 million population), ages 0–22 years; Pneumococcal Serotypes (1998) and Meningococcal Serogroups (mean annual cases 1990–1998). NM, *N. meningitides*; SP, *Streptococcus pneumoniae*. Data adapted from **refs.** ***3*** and ***9*** and CDC unpublished data.

ticularly problematic. Moreover, because of the broad age distribution of meningococcal disease, it would be difficult to have a major impact on disease incidence through only infant immunization.

The serogroup distribution of meningococcal disease in the US is unlike that in the UK, where a monovalent serogroup C meningococcal vaccine has been recently introduced ***(61)***. This complicates vaccine planning in the US, where any vaccine for universal use would probably need to include at least serogroups C and Y ***(66)***. The recent outbreak of W135 disease associated with the Hajj pilgrimage suggests that based on current understanding of *N. meningitidis*, the broadest possible approach may be the best choice ***(66)***. There is also a strong argument for inclusion of a serogroup A polysaccharide-protein conjugate in any future meningococcal vaccines for North America for use by travelers in order to facilitate development of this combination vaccine for use in sub-Saharan Africa ***(66)***.

4.3. Future Introduction of Meningococcal Vaccines in North America

A number of arguments can be made in favor of introducing routine use meningococcal conjugate vaccines in North America. The high morbidity and mortality from the disease, the outbreak potential and the complexity and expense of the public-health response, all argue in favor of vaccination. Against such a policy is the low rate of disease, the lack of efficacy data (although early information from the UK is encouraging), the anticipated cost of the vaccine, the fact that the vaccine will probably not be cost "sparing" and the contribution of serogroups not contained in the vaccine, such as B, to disease prevalence. In the US, crowding of the routine infant immunization schedule and the need to target a broad age range will impact on a decision.

Vaccine policy is made by the ACIP in the United States and by the National Advisory Committee on Immunization (NACI) in Canada. However, policy is not usually decided by these committees in advance of a license application and no polysaccharide-conjugate vaccine has yet been licensed in North America. Neverthless, meningococcal conjugate vaccines offer the first opportunity to have a significant impact on the burden of meningococcal disease across the continent.

4.4. Serogroup B Vaccines

If vaccination against serogroups A,C,Y, and W135 meningococci could be implemented, it is likely that disease caused by these organisms could be reduced to very low levels ***(67)***. However, these vaccines would not target the significant proportion of disease owing to serogroup B. There also remains a concern that nonvaccine strains of meningococci, and particularly serogroup B, could take up the ecological niche vacated by the vaccine strains ("strain-replacement") and reduce the impact on overall disease rates ***(68)***. Unfortunately, the polysaccharide capsule of serogroup B meningocococci is poorly immunogenic ***(69)*** and cannot be included in a combination meningococcal conjugate vaccine in its native form. For this reason, most vaccine development for serogroup B disease has focused on antigenic proteins in the outer membrane of the organism ***(70)***. Vaccine efficacy in those most at risk of group B disease, children under 4 yr of age, has not been demonstrated. In addition, these vaccines may be strain-specific and the variability in OMPs may limit their usefulness in control of endemic disease ***(71,72)***. Development of a safe and immunogenic serogroup B vaccine in combination with A, C, Y, and W135 polysaccharide-protein conjugate vaccines is probably the key to vaccine prevention of meningococcal disease in the future. The recent delineation of the meningococcal genome ***(73,74)*** may facilitate development of an effective serogroup B meningococcal vaccine and increase the potential for widespread prevention of meningococcal disease.

Acknowledgments

This chapter is adapted from an article first published in Journal of Pediatrics and Child Health and is reproduced here with permission from the publishers. AJP is funded by the Paediatric Infectious Disease Society (USA) through an educational grant from Pfizer Inc. The authors are grateful to the following individuals who were available to discuss meningococcal epidemiology and vaccine policy in North America prior to the oral presentation of this review at the Meningococcal Workshop in Sydney, Australia, 2000: John Modlin, David Fleming, Victor Marchessault, Susan Squires, Theresa Tam, Francoise Collins, and Philippe De Wals.

References

1. Hoyert, D. L., Kochaneck, K. D., and Murpht, S. L. (1999) Deaths: Final Data for 1997, National Vital Statistics Reports vol. 47. Centers for Disease Control and Prevention, Atlanta, GA, pp. 55–57.
2. Deeks, S., Kertesz, D., Ryan, A., Johnson, W., and Ashton, F. (1997) Surveillance of invasive meningococcal disease in Canada, 1995–1996. *Can. Commun. Dis. Rep.* **23,** 121–125.
3. Rosenstein, N. E., Perkins, B. A., Stephens, D. S., Lefkowitz, L., Cartter, M. L., Danila, R., et al. (1999) The changing epidemiology of meningococcal disease in the United States, 1992–1996. *J. Infect. Dis.* **180,** 1894–1901.
4. Noah, N. and Conolly, M. (1996) *Surveillance of Bacterial Meningitis in Europe 1995.* King's European Meningitis Surveillance Unit, London, UK.
5. Kieft, C., Martin, D., and Baker, M. (2000) *The Epidemiology of Meningococcal Disease in New Zealand in 1999.* Ministry of Health, Wellington, New Zealand, Wellington, pp. 1–39.
6. Caugant, D. A., Høiby, E. A., Magnus, P., Scheel, O., Hoel, T., Bjune, G., et al. (1994) Asymptomatic carriage of Neisseria meningitidis in a randomly sampled population. *J. Clin. Microbiol.* **32,** 323–330.
7. Davis, B. D., Dulbecco, R., Eisen, H. N., and Ginsberg, H. S. (1980) The Neisseriae, in *Microbiology* (Gotschlich, E. C., ed.), Harper, New York, NY, pp. 635–644.
8. Achtman, M. (1995) Global epidemiology of meningococcal disease, in *Meningococcal Disease* (Cartwright, K. A. V., ed.), John Wiley and Sons, Chichester, UK, pp. 159–175.
9. Centers for Disease Control and Prevention (2000) *Neisseria meningitidis. Active bacterial core surveillance reports.* http://www.cdc.gov/ncidod/dbmd/abcs.
10. Anonymous (1991) Canadian communicable disease surveillance system. Disease specific case definitions and surveillance methods. *Can. Dis. Wkly Rep.* **17,** 1–55.
11. Centers for Disease Control and Prevention (1997) Case definitions for infectious conditions under public health surveillance. *Morb. Mortal. Wkly Rep.* **46,** 1–55.
12. Varughese, P. V. (1989) Meningococcal disease in Canada: surveillance summary to 1987. *CMAJ* **141,** 567–569.
13. Centers for Disease Control and Prevention (1999) Notifiable diseases: Summary of reported cases per 100,000 population, United States. *Morb. Mortal. Wkly Rep.* **47,** 77–83.

14. Centers for Disease Control and Prevention (1993) Summary of notifiable diseases, United States, 1993. *Morb. Mortal. Wkly Rep.* **42,** 1–73.
15. Anonymous (1976) Analysis of endemic meningococcal disease by serogroup and evaluation of chemoprophylaxis. *J. Infect. Dis.* **134,** 201–204.
16. Moore, P. S., Hierholzer, J., De Witt, W., Gouan, K., Djore, D., Lippeveld, T., et al. (1990) Respiratory viruses and mycoplasma as cofactors for epidemic group A meningococcal meningitis. *JAMA* **264,** 1271–1275.
17. Cartwright, K. A., Jones, D. M., Smith, A. J., Stuart, J. M., Kaczmarski, E. B., and Palmer, S. R. (1991) Influenza A and meningococcal disease. *Lancet* **338,** 554–557.
18. Stanwell-Smith, R. E., Stuart, J. M., Hughes, A. O., Robinson, P., Griffin, M. B., and Cartwright, K. (1994) Smoking, the environment and meningococcal disease: a case control study. *Epidemiol. Infect.* **112,** 315–328.
19. Fischer, M., Hedberg, K., Cardosi, P., Plikaytis, B. D., Hoesly, F. C., Steingart, K. R., et al. (1997) Tobacco smoke as a risk factor for meningococcal disease. *Pediatr. Infect. Dis. J.* **16,** 979–983.
20. Haneberg, B., Tonjum, T., Rodahl, K., and Gedde-Dahl, T. W. (1983) Factors preceding the onset of meningococcal disease, with special emphasis on passive smoking, symptoms of ill health. *NIPH Ann.* **6,** 169–173.
21. Yusuf, H. R., Rochat, R. W., Baughman, W. S., Gargiullo, P. M., Perkins, B. A., Brantley, M. D., and Stephens, D. S. (1999) Maternal cigarette smoking and invasive meningococcal disease: a cohort study among young children in metropolitan Atlanta, 1989–1996. *Am. J. Public Health* **89,** 712–717.
22. Imrey, P. B., Jackson, L. A., Ludwinski, P. H., England, A. C., 3rd, Fella, G. A., Fox, B. C., et al. (1995) Meningococcal carriage, alcohol consumption, and campus bar patronage in a serogroup C meningococcal disease outbreak. *J. Clin. Micriobiol.* **33,** 3133–3137.
23. Imrey, P. B., Jackson, L. A., Ludwinski, P. H., England, A. C., 3rd, Fella, G. A., Fox, B. C., et al. (1996) Outbreak of serogroup C meningococcal disease associated with campus bar patronage. *Am. J. Epidemiol.* **143,** 624–630.
24. Cookson, S. T., Corrales, J. L., Lotero, J. O., Regueira, M., Binsztein, N., Reeves, M. W., et al. (1998) Disco fever: epidemic meningococcal disease in northeastern Argentina associated with disco patronage. *J. Infect. Dis.* **178,** 266–269.
25. Petersen, B. H., Lee, T. J., Snyderman, R., and Brooks, G. F. (1979) Neisseria meningitidis and Neisseria gonorrhoeae bacteremia associated with C6, C7, or C8 deficiency. *Ann. Intern. Med.* **90,** 917–920.
26. Figueroa, J., Andreoni, J., and Densen, P. (1993) Complement deficiency states and meningococcal disease. *Immunol. Res.* **12,** 295–311.
27. Salit, I. E. (1981) Meningococcemia caused by serogroup W135. Association with hypogammaglobulinemia. *Arch. Intern. Med.* **141,** 664–665.
28. Hobbs, J. R., Milner, R. D., and Watt, P. J. (1967) Gamma-M deficiency predisposing to meningococcal septicaemia. *BMJ* **4,** 583–586.
29. Ellison, E. C. and Fabri, P. J. (1983) Complications of splenectomy. Etiology, prevention and management. *Surg. Clin. North Am.* **63,** 1313–1330.

30. Fischer, M., Harrison, L., Farley, M., et al. (1998) *Risk Factors for Sporadic Meningococcal Disease in North America.* Infectious Diseases Society of America, Denver, Colorado, p. 180.
31. Mitchell, S. R., Nguyen, P. Q., and Katz, P. (1990) increased risk of neisserial infections in systemic lupus erythematosus. *Semin. Arthritis Rheum.* **20,** 174–184.
32. Stephens, D. S., Hajjeh, R. A., Baughman, W. S., Harvey, R. C., Wenger, J. D., and Farley, M. M. (1995) Sporadic meningococcal disease in adults: results of a 5-year population-based study. *Ann. Intern. Med.* **123,** 937–940.
33. Jackson, L. A. and Wenger, J. D. (1993) Laboratory-based surveillance for meningococcal disease in selected areas, United States, 1989–1991. *Morb. Mortal. Wkly Rep. CDC Surveill. Summ.* **42,** 21–30.
34. Kirsch, E. A., Barton, R. P., Kitchen, L., and Giroir, B. P. (1996) Pathophysiology, treatment and outcome of meningococcemia: a review and recent experience. *Pediatr. Infect. Dis. J.* **15,** 967–978.
35. Edwards, M. S. and Baker, C. J. (1981) Complications and sequelae of meningococcal infections in children. *J. Pediatr.* **99,** 540–545.
36. Jackson, L. A., Schuchat, A., Reeves, M. W., and Wenger, J. D. (1995) Serogroup C meningococcal outbreaks in the United States. An emerging threat. *JAMA* **273,** 383–389.
37. Woods, C. R., Rosenstein, N., and Perkins, B. A. (1998) *Neisseria meningitidis Outbreaks in the United States, 1994–1997.* Denver, CO, p. 125FR.
38. Centers for Disease Control and Prevention (1997) Control and prevention of serogroup C meningococcal disease: evaluation and management of suspected outbreaks: recommendations of the Advisory Committee on Immunization Practices (ACIP). *MMWR Morb. Mortal. Wkly Rep.* **46,** 13–21.
39. Anonymous (2000) Prevention and Control of meningococcal disease. *MMWR Rec. Rep.* **49,** 1–20.
40. Diermayer, M., Hedberg, K., Hoesly, F., Fischer, M., Perkins, B., Reeves, M., and Fleming, D. (1999) Epidemic serogroup B meningococcal disease in Oregon: the evolving epidemiology of the ET-5 strain. *JAMA* **281,** 1493–1497.
41. Sullivan, A., Hedberg, K., Reeves, M., et al. (2000) *Natural history of epidemic serogroup B meningococcal disease, Oregon 1998 and 1999.* Atlanta, GA, p. 143.
42. Ashton, F. E., Ryan, J. A., Borczyk, A., Caugant, D. A., Mancino, L., and Huang, D. (1991) Emergence of a virulent clone of Neisseria meningitidis serotype 2a that is associated with meningococcal group C disease in Canada. *J. Clin. Microbiol.* **29,** 2489–2493.
43. Whalen, C. M., Hockin, J. C., Ryan, A., and Ashton, F. (1995) The changing epidemiology of invasive meningococcal disease in Canada, 1985 through 1992. Emergence of a virulent clone of Neisseria meningitidis. *JAMA* **273,** 390–394.
44. Anon (2000) Vaccination program launched. *Alberta Health and Wellness News Release.* http://www.health.gov.ab.ca/whatsnew/Releases%202000/feb28-2000.htm.
45. Woods, C. R., Rosenstein, N., and Perkins, B. A. (1998) *Neisseria meningitidis Outbreaks in the United States 1994–97*, Denver, CO, p. 125FR.

46. Anon (1996) Serogroup Y meningococcal disease—Illinois, Connecticut, and selected areas, United States, 1989–1996. *MMWR Morb. Mortal. Wkly Rep.* **45,** 1010–1013.
47. Varughese, P. and Acres, S. (1983) Meningococcal disesae in Canada and serogroup distribution. *Can. Dis. Wkly Rep.* **9,** 177–180.
48. Squires, S. G., Pelletier, L., Mungai, M., Tsang, R., Collins, F., and Stoltz, J. (2000) Invasive meningococcal disease in Canada, 1 January 1997 to 31 December 1998. *CCDR* **26–21,** 177–182.
49. Centers for Disease Control and Prevention (2000) Serogroup W-135 meningococcal disease among travelers returning from Saudi Arabia—United States, 2000. *MMWR Morb. Mortal. Wkly Rep.* **49,** 345–346.
50. Rosenstein, N., Levine, O., Taylor, J. P., Evans, D., Plikaytis, B. D., Wenger, J. D., and Perkins, B. A. (1998) Efficacy of meningococcal vaccine and barriers to vaccination. *JAMA* **279,** 435–439.
51. MacLennan, J., Obaro, S., Deeks, J., Williams, D., Pais, L., Carlone, G., et al. (1999) Immune response to revaccination with meningococcal A and C polysaccharides in Gambian children following repeated immunisation during early childhood. *Vaccine* **17,** 3086–3093.
52. Anonymous (1994) Guidelines for control of meningococcal disease. Laboratory Centre for Disease Control. Canadian Consensus Conference on Meningococcal Disease. *CMAJ* **150,** 1825–1839.
53. Immunization, N.A.C.o. (1998) Meningococcal vaccine, in *Canadian Immunization Guide Fifth Edition, 1998* (Scheifele, D., ed.), Canadian Medical Association, Ottawa, pp. 125–129.
54. Anonymous (1996) Meningococcal disease prevention and control strategies for practice-based physicians. Committee on Infectious Diseases, American Academy of Pediatrics. Infectious Diseases and Immunization Committee, Canadian Paediatric Society. *Pediatrics* **97,** 404–412.
55. Birk, H. (1999) An Advisory Committee Statement (ACS). Committee to Advise on Tropical Medicine and Travel (CATMAT). Statement on meningococcal vaccination for travellers. *Can. Commun. Dis. Rep.* **25,** 1–12.
56. Centers for Disease Control and Prevention (1999) Change in recommendation for meningococcal vaccine for travelers. *MMWR Morb. Mortal. Wkly Rep.* **48,** 104.
57. Center for Disease Control and Prevention (1997) *Health Information for International Travel 1996–1997.* U.S. Department of Health and Human Services, Atlanta, GA.
58. Harrison, L. H., Dwyer, D. M., Maples, C. T., and Billmann, L. (1999) Risk of meningococcal infection in college students. *JAMA* **281,** 1906–1910.
59. Jackson, L. A., Schuchat, A., Gorsky, R. D., and Wenger, J. D. (1995) Should college students be vaccinated against meningococcal disease? A cost-benefit analysis. *Am. J. Public Health* **85,** 843–845.

60. Pollard, A. J., Bigham, J. M., Bhachu, K., Shaw, C., Isaac-Renton, J., Tan, R., and Thomas, E. (2001) Meningococcal disease in British Columbia. *Br. Columb. Med. J.* **43,** 9–15.
61. Anonymous (2000) Meningococcal disease falls in vaccine recipients. *Comm. Dis. Rev. Wkly* **10,** 133,136.
62. McDougal, L. K., Rasheed, J. K., Biddle, J. W., and Tenover, F. C. (1995) Identification of multiple clones of extended-spectrum cephalosporin-resistant Streptococcus pneumoniae isolates in the United States. *Antimicrob. Agents Chemother.* **39,** 2282–2288.
63. Scheifele, D., Halperin, S., Pelletier, L., and Talbot, J. (2000) Invasive pneumococcal infections in Canadian children, 1991–1998: implications for new vaccination strategies. *Clin. Infect. Dis.* **31,** 58–64.
64. Black, S., Shinefield, H., Fireman, B., Lewis, E., Ray, P., Hansen, R. J., et al. (2000) Efficacy, safety and immunogenicity of heptavalent pneumococcal conjugate vaccine in children. Northern California Kaiser Permanente Vaccine Study Center Group [see comments]. *Pediatr. Infect. Dis. J.* **19,** 187–195.
65. Advisory Committee on Immunization Practices Vaccines for Children Programme (2000) Pneumococcal. *http://www.cdc.gov/nip/vfc/acip.htm* Resolution No. 6/00-1.
66. Perkins, B. A. (2000) New opportunities for prevention of meningococcal disease. *JAMA* **283,** 2842–2843.
67. Booy, R., Hodgson, S., Carpenter, L., Mayon-White, R. T., Slack, M. P. E., Macfarlane, J. A., et al. (1994) Efficacy of Heamophilus influenzae type b conjugate vaccine PRP-T. *Lancet* **344,** 362–366.
68. Maiden, M. C. and Spratt, B. G. (1999) Meningococcal conjugate vaccines: new opportunities and new challenges. *Lancet* **354,** 615–616.
69. Wyle, F. A., Artenstein, M. S., Brandt, B. L., Tramont, E. C., Kasper, D. L., Altieri, P. L., et al. (1972) Immunologic response of man to group B meningococcal polysaccharide vaccines. *J. Infect. Dis.* **126,** 514–521.
70. Pollard, A. J. and Levin, M. (2000) Vaccines for prevention of meningococcal disease. *Pediatr. Infect. Dis. J.* **19,** 333–345.
71. Tondella, M. L., Popovic, T., Rosenstein, N. E., Lake, D. B., Carlone, G. M., Mayer, L. W., and Perkins, B. A. (2000) Distribution of *Neisseria meningitidis* serogroup B serosubtypes and serotypes circulating in the united states. *J. Clin. Microbiol.* **38,** 3323–3328.
72. Sacchi, C. T., Whitney, A. M., Popovic, T., Beall, D. S., Reeves, M. W., Plikaytis, B. D., et al. (2000) Diversity and prevalence of PorA types in *Neisseria meningitidis* serogroup B in the united states, 1992–1998. *J. Infect. Dis.* **182,** 1169–1176.
73. Parkhill, J., Achtman, M., James, K. D., Bentley, S. D., Churcher, C., Klee, S. R., et al. (2000) Complete DNA sequence of a serogroup A strain of Neisseria meningitidis Z2491 [see comments]. *Nature* **404,** 502–506.

74. Tettelin, H., Saunders, N. J., Heidelberg, J., Jeffries, A. C., Nelson, K. E., Eisen, J. A., et al. (2000) Complete genome sequence of *Neisseria meningitidis* serogroup B strain MC58. *Science* **287,** 1809–1815.
75. Anon (2000) Notifiable diseases on-line. *Health protection branch—laboratory center for disease control, Health Canada,* http://cythera.ic.gc.ca/spansweb/ndis/index_e.html.
76. Perkins, B. A. (1999) In James, W. E. (ed.) *Public Health Perspective on Meningococcal Disease in the US.* Postgraduate Institute for Medicine, Englewood, CO, pp. 3–6.
77. Varughese, P. V. and Carter, A. O. (1989) Meningococcal disease in Canada. Surveillance summary to 1987. *Can. Dis. Wkly. Rep.* **15,** 89–96.

23

Computational Methods for Meningococcal Population Studies

Keith A. Jolley and Rachel Urwin

1. Introduction

The complementary fields of molecular evolution and population genetics are both complex and wide-ranging. In this chapter we review some of the basic concepts and describe the methods used to investigate bacterial population biology in general and *Neisseria* populations in particular. A number of recently published textbooks can be referred to for more comprehensive descriptions of general evolutionary theory and methods of gene-sequence analysis ***(1–3)***.

1.1. Sampling Bacterial Populations

In order to make meaningful evolutionary or epidemiological inferences about any bacterial species, it is essential that the data collected is from a representative sample of the whole population that is under investigation. Until recently, most strain collections used for population analyses of *Neisseria meningitidis* consisted of isolates that had caused invasive disease, as these were most readily available from public health and reference laboratories. Although the study of these organisms is undoubtedly necessary to provide essential epidemiological information for monitoring meningococcal infection, disease-causing strains represent only a small fraction of the total population and consequently characterization of only these isolates gives an unrepresentative picture of the genetic and phenotypic diversity present within the whole species. To redress the bias that exists in most *N. meningitidis* strain collections, it is necessary to also isolate and examine noninvasive meningococci because these provide important information about population structure as well as the role of carriage and the mechanisms of pathogenicity.

From: *Methods in Molecular Medicine, vol. 67: Meningococcal Disease: Methods and Protocols*
Edited by: A. J. Pollard and M. C. J. Maiden © Humana Press Inc., Totowa, NJ

1.2. The Structure of Bacterial Populations

Bacterial population structure is determined by a number of genetic processes such as mutation, recombination, natural selection, and the degree of population sub-division. Recombination is particularly important because it can result in two extreme population types: clonal (nonrecombining) and nonclonal (recombining) ***(4,5)***. In strictly clonal populations, new alleles arise only as a result of mutations that are accumulated by vertical transmission of genetic material from mother cell to daughter cell without genetic exchange taking place. Consequently, the population will comprise of a limited number of groups or clones of closely related bacteria ***(6)***. Because of the lack of recombination, clonal populations are said to exhibit linkage disequilibrium, or the nonrandom assortment of alleles ***(4,7)***. Recombination among bacteria that do not share a mother cell provides an opportunity for exchange of genetic material, leading to the reassortment of alleles among strains and an increase in the diversity of the species ***(8,9)***. If recombination occurs at a high frequency, alleles within a population will be reassorted to the extent that distinct clones can no longer be recognized. This random assortment of alleles results in a nonclonal population structure. It has, however, been suggested that these extreme population structures are found rarely in bacterial species and rather, that a spectrum of bacterial population structure exists depending on the ratio of recombination relative to mutation ***(10,11)***.

The population structure of *Neisseria meningitidis* was first investigated by multi-locus enzyme electrophoresis (MLEE), isolates with the same electrophoretic patterns being classified as a single electrophoretic type (ET) ***(12–16)***. Groups of related ETs, defined by UPGMA cluster analyses, were postulated to consist of bacteria that had descended from a single ancestral cell and were often referred to as clones, clonal groups, or genetic lineages. Although proving invaluable for identifying meningococci belonging to hypervirulent lineages, variation recognized by MLEE within and among clonal groups could not be ascribed to recombination or mutation on the basis of differences in electrophoretic mobility alone.

A direct method for identifying the allelic variation at multiple housekeeping loci is by nucleotide sequence determination. Multi-locus sequence typing (MLST), where fragments of 7 housekeeping genes are sequenced and the sequence type (ST) of an isolate assigned according to the combination of alleles identified, is now used widely for epidemiological and population studies of *N. meningitidis* ***(17–20)*** (Chapter 12). These data, along with the sequences from other genes of interest—for example, antigen genes (Chapter 11), genes encoding antibiotic resistance (Chapter 7) and virulence—can be subjected to a variety of evolutionary analyses in order to determine the genetic processes and evolutionary forces that are contributing to meningococcal population structure.

1.3. Identifying Clonal Complexes

Both MLEE and nucleotide-sequence data obtained from collections of meningococcal isolates have been subject to cluster analyses. In an early survey of *N. meningitidis* populations, 688 world-wide isolates were subject to MLEE and were analyzed by UPGMA cluster analysis ***(16)***. A total of 331 distinct ETs were identified that belonged to 14 major clonal lineages, many of which—for example, the ET-5 complex, ET-37 complex, and the A4 cluster—were identified as the common causes of serogroup B and C disease ***(15,21,22)***. In studies of over 500 serogroup A meningococcal isolates, chosen to be representative of all epidemic disease-causing strains isolated since 1960, MLEE defined 84 unique ETs, within which 9 clonal subgroups were identified by cluster analysis ***(14,23)***.

When the allelic profiles obtained from a collection of 107 global meningococcal isolates by MLST were subject to UPGMA cluster analyses, the clonal groupings assigned by MLEE were confirmed ***(17)***. These and MLST data from other collections of meningococci have also been examined using cluster analysis methods such as split decomposition ***(20)*** and BURST (E. J. Feil, http://www.mlst.net). In a study of 156 carried meningococci isolated in the Czech Republic, 71 different sequence types that belonged to 34 distinct clonal complexes were identified using Split Decomposition ***(20)***. Only three of the hypervirulent lineages were identified in this data set, revealing the extent of meningococcal strain diversity within a carrier population.

1.4. Detecting Recombination

There are a variety of ways in which recombination can be detected from gene sequences. A simple indication of a recombining organism is the incongruence of phylogenetic trees obtained from different loci. This method has been presented as evidence for inter- and intra-species recombination within housekeeping and antigen genes of *N. meningitidis* ***(24–27)***. In an analysis of gene fragments from 12 housekeeping loci, maximum likelihood phylogenetic trees were constructed that showed that different combinations of loci gave distinct incongruent phylogenetic trees that were all well-supported by bootstrap analysis and therefore sequences at all loci were incompatible with a bifurcating tree-like phylogeny ***(27)***. These data were instead represented graphically by Split Decomposition ***(28)*** using the program SplitsTree ***(29)***, a program that will draw a tree if the data support one (for example, in the absence of recombination) or an interconnected "network" of sequences if this is a more appropriate visualization of the data (for example, if recombination is frequent).

Where candidate recombinant sequences and putative "parental" alleles have been identified, statistical tests can be performed to locate crossover points, where blocks of sequence have been replaced, resulting in mosaic gene structures with regions that have different evolutionary histories. The Maximum Chi-Squared Test uses the distribution of polymorphic sites to locate recombination junctions ***(30)*** and has been used to identify different mosaic sequences in the penicillin-binding protein gene, *penA*, of penicillin-resistant meningococci ***(31)***. Commensal *Neisseria* species, which are naturally more resistant to penicillin than the pathogenic *Neisseriae*, were identified as the sequence "donors" in these genetic-exchange events. Intra-species DNA exchange among meningococcal antigen and housekeeping genes has also been detected using the Maximum Chi-Squared Test ***(32)***.

1.5. Determining the Extent of Recombination in Meningococcal Populations

Quantifying the extent of recombination occurring in a bacterial population is important for predicting the diversity and structure of that population. MLEE and MLST data have been used to calculate the index of association (I_A), a statistical test designed to detect associations among alleles at different loci ***(4)***. If there is linkage equilibrium, as a consequence of frequent recombination events, the expected value of I_A is zero. Clonal populations are identified by an I_A value that differs significantly from zero. When Maynard Smith et al. calculated the I_A from MLEE data from a world-wide collection of meningococci (which consisted largely serogroup B and C strains), they found a high value (1.96 ± 0.05) obtained when all isolates were included in the analyses, indicative of clonality. This I_A value was greatly reduced when only one isolate from each ET was used (I_A = 0.21 ± 0.08) and virtually disappeared when one representative from each of the 37 ET clusters were compared (I_A = –0.14 ± 0.17), suggesting an underlying nonclonal population structure ***(4)***. A reduction in the I_A value is consistent with the "epidemic" population structure of serogroup B and C *N. meningitidis* organisms. That is, the frequently recombining, nonclonal population appears artificially to be in linkage disequilibrium by the over-representation (clonal expansion) of successful, but transient, genetically related strains. In the study of carried meningococci in the Czech republic, the I_A calculated for the whole data set was 2.47, which decreased to 0.132 when one representative of each lineage was included ***(20)***. In contrast to serogroup B and C populations, the I_A value calculated from the MLEE data obtained from isolates in a population of 292 serogroup A meningococci was high and remained so when ETs were treated as single units *(33)*, suggesting that these organisms are more clonal and recombine less frequently.

The relative contributions of recombination and mutation to the evolution of meningococcal clones has been estimated using MLST allele sequence data obtained from 126 meningococcal isolates using "tips of trees" analysis *(10)*. Allelic variation within the 10 clonal complexes identified was examined visually and classified as having arisen either as the result of recombination or point mutation. In this data set it was calculated that a single base-change in a meningococcal housekeeping gene was at least 80-fold more likely to be the result of recombination than point mutation, a value that is not substantially different to those estimated for *Escherichia coli* and *Streptococcus pneumoniae*. The importance of recombination in determining variation in meningococcal populations has also been supported using the homoplasy test *(34)*. In this test, a parsimony tree is constructed from the data and the number of homoplasies (repeated base-changes) observed is compared to that number expected by chance. An excess of homoplasies is an indication of recombination.

1.6. Detecting Natural Selection

Determining which sequences or sites are subject to positive selection is important for understanding gene function. It is also a useful tool in phylogenetic and population studies for identifying neutrally evolving loci for analysis and for detecting positive selection for change from, for example, the immune response or antibiotics. An indicator of positive selection is an excess of nonsynonymous (d_N) over synonymous (d_S) substitutions per nucleotide site. In most genes, an overall d_N/d_S ratio <1 is observed, which shows that nonsynonymous changes are usually deleterious and therefore selected out of the population. A d_N/d_S ratio of 1 implies that sequences are evolving neutrally—that is, both synonymous and nonsynonymous substitutions have no effect on fitness—so their frequency depends only on how often they are produced by mutation. A d_N/d_S ratio >1 suggests that nonsynonymous changes are being fixed faster than they occur by mutation, which can only occur if there is positive selection for particular amino acids.

Among the 7 meningococcal housekeeping genes chosen for MLST, the d_N/d_S ratios are considerably less than 1 *(20)*, suggesting that the proteins they encode are well-conserved, probably owing to strong functional constraints. Conversely, a mutation in a surface antigen that is exposed to the host immune system may confer a selective advantage to the bacterium with that mutation. Calculation of the d_N/d_S ratios for the *porB* porin genes of the pathogenic *Neisseria* showed there was positive selection for amino acid change in the surface loops of the protein while the membrane-spanning structural regions were highly conserved *(35)*. In the data set examined, the gonococcal *porB* gene appears to be under stronger positive selection than that of the meningococcus, possibly owing to the absence of PorA in gonococci. PorA is the immunodominant surface antigen in meningococci: examination of the nucleotide sequences that encode the surface exposed variable epitopes of PorA has shown that virtually every nucleotide change in these regions is nonsynonymous (J. Russell, personal communication).

In the next section, we describe many of the programs used in our laboratory for examining the population structure and evolution of the meningococcus.

2. Methods

2.1. Analysis of Nucleotide Sequences and Allelic Profiles

2.1.1. Phylogenetic Analysis

As recombination is an important factor in the evolution of meningococci, tree-building methods that assume characteristics are independently and stably inherited are not appropriate models for phylogenetic reconstruction for this organism. Phylogenies can still be used to test for congruence at different loci *(27)* in order to demonstrate nonclonal descent of sequences, or for cluster analysis, where very closely related sequences or allelic profiles can be identified but deep branches are considered less informative. Phylogenetic reconstruction is a subject of some complexity, with the accuracy of any analysis dependent on: the genes and population sampled; the genetic diversity within the sample; the model of DNA substitution used; and the tree-building method chosen for the analysis.

Distance models, which estimate numbers of nucleotide and amino acid substitutions among sequences, range in complexity from simple calculation of the number, or proportion, of nucleotide or amino acid differences between sequences to multi-parameter models that attempt to correct for variable rates of substitution along the sequence, multiple substitutions at single sites, rates of transition and tranversion, and nucleotide frequencies. The HKY85 model, which takes into account base frequencies and transition and tranversion rates, is regarded as a realistic model of DNA substitution, although more simplistic models such as the Jukes-Cantor model have also been utilized in our laboratory. DNA substitution models are employed with tree-building methods to construct phylogenies. A wide range of tree-building methods are also available, from the simple and fast neighbor-joining (NJ) clustering method to the more accurate but very computationally intensive maximum likelihood (ML) method.

If phylogenetic trees are to be constructed, we recommend that a NJ tree is initially constructed, using a model of DNA substitution such as HKY85. The reliability of the NJ trees obtained can then be tested using bootstrap analysis. Briefly, in bootstrap tests, nucleotides (equal in number to those used to construct the initial tree) are randomly sampled with replacement from the original data set and used to construct another phylogeny. The branching patterns observed in this tree are then stored. This process of sampling the data with replacement and constructing NJ trees is repeated several hundred times. The bootstrap confidence level (BCL) of a branch represents the percentage of times that each branch is found throughout the replicate samples: the more often it is found, the better the support for that branch. Branches with BCL values ≥90% are regarded as well-supported. Finally, if powerful computers are available, ML phylogenetic trees can be constructed, using the same model of DNA substitution as before. A range of substitution models and phylogenetic methods can be found in phylogenetic analysis packages such as MEGA, PAUP*, and PHYLIP (*see* **Note 1**).

2.1.2. Split Decomposition Analysis of Sequences and Allelic Profiles

As evolutionary relationships in *Neisseria* species can be obscured by inter- and intra- specific recombination events, the relationships among meningococcal gene sequences are better represented as a network of interconnected branches rather than a tree-like phylogeny. Split decomposition ***(28,36)*** does not force data into a tree structure, but will instead link strains to create a network if that is more appropriate, producing a tree only if the data support it.

The program SplitsTree ***(29)***, available for 32-bit Windows, Macintosh, and UNIX operating systems along with a WWW version running at http://bibiserv.techfak.uni-bielefeld.de/splits/, produces splits-graphs from distance matrices or sequence data. Files containing aligned allele sequences must be in NEXUS format ***(37)*** before they can be opened in SplitsTree. Most phylogenetic analysis packages (MEGA, PAUP*, PHYLIP) will reformat sequence alignments into NEXUS files. The defined scale used to draw splits-graphs means that if distantly related taxa or large numbers of taxa are analyzed, the small networks that link sequences cannot be depicted and are represented as unresolved star-shaped phylogenies. To decipher any unresolved regions of a splits-graph, it is therefore necessary to deconstruct the data set carefully by removing from the Taxa window both distantly related sequences and resolved networks for any further analyses. This, in effect, increases the scale of the graph, magnifying one particular region of the original drawing. This process also improves the "Fit" value of the splits-graph, which is listed in the Log window and is an indication of how well the displayed splits-graph represents the distance matrix from which it was computed, where 100% indicates a perfect fit.

Split decomposition can be performed with MLST data, using just the allelic profiles, for initial cluster analysis (lineage assignment) and subsequent within lineage analysis. The first step is to produce a distance matrix, where each isolate is compared with every other isolate and distances are calculated from the number of shared alleles. The program START (*see* **Subheading 3.1.**) creates such a distance matrix from MLST profiles with output in the NEXUS file. All changes in alleles between isolates are treated identically, i.e., the sequences of the alleles are not compared as alleles with multiple nucleotide differences may occur from a single recombination event, and may in fact be phylogenetically closer than alleles with two nucleotide differences brought about by mutation.

Assigning isolates to lineages using split decomposition is a fairly subjective process. It is likely that upon first loading a diverse meningococcal dataset into SplitsTree, with the "equal edges" option selected, a star-like phylogeny will be indicated showing little relatedness between the majority of isolates. At the center of this star-burst will be unresolved strains, which are more closely related to each other. Immediately from this, one can assign strains found on long "spokes" emanating from the center to individual lineages, as these will all be very different from those found on other similar spokes. To resolve further, isolates can be gradually removed from the analysis, starting from those furthest from the center and leaving isolates that fall within the next concentric circle. At this stage, it becomes necessary to relate isolates to their allelic profiles (sequence type) so that sense can be made of the groupings. We have found that a useful definition of a lineage is when all members share at least four alleles with at least one other member of the lineage.

Once strains have been assigned to lineages, the relationships within each lineage can be determined by including just those strains within the analysis. In some lineages, a central sequence type will be obvious, with variants branching off from it. This may represent the founder sequence type, i.e., the clone from which all variants have descended.

2.1.2. UPGMA Cluster Analysis

UPGMA (Unweighted Pair Group Method with Arithmetic Mean) *(38)* is a simple method of tree construction. Its original purpose was to construct phenograms: trees that reflect the phenotypic similarities between operational taxonomic units (OTUs). It is generally not considered a good algorithm for construction of phylogenetic trees as it assumes equal rates of evolutionary changes among different lineages. In the study of bacterial population biology, this is likely not to be the case, so the method should not be used to construct reliable phylogenies. The method uses a sequential clustering algorithm, in which local homology between OTUs is identified in order of similarity, and the tree is built in a stepwise manner. The two OTUs that are most similar to each other are first determined and then these are treated as a new single "composite" OTU. Subsequently from among the new group of OTUs (composite and simple), the pair with the highest similarity is identified and clustered. This continues until only two OTUs are left. The algorithm assumes that the two most closely related OTUs are more similar to each other than they are to any other. Slightly different clustering may also be seen when the data is presented to the algorithm in a different order. It is important, therefore, not to draw phylogenetic inferences from the clustering pattern seen with this method, although it may prove useful as a quick guide to identifying similar isolates.

UPGMA can be performed on allelic profile data, such as MLST or MLEE, using the program START for 32-bit Windows (*see* **Subheading 3.1.**).

2.1.3. BURST

BURST (Based Upon Related Sequence Types) is a new clustering algorithm, developed by E.J. Feil, for use with multi-locus data. The procedure separates isolates into clonal complexes, where every allelic profile shares at least five loci with at least one other member of the group. More distant relationships among complexes are not determined because they are not meaningful within a recombining population. The most likely ancestral genotype is assigned as the one with the highest number of single-locus variants (SLVs) within the complex. If two or more genotypes have an equal number of SLVs then the number of double-locus variants (DLVs) are taken into consideration. In data sets representative of a population, this ancestral genotype is commonly found to be present at the highest frequency. Likely patterns of descent within each group are then inferred and a graphical representation produced. In a recent study of carried meningococcal strains in the Czech Republic *(20)*, lineages assigned by split decomposition and BURST analysis were in close agreement.

A web-based version of BURST is available (http://www.mlst.net) and the method is included in the sequence type analysis package, START (*see* **Subheading 3.1.**).

2.2. Tests for Recombination

2.2.1. Index of Association

This statistical test attempts to measure the extent of linkage equilibrium within a population by quantifying the amount of recombination among a set of sequences and detecting associations between alleles at different loci. The index of association (I_A) is calculated as:

$$I_A = V_O/V_E - 1,$$

if V_O is the observed variance of K and V_E is the expected variance of K, where K is the number of loci at which two individuals differ. If there is linkage equilibrium because of frequent recombination events, the expected value of I_A is zero. Clonal populations are identified by an I_A value that differs significantly from zero. This analysis can be performed using the START package (*see* **Subheading 3.1.**).

2.2.2. PLATO (Partial Likelihoods Assessed Through Optimisation)

This program can be used to detect "anomalously" evolving regions of sequence that could be owing to either natural selection, which will increase the rate of substitution in this region, or recombination, which will give the region a different evolutionary history to the rest of the sequence ***(39)***. The input file should consist of a PHYLIP formatted (i.e., saved in "flat ASCII" or "text only" format) alignment of sequences together with their maximum likelihood phylogeny (the "null" phylogenetic hypothesis). Using a sliding window analysis and Monte Carlo simulation, PLATO finds regions of the sequence alignment that do not resemble the null phylogeny and calculates the significance of this departure. A PLATO output file lists regions of the sequence alignment where phylogenetic signal differs significantly from that expected, giving a Z-value or significance level for each region. Regions identified can then be examined further for evidence of either recombination or selection. PLATO Version 2.11 is available free for download from http://evolve.zps.ox.ac.uk and can be run on UNIX or Macintosh operating systems.

2.2.3. Homoplasy Test

The homoplasy test ***(34)*** aims to measure the degree of recombination between members of a population. It is only valid where sequences differ by ~5% of nucleotides or less. The test tries to determine if there is a statistically significant excess of homoplasies (shared similarities found in different branches of a phylogenetic tree not inherited directly from an ancestor), compared to an estimate of the number of homoplasies expected by mutation in the absence of recombination. An excess of homoplasies is likely to have been brought about by recombination. The test requires at least six sequences containing 10 or more "informative sites" (sites at which the rarer of two alternative bases is present at least twice). A "homoplasy ratio" is calculated that should range from zero, for a clonal population, to one, for a population under free recombination.

The original homoplasy test program, written by John Maynard-Smith, runs using QBasic under MS-DOS and can be downloaded from http://www.biols.susx.ac.uk/Home/John_Maynard_Smith/. This code has been implemented in the START package for 32-bit Windows (*see* **Subheading 3.1.**).

To calculate the expected homoplasies if the data set was from a clonal population, an estimate of the number of effective sites is required. An effective site is one that is free to change, rather than being selectively constrained. The most reliable method of estimating effective sites is to use an outgroup sequence from a more distantly related species that has the same GC ratio and codon bias ***(34)***. This may not always be possible, so you can set the effective sites to be a proportion of the total sites analyzed, S. A value of $0.6 \times S$ is conservative and is unlikely to indicate recombination unless it really exists.

2.2.4. Sawyer's Runs Test

This test looks for evidence of recombinational exchanges within a set of aligned sequences by determining if regions of sequence pairs have more consecutive identical polymorphic sites in common than would be expected by chance ***(40,41)***. Pair-wise comparisons of derived sequences containing only silent polymorphic sites (condensed sequences) are made. Each pair of sequences is partitioned into fragments containing runs of identical sites. The lengths of all the fragments found between every pair-wise comparison are used to obtain two values: the sum of the squares of condensed fragments (SSCF) and the maximum condensed fragment (MCF). A gene conversion event tends to increase the values of SSCF and MCF because it results in an identical region within two sequences and may produce an unusually long fragment. Provided the mutation rate is constant across sequences, SSCF and MCF are not significantly influenced by mutational hot and cold spots.

Alternative measures of the sizes of conserved segments are obtained by performing the tests on all nucleotide sites (uncondensed sequences). For each pair-wise partition, fragment boundaries are defined by the presence of a discordant silent polymorphic site. The corresponding uncondensed fragment statistics, SSUF and MUF, are more likely to resolve large conversion events but do not control for mutational hot and cold spots. The tests can be performed using the "Sawyer's Runs Test" program for MS-DOS, available free for download from http://www.biols.susx.ac.uk/Biochem/Molbiol/, or using START for 32-bit Windows (*see* **Subheading 3.1.**). Along with the values described, both packages identify the largest fragments. Recombinational end-points may then be identified using the Maximum Chi-Squared Test.

2.2.5. Maximum Chi-Squared Test

The Maximum Chi-Squared (χ^2) Test is used to identify potential recombination events ***(30)***. Briefly, by comparing the distribution of polymorphic sites between "parental" sequences and a putative recombinant sequence, the maximum chi-squared method identifies potential mosaic gene structures and tests the statistical significance of this sequence arising as a result of the import of a diverged block of sequence from one allele to another. Up to 3 sequences of equal length (with no gaps or ambiguous characters, such as N, -, ?) are examined. The location along the sequence of the putative imported block (identified by visual inspection or by using programs such as PLATO or Sawyer's Runs Test) may also be entered. Following several thousand simulations of the data, the test will output all of the potential mosaic structures across the sequence, along with the level of significance of each mosaic. The test can be performed using the programs "maximum chi-squared" (Macintosh) (http://www.biols.susx.ac.uk/Biochem/Molbiol/) or the START package (32-bit Windows) (*see* **Subheading 3.1.**).

2.3. Analysis of Selection Pressure

2.3.1. d_N/d_S ratio

The number of substitutions per synonymous (d_S) and nonsynonymous (d_N) site can be calculated for the gene of interest using the method of Nei and Gojobori ***(42)*** as implemented in the MEGA ***(43)*** (*see* **Subheading 3.2.**) and START software packages (*see* **Subheading 3.1.**), and the d_N/d_S ratio, a marker of selection pressure, can therefore be determined. The method described earlier undertakes multiple pair-wise comparisons of entire sequences or regions. This is not always ideal, as very localized selection pressures may not be identified. There are methods available that examine differences in d_N and d_S at every codon along the sequence. The Synonymous/Non-synonymous Analysis Program (SNAP) calculates pair-wise codon-by-codon substitution rates among a set of aligned sequences. The output data generated by SNAP can be plotted graphically either for each codon or by using a sliding window of a defined number of codons. The SNAP program can be used at http://www.hiv.lanl.gov/ or downloaded free for UNIX and Windows operating systems from the same web-site.

3. Software Packages

3.1. START

START (Sequence Type Analysis and Recombinational Tests), written by K.A. Jolley, is a program for 32-bit Windows operating systems that attempts to combine many of the techniques referred to in this chapter for analysing multi-locus sequence data into a single package. It uses both allelic profile and allele sequence data to perform tests and analyses that can be split into four categories: 1) data summary, 2) lineage assignment, 3) tests for recombination, and 4) tests for selection.

Data summary analyses present the data in a number of ways, such as allele and profile frequencies, identification and quantification of polymorphic sites, codon usage, and GC content. Lineage assignment methods included are UPGMA clustering and tree drawing, BURST analysis, and creation of distance matrices for use with SplitsTree. Tests for Recombination are the Sawyer's Runs Tests for the identification of recombinational exchanges, the maximum chi-squared test that can be used to identify recombination cut-points, the homoplasy test, and the index of association. The test for selection is determination of d_N/d_S ratios.

The program is available free for download from the MLST web-site (http://mlst.zoo.ox.ac.uk).

3.2. MEGA

The Molecular Evolutionary Genetics Analysis (MEGA) program is used for comparative analyses of nucleotide or amino acid sequence data. A recently updated and improved version of the program for 32-bit Windows operating systems (MEGA2) is available free for download for use in research and education from http://www.megasoftware.net, as is the earlier MEGA version 1.02 for DOS. The tests and analyses performed in MEGA2 include: data summary; evolutionary distance estimation; phylogenetic reconstruction and tests.

3.2.1. Data Summary

The aligned sequences can be viewed using the Data Explorer option. Variable (or conserved) sites in the sequence can be identified and basic sequence statistics such as nucleotide composition, nucleotide pair frequencies, and codon usage can be calculated.

3.2.2. Distance Estimation

Many of the widely used estimates of evolutionary distance between sequences can be determined in MEGA. Included are a range of substitution models, from calculation of the proportion of nucleotide or amino acid differences between sequences (*p*-distance) to the multi-parameter Tamura-Nei model. Furthermore, there are several models included that can be used to calculate rates of synonymous and nonsynonymous substitution.

3.2.3. Phylogenetic Reconstruction and Tests

MEGA offers several tree-building methods including the NJ method, a distance based tree-building method ***(44)***, which searches for an estimate of the minimum amount of evolutionary change linking sequences, and UPGMA. Bootstrap-resampling analysis can also provide information about which groupings in a phylogeny are more robust.

3.3. Wisconsin Package

The Wisconsin Package Version 10.1 is a UNIX-based package produced by Genetics Computer Group (GCG) for the management and analysis of DNA and amino acid sequence data. Included in the package is SeqLab, an X Windows-based graphical user interface used for compiling, editing, and annotating multiple-sequence alignments, which can then be subject to evolutionary analyses. The nucleotide-sequence and protein-sequence databases GenBank, EMBL, SP-TREMBL, and SWISS-PROT can be accessed and sequences from these databases can be imported directly into SeqLab, as can locally stored sequence files. The sequence databases can also be interrogated using BLAST searching. As well as the calculation of basic sequence statistics, such as codon usage and base composition, there are programs included in SeqLab for sequence mapping, oligonucleotide primer design, and the prediction of secondary structure in nucleic acid and peptide sequences. The evolutionary analyses performed in SeqLab on aligned sequences include: several models for distance estimation; a GCG interface to the comprehensive tree-searching, manipulation, and display options in PAUP (Phylogenetic Analysis Using Parsimony: *see* Appendix); and calculation of synonymous and nonsynonymous substitution rates.

Further information about system requirements and cost of the Wisconsin Package can be found at http://www.gcg.com/products/wis-package.html.

4. Notes

1. Phylogenetic analysis software. There are additional programs available for gene-sequence analysis that are worthy of mention.

   PHYLIP (Phylogeny Inference Package): PHYLIP is a suite of programs used to infer evolutionary trees from DNA sequence, amino acid sequences, gene-frequency data, and distance matrices. The package has been written for Windows, DOS, PowerMac, and 68k Macintosh systems and can be downloaded free from http://evolution.genetics.washington.edu/phylip.html.

   PAUP* (Phylogenetic Analysis Using Phylogeny): This phylogenetic analysis software is available for Macintosh, DOS, UNIX, and Windows operating systems. Further details and information about ordering the program can be found at http://www.lms.si.edu/PAUP/.
2. Useful Web-sites:

   http://phylogeny.arizona.edu/tree/programs/programs.html: information about a large number of phylogenetic analysis packages.

   http://evolve.zoo.ox.ac.uk: sequence analysis programs and useful links.

   http://grinch.zoo.ox.ac.uk/RAP_links.html: lists programs that can be used for detecting and analysing recombination.

   http://taxonomy.zoology.gla.ac.uk/rod/rod.html: includes programs for displaying and comparing phylogenetic trees.

References

1. Hillis, D. M., Moritz, C., and Mable, B.K. (1996) *Molecular Systematics*. Sinauer Associates, Sunderland, MA.
2. Li, W.-H. (1997) *Molecular Evolution*. Sinauer Associates, Sunderland, MA.
3. Page, R. D. M. and Holmes, E. C. (1998) *Molecular Evolution: A Phylogenetic Approach*. Blackwell Science Inc., Oxford, UK.
4. Maynard Smith, J., Smith, N. H., O'Rourke, M., and Spratt, B.G. (1993) How clonal are bacteria? *Proc. Natl. Acad. Sci. USA* **90,** 4384–4388.
5. Maynard Smith, J. (1995) Do bacteria have population genetics?, in *Population Genetics of Bacteria* (Baumberg, S., Young, J. P. W., Wellington, E. M. H., and Saunders, J. R., eds.), Cambridge University Press, Cambridge, UK, pp. 1–12.
6. Maiden, M. C. J. and Feavers, I. M. (1995) Population genetics and global epidemiology of the human pathogen *Neisseria meningitidis*, in *Population Genetics of Bacteria* (Baumberg, S., Young, J. P. W., Wellington, E. M. H., and Saunders, J. R., eds.), Cambridge University Press, Cambridge, UK, pp. 269–293.
7. Selander, R. K., Caugant, D. A., Ochman, H., Musser, J. M., Gilmour, M. N., and Whittam, T. S. (1986) Methods of multilocus enzyme electrophoresis for bacterial population genetics and systematics. *Appl. Environ. Microbiol.* **51,** 837–884.
8. Achtman, M. and Hakenbeck, R. (1992) Recent developments regarding the evolution of pathogenic bacteria, in *Molecular Biology of Bacterial Infection: Current Status and Future Perspectives* (Hormaeche, C., Penn, C. W., and Smyth, C. J., eds.), Cambridge University Press, Cambridge, UK, pp. 13–31.
9. Ochman, H., Lawrence, J. G., and Groisman, E.A. (2000) Lateral gene transfer and the nature of bacterial innovation. *Nature* **405,** 299–304.
10. Feil, E. J., Maiden, M. C. J., Achtman, M., and Spratt, B. G. (1999) The relative contribution of recombination and mutation to the divergence of clones of *Neisseria meningitidis*. *Mol. Biol. Evol.* **16,** 1496–1502.
11. Spratt, B. G. and Maiden, M. C. (1999) Bacterial population genetics, evolution and epidemiology. *Proc. R. Soc. Lond. B Biol. Sci.* **354,** 701–710.
12. Achtman, M. (1990) Molecular epidemiology of epidemic bacterial meningitis. *Rev. Med. Microbiol.* **1,** 29–38.
13. Olyhoek, T., Crowe, B. A., and Achtman, M. (1987) Clonal Population Structure of *Neisseria meningitidis* Serogroup A Isolated from Epidemics and pandemics Between 1915 and 1983. *Rev. Infect. Dis* **9,** 665–682.
14. Wang, J.-F., Caugant, D. A., Li, X., Hu, X., Poolman, J. T., Crowe, B. A., and Achtman, M. (1992) Clonal and antigenic analysis of serogroup A *Neisseria meningitidis* with particular reference to epidemiological features of epidemic meningitis in China. *Infect. Immun.* **60,** 5267–5282.
15. Caugant, D. A., Froholm, L. O., Bovre, K., Holten, E., Frasch, C. E., Mocca, L. F., et al. (1986) Intercontinental spread of a genetically distinctive complex of clones of *Neisseria meningitidis* causing epidemic disease. *Proc. Natl. Acad. Sci. USA* **83,** 4927–4931.
16. Caugant, D. A., Mocca, L. F., Frasch, C. E., Froholm, L. O., Zollinger, W. D., and Selander, R. K. (1987) Genetic structure of *Neisseria meningitidis* populations in

relation to serogroup, serotype, and outer membrane protein pattern. *J. Bacteriol.* **169,** 2781–2792.

17. Maiden, M. C. J., Bygraves, J. A., Feil, E., Morelli, G., Russell, J. E., Urwin, R., et al. (1998) Multilocus sequence typing: a portable approach to the identification of clones within populations of pathogenic microorganisms. *Proc. Natl. Acad. Sci. USA* **95,** 3140–3145.
18. Feavers, I. M., Gray, S. J., Urwin, R., Russell, J. E., Bygraves, J. A., Kaczmarski, E. B., and Maiden, M. C. J. (1999) Multilocus sequence typing and antigen gene sequencing in the investigation of a meningococcal disease outbreak. *J. Clin. Microbiol.* **37,** 3883–3887.
19. Bygraves, J. A., Urwin, R., Fox, A. J., Gray, S. J., Russell, J. E., Feavers, I. M., and Maiden, M. C. J. (1999) Population genetic and evolutionary approaches to the analysis of *Neisseria meningitidis* isolates belonging to the ET-5 complex. *J. Bacteriol.* **181,** 5551–5556.
20. Jolley, K. A., Kalmusova, J., Feil, E. J., Gupta, S., Musilek, M., Kriz, P., and Maiden, M. C. J. (2000) Carried meningococci in the Czech Republic: a diverse recombining population. *J. Clin. Microbiol.* **38,** 4492–4498.
21. Caugant, D. A., Froholm, L. O., Bovre, K., Holten, E., Frasch, C. E., Mocca, L. F., et al. (1987) Intercontinental spread of *Neisseria meningitidis* clones of the ET-5 complex. *Antonie van Leeuwenhoek J. Microbiol.* **53,** 389–394.
22. Wang, J.-F., Caugant, D. A., Morelli, G., Koumaré, B., and Achtman, M. (1993) Antigenic and epidemiological properties of the ET-37 complex of *Neisseria meningitidis*. *J. Infect. Dis.* **167,** 1320–1329.
23. Achtman, M. (1994) Clonal spread of serogroup A meningococci. A paradigm for the analysis of microevolution in bacteria. *Mol. Microbiol.* **11,** 15–22.
24. Feil, E., Zhou, J., Maynard Smith, J., and Spratt, B. G. (1996) A comparison of the nucleotide sequences of the *adk* and *recA* genes of pathogenic and commensal *Neisseria* species: evidence for extensive interspecies recombination within *adk*. *J. Mol. Evol.* **43,** 631–640.
25. Vazquez, J., Berron, S., O'Rourke, M., Carpenter, G., Feil, E., Smith, N. H., and Spratt, B. G. (1995) Interspecies recombination in nature: a meningococcus that has acquired a gonococcal PIB porin. *Mol. Microbiol.* **15,** 1001–1007.
26. Bash, M. C., Lesiak, K. B., Banks, S. D., and Frasch, C. E. (1995) Analysis of *Neisseria meningitidis* class 3 outer membrane protein gene variable regions and type identification using genetic techniques. *Infect. Immun.* **63,** 1484–1490.
27. Holmes, E. C., Urwin, R., and Maiden, M. C. J. (1999) The influence of recombination on the population structure and evolution of the human pathogen *Neisseria meningitidis*. *Mol. Biol. Evol.* **16,** 741–749.
28. Bandelt, H. J. and Dress, A. W. (1992) Split decomposition: a new and useful approach to phylogenetic analysis of distance data. *Mol. Phylogenet. Evol.* **1,** 242–252.
29. Huson, D. H. (1998) SplitsTree: a program for analysing and visualising evolutionary data. *Bioinformatics* **14,** 68–73.

30. Maynard Smith, J. (1992) Analysing the mosaic structure of genes. *J. Mol. Evol.* **34,** 126–129.
31. Spratt, B. G., Bowler, L. D., Zhang, Q. Y., Zhou, J., and Smith, J. M. (1992) Role of interspecies transfer of chromosomal genes in the evolution of penicillin resistance in pathogenic and commensal *Neisseria* species. *J. Mol. Evol.* **34,** 115–125.
32. Urwin, R. (1998) *Variation in Meningococcal PorB Proteins.* University of Staffordshire, Stoke-on-Trent, UK.
33. Spratt, B. G., Smith, N. H., Zhou, J., O'Rourke, M., and Feil, E. (1995) The population genetics of the pathogenic *Neisseria*, in *Population Genetics of Bacteria* (Baumberg, S., Young, J. P. W., Wellington, E. M. H., and Saunders, J. R., eds.), Cambridge University Press, Cambridge, UK, pp. 143–160.
34. Maynard Smith, J. and Smith, N. H. (1998) Detecting recombination from gene trees. *Mol. Biol. Evol.* **15,** 590–599.
35. Maynard Smith, J. (1994) Estimating selection by comparing synonymous and substitutional changes. *J. Mol. Evol.* **39,** 123–128.
36. Bandelt, H.-J. and Dress, A. (1992) A canonical decomposition theory for metrics on a finite set. *Adv. Math.* **92,** 47–105.
37. Maddison, D. R., Swofford, D. L., and Maddison, W. P. (1997) Nexus: An extensible file format for systematic information. *System. Biol.* **46,** 590–621.
38. Sneath, P. H. A. and Sokal, R. R. (1973) *Numerical Taxonomy.* Freeman, San Francisco.
39. Grassly, N. C. and Holmes, E. C. (1997) A likelihood method for the detection of selection and recombination using nucleotide sequences. *Mol. Biol. Evol.* **14,** 239–247.
40. Sawyer, S. (1989) Statistical tests for detecting gene conversion. *Mol. Biol. Evol.* **6,** 526–538.
41. Drouin, G., Prat, F., Ell, M., and Clarke, G. D. B. (1999) Detecting and characterizing gene conversions between multigene family members. *Mol. Biol. Evol.* **16,** 1369–1390.
42. Nei, M. and Gojobori, T. (1986) Simple methods for estimating the numbers of synonymous and nonsynonymous nucleotide substitutions. *Mol. Biol. Evol.* **3,** 418–426.
43. Kumar, S., Tamura, K., and Nei, M. (1994) MEGA: molecular evolutionary genetics analysis software for microcomputers. *Comput. Appl. Biosci.* **10,** 189–191.
44. Saitou, N. and Nei, M. (1987) The neighbor-joining method: a new method for reconstructing phylogenetic trees. *Mol. Biol. Evol.* **4,** 406–425.

24

Clinical Studies

An Overview

F. Andrew I. Riordan and Andrew J. Pollard

1. Introduction

Disease caused by *Neisseria meningitidis* is a worldwide problem *(1)*. Epidemics of meningococcal disease regularly occur in the "meningitis belt" of sub-Saharan Africa and in Asia *(2–5)* and high or increasing levels of endemic meningococcal disease have been reported recently in the UK *(6)*, New Zealand *(7)*, Cuba *(8)*, Brazil *(9)*, Norway *(10)*, and the Pacific Northwest of the United States *(11)*. Meningococcal disease predominantly affects children and has a high mortality, which has remained unchanged for 30 years, despite advances in antibiotics and intensive care *(12)*. Efforts have therefore been made to understand the pathophysiology of the disease and use this knowledge to improve treatment and develop novel therapies.

This chapter precedes a series of chapters that discuss clinical measurements in meningococcal infection including disease severity using clinical scoring systems, endotoxin and cytokine levels, examination of the coagulation cascade, and the conduct of trials of new therapies. The aim of this chapter is to describe the clinical setting in which these measurements are undertaken and to provide a brief overview of the background to the pathophysiology of meningococcal meningitis and septic shock.

2. Epidemiology of Meningococcal disease

The incidence of meningococcal disease varies with age, location, and season.

2.1. Age Distribution and Strain Differences

In the industrialized countries during nonepidemic conditions, meningococcal disease is most common in pre-school children *(1)*. However the case-

From: *Methods in Molecular Medicine, vol. 67: Meningococcal Disease: Methods and Protocols*
Edited by: A. J. Pollard and M. C. J. Maiden © Humana Press Inc., Totowa, NJ

fatality ratio is highest in teenagers with serogroup C disease *(13)*, particularly where ET-37 complex organisms predominate, as these organisms are associated with higher fatality rates *(14)*. Immunity to most strains of meningococci is probably conferred by bactericidal antibodies, susceptibility to the disease being inversely proportional to the level of antibody *(15)*. However, it is not certain if the primary mechanism of protection against serogroup B meningococci is complement-mediated bacterial lysis. At birth, neonates have high levels of anti-meningococcal antibodies, acquired transplacentally. Antibody levels fall during the first 3 mo of life, making the young infant particularly at risk, the peak attack rate being 7 mo *(16)*. During childhood, antibodies are stimulated by carriage of the meningococcus in the nasopharynx, but only 2% of children aged 1–4 yr carry meningococci, thus children under 4 are most susceptible to meningococcal disease.

Different strains may affect different age groups, however. Only 20% of group A infections occur in children under 4 in the northern hemisphere *(12)*. Group C disease is less common than group B in infants, but causes many of the cases in teenagers and almost all of the outbreaks of disease in this age group *(17)*. A majority of the cases of Group Y disease in the US affect adults and particularly the elderly *(18)*. Furthermore, the age of children with meningococcal disease shifts upwards at the start of an epidemic *(19)*.

The prevalence of meningococcal disease in children of different ages thus depends on the prevailing serogroups and probably serotypes, on population immunity (endemic or epidemic conditions) and other social factors.

2.2. Geographical Distribution

Meningococcal disease is known on all continents with 500,000 cases occurring globally every year *(20)* and attack rates of 1–20 per 100,000 in most developed countries. The classical epidemic area is the Subsaharan meningitis belt of Africa *(5)*, where the estimated annual incidence is 70 cases per 100,000 persons and may rise to as high as 1000/100,000 in an epidemic year *(1)*. There is probably no other comparable epidemic area, but large epidemics of meningococcal disease have occurred in practically all areas of the world.

2.3. Seasonal Variation

In the meningitis belt of Africa, epidemics start at the end of the hot, dry season and end abruptly with the onset of the rains *(5)*. Conversely the highest incidence of meningococcal disease in temperate climates is in winter, the first 3 mo of the year *(12)*. This may reflect more overcrowding, close personal contact, and intercurrent infections during the winter months. Season does not appear to affect the number of meningococcal carriers, but it may affect the carrier-to-case ratio *(21)*.

The likelihood of certain groups developing meningococcal disease can be influenced by their age, season, geographical location, exposure to tobacco smoke, recent viral infection, overcrowding, and the prevailing organism. Mortality may also be affected by these factors. However, in most people the meningococcus colonizes the nasopharynx and is eliminated after a few weeks or months with no ill effects. In a small number of individuals, an invasive infection develops that can kill them in a matter of hours.

3. Spectrum of Disease

3.1. Nasopharyngeal Colonization

Humans are the only natural hosts for the meningococcus and thus the human nasopharynx acts as a reservoir for the organism, which is passed on by droplet spread during coughing, sneezing, kissing, and so on. Airborne organisms are able to adhere to the nasopharyngeal epithelium by means of pili *(22)* and other surface structures *(23)* and establish colonies *(24)*. Some of the mechanisms for studying host-pathogen interactions on the nasopharyngeal mucosa are discussed in Chapters 34 and 35. The host begins developing antibodies against meningococci within 7–10 d of colonization. Invasive disease, if it occurs, usually does so within 10 d of acquisition of the organism *(25)*.

Rates of carriage vary within populations. Carriage is low in young children and the elderly and peaks at 15–20 yr of age *(26)*. Carriage can be influenced by secretor status *(27)* or smoking *(28)*. However the rate of infection is not related to the carriage rate *(29)*, with a low carriage rate of invasive strains found even during outbreaks *(30)*. The development of meningococcal disease depends on both the hosts' resistance and the virulence of the organism *(31)*.

3.2. Invasion of the Nasopharyngeal Epithelium

Meningococcal disease mostly affects previously healthy people. Those with deficiencies of complement C5-9 or properdin *(32)* are particularly susceptible to the disease, but these patients are in the minority. Polymorphisms in the genes for the plasma opsonins that activate complement (mannose-binding lectin) may also increase susceptibility to meningococcal disease *(33)*. Recent Influenza A or other respiratory infections may pre-dispose individuals to meningococcal disease *(34–36)*. Invasive disease is also more likely in those exposed to passive smoking *(37)* and in those of lower socioeconomic status *(38)*.

Once meningococci have invaded through the mucosal barrier and gained access to the blood stream, they may cause a variety of infections. Rarely, they may remain within the circulation and cause little systemic effect (occult and benign meningococcaemia). More often they cause systemic inflammation (septicemia), but mostly they seed to parts of the body and cause local infection (meningitis, arthritis, etc.). The highest mortality is in those who present with a predominant picture of septicemia ***(39–41)*** and amongst these patients, polymorphisms in the tumor necrosis factor (TNF)-α promoter region are associated with a worse outcome ***(42)***.

3.3. Local Infection

The most common local infection is meningitis. Meningococci gain entry to the cerebrospinal fluid (CSF) from the blood stream, probably via the choroid plexus ***(43)***. Methods used in the study of central nervous system (CNS) invasion by meningococci are described in Chapter 36. The clinical presentation of meningococcal meningitis is similar to other forms of bacterial meningitis, with fever, irritability, vomiting, headache, and neck stiffness. Occasionally meningoencephalitis with a rapidly deteriorating conscious level is present. Without antibiotic treatment, this infection is invariably fatal; however, mortality with antibiotic treatment is only 2–10% ***(1)***.

Meningococci may also cause pneumonia, arthritis, opthalmitis, or pericarditis ***(1)***; these other focal infections are rare and mortality is low.

3.4. Septicemia

Septicemia is the presentation with the highest mortality as a result of cardiovascular shock ***(41)***. A rash occurs in over 60% of cases ***(44)*** that may be maculopapular ***(45)***, but the hallmark of meningococcal septicemia is a petechial or purpuric rash, with the larger lesions being seen in those with the most severe disease ***(46)***. The highest mortality in septicemia is in those with shock.

3.5. Meningitis Plus Septicemia

Despite the classification into either meningitis or septicemia ***(47)***, there is a marked overlap between the two clinical presentations. Many children with "meningitis" have the petechial rash of septicemia and/or positive blood cultures. This group have clinical features of both meningitis and septicemia and constitute the largest clinical group. Mortality in these individuals falls between that of meningitis alone and septicemia alone ***(41)***.

3.6. Septic Shock

Understanding the pathological mechanisms that lead to septic shock, may suggest ways in which mortality could be decreased. In septic shock there is endothelial damage and capillary leak, intravascular thrombosis ***(48)***, abnormal vascular tone, and myocardial dysfunction ***(49)***. These processes lead to decreased systemic and cutaneous perfusion, focal thrombosis, and tissue edema, which can cause multi-organ failure and shock ***(50)***.

4. Pathophysiology of Meningococcal Septic Shock

The outer membrane of the meningococcus contains and releases endotoxin (lipopolysaccharide or LPS) into the bloodstream continuously during growth. The endotoxin is contained in "blebs" of outer membrane and in the bacterial outer membrane from which the blebs are released. Endotoxin is the primary bacterial mediator of Gram-negative sepsis. It triggers a cascade of events that ultimately produce the clinical features of meningococcal septic shock. High levels of meningococcal endotoxin are found in severe meningococcal disease and levels correlate strongly with mortality ***(51)***. Measurement of endotoxin levels in clinical specimens is described in Chapter 25 and isolation of purified meningococcal LPS is described in Chapter 26. It is conceivable that those with high levels of plasma endotoxin may benefit from anti-endotoxin therapies. It has become clear that host-derived factors (cytokines) are responsible for the progression of septic shock ***(52)***.

4.1. Cytokines

Cytokines are low molecular weight glycoproteins. The pro-inflammatory cytokines (Interleukin [IL]-1, TNF, IL-8, Interferon-γ [IFN-γ]) promote inflammation. Their production is blocked by the regulatory cytokines (IL-4, IL-10, transforming growth factor β [TGF-β]) ***(53)*** or by inhibitors IL-1ra ***(53)***, and soluble TNF receptors ***(54)***.

LPS (endotoxin) may be the most important stimulus of inflammation in meningococcal disease (*see* **Fig. 1**) ***(55–60)***. The binding of LPS molecule to CD14 on macrophages induces the release of TNF-α and IL-1, which in turn induce the release of IL-6 and IL-8 and other cytokines, and upregulate the expression of adhesion molecules including endothelial ICAM-1, allowing neutrophil adherence, and together they mediate the clinical features of sepsis ***(53,61,62)***. At the same time, anti-inflammatory mediators (IL-4, IL-10, PGE2, sTNFR, and IL-1ra) are released and presumably modulate the inflammatory response ***(63–65)***. During acute infection with *N. meningitidis*, plasma levels of TNF-α, IL-6, IL-8, and IL-10 levels are similar in children, irrespective of age ***(66)***. Measurement of cytokines in meningococcal disease provides insight into the pathophysiology of the disease and is helpful in the evaluation of the response to new therapies (*see* Chapters 27 and 28).

In the acute response to invasive meningococcal disease, high levels of TNF-α, sTNFR, IL-1, IL-1ra, IL-1β, IL-6, IL-8, IL-10, and plasminogen activator inhibitor (PAI-1), leukaemia inhibitory factor ***(67)*** are detectable in blood and levels of most have been associated with either disease severity or fatality from the disease ***(66,68–80)***. Indeed, the balance between these cytokines and their antagonists may influence the outcome of meningococcal disease ***(68)***.

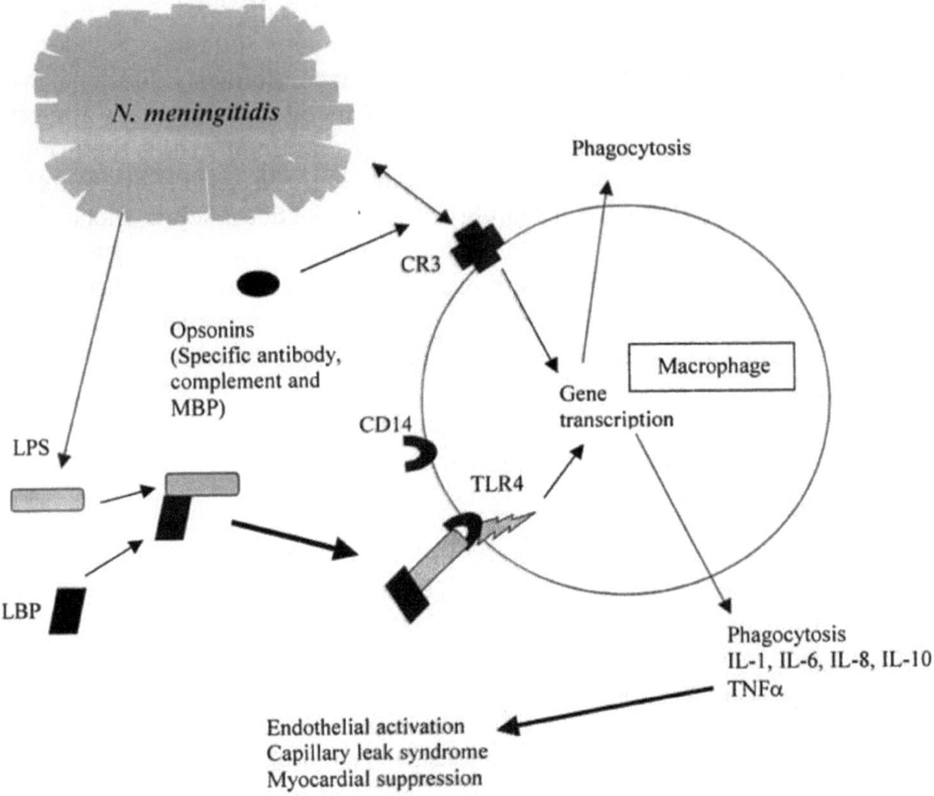

Fig. 1. Binding of LPS to macrophage surface receptors induces cytokine release and starts the roller-coaster inflammatory cascade to produce septic shock. CR3, complement receptor 3; LPS, lipopolysaccharide; TLR, Toll receptor; MBP, mannose-binding lectin.

Some suggest that excessive production of IL-10, an anti-inflammatory cytokine, may be associated with higher mortality ***(81)***. Studies of cytokine gene polymorphisms that may explain individual differences in susceptibility to meningococcal infection or severity of disease are discussed in Chapter 29.

4.2. Cytokines in Meningitis

The inflammatory cascade of cytokines also occurs within the subarachnoid space during meningitis *(73)*. However the systemic circulation and the subarachnoid space are functionally separate compartments with respect to the production and effects of these cytokines. High levels in CSF are not associated with death and do not cross into the bloodstream *(73)*.

5. Early Management

Death in meningococcal disease is usually from shock and occasionally from raised intracranial pressure. The priority in managing patients with this disease is early recognition and treatment to prevent progression to shock. Once shock is established, the clinical priority is aggressive replacement of intravascular volume and myocardial support.

With the increased understanding of the pathophysiology of septic shock, the leading cause of death in meningococcal disease, new forms of treatment may become available. However for these therapies to be effective, it is likely that they will need to be given early in the course of the disease. Decreasing the mortality from meningococcal disease will thus not only require new treatments, but also early recognition and appropriate treatment of cases and early identification of life-threatening disease that may benefit from novel therapies. Of course, vaccination is the most rational approach to reducing mortality from meningococcal disease and is reviewed in *(82)*.

5.1. Recognition by Parents

Parents of children with meningococcal disease may delay seeking medical advice because they do not recognize the severity of the illness ***(83)***. Parents thus require accurate and appropriate information about meningococcal disease. In contrast to classic signs of meningitis, the rash of septicemia is one of the most common reasons for seeking medical advice ***(84)*** in this patient group.

5.2. Recognition and Treatment in Primary Care

Prompt treatment requires doctors to recognize meningococcal disease in its early stages. The difficulty for primary-care doctors is to differentiate the two or three cases of meningococcal disease they may see in a lifetime, from the majority of febrile children with less serious illnesses ***(85)***.

General practitioners correctly diagnose meningococcal disease in 70–80% of the cases that they admit ***(85–88)***. However, around 50% of cases are seen by a doctor, but not sent for admission during the early stages of their illness ***(84,86)***, because the symptoms are nonspecific ***(89)***. A general practitioner is significantly more likely to make a diagnosis if specific signs such as neck stiffness or petechiae are present ***(86,88)***. However only 50% of cases have a hemorrhagic rash when seen by a general practitioner ***(88,89)***. If these signs are not recognized, the delay in diagnosis may contribute to a fatal outcome ***(90,91)***.

In the UK, all doctors are advised to consider giving parenteral penicillin in cases of suspected meningococcal disease before transfer to hospital ***(92)***. A meta-analysis of studies showed a significant benefit from pre-admission penicillin ***(93)***.

By contrast, a study from Denmark found a significantly higher mortality among those given early penicillin *(94)*. However, this study may have been flawed as the authors suggest that this increased mortality was because those with fulminant disease were most likely to receive penicillin. Data is not available to support this hypothesis, but this highlights the confounding variable of disease severity. The theoretical concern that pre-admission penicillin may cause a release of endotoxin leading to septic shock *(95)*, has not been found in clinical practice *(51)* and these data support the use of pre-admission antibiotics *(96)*. In the many countries that have not adopted urgent community antibiotic administration at the first medical contact, it is possible that a reduction in mortality might occur if this policy were now to be introduced.

5.3. Diagnosis in Hospital

The diagnosis of meningococcal disease, and thus appropriate treatment, is delayed following admission to hospital in 8–12% of cases *(97,98)* and in 15–20% of those who die *(90,91)*. These delays in treatment result from diagnostic uncertainty or for no obvious reason *(90,99)*.

5.4. Severity Assessment

Once the child is admitted to hospital, mortality may be decreased by appropriate early management. This requires early recognition of the signs of shock and/or raised intracranial pressure, as outlined in **Fig. 2**. Various clinical scores have been developed as an aid to the assessment of disease severity and may allow individuals with life-threatening disease to be recognized and given early optimal management. These scores are also essential tools in the evaluation of new therapies where the recording of mortality data in isolation is a blunt outcome measure.

5.4.1. Severity Scores

To be clinically useful, disease-severity scores should be simple, made up from rapidly available data, and easy to compute. Scoring systems are reviewed

---

Fig. 2. *(opposite page)* Algorithm describing initial emergency management of meningococcal disease. Copies of this algorithm are available in poster and leaflet format from Meningitis Research Foundation (MRF; info@meningitis.org), a registered UK-based charity that supports an international programme of independently peer-reviewed research into the prevention, detection, and treatment of meningitis and septicemia through public donations. MRF also provides information for the public and health professionals, runs medical and scientific meetings, and provides support to people affected by meningitis and septicemia.

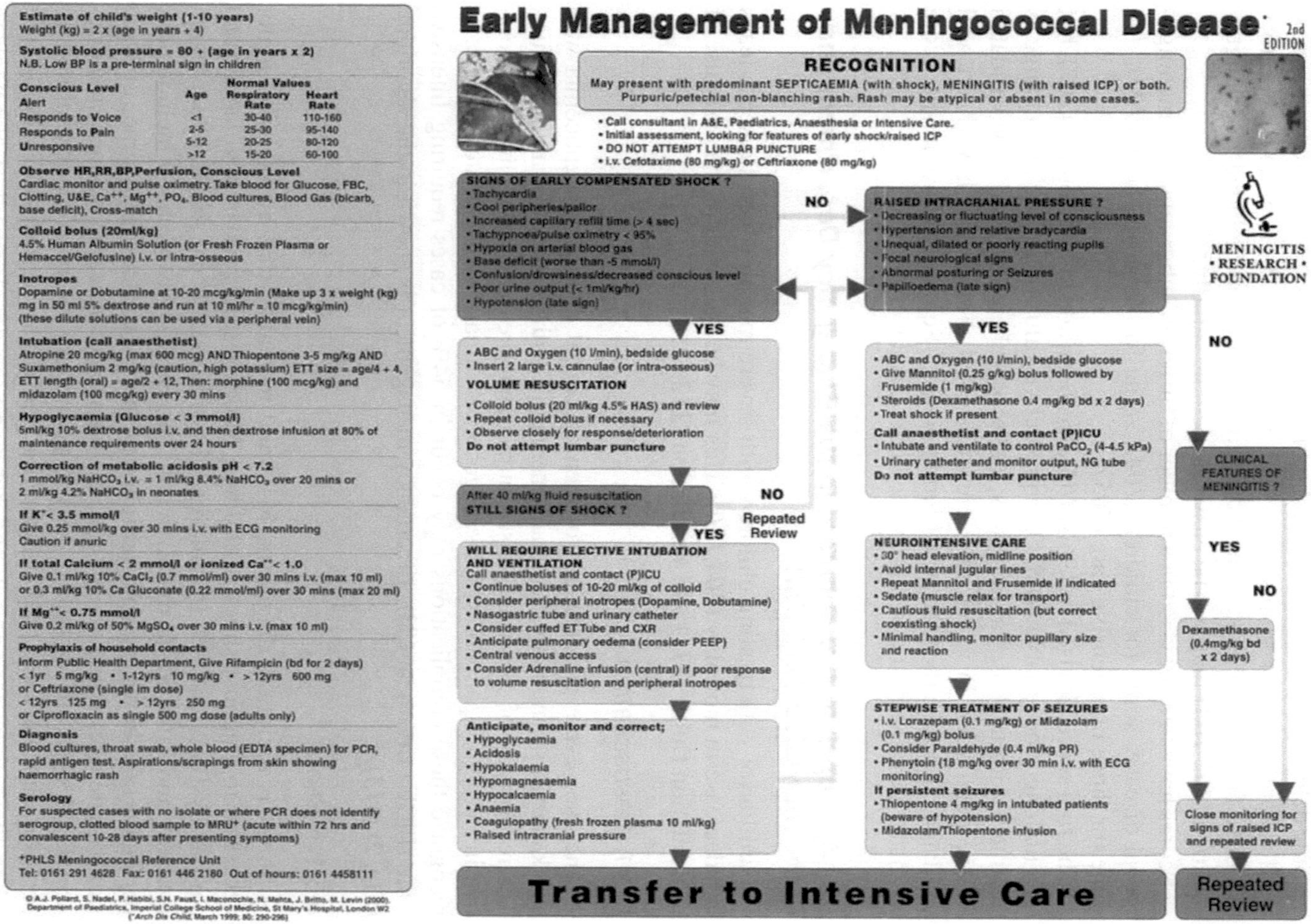
Estimate of child's weight (1-10 years)
Weight (kg) = 2 x (age in years + 4)
Systolic blood pressure = 80 + (age in years x 2)
N.B. Low BP is a pre-terminal sign in children
Conscious Level
Alert
Responds to Voice
Responds to Pain
Unresponsive
Normal Values
Age | Respiratory Rate | Heart Rate
<1 | 30-40 | 110-160
2-5 | 25-30 | 95-140
5-12 | 20-25 | 80-120
>12 | 15-20 | 60-100
Observe HR,RR,BP,Perfusion, Conscious Level
Cardiac monitor and pulse oximetry. Take blood for Glucose, FBC, Clotting, U&E, Ca++, Mg++, PO4, Blood cultures, Blood Gas (bicarb, base deficit), Cross-match
Colloid bolus (20ml/kg)
4.5% Human Albumin Solution (or Fresh Frozen Plasma or Hemaccel/Gelofusine) i.v. or intra-osseous
Inotropes
Dopamine or Dobutamine at 10-20 mcg/kg/min (Make up 3 x weight (kg) mg in 50 ml 5% dextrose and run at 10 ml/hr = 10 mcg/kg/min) (these dilute solutions can be used via a peripheral vein)
Intubation (call anaesthetist)
Atropine 20 mcg/kg (max 600 mcg) AND Thiopentone 3-5 mg/kg AND Suxamethonium 2 mg/kg (caution, high potassium) ETT size = age/4 + 4, ETT length (oral) = age/2 + 12, Then: morphine (100 mcg/kg) and midazolam (100 mcg/kg) every 30 mins
Hypoglycaemia (Glucose < 3 mmol/l)
5ml/kg 10% dextrose bolus i.v. and then dextrose infusion at 80% of maintenance requirements over 24 hours
Correction of metabolic acidosis pH < 7.2
1 mmol/kg NaHCO3 i.v. = 1 ml/kg 8.4% NaHCO3 over 20 mins or 2 ml/kg 4.2% NaHCO3 in neonates
If K+ < 3.5 mmol/l
Give 0.25 mmol/kg over 30 mins i.v. with ECG monitoring
Caution if anuric
If total Calcium < 2 mmol/l or ionized Ca++ < 1.0
Give 0.1 ml/kg 10% CaCl2 (0.7 mmol/ml) over 30 mins i.v. (max 10 ml) or 0.3 ml/kg 10% Ca Gluconate (0.22 mmol/ml) over 30 mins (max 20 ml)
If Mg++ < 0.75 mmol/l
Give 0.2 ml/kg of 50% MgSO4 over 30 mins i.v. (max 10 ml)
Prophylaxis of household contacts
Inform Public Health Department, Give Rifampicin (bd for 2 days)
< 1yr 5 mg/kg • 1-12yrs 10 mg/kg • > 12yrs 600 mg
or Ceftriaxone (single im dose)
< 12yrs 125 mg • > 12yrs 250 mg
or Ciprofloxacin as single 500 mg dose (adults only)
Diagnosis
Blood cultures, throat swab, whole blood (EDTA specimen) for PCR, rapid antigen test. Aspirations/scrapings from skin showing haemorrhagic rash
Serology
For suspected cases with no isolate or where PCR does not identify serogroup, clotted blood sample to MRU+ (acute within 72 hrs and convalescent 10-28 days after presenting symptoms)
+PHLS Meningococcal Reference Unit
Tel: 0161 291 4628 Fax: 0161 446 2180 Out of hours: 0161 4458111
© A.J. Pollard, S. Nadel, P. Habibi, S.N. Faust, I. Maconochie, N. Mehta, J. Britto, M. Levin (2000).
Department of Paediatrics, Imperial College School of Medicine, St Mary's Hospital, London W2
(*Arch Dis Child, March 1999; 80: 290-296)
Early Management of Meningococcal Disease* 2nd EDITION
RECOGNITION
May present with predominant SEPTICAEMIA (with shock), MENINGITIS (with raised ICP) or both.
Purpuric/petechial non-blanching rash. Rash may be atypical or absent in some cases.
• Call consultant in A&E, Paediatrics, Anaesthesia or Intensive Care.
• Initial assessment, looking for features of early shock/raised ICP
• DO NOT ATTEMPT LUMBAR PUNCTURE
• i.v. Cefotaxime (80 mg/kg) or Ceftriaxone (80 mg/kg)
MENINGITIS • RESEARCH • FOUNDATION
SIGNS OF EARLY COMPENSATED SHOCK ?
• Tachycardia
• Cool peripheries/pallor
• Increased capillary refill time (> 4 sec)
• Tachypnoea/pulse oximetry < 95%
• Hypoxia on arterial blood gas
• Base deficit (worse than -5 mmol/l)
• Confusion/drowsiness/decreased conscious level
• Poor urine output (< 1ml/kg/hr)
• Hypotension (late sign)
NO
RAISED INTRACRANIAL PRESSURE ?
• Decreasing or fluctuating level of consciousness
• Hypertension and relative bradycardia
• Unequal, dilated or poorly reacting pupils
• Focal neurological signs
• Abnormal posturing or Seizures
• Papilloedema (late sign)
NO
YES
• ABC and Oxygen (10 l/min), bedside glucose
• Insert 2 large i.v. cannulae (or intra-osseous)
VOLUME RESUSCITATION
• Colloid bolus (20 ml/kg 4.5% HAS) and review
• Repeat colloid bolus if necessary
• Observe closely for response/deterioration
Do not attempt lumbar puncture
YES
• ABC and Oxygen (10 l/min), bedside glucose
• Give Mannitol (0.25 g/kg) bolus followed by Frusemide (1 mg/kg)
• Steroids (Dexamethasone 0.4 mg/kg bd x 2 days)
• Treat shock if present
Call anaesthetist and contact (P)ICU
• Intubate and ventilate to control PaCO2 (4-4.5 kPa)
• Urinary catheter and monitor output, NG tube
Do not attempt lumbar puncture
CLINICAL FEATURES OF MENINGITIS ?
After 40 ml/kg fluid resuscitation
STILL SIGNS OF SHOCK ?
NO
Repeated Review
YES
WILL REQUIRE ELECTIVE INTUBATION AND VENTILATION
Call anaesthetist and contact (P)ICU
• Continue boluses of 10-20 ml/kg of colloid
• Consider peripheral inotropes (Dopamine, Dobutamine)
• Nasogastric tube and urinary catheter
• Consider cuffed ET Tube and CXR
• Anticipate pulmonary oedema (consider PEEP)
• Central venous access
• Consider Adrenaline infusion (central) if poor response to volume resuscitation and peripheral inotropes
NEUROINTENSIVE CARE
• 30° head elevation, midline position
• Avoid internal jugular lines
• Repeat Mannitol and Frusemide if indicated
• Sedate (muscle relax for transport)
• Cautious fluid resuscitation (but correct coexisting shock)
• Minimal handling, monitor pupillary size and reaction
YES
NO
Dexamethasone (0.4mg/kg bd x 2 days)
Anticipate, monitor and correct;
• Hypoglycaemia
• Acidosis
• Hypokalaemia
• Hypomagnesaemia
• Hypocalcaemia
• Anaemia
• Coagulopathy (fresh frozen plasma 10 ml/kg)
• Raised intracranial pressure
STEPWISE TREATMENT OF SEIZURES
• i.v. Lorazepam (0.1 mg/kg) or Midazolam (0.1 mg/kg) bolus
• Consider Paraldehyde (0.4 ml/kg PR)
• Phenytoin (18 mg/kg over 30 min i.v. with ECG monitoring)
If persistent seizures
• Thiopentone 4 mg/kg in intubated patients (beware of hypotension)
• Midazolam/Thiopentone infusion
Close monitoring for signs of raised ICP and repeated review
Transfer to Intensive Care
Repeated Review

in some detail in Chapter 24. Clinical scores ***(100,101)*** are likely to be the most rapidly applied. Most scores consist of a mixture of clinical and laboratory features. Those scores requiring laboratory data to be included in a lengthy equation ***(102,103)*** may not be easy to calculate rapidly.

Scores have been devised in a number of different subgroups with meningococcal disease, some for children ***(104)***, some for those in shock ***(102)***, and some for those on intensive care ***(105)***.

The first score, devised in 1966 ***(106)***, has been added to by others ***(107)***, but may no longer be reliable ***(108)***. The predictive value of a score may change as treatment within a hospital improves, and scores therefore need to be validated for the population in which they are to be used. Few scores have been well validated, although the Glasgow Meningococcal Septicemia Prognostic Score seems to have the best performance characteristics ***(109)***.

5.5. Appropriate Management in the Emergency Department and in the Intensive Care Unit

Familiarity with treating children with severe meningococcal disease leads to a decrease in mortality ***(104,110)***. This may be the result of the early use of resuscitation fluids ***(111)*** and ventilation ***(112)***.

5.5.1. Resuscitation

The two severe presentations of meningococcal disease are septicemia with shock and, less commonly, fulminant meningitis with raised intracranial pressure. The recognition of shock and raised intracranial pressure is the clinical imperative in managing patients with meningococcal disease. Unfortunately, failure to recognize these complications may occur in 54% of cases requiring Intensive Care (PICU) treatment ***(83)***. Emergency management is shown in the algorithm (**Fig. 2**) ***(113)***.

5.5.1.1. Shock

Shock is a clinical diagnosis. It is vital to realize that hypotension is not necessary to diagnose shock in children. Shock results from hypovolaemia and cardiac dysfunction ***(49)***. In children with meningococcal shock, hypotension is a late, and often the terminal, event. The early signs of shock include poor perfusion (as shown by cool peripheries, poor capillary refill time, or wide skin-core temperature gap, lactic acidosis), tachycardia, tachypnoea, and oliguria. Later signs are hypoxia (owing to pulmonary edema and poor pulmonary perfsion) and confusion (reduced cerebral perfusion). Resuscitation should start when these signs are present, and not await the development of hypotension (*see* **Fig. 2**).

Table 1
Symptoms and Signs of Cerebral Herniation

Feature	Comment
Glasgow Coma Score <8	
Abnormal pupil size and reaction	(Unilateral or bilateral)
Absent Doll's eye movements	
Abnormal tone	(Decerebrate/decorticate posturing, flaccidity)
Tonic posturing	
Respiratory abnormalities	(Hyperventilation, Cheyne-Stokes breathing, apnoea, respiratory arrest)
Papilloedema	(Rare, especially in infants)

Hypovolaemia is principally due to capillary leak and its correction may require infusion of several times the blood volume in replacement fluid. Failure to correct hypovolaemia is associated with increased mortality ***(49)***.

Rapid correction with 20–40 mL/kg of colloid is recommended as soon as the clinical diagnosis of shock is made ***(50,114)***. Human 4.5% albumin has been commonly used as the initial volume expander in pediatrics and remains the resuscitation fluid of choice. Although a recent meta-analysis has suggested the use of human albumin may increase mortality in critically ill patients ***(115)***, no studies of children with meningococcal sepsis were included. Indeed, claims of reduced mortality in meningococcal disease have been made against a background of increased use of albumin ***(116,117)*** and 4.5% albumin remains the recommended resuscitation fluid in many centers ***(117)***. Where there is an initial response to therapy, repeated reassessment is required as the response may be temporary, even after the appropriate antibiotic therapy, as capillary-leak syndrome and myocardial suppression may continue. If shock persists despite 40 mL/kg volume resuscitation then management should continue as outlined in **Fig. 2** and **Subheading 5.6.1.**

5.5.1.2. Raised Intracranial Pressure

Clinically significant raised intracranial pressure is an uncommon presenting feature of meningococcal disease. The symptoms and signs of raised intracranial pressure have a rapid onset (**Table 1**) and are particularly suggested by rapid progression to coma. Herniation, or coning, of the brain is the usually cause of death from meningococcal meningitis; it is commonly found at post-mortem and can occur in cases where a lumbar puncture has not been performed ***(118)***. Lumbar puncture should not be performed if there are any signs of impending cerebral herniation (*see* **Table 1**), because this may lead to, or exacerbate, coning and death. Cranial imaging will not identify most cases of meningitis with raised intracranial pressure ***(119–123)***, such that a normal computed tomography (CT) scan does not mean that it is safe to perform a lumbar puncture.

Patients with raised intracranial pressure need aggressive but careful correction of hypovolaemia, elective ventilation, and antibiotic treatment. In children with impending cerebral herniation, an infusion of mannitol (0.25–1 g/kg) may be life-saving and may be combined with furosemide. Because the diuresis caused by these treatments for raised intracranial pressure may exacerbate hypovlaemia, the management of the combination of raised intracranial pressure and septic shock in an individual is particularly challenging.

Neurointensive care should be instituted using 30° head-up positioning, head midline, minimal suction, deep sedation, and avoidance of hypercapnia. The use of hyperventilation to manage raised intracranial pressure is no longer acceptable ***(50,113)*** as the decrease in cerebral blood flow produced may reduce the oxygen delivery to critically dependant areas and current practice is to maintain normocapnia (4–4.5 Kpa).

Seizures should be controlled as these may further raise intracranial pressure. Acute seizures can be controlled with diazepam, while further seizure may be prevented by phenytoin or phenobarbitone ***(43)***. There are no studies showing proven benefit of measuring intracranial pressure in meningitis. Emergency management of raised intracranial pressure is outlined in **Fig. 2** ***(113)***.

5.6. Complications of Shock

5.6.1. Refractory Shock

Shock that persists despite correction of hypovolaemia has a poor prognosis. Children and adults with refractory shock may have different hemodynamic states requiring different treatments ***(124)***.

When there has been no response to volume replacement of 40 mL/kg, inotropes may be given. Peripheral venous or intra-osseous administration is often necessary, until central venous access is available. Dobutamine, dopamine, or adrenaline (epinephrine) may be used ***(50,113)***. Downregulation of adrenergic receptors occurs when large doses of inotropes are used and particularly after sustained use ***(125)***. The lowest possible dose of adrenaline (epinephrine) should therefore be used, although this is not a major consideration during initial resuscitation.

5.6.2. Respiratory Failure

Elective ventilation can improve outcome in septic shock and severe meningitis ***(112,126)***. It is recommended that intubation is performed if shock persists despite replacement of 40 mL/kg colloid in order to reduce the work of breathing and to control imminent pulmonary edema. Early problems with pulmonary edema and later the adult respiratory distress syndrome will require ventilatory support as well as careful fluid management.

5.6.3. Coagulopathy

The inflammatory response in meningococcal disease strips the anticoagulant lining of the epithelium ***(127)***. The released anticoagulant impairs clotting, but trombus formation occurs on the denuded epithelium. Both the coagulation and fibrinolytic systems are activated by LPS, cytokines, and other mediators released during meningococcal sepsis (*see* **Fig. 1**). Low levels of the natural inhibitors of coagulation—anti-thrombin III, Protein S, and Protein C—are found in meningococcal disease ***(128)***. These low levels are associated with poor outcome. High levels of the fibrinolytic inhibitor, PAI-1 also occur in meningococcal sepsis ***(129)*** and these high levels are also associated with poor outcome.

Attempts to correct this imbalance systemically or lessen its effect locally have been reported ***(130–132)*** and a recent trial of activated protein C replacement in adult sepsis is reported to have had promising results ***(132a)***. As with the cytokine network, manipulating one component of the complex coagulation cascade may not necessarily be beneficial.

Children who develop skin necrosis or limb ischemia after meningococcal septic shock have lower factor VII levels than those without these sequelae ***(133)***. This suggests that inhibition of the intrinsic pathway might decrease the need for skin grafts and amputations.

Combinations of heparin, anti-thrombin III, and fresh frozen plasma may improve survival in children with moderately severe meningococcal disease, but not fulminant disease ***(134)***. Further trials will be needed.

Evaluation of coagulation disturbances in meningococcal disease is described in Chapter 30.

5.6.4. Renal Failure

Renal failure may be managed by dialysis or hemofiltration.

5.6.5. Metabolic Problems

Low serum potassium, calcium, phosphate, and glucose are common in meningococcal disease. The hypokalemia is particularly striking in the face of acidosis and requires aggressive correction. These metabolic derangements may contribute to myocardial depression, and should be corrected (**Fig. 2**).

5.7. Novel Therapies

5.7.1. Corticosteroids

Steroids have been suggested as therapy in meningococcal disease for 3 reasons; 1) as replacement in adrenal insufficiency, 2) as an anti-inflammatory agent in septic shock, and 3) as an anti-inflammatory agent in meningitis *(135,136)*. There is little evidence to support their use in any of these situations.

5.7.2. Replacement Steroids

Low cortisol levels have been documented in some children with meningococcal disease, with lower levels seen in those who die *(137)*. However the interpretation of cortisol levels in these critically ill children may be complicated by a number of factors. Adrenal insufficiency may contribute to hypotension and steroid replacement is still often used in meningococcal septic shock *(50)*.

5.7.3. Corticosteroids in Meningococcal Septic Shock

Controlled trials did not show a significant reduction in mortality in adults with septic shock given steroids *(136,138)*. These trials did not include patients with meningococcal septic shock. No trials of high-dose steroids in meningococcal septic shock have been performed.

5.7.4. Cytokines and Anti-Endotoxin Therapy

The mortality from meningococcal septic shock has remained high despite conventional treatments *(12)*. This has stimulated research into novel methods of treatment, most aimed at decreasing the levels of endotoxin or the circulating inflammatory mediators.

As described earlier, although during in vitro experiments the effects of individual cytokines can be studied, a large array of cytokines are produced in meningococcal disease *(74)*. Because the pattern of cytokines in meningococcal disease is so complicated, attempts at improving the outcome by blocking just one cytokine may not be successful or even desirable. There is probably a critical balance between pro- and anti-inflammatory mediators that allows control of infection without severe cardiovascular compromise, and it is probably naïve to expect that monotherapy, at some point after the cascade has been activated, would be successful in such a complex process. Achieving the appropriate balance of mediators through use of multiple pharmacological agents may not be a realistic goal without a better understanding of the process. This has led to enthusiasm for removal of soluble mediators by plasmapheresis or hemofiltration *(139)* but this approach also remains unproven and could be detrimental and should be subject to controlled trials.

Despite initial enthusiasm for anti-endotoxin monoclonal antibodies (MAbs) that might block the inflammatory response, a number of clinical trials have failed to demonstrate benefit in clinical practice (reviewed in **refs.** ***140*** and ***141*** and Chapter 32), probably because the inflammatory cascade has already been activated by the time of enrollment of the patient, and because these antibodies have only weak affinities for lipid A. If there was an intrinsic problem with these MAbs, alternative antibodies with higher binding affinity or different specificity may be more successful and several are under development ***(140,141)***. An attractive alternative strategy is to induce anti-endotoxin antibodies through immunization in childhood and thus prevent LPS-mediated shock ***(140)***.

Although there are many exciting case reports and small uncontrolled series reporting novel therapies, none have yet been shown to be safe and effective in randomized controlled trials ***(140)*** as is discussed in detail in Chapter 32. One promising agent, bactericidal permeability increasing protein (BPI), has recently completed its first large-scale clinical trial. However, the Food and Drug Administration (FDA) was not satisfied with the data presented by the study group and has requested further phase III clinical trials before considering licensure ***(142)***. Mortality from meningococcal disease may also be decreasing in some regions, because of increasing familiarity with the disease and improved delivery of initial management ***(110)***.

6. Outcomes

6.1. Mortality

In children with meningococcal meningitis, mortality with antibiotic treatment is only 2% rising to 11% in those with meningitis and septicemia ***(41)***. The mortality from septicemia is 19%, and this increases to 40–50% if the patient is shocked ***(50)***. Lower mortality has been described in intensive care units that are familiar with the disease and where the local emergency departments have adopted aggressive resuscitation protocols for these patients ***(110)***.

6.2. Sequelae

Serious sequelae occur in 8.5% of survivors ***(143)***, and may occur more frequently with serogroup C disease compared to group B disease ***(13)***.

6.2.1. Meningitis

Following meningitis, patients may suffer sequelae such as sensorineural deafness (6.4%), psychomotor retardation (2.1%), and seizures (1.4%) ***(144)***, but these are uncommon compared with other forms of bacterial meningitis.

6.2.2. Septicemia

Sequelae following meningococcal septicemia result from thrombosis and reduced peripheral perfusion and include skin necrosis and peripheral ischemia. Survivors of septicemia may need limb amputations (3–4%) or skin grafting (5%) ***(44,145,146)***. This proportion increases to 14–39% of those with shock ***(139,147)***. Neurological and audiological sequelae can also occur in those who had septicemia without apparent meningitis ***(148,149)***.

7. Conclusion

The early management of patients with severe meningococcal disease is challenging even for the most experienced clinician, but it seems likely that an aggressive approach to this management can reduce mortality from the disease. Understanding the pathophysiology of septic shock may hold the key to the development of new therapies that will be active even in real-life clinical situations where the process is already well underway. The study of septic shock and its manipulation by new therapies requires measurement of the clinical process using disease scores and also quantitation of the molecules responsible for the process: bacterial products, cytokines, and coagulation-pathways mediators. A methodological approach to quantifying these is considered in the chapters that follow.

8. Appendix to Chapter 24

8.1. Cytokine Structure and Function

8.1.1. TNF-α

TNF-α is a 17 kDa homotrimer ***(150)*** that is encoded by a gene in the MHC on chromosome 6 ***(151)***. Many cell types can be induced to produce TNF-α in vitro but the major sources are monocytes and macrophages ***(152)***. The major stimulus to TNF-α release is LPS, but C5a, viral, parasitic, and fungal antigens, immune complexes, IL-1, IL-2, and TNF-α itself may all stimulate its release ***(151)***. LPS binds to CD14 (and other receptors) on macrophages causing macrophage activation and stimulating the release of TNF-α both in vivo and in vitro ***(153–155)***, although there is wide variation in responses between individuals ***(156)***. TNF-α release is mediated by interaction of LPS with the serum protein lipoprotein-binding protein (LBP) ***(157–161)***.

TNF-α is the key pro-inflammatory mediator. It induces release of IL-1, IL-6, IL-8, PGE2, and NO ***(73,151,162,163)*** and acts with them to mediate the features of sepsis including hypotension, fever, catecholamine release, and cortisol production ***(74,153)***.

TNF-α plays a central role in the physiology of Gram-negative sepsis. Certain polymorphisms in the promoter region of the TNF-α gene seem to be associated with death from meningococcal disease ***(42)*** and other forms of sepsis ***(164)***. High levels of TNF-α are found in meningococcal infection and correlate with fatal outcome from the disease ***(72)***. However, Westendorp et al. (1997) has suggested that low producers of TNF-α have an increased risk of fatal outcome from meningococcal infection ***(81)***, but this has been disputed ***(165)***. Contrary to Westendorp's findings, pre-treatment with rTNF-α protects animals from lethal sepsis with Gram-negative bacteria and knockout mice lacking TNF-α receptors are more susceptible to infection ***(166,167)***. Conversely, blockade of TNF-α using anti-TNF antibodies protects animals against experimental Gram-negative sepsis ***(168)***. Trials of rTNF-α receptors or anti-TNF antibodies or other anti-inflammatory agents in established sepsis in humans have failed to show a consistently beneficial effect ***(169–172)***.

8.1.2. TNF-β (Lymphotoxin)

The TNF-β gene is also located in the MHC on chromosome 6 and encodes a 25 kDa homotrimer ***(150)***. TNF-β is produced almost exclusively by CD4 or CD8 positive T cells following antigenic stimulation in the context of MHC class I or class II restriction ***(173)***. In vitro activities of TNF-β are similar to TNF-α, but TNF-β probably has less pro-inflammatory activity ***(151)***.

8.1.3. IL-12

IL-12 is a 70 kDa heterodimer of 2 subunits, p35 and p40, which are encoded by separate genes on chromosome 3 and 5, respectively ***(174)***. The two subunits are co-expressed to form IL-12 ***(175)***. IL-12 is produced by macrophages, and B cells ***(176)***. LPS and mycobacteria are potent stimuli for production in vitro ***(177)***, although IL-12 production does not seem to be induced by a wide range of other cytokines ***(177)***. However, production of IL-12 following LPS stimulation of human monocytes is enhanced by IFN-γ and inhibited by IL-4 and IL-10 ***(178)***. IL-12 activates NK cells and lymphokine-activated killer (LAK) cells and induces T cell and natural killer (NK) cell proliferation ***(179–182)***. IL-12 induces production of IFN-γ from protein-bound monocytes (PBMC)s and regulates induction of T_H1 cell activity by switching T_H2 cells to a T_H1 or Th0 phenotpye and T_H1 cells to a Th0 phenotype ***(183–186)***. IL-12 is a potent inhibitor of IgE production by B cells ***(187)*** but does not prevent secretion by IgE dedicated B cells ***(188)***. In animal models, exogenous IL-12 enhances T_H1 activity against intracellular parasites ***(178,189–191)***. Circulating levels of IL-12 are elevated in children with meningococcal septic shock, and correlate with disease outcome and severity ***(192)***.

8.1.4. IFN-γ

IFN-γ is encoded by a gene situated on chromosome 12 to produce a 20-25 kDa protein, which forms a dimer ***(193)***. IFN-y produced by T cells and NK cells and defines the phenotype of T_H1 cells ***(194–196)***.

IFN-γ induces MHC class II expression on the surface of macrophages and B cells, activates NK cells, induces macrophage NO production and stimulates macrophages to kill intracellular organisms such as *Toxoplasma* and mycobacteria ***(197–199)***.

8.1.5. IL-4

Interleukin-4 is the 18 kDa product of a gene on chromosome 5 ***(200,201)*** and is mainly produced by T cells, mast cells and basophils ***(202)***. The major source of IL-4 is CD4+ CD45RO memory T cells ***(203)*** and synthesis is induced following activation of the T-cell receptor by antigen. IL-4 defines the T_H2 cell phenotype and acts as a co-factor for B-cell proliferation and induces expression of surface IgM, Fc receptors, and CD40 ***(202,204,205)***. IL-4 plays an important role in inducing switching to Ig class and subclass production. In conjunction with CD4+ T cells and other co-factors, IL-4 can induce production of IgE and IgG4 ***(206–211)***. IL-4 inhibits the release of many macrophage-derived cytokines including TNF-α, IL-1, IL-2, IL-3, IL-8, and PGE2 ***(212–214)***. Elevated levels of IL-4 are present in allergic disease ***(215)***.

8.1.6. IL-10

IL-10 is a 36 kDa homodimer that is produced by T cells, B cells, and macrophages ***(216–218)***. TNF-α enhances IL-10 expression ***(219,220)*** but IFN-γ IL-4, IL-13, and IL-10 itself reduces IL-10 production ***(221–223)***. The IL-10 gene is located on chromosome 1q ***(224)*** and polymorphisms in the promoter region of this gene correlate with levels of IL-10 production in vitro ***(225)***.

IL-10 stimulates B cells to proliferate and differentiate and to increase their expression of MHC class II antigens ***(226,227)***. It also increases expression of Fcγ receptors on monocytes ***(228)***, so enhancing ADCC. IL-10 may be involved in switching of B cells to produce IgA or IgG1 and IgG3 ***(229–231)***. On the other hand, IL-10 downregulates expression of MHC class II, ICAM-1, and B7 on monocytes, thereby reducing antigen presentation and attenuating T-cell activation and proliferation ***(216,232–234)***. IL-10 inhibits secretion of TNF-α IL-1, IL-6, IL-8, and IL-12 from monocytes and macrophages ***(223,232,235)*** and inhibits release of IFN-γ, TNF-β, and IL-2 from T cells ***(236,237)***, probably via decreasing IL-12 synthesis ***(235)***. Although IL-10 is produced by both T_H1 and T_H2 T cells, it seems that the level of IL-10 produced relative to IFN-γ and IL-2 determines whether T-cell proliferation and macrophage activation are enhanced (T_H1) or inhibited (T_H2) ***(238)***.

In vitro, IL-10 has major anti-inflammatory activities and there is evidence in vivo that this activity is important in the pathogenesis of leishmaniasis, filariasis, leprosy, and tuberculosis in humans ***(239–244)***.

In contrast to the effects of TNF-α infusion, which mimics endotoxemia, IL-10 infusion in healthy individuals seems to be without adverse effects ***(218)***, but it impairs defense against infection in animal models ***(65,220,245)***.

The highest levels of IL-10 in an individual during acute infection with *N. meningitidis* are found on presentation to hospital and the highest levels among patients have been associated with fatality from meningococcal disease ***(69,70,77,246)***. In survivors, IL-10 levels rapidly fall following admission to hospital but raised levels persist in nonsurvivors ***(65)***.

8.1.7. IL-13

IL-13 is an anti-inflammatory cytokine of 17 kDa encoded by a gene on chromosome 5 ***(247)***. It is produced by T cells ($CD4^+$ and $CD8^+$) following both antigenic and mitogenic stimulation, B cells, and mast cells ***(247–251)***. The action on B cells is similar to that of IL-4 with increased expression of IgM and MHC class II, B-cell proliferation, and IgE/IgG4 heavy-chain switching ***(252–254)***. IL-13 downregulates the expression of many macrophage-surface receptors (including CD14) and upregulates others ***(255,256)***. The production of LPS-induced pro-inflammatory cytokines, NO and ADCC activity is inhibited by IL-13 ***(247,255,256)***. However, IL-13 could not be detected during acute clinical sepsis or experimental endotoxemia ***(65)***. IL-13 is produced at high levels in mononuclear-cell preparations from allergic patients ***(257,258)***.

References

1. Peltola, H. (1983) Meningococcal disease: still with us. *Rev. Infect. Dis.* **5,** 71–91.
2. Zhen, H. (1987) Prevalence of CSM over 30-Year period: overview, in *Evolution of Meningococcal Disease* (Vedros, N. A., ed.), CRC Press Inc., Boca Raton, FL, pp. 20–21.
3. Hu, X. (1991) [Study on periodically prevalent feature for epidemic cerebrospinal meningitis in China]. *Chung Hua Liu Hsing Ping Hsueh Tsa Chih* **12,** 136–139.
4. Wang, J. F., Caugant, D. A., Li, X., Hu, X., Poolman, J. T., Crowe, B. A., and Achtman, M. (1992) Clonal and antigenic analysis of serogroup A Neisseria meningitidis with particular reference to epidemiological features of epidemic meningitis in the People's Republic of China. *Infect. Immun.* **60,** 5267–5282.
5. Lapeyssonnie, L. (1963) La meningite cerebro-spinale en Afrique. *Bull. WHO* **28,** 3–114.
6. Ramsay, M., Kaczmarski, E., Rush, M., Mallard, R., Farrington, P., and White, J. (1997). Changing patterns of case ascertainment and trends in meningococcal disease in England and Wales. *Commun. Dis. Rep. CDR Rev.* **7,** R49–R54.
7. Wilson, N., Baker, M., Martin, D., Lennon, D., O'Hallahan, J., Jones, N., et al. (1995) Meningococcal disease epidemiology and control in New Zealand. *N. Z. Med. J.* **108,** 437–442.
8. Terry Molinert, G., Demina, A. A., and Valcarcel Novo, M. (1986) [Epidemiological characteristics of meningococcal infection in Cuba]. *Zh. Mikrobiol. Epidemiol. Immunobiol.* 54–59.
9. Gama, S. G., Marzochi, K. B., and da Siveira Filho, G. B. (1997) [Epidemiological characterization of meningococcal disease in a metropolitan area in Southeastern Brazil, 1976-1994]. *Rev. Saude Publica* **31,** 254–262.
10. Lystad, A. and Aasen, S. (1991) The epidemiology of meningococcal disease in Norway 1975-91. *NIPH Ann.* **14,** 57–65, 65–66.

11. Diermayer, M., Hedberg, K., Hoesly, F., Fischer, M., Perkins, B., Reeves, M., and Fleming, D. (1999) Epidemic serogroup B meningococcal disease in Oregon: the evolving epidemiology of the ET-5 strain. *JAMA* **281,** 1493–1497.
12. Abbott, J. D., Jones, D. M., Painter, M. J., and Young, S. E. (1985) The epidemiology of meningococcal infections in England and Wales, 1912–1983. *J. Infect.* **11,** 241–257.
13. Erickson, L. and De Wals, P. (1998) Complications and sequelae of meningococcal disease in Quebec, Canada, 1990-1994. *Clin. Infect. Dis.* **26,** 1159–1164.
14. Whalen, C. M., Hockin, J. C., Ryan, A., and Ashton, F. (1995) The changing epidemiology of invasive meningococcal disease in Canada, 1985 through 1992. Emergence of a virulent clone of Neisseria meningitidis. *JAMA* **273,** 390–394.
15. Goldschneider, I., Gotschlich, E. C., and Artenstein, M. S. (1969) Human immunity to the meningococcus. I. The role of humoral antibodies. *J. Exp. Med.* **129,** 1307–1326.
16. Jones, D. M. and Mallard, R. H. (1993) Age incidence of meningococcal infection England and Wales, 1984–1991. *J. Infect.* **27,** 83–88.
17. Baker, C. J. and Griffiss, J. M. (1983) Influence of age on serogroup distribution of endemic meningococcal disease. *Pediatrics* **71,** 923–926.
18. Rosenstein, N. E., Perkins, B. A., Stephens, D. S., Lefkowitz, L., Cartter, M. L., Danila, R., et al. (1999) The changing epidemiology of meningococcal disease in the United States, 1992–1996. *J. Infect. Dis.* **180,** 1894–1901.
19. Peltola, H., Kataja, J. M., and Makela, P. H. (1982) Shift in the age-distribution of meningococcal disease as predictor of an epidemic? *Lancet* **2,** 595–597.
20. Tikhomirov, E., Santamaria, M., and Esteves, K. (1997) Meningococcal disease: public health burden and control. *World Health Stat. Q.* **50,** 170–176.
21. Greenwood, B. M., Blakebrough, I. S., Bradley, A. K., Wali, S., and Whittle, H. C. (1984) Meningococcal disease and season in sub-Saharan Africa. *Lancet* **1,** 1339–1342.
22. Virji, M., Saunders, J. R., Sims, G., Makepeace, K., Maskell, D., and Ferguson, D. J. (1993) Pilus-facilitated adherence of Neisseria meningitidis to human epithelial and endothelial cells: modulation of adherence phenotype occurs concurrently with changes in primary amino acid sequence and the glycosylation status of pilin. *Mol. Microbiol.* **10,** 1013–1028.
23. Virji, M., Makepeace, K., Ferguson, D. J., Achtman, M., and Moxon, E. R. (1993) Meningococcal Opa and Opc proteins: their role in colonization and invasion of human epithelial and endothelial cells. *Mol. Microbiol.* **10,** 499–510.
24. DeVoe, I. W. (1982) The meningococcus and mechanisms of pathogenicity. *Microbiol. Rev.* **46,** 162–190.
25. Edwards, E. A., Devine, L. F., Sengbusch, G. H., and Ward, H. W. (1977) Immunological investigations of meningococcal disease. III. Brevity of group C acquisition prior to disease occurrence. *Scand. J. Infect. Dis.* **9,** 105–110.
26. Gold, R., Goldschneider, I., Lepow, M. L., Draper, T. F., and Randolph, M. (1978) Carriage of Neisseria meningitidis and Neisseria lactamica in infants and children. *J. Infect. Dis.* **137,** 112–121.

27. Blackwell, C. C., Weir, D. M., James, V. S., Cartwright, K. A., Stuart, J. M., and Jones, D. M. (1989) The Stonehouse study: secretor status and carriage of Neisseria species. *Epidemiol. Infect.* **102,** 1–10.
28. Stuart, J. M., Cartwright, K. A., Robinson, P. M., and Noah, N. D. (1989) Effect of smoking on meningococcal carriage. *Lancet* **2,** 723–725.
29. Wenzel, R. P., Davies, J. A., Mitzel, J. R., and Beam, W. E., Jr. (1973) Non-usefulness of meningococcal carriage-rates. *Lancet* **2,** 205.
30. Cartwright, K. A., Stuart, J. M., and Noah, N. D. (1986) An outbreak of meningococcal disease in Gloucestershire. *Lancet* **2,** 558–561.
31. Frasch, C. E. and Mocca, L. F. (1982) Strains of Neisseria meningitidis isolated from patients and their close contacts. *Infect. Immun.* **37,** 155–159.
32. Ross, S. C. and Densen, P. (1984) Complement deficiency states and infection: epidemiology, pathogenesis and consequences of neisserial and other infections in an immune deficiency. *Medicine (Baltimore)* **63,** 243–273.
33. Hibberd, M. L., Sumiya, M., Summerfield, J. A., Booy, R., and Levin, M. (1999) Association of variants of the gene for mannose-binding lectin with susceptibility to meningococcal disease. Meningococcal Research Group. *Lancet* **353,** 1049–1053.
34. Moore, P. S., Hierholzer, J., DeWitt, W., Gouan, K., Djore, D., Lippeveld, T., et al. (1990) Respiratory viruses and mycoplasma as cofactors for epidemic group A meningococcal meningitis. *JAMA* **264,** 1271–1275.
35. Cartwright, K. A., Jones, D. M., Smith, A. J., Stuart, J. M., Kaczmarski, E. B., and Palmer, S. R. (1991) Influenza A and meningococcal disease. *Lancet* **338,** 554–557.
36. Hubert, B., Watier, L., Garnerin, P., and Richardson, S. (1992) Meningococcal disease and influenza-like syndrome: a new approach to an old question. *J. Infect. Dis.* **166,** 542–545.
37. Haneberg, B., Tonjum, T., Rodahl, K., and Gedde-Dahl, T. W. (1983) Factors preceding the onset of meningococcal disease, with special emphasis on passive smoking, symptoms of ill health. *NIPH Ann.* **6,** 169–173.
38. De Wals, P., Hertoghe, L., Reginster, G., Borlee, I., Bouckaert, A., Dachy, A., and Lechat, M. F. (1984) Mortality in meningococcal disease in Belgium. *J. Infect.* **8,** 264–273.
39. Andersen, B. M. (1978) Mortality in meningococcal infections. *Scand. J. Infect. Dis.* **10,** 277–282.
40. Fallon, R. J., Brown, W. M., and Lore, W. (1984) Meningococcal infections in Scotland 1972-82. *J. Hyg. (Lond.)* **93,** 167–180.
41. Riordan, F. A., Marzouk, O., Thomson, A. P., Sills, J. A., and Hart, C. A. (1995) The changing presentations of meningococcal disease. *Eur. J. Pediatr.* **154,** 472–474.
42. Nadel, S., Newport, M. J., Booy, R., and Levin, M. (1996) Variation in the tumor necrosis factor-alpha gene promoter region may be associated with death from meningococcal disease. *J. Infect. Dis.* **174,** 878–880.
43. Feigin, R. D., McCracken, G. H., Jr., and Klein, J. O. (1992) Diagnosis and management of meningitis. *Pediatr. Infect. Dis. J.* **11,** 785–814.
44. Wong, V. K., Hitchcock, W., and Mason, W. H. (1989) Meningococcal infections in children: a review of 100 cases. *Pediatr. Infect. Dis. J.* **8,** 224–227.

45. Marzouk, O., Thomson, A. P., Sills, J. A., Hart, C. A., and Harris, F. (1991) Features and outcome in meningococcal disease presenting with maculopapular rash. *Arch. Dis. Child.* **66,** 485–487.
46. Toews, W. H. and Bass, J. W. (1974) Skin manifestations of meningococcal infection; an immediate indicator of prognosis. *Am. J. Dis. Child.* **127,** 173–176.
47. Niklasson, P. M., Lundbergh, P., and Strandell, T. (1971) Prognostic factors in meningococcal disease. *Scand. J. Infect. Dis.* **3,** 17–25.
48. Heyderman, R. S., Klein, N. J., Shennan, G. I., and Levin, M. (1991) Deficiency of prostacyclin production in meningococcal shock. *Arch. Dis. Child.* **66,** 1296–1299.
49. Mercier, J. C., Beaufils, F., Hartmann, J. F., and Azema, D. (1988) Hemodynamic patterns of meningococcal shock in children. *Crit. Care Med.* **16,** 27–33.
50. Nadel, S., Levin, M., and Habibi, P. (1995) Treatment of meningococcal disease in childhood, in *Meningococcal Disease* (Cartwright, K., ed.), John Wiley and Sons, Chichester, UK, pp. 207–243.
51. Brandtzaeg, P., Kierulf, P., Gaustad, P., Skulberg, A., Bruun, J. N., Halvorsen, S., and Sorensen, E. (1989) Plasma endotoxin as a predictor of multiple organ failure and death in systemic meningococcal disease. *J. Infect. Dis.* **159,** 195–204.
52. Tracey, K. J. and Cerami, A. (1993) Tumor necrosis factor, other cytokines and disease. *Annu. Rev. Cell Biol.* **9,** 317–343.
53. Dinarello, C. A. and Cannon, J. G. (1993) Cytokine measurements in septic shock. *Ann. Intern. Med.* **119,** 853–854.
54. Spinas, G. A., Keller, U., and Brockhaus, M. (1992) Release of soluble receptors for tumor necrosis factor (TNF) in relation to circulating TNF during experimental endotoxinemia. *J. Clin. Invest.* **90,** 533–536.
55. Wilson, M., Seymour, R., and Henderson, B. (1998) Bacterial perturbation of cytokine networks. *Infect. Immun.* **66,** 2401–2409.
56. Henderson, B. and Wilson, M. (1995) Modulins: a new class of cytokine-inducing, pro-inflammatory bacterial virulence factor. *Inflamm. Res.* **44,** 187–197.
57. Henderson, D. C. and Rippin, J. J. (1995) Stimulus-dependent production of cytokines and pterins by peripheral blood mononuclear cells. *Immunol. Lett.* **45,** 29–34.
58. Henderson, B., Poole, S., and Wilson, M. (1996) Microbial/host interactions in health and disease: who controls the cytokine network? *Immunopharmacology* **35,** 1–21.
59. Henderson, B., Poole, S., and Wilson, M. (1996) Bacterial modulins: a novel class of virulence factors which cause host tissue pathology by inducing cytokine synthesis. *Microbiol. Rev.* **60,** 316–341.
60. Henderson, B. and Wilson, M. (1996) Cytokine induction by bacteria: beyond lipopolysaccharide. *Cytokine* **8,** 269–282.
61. Beutler, B. A. (1989). Orchestration of septic shock by cytokines: the role of cachectin (tumor necrosis factor). *Prog. Clin. Biol. Res.* **286,** 219–235.
62. Gutierrez-Ramos, J. C. and Bluethmann, H. (1997) Molecules and mechanisms operating in septic shock: lessons from knockout mice. *Immunol. Today* **18,** 329–334.

63. Bone, R. C. (1996) Immunologic dissonance: a continuing evolution in our understanding of the systemic inflammatory response syndrome (SIRS) and the multiple organ dysfunction syndrome (MODS). *Ann. Intern. Med.* **125,** 680–687.
64. Astiz, M. E. and Rackow, E. C. (1998) Septic shock. *Lancet* **351,** 1501–1505.
65. van der Poll, T., de Waal Malefyt, R., Coyle, S. M., and Lowry, S. F. (1997) Antiinflammatory cytokine responses during clinical sepsis and experimental endotoxemia: sequential measurements of plasma soluble interleukin (IL)-1 receptor type II, IL-10, and IL-13. *J. Infect. Dis.* **175,** 118–122.
66. Hazelzet, J. A., Risseeuw-Appel, I. M., Kornelisse, R. F., Hop, W. C., Dekker, I., Joosten, K. F., et al. (1996) Age-related differences in outcome and severity of DIC in children with septic shock and purpura. *Thromb. Haemost.* **76,** 932–938.
67. Waring, P. M., Waring, L. J., and Metcalf, D. (1994) Circulating leukemia inhibitory factor levels correlate with disease severity in meningococcemia. *J. Infect. Dis.* **170,** 1224–1228.
68. Girardin, E., Roux-Lombard, P., Grau, G. E., Suter, P., Gallati, H., and Dayer, J. M. (1992) Imbalance between tumour necrosis factor-alpha and soluble TNF receptor concentrations in severe meningococcemia. The J5 Study Group. *Immunology* **76,** 20–23.
69. Derkx, B., Marchant, A., Goldman, M., Bijlmer, R., and van Deventer, S. (1995) High levels of interleukin-10 during the initial phase of fulminant meningococcal septic shock. *J. Infect. Dis.* **171,** 229–232.
70. Lehmann, A. K., Halstensen, A., Sornes, S., Rokke, O., and Waage, A. (1995) High levels of interleukin 10 in serum are associated with fatality in meningococcal disease. *Infect. Immun.* **63,** 2109–2112.
71. Halstensen, A., Ceska, M., Brandtzaeg, P., Redl, H., Naess, A., and Waage, A. (1993) Interleukin-8 in serum and cerebrospinal fluid from patients with meningococcal disease. *J. Infect. Dis.* **167,** 471–475.
72. Waage, A., Halstensen, A., and Espevik, T. (1987) Association between tumour necrosis factor in serum and fatal outcome in patients with meningococcal disease. *Lancet* **1,** 355–357.
73. Waage, A., Halstensen, A., Shalaby, R., Brandtzaeg, P., Kierulf, P., and Espevik, T. (1989) Local production of tumor necrosis factor alpha, interleukin 1, and interleukin 6 in meningococcal meningitis. Relation to the inflammatory response. *J. Exp. Med.* **170,** 1859–1867.
74. Waage, A., Brandtzaeg, P., Halstensen, A., Kierulf, P., and Espevik, T. (1989) The complex pattern of cytokines in serum from patients with meningococcal septic shock. Association between interleukin 6, interleukin 1, and fatal outcome. *J. Exp. Med.* **169,** 333–338.
75. Kornelisse, R. F., Hazelzet, J. A., Savelkoul, H. F., Hop, W. C., Suur, M. H., Borsboom, A. N., et al. (1996) The relationship between plasminogen activator inhibitor-1 and proinflammatory and counterinflammatory mediators in children with meningococcal septic shock. *J. Infect. Dis.* **173,** 1148–1156.

76. van Deuren, M., van der Ven-Jongekrijg, J., Demacker, P. N., Bartelink, A. K., van Dalen, R., Sauerwein, R. W., et al. (1994) Differential expression of proinflammatory cytokines and their inhibitors during the course of meningococcal infections. *J. Infect. Dis.* **169,** 157–161.
77. van Deuren, M., van der Ven-Jongekrijg, J., Bartelink, A. K., van Dalen, R., Sauerwein, R. W., and van der Meer, J. W. (1995) Correlation between proinflammatory cytokines and antiinflammatory mediators and the severity of disease in meningococcal infections. *J. Infect. Dis.* **172,** 433–439.
78. van Deuren, M., van der Ven-Jongekrijg, J., Vannier, E., van Dalen, R., Pesman, G., Bartelink, A. K., et al. (1997) The pattern of interleukin-1beta (IL-1beta) and its modulating agents IL-1 receptor antagonist and IL-1 soluble receptor type II in acute meningococcal infections. *Blood* **90,** 1101–1108.
79. van Deuren, M., Frieling, J. T., van der Ven-Jongekrijg, J., Neeleman, C., Russel, F. G., van Lier, H. J., et al. (1998) Plasma patterns of tumor necrosis factor-alpha (TNF) and TNF soluble receptors during acute meningococcal infections and the effect of plasma exchange. *Clin. Infect. Dis.* **26,** 918–923.
80. Gardlund, B., Sjolin, J., Nilsson, A., Roll, M., Wickerts, C. J., and Wretlind, B. (1995) Plasma levels of cytokines in primary septic shock in humans: correlation with disease severity. *J. Infect. Dis.* **172,** 296–301.
81. Westendorp, R. G., Langermans, J. A., Huizinga, T. W., Elouali, A. H., Verweij, C. L., Boomsma, D. I., et al. (1997) Genetic influence on cytokine production and fatal meningococcal disease. *Lancet* **349,** 170–173.
82. Pollard, A. J. and Levin, M. (2000) Vaccines for prevention of meningococcal disease. *Pediatr. Infect. Dis. J.* **19,** 333–345.
83. Nadel, S., Britto, J., Booy, R., Maconochie, I., Habibi, P., and Levin, M. (1998). Avoidable deficiencies in the delivery of health care to children with meningococcal disease. *J. Accid. Emerg. Med.* **15,** 298–303.
84. Riordan, F. A., Thomson, A. P., Sills, J. A., and Hart, C. A. (1996) Who spots the spots? Diagnosis and treatment of early meningococcal disease in children. *BMJ* **313,** 1255–1256.
85. Strang, J. R. and Pugh, E. J. (1992) Meningococcal infections: reducing the case fatality rate by giving penicillin before admission to hospital. *BMJ* **305,** 141–143.
86. Sorensen, H. T., Moller-Petersen, J., Krarup, H. B., Pedersen, H., Hansen, H., and Hamburger, H. (1992) Diagnostic problems with meningococcal disease in general practice. *J. Clin. Epidemiol.* **45,** 1289–1293.
87. Mathiassen, B., Thomsen, H., and Landsfeldt, U. (1989) An evaluation of the accuracy of clinical diagnosis at admission in a population with epidemic meningococcal disease. *J. Intern. Med.* **226,** 113–116.
88. Granier, S., Owen, P., Pill, R., and Jacobson, L. (1998) Recognising meningococcal disease in primary care: qualitative study of how general practitioners process clinical and contextual information. *BMJ* **316,** 276–279.
89. Tonjum, T., Nilsson, F., Bruun, J. N., and Haneberg, B. (1983) The early phase of meningococcal disease. *NIPH Ann.* **6,** 175–181.

90. Slack, J. (1982) Deaths from meningococcal infection in England and Wales in 1978. *J. R. Coll. Physicians Lond.* **16,** 40–44.
91. Oakley, J. R. and Stanton, A. N. (1979) Meningococcal infections during infancy: confidential inquiries into 10 deaths. *BMJ* **2,** 468–469.
92. Donaldson, L. (1999) Meningococcal infection, in Department of Health, London PL.CM0/99/1.
93. Cartwright, K., Strang, J., Gossain, S., and Begg, N. (1992) Early treatment of meningococcal disease. *BMJ* **305,** 774.
94. Sorensen, H. T., Moller-Petersen, J., Krarup, H. B., Pedersen, H., Hansen, H., and Hamburger, H. (1992). Early treatment of meningococcal disease. *BMJ* **305,** 774.
95. Hopkin, D. A. (1978) Frapper fort ou frapper doucement: a gram-negative dilemma. *Lancet* **2,** 1193–1194.
96. Kirsch, E. and Giroir, B. (1997) Timing of therapy for meningococcal infection. *Pediatr. Infect. Dis. J.* **16,** 541–542.
97. Borchsenius, F., Bruun, J. N., and Tonjum, T. (1991) Systemic meningococcal disease: the diagnosis on admission to hospital. *NIPH Ann.* **14,** 11–22.
98. Olcen, P., Barr, J., and Kjellander, J. (1979) Meningitis and bacteremia due to Neisseria meningitidis: clinical and laboratory findings in 69 cases from Orebro county, 1965 to 1977. *Scand. J. Infect. Dis.* **11,** 111–119.
99. Wilks, D. and Lever, A. M. (1996) Reasons for delay in administration of antibiotics to patients with meningitis and meningococcemia. *J. Infect.* **32,** 49–51.
100. Bjark, P., Gedde-Dahl, T. W., Høiby, E. A., and Bruun, J. N. (1987) Prognosis ofmeningococcal septicemia. *Lancet* **ii,** 861–862.
101. Stokland, T., Flægstad, T., and Gutteberg, T. J. (1985) A clinical score for the prediction of outcome of patients with meningococcal infection. *Acta Paediatr. Scand.* **(Suppl. 322),** 12.
102. Leclerc, F., Beuscart, R., Guillois, B., Diependaele, J. F., Krim, G., Devictor, D., et al. (1985) Prognostic factors of severe infectious purpura in children. *Intensive Care Med.* **11,** 140–143.
103. Emparanza, J. I., Aldamiz-Echevarria, L., Perez-Yarza, E. G., Larranaga, P., Jiminez, J. L., Labiano, M., and Ozcoidi, I. (1988) Prognostic score in acute meningococcemia. *Crit. Care Med.* **16,** 168–169.
104. Sinclair, J. F., Skeoch, C. H., and Hallworth, D. (1987) Prognosis of meningococcal septicemia. *Lancet* **2,** 38.
105. Kahn, A. and Blum, D. (1978) Factors for poor prognosis in fulminating meningococcemia. Conclusions from observations of 67 childhood cases. *Clin. Pediatr. (Phila)* **17,** 680–682, 687.
106. Stiehm, E. R. and Damrosch, D. S. (1966) Factors in the prognosis of meningococcal infection. Review of 63 cases with emphasis on recognition and management of the severely ill patient. *J. Pediatr.* **68,** 457–467.
107. Ansari, B. M., Davies, D. B., and Boyce, J. M. (1979) A comparative study of adverse factors in meningococcemia and meningococcal meningitis. *Postgrad. Med. J.* **55,** 780–783.

108. Tesoro, L. J. and Selbst, S. M. (1991) Factors affecting outcome in meningococcal infections. *Am. J. Dis. Child.* **145,** 218–220.
109. Derkx, H. H., van den Hoek, J., Redekop, W. K., Bijlmer, R. P., van Deventer, S. J., and Bossuyt, P. M. (1996) Meningococcal disease: a comparison of eight severity scores in 125 children. *Intensive Care Med.* **22,** 1433–1441.
110. Levin, M., Galassini, R., de Munter, C., Nadel, S., Habibi, P., Britto, J., and Booy, R. (1998) Improved survival in children admitted to intensive care with meningococcal disease, in *2nd Annual Spring Meeting of the Royal College of Paediatrics and Child Health,* Royal College of Paediatric and Child Health, University of York, p. 98.
111. Carcillo, J. A., Davis, A. L., and Zaritsky, A. (1991) Role of early fluid resuscitation in pediatric septic shock. *JAMA* **266,** 1242–1245.
112. Rasmussen, N., Hansen, B., Bohr, V., and Kristensen, H. S. (1988) Artificial ventilation and prognostic factors in bacterial meningitis. *Infection* **16,** 158–162.
113. Pollard, A. J., Britto, J., Nadel, S., DeMunter, C., Habibi, P., and Levin, M. (1999) Emergency management of meningococcal disease. *Arch. Dis. Child.* **80,** 290–296.
114. Kennedy, N. J. and Duncan, A. W. (1996) Acute meningococcemia: recent advances in management (with particular reference to children). *Anaesth. Intensive Care* **24,** 197–216.
115. Cochrane Injuries Group Albumin Reviewers (1998) Human albumin administration in critically ill patients: systematic review of randomised controlled trials. *BMJ* **317,** 225–240.
116. Nadel, S., Marriage, S., De Munter, C., Britto, J., Habibi, P., and Levin, M. (1998) Human albumin administration in critically ill patients. Review did not provide recommendations for alternative treatment. *BMJ* **317,** 882–883.
117. Nadel, S., De Munter, C., Britto, J., Levin, M., and Habibi, P. (1998) Albumin: saint or sinner. *Arch. Dis. Child.* **79,** 384–385.
118. Slack, J. (1980) Coning and lumbar puncture. *Lancet* **2,** 474–475.
119. Cabral, D. A., Flodmark, O., Farrell, K., and Speert, D. P. (1987) Prospective study of computed tomography in acute bacterial meningitis. *J. Pediatr.* **111,** 201–205.
120. Heyderman, R. S., Robb, S. A., Kendall, B. E., and Levin, M. (1992) Does computed tomography have a role in the evaluation of complicated acute bacterial meningitis in childhood? *Dev. Med. Child. Neurol.* **34,** 870–875.
121. Kline, M. W. and Kaplan, S. L. (1988) Computed tomography in bacterial meningitis of childhood. *Pediatr. Infect. Dis. J.* **7,** 855–857.
122. Friedland, I. R., Paris, M. M., Rinderknecht, S., and McCracken, G. H., Jr. (1992) Cranial computed tomographic scans have little impact on management of bacterial meningitis. *Am. J. Dis. Child.* **146,** 1484–1487.
123. Riordan, F. A., Thomson, A. P., Sills, J. A., and Hart, C. A. (1993) Does computed tomography have a role in the evaluation of complicated acute bacterial meningitis in childhood? *Dev. Med. Child. Neurol.* **35,** 275–276.
124. Ceneviva, G., Paschall, J. A., Maffei, F., and Carcillo, J. A. (1998) Hemodynamic support in fluid-refractory pediatric septic shock. *Pediatrics* **102,** e19.

125. Motulsky, H. J. and Insel, P. A. (1982). Adrenergic receptors in man: direct identification, physiologic regulation, and clinical alterations. *N. Engl. J. Med.* **307,** 18–29.
126. Ledingham, I. M. and McArdle, C. S. (1978) Prospective study of the treatment of septic shock. *Lancet* **1,** 1194–1197.
127. Heyderman, R. S. (1993) Sepsis and intravascular thrombosis. *Arch. Dis. Child.* **68,** 621–623.
128. Leclerc, F., Hazelzet, J., Jude, B., Hofhuis, W., Hue, V., Martinot, A., and Van der Voort, E. (1992) Protein C and S deficiency in severe infectious purpura of children: a collaborative study of 40 cases. *Intensive Care Med.* **18,** 202–205.
129. Brandtzaeg, P., Joo, G. B., Brusletto, B., and Kierulf, P. (1990) Plasminogen activator inhibitor 1 and 2, alpha-2-antiplasmin, plasminogen, and endotoxin levels in systemic meningococcal disease. *Thromb. Res.* **57,** 271–278.
130. Rintala, E., Seppala, O. P., Kotilainen, P., Pettila, V., and Rasi, V. (1998) Protein C in the treatment of coagulopathy in meningococcal disease. *Crit. Care Med.* **26,** 965–968.
131. de Jonge, E., Levi, M., Stoutenbeek, C. P., and van Deventer, S. J. (1998) Current drug treatment strategies for disseminated intravascular coagulation. *Drugs* **55,** 767–777.
132. Smith, O. P., White, B., Vaughan, D., Rafferty, M., Claffey, L., Lyons, B., and Casey, W. (1997) Use of protein-C concentrate, heparin, and haemodiafiltration in meningococcus-induced purpura fulminans. *Lancet* **350,** 1590–1593.
132a. Bernard GR, Vincent J-L, Laterre P-F, et al. (2001) Efficacy and safety of recombinant human activated Protein C in severe sepsis. *N Eng J Med* **344,** 699-709.
133. Cremer, R., Leclerc, F., Jude, B., Sadik, A., Leteurtre, S., Fourier, C., et al. (1999) Are there specific haemostatic abnormalities in children surviving septic shock with purpura and having skin necrosis or limb ischaemia that need skin grafts or limb amputations? *Eur. J. Pediatr.* **158,** 127–132.
134. Nurnberger, W., v. Kries, R., Bohm, O., and Gobel, U. (1999) Systemic meningococcal infection: which children may benefit from adjuvant haemostatic therapy? Results from an observational study. *Eur. J. Pediatr.* **158(Suppl. 3),** S192–S196.
135. McIntyre, P. B., Berkey, C. S., King, S. M., Schaad, U. B., Kilpi, T., Kanra, G. Y., and Perez, C. M. (1997) Dexamethasone as adjunctive therapy in bacterial meningitis. A meta-analysis of randomized clinical trials since 1988. *JAMA* **278,** 925–931.
136. Veterans Administration Systemic Sepsis Cooperative Study Group (1987) Effect of high dose glucocorticoid therapy on mortality in patients with clinical signs of systemic sepsis. *N. Engl. J. Med.* **317,** 659–665.
137. Riordan, F. A., Thomson, A. P., Ratcliffe, J. M., Sills, J. A., Diver, M. J., and Hart, C. A. (1999) Admission cortisol and adrenocorticotrophic hormone levels in children with meningococcal disease: evidence of adrenal insufficiency? *Crit. Care Med.* **27,** 2257–2261.
138. Bone, R. C., Fisher, C. J., Jr., Clemmer, T. P., Slotman, G. J., Metz, C. A., and Balk, R. A. (1987) A controlled clinical trial of high-dose methylprednisolone in the treatment of severe sepsis and septic shock. *N. Engl. J. Med.* **317,** 653–658.

139. Mok, Q. and Butt, W. (1996) The outcome of children admitted to intensive care with meningococcal septicemia. *Intensive Care Med.* **22,** 259–263.
140. Hellman, J. and Warren, H. S. (1999) Antiendotoxin strategies. *Infect. Dis. Clin. North. Am.* **13,** 371–386, ix.
141. Bhattacharjee, A. K. and Cross, A. S. (1999) Vaccines and antibodies in the prevention and treatment of sepsis. *Infect. Dis. Clin. North Am.* **13,** 355–369, vii.
142. Anonymous (2000) http://www.xoma.com/news/pressrel/00_04_25.html. In. Xoma.
143. Schildkamp, R. L., Lodder, M. C., Bijlmer, H. A., Dankert, J., and Scholten, R. J. (1996) Clinical manifestations and course of meningococcal disease in 562 patients. *Scand. J. Infect. Dis.* **28,** 47–51.
144. Baraff, L. J., Lee, S. I., and Schriger, D. L. (1993) Outcomes of bacterial meningitis in children: a meta-analysis. *Pediatr. Infect. Dis. J.* **12,** 389–394.
145. Herrera, R., Hobar, P. C., and Ginsburg, C. M. (1994) Surgical intervention for the complications of meningococcal-induced purpura fulminans. *Pediatr. Infect. Dis. J.* **13,** 734–737.
146. Malley, R., Huskins, W. C., and Kuppermann, N. (1996) Multivariable predictive models for adverse outcome of invasive meningococcal disease in children. *J. Pediatr.* **129,** 702–710.
147. Cremer, R., Leclerc, F., Martinot, A., Sadik, A., and Fourier, C. (1997) Adverse outcome in children with meningococcemia. *J. Pediatr.* **131,** 649–651.
148. Naess, A., Halstensen, A., Nyland, H., Pedersen, S. H., Moller, P., Borgmann, R., et al. (1994) Sequelae one year after meningococcal disease. *Acta Neurol. Scand.* **89,** 139–142.
149. Thomson, A. and Marzouk, O. (1991) Endotoxin induced cochlear damage. *Arch. Dis. Child.* **66,** 907–908.
150. Wingfield, P., Pain, R. H., and Craig, S. (1987) Tumour necrosis factor is a compact trimer. *FEBS Lett.* **211,** 179–184.
151. Beyaert, R. and Fiers, W. (1998). Tumour necrosis factor and lymphotoxin, in *Cytokines* (Mire-Sluis, A. R. and Thorpe, R., eds.), Academic Press, London, p. 335–360.
152. Sidhu, R. S. and Bollon, A. P. (1993) Tumor necrosis factor activities and cancer therapy: a perspective. *Pharmacol. Ther.* **57,** 79–128.
153. Michie, H. R., Spriggs, D. R., Manogue, K. R., Sherman, M. L., Revhaug, A., O'Dwyer, S. T., et al. (1988) Tumor necrosis factor and endotoxin induce similar metabolic responses in human beings. *Surgery* **104,** 280–286.
154. Weingarten, R., Sklar, L. A., Mathison, J. C., Omidi, S., Ainsworth, T., Simon, S., et al. (1993) Interactions of lipopolysaccharide with neutrophils in blood via CD14. *J. Leukoc. Biol.* **53,** 518–524.
155. Heumann, D., Gallay, P., Barras, C., Zaech, P., Ulevitch, R. J., Tobias, P. S., et al. (1992) Control of lipopolysaccharide (LPS) binding and LPS-induced tumor necrosis factor secretion in human peripheral blood monocytes. *J. Immunol.* **148,** 3505–3512.
156. Desch, C. E., Kovach, N. L., Present, W., Broyles, C., and Harlan, J. M. (1989) Production of human tumor necrosis factor from whole blood ex vivo. *Lymphokine Res.* **8,** 141–146.

157. Schumann, R. R., Leong, S. R., Flaggs, G. W., Gray, P. W., Wright, S. D., Mathison, J. C., et al. (1990) Structure and function of lipopolysaccharide binding protein. *Science* **249,** 1429–1431.
158. Wright, S. D., Ramos, R. A., Tobias, P. S., Ulevitch, R. J., and Mathison, J. C. (1990) CD14, a receptor for complexes of lipopolysaccharide (LPS) and LPS binding protein. *Science* **249,** 1431–1433.
159. Couturier, C., Haeffner-Cavaillon, N., Caroff, M., and Kazatchkine, M. D. (1991) Binding sites for endotoxins (lipopolysaccharides) on human monocytes. *J. Immunol.* **147,** 1899–1904.
160. Gallay, P., Barras, C., Tobias, P. S., Calandra, T., Glauser, M. P., and Heumann, D. (1994) Lipopolysaccharide (LPS)-binding protein in human serum determines the tumor necrosis factor response of monocytes to LPS. *J. Infect. Dis.* **170,** 1319–1222.
161. Gallay, P., Heumann, D., Le Roy, D., Barras, C., and Glauser, M. P. (1994) Mode of action of anti-lipopolysaccharide-binding protein antibodies for prevention of endotoxemic shock in mice. *Proc. Natl. Acad. Sci. USA* **91,** 7922–7926.
162. Kettelhut, I. C., Fiers, W., and Goldberg, A. L. (1987) The toxic effects of tumor necrosis factor in vivo and their prevention by cyclooxygenase inhibitors. *Proc. Natl. Acad. Sci. USA* **84,** 4273–4277.
163. Kilbourn, R. G. and Belloni, P. (1990) Endothelial cell production of nitrogen oxides in response to interferon gamma in combination with tumor necrosis factor, interleukin-1, or endotoxin. *J. Natl. Cancer Inst.* **82,** 772–776.
164. Stuber, F., Petersen, M., Bokelmann, F., and Schade, U. (1996) A genomic polymorphism within the tumor necrosis factor locus influences plasma tumor necrosis factor-alpha concentrations and outcome of patients with severe sepsis. *Crit. Care Med.* **24,** 381–384.
165. Booy, R., Nadel, S., Hibberd, M., Levin, M., and Newport, M. J. (1997) Genetic influence on cytokine production in meningococcal disease. *Lancet* **349,** 1176.
166. Alexander, H. R., Sheppard, B. C., Jensen, J. C., Langstein, H. N., Buresh, C. M., Venzon, D., et al. (1991) Treatment with recombinant human tumor necrosis factor-alpha protects rats against the lethality, hypotension, and hypothermia of gram- negative sepsis. *J. Clin. Invest.* **88,** 34–39.
167. Rothe, J., Lesslauer, W., Lotscher, H., Lang, Y., Koebel, P., Kontgen, F., et al. (1993) Mice lacking the tumour necrosis factor receptor 1 are resistant to TNF-mediated toxicity but highly susceptible to infection by Listeria monocytogenes. *Nature* **364,** 798–802.
168. Silva, A. T., Appelmelk, B. J., Buurman, W. A., Bayston, K. F., and Cohen, J. (1990) Monoclonal antibody to endotoxin core protects mice from Escherichia coli sepsis by a mechanism independent of tumor necrosis factor and interleukin-6. *J. Infect. Dis.* **162,** 454–459.
169. Abraham, E., Wunderink, R., Silverman, H., Perl, T. M., Nasraway, S., Levy, H., et al. (1995) Efficacy and safety of monoclonal antibody to human tumor necrosis factor alpha in patients with sepsis syndrome. A randomized, controlled,

double-blind, multicenter clinical trial. TNF-alpha MAb Sepsis Study Group. *JAMA* **273,** 934–941.

170. Zeni, F., Freeman, B., and Natanson, C. (1997) Anti-inflammatory therapies to treat sepsis and septic shock: a reassessment. *Crit. Care Med.* **25,** 1095–1100.
171. Fisher, C. J., Jr., Agosti, J. M., Opal, S. M., Lowry, S. F., Balk, R. A., Sadoff, J. C., et al. (1996) Treatment of septic shock with the tumor necrosis factor receptor:Fc fusion protein. The Soluble TNF Receptor Sepsis Study Group. *N. Engl. J. Med.* **334,** 1697–1702.
172. Fisher, C. J., Jr. and Zheng, Y. (1996) Potential strategies for inflammatory mediator manipulation: retrospect and prospect. *World J. Surg.* **20,** 447–453.
173. Paul, N. L. and Ruddle, N. H. (1988) Lymphotoxin. *Ann. Rev. Immunol.* **6,** 407–438.
174. Sieburth, D., Jabs, E. W., Warrington, J. A., Li, X., Lasota, J., LaForgia, S., et al. (1992) Assignment of genes encoding a unique cytokine (IL12) composed of two unrelated subunits to chromosomes 3 and 5. *Genomics* **14,** 59–62.
175. Gubler, U., Chua, A. O., Schoenhaut, D. S., Dwyer, C. M., McComas, W., Motyka, R., et al. (1991) Coexpression of two distinct genes is required to generate secreted bioactive cytotoxic lymphocyte maturation factor. *Proc. Natl. Acad. Sci. USA* **88,** 4143–4147.
176. Trinchieri, G. and Scott, P. (1995) Interleukin-12: a proinflammatory cytokine with immunoregulatory functions. *Res. Immunol.* **146,** 423–431.
177. D'Andrea, A., Rengaraju, M., Valiante, N. M., Chehimi, J., Kubin, M., Aste, M., et al. (1992) Production of natural killer cell stimulatory factor (interleukin 12) by peripheral blood mononuclear cells. *J. Exp. Med.* **176,** 1387–1398.
178. Chizzonite, R., Gubler, U., Magram, J., and Stern, A. S. (1998) IL-12, in *Cytokines* (Mire-Sluis, A. R. and Thorpe, R., eds.), Academic Press, London, pp. 183–204.
179. Naume, B., Gately, M., and Espevik, T. (1992) A comparative study of IL-12 (cytotoxic lymphocyte maturation factor)-, IL-2-, and IL-7-induced effects on immunomagnetically purified CD56+ NK cells. *J. Immunol.* **148,** 2429–2436.
180. Chehimi, J., Starr, S. E., Frank, I., Rengaraju, M., Jackson, S. J., Llanes, C., et al. (1992) Natural killer (NK) cell stimulatory factor increases the cytotoxic activity of NK cells from both healthy donors and human immunodeficiency virus-infected patients. *J. Exp. Med.* **175,** 789–796.
181. Kobayashi, M., Fitz, L., Ryan, M., Hewick, R. M., Clark, S. C., Chan, S., et al. (1989) Identification and purification of natural killer cell stimulatory factor (NKSF), a cytokine with multiple biologic effects on human lymphocytes. *J. Exp. Med.* **170,** 827–845.
182. Gately, M. K., Desai, B. B., Wolitzky, A. G., Quinn, P. M., Dwyer, C. M., Podlaski, F. J., et al. (1991) Regulation of human lymphocyte proliferation by a heterodimeric cytokine, IL-12 (cytotoxic lymphocyte maturation factor). *J. Immunol.* **147,** 874–882.
183. Romagnani, S. (1992) Human TH1 and TH2 subsets: regulation of differentiation and role in protection and immunopathology. *Int. Arch. Allergy Immunol.* **98,** 279–285.

184. Manetti, R., Parronchi, P., Giudizi, M. G., Piccinni, M. P., Maggi, E., Trinchieri, G., and Romagnani, S. (1993) Natural killer cell stimulatory factor (interleukin 12 [IL-12]) induces T helper type 1 (Th1)-specific immune responses and inhibits the development of IL-4-producing Th cells. *J. Exp. Med.* **177,** 1199–1204.
185. Trinchieri, G., Kubin, M., Bellone, G., and Cassatella, M. A. (1993) Cytokine cross-talk between phagocytic cells and lymphocytes: relevance for differentiation/activation of phagocytic cells and regulation of adaptive immunity. *J. Cell Biochem.* **53,** 301–308.
186. Lamont, A. G. and Adorini, L. (1996) IL-12: a key cytokine in immune regulation. *Immunol. Today* **17,** 214–217.
187. Kiniwa, M., Gately, M., Gubler, U., Chizzonite, R., Fargeas, C., and Delespesse, G. (1992) Recombinant interleukin-12 suppresses the synthesis of immunoglobulin E by interleukin-4 stimulated human lymphocytes. *J. Clin. Invest.* **90,** 262–266.
188. Morris, S. C., Madden, K. B., Adamovicz, J. J., Gause, W. C., Hubbard, B. R., Gately, M. K., and Finkelman, F. D. (1994) Effects of IL-12 on in vivo cytokine gene expression and Ig isotype selection. *J. Immunol.* **152,** 1047–1056.
189. Heinzel, F. P., Schoenhaut, D. S., Rerko, R. M., Rosser, L. E., and Gately, M. K. (1993) Recombinant interleukin 12 cures mice infected with Leishmania major. *J. Exp. Med.* **177,** 1505–1509.
190. Khan, I. A., Matsuura, T., and Kasper, L. H. (1994) Interleukin-12 enhances murine survival against acute toxoplasmosis. *Infect. Immun.* **62,** 1639–1642.
191. Clemons, K. V., Brummer, E., and Stevens, D. A. (1994) Cytokine treatment of central nervous system infection: efficacy of interleukin-12 alone and synergy with conventional antifungal therapy in experimental cryptococcosis. *Antimicrob. Agents Chemother.* **38,** 460–464.
192. Hazelzet, J. A., Kornelisse, R. F., van der Pouw Kraan, T. C., Joosten, K. F., van der Voort, E., van Mierlo, G., et al. (1997) Interleukin 12 levels during the initial phase of septic shock with purpura in children: relation to severity of disease. *Cytokine* **9,** 711–716.
193. Yip, Y. K., Barrowclough, B. S., Urban, C., and Vilcek, J. (1982) Purification of two subspecies of human gamma (immune) interferon. *Proc. Natl. Acad. Sci. USA* **79,** 1820–1824.
194. Mosmann, T. R., Cherwinski, H., Bond, M. W., Giedlin, M. A., and Coffman, R. L. (1986) Two types of murine helper T cell clone. I. Definition according to profiles of lymphokine activities and secreted proteins. *J. Immunol.* **136,** 2348–2357.
195. Parronchi, P., Macchia, D., Piccinni, M. P., Biswas, P., Simonelli, C., Maggi, E., et al. (1991) Allergen- and bacterial antigen-specific T-cell clones established from atopic donors show a different profile of cytokine production. *Proc. Natl. Acad. Sci. USA* **88,** 4538–4542.
196. Salgame, P., Abrams, J. S., Clayberger, C., Goldstein, H., Convit, J., Modlin, R. L., and Bloom, B. R. (1991) Differing lymphokine profiles of functional subsets of human CD4 and CD8 T cell clones. *Science* **254,** 279–282.

197. Flesch, I. E. and Kaufmann, S. H. (1991) Mechanisms involved in mycobacterial growth inhibition by gamma interferon-activated bone marrow macrophages: role of reactive nitrogen intermediates. *Infect. Immun.* **59,** 3213–3218.
198. Nathan, C. F., Kaplan, G., Levis, W. R., Nusrat, A., Witmer, M. D., Sherwin, S. A., et al. (1986) Local and systemic effects of intradermal recombinant interferon-gamma in patients with lepromatous leprosy. *N. Engl. J. Med.* **315,** 6–15.
199. De Maeyer, E. and De Maeyer-Guignard, J. (1998) Interferon-Gamma, in *Cytokines* (Mire-Sluis, A. R. and Thorpe, R., eds.), Academic Press, London, pp. 391–400.
200. Carballido, J. M., Schols, D., Namikawa, R., Zurawski, S., Zurawski, G., Roncarolo, M. G., and de Vries, J. E. (1995) IL-4 induces human B cell maturation and IgE synthesis in SCID-hu mice. Inhibition of ongoing IgE production by in vivo treatment with an IL- 4/IL-13 receptor antagonist. *J. Immunol.* **155,** 4162–4170.
201. Arai, N., Nomura, D., Villaret, D., DeWaal Malefijt, R., Seiki, M., Yoshida, M., et al. (1989) Complete nucleotide sequence of the chromosomal gene for human IL-4 and its expression. *J. Immunol.* **142,** 274–282.
202. Mire-Sluis, A. R. (1998) IL-4, in *Cytokines* (Mire-Sluis, A. R. and Thorpe, R., eds.), Academic Press, London, pp. 53–68.
203. DeKruyff, R. H., Fang, Y., Secrist, H., and Umetsu, D. T. (1995) IL-4 synthesis by in vivo-primed memory CD4+ T cells: II. Presence of IL-4 is not required for IL-4 synthesis in primed CD4+ T cells. *J. Clin. Immunol.* **15,** 105–115.
204. Conrad, D. H., Waldschmidt, T. J., Lee, W. T., Rao, M., Keegan, A. D., Noelle, R. J., et al. (1987) Effect of B cell stimulatory factor-1 (interleukin 4) on Fc epsilon and Fc gamma receptor expression on murine B lymphocytes and B cell lines. *J. Immunol.* **139,** 2290–2296.
205. Howard, M., Farrar, J., Hilfiker, M., Johnson, B., Takatsu, K., Hamaoka, T., and Paul, W. E. (1982) Identification of a T cell-derived b cell growth factor distinct from interleukin 2. *J. Exp. Med.* **155,** 914–923.
206. Callard, R. E., Smith, S. H., and Scott, K. E. (1991) The role of interleukin 4 in specific antibody responses by human B cells. *Int. Immunol.* **3,** 157–163.
207. Schultz, C. L., Rothman, P., Kuhn, R., Kehry, M., Muller, W., Rajewsky, K., et al. (1992) T helper cell membranes promote IL-4-independent expression of germ-line C gamma 1 transcripts in B cells. *J. Immunol.* **149,** 60–64.
208. Vercelli, D., Jabara, H. H., Lee, B. W., Woodland, N., Geha, R. S., and Leung, D. Y. (1988) Human recombinant interleukin 4 induces Fc epsilon R2/CD23 on normal human monocytes. *J. Exp. Med.* **167,** 1406–1416.
209. Pene, J., Rousset, F., Briere, F., Chretien, I., Bonnefoy, J. Y., Spits, H., et al. (1988) IgE production by normal human lymphocytes is induced by interleukin 4 and suppressed by interferons gamma and alpha and prostaglandin E2. *Proc. Natl. Acad. Sci. USA* **85,** 6880–6884.
210. Jabara, H. H., Ackerman, S. J., Vercelli, D., Yokota, T., Arai, K., Abrams, J., et al. (1988) Induction of interleukin-4-dependent IgE synthesis and interleukin-5-dependent eosinophil differentiation by supernatants of a human helper T-cell clone. *J. Clin. Immunol.* **8,** 437–446.

211. Lundgren, M., Persson, U., Larsson, P., Magnusson, C., Smith, C. I., Hammarstrom, L., and Severinson, E. (1989) Interleukin 4 induces synthesis of IgE and IgG4 in human B cells. *Eur. J. Immunol.* **19,** 1311–1315.
212. Hart, P. H., Whitty, G. A., Piccoli, D. S., and Hamilton, J. A. (1989) Control by IFN-gamma and PGE2 of TNF alpha and IL-1 production by human monocytes. *Immunology* **66,** 376–383.
213. Standiford, T. J., Strieter, R. M., Chensue, S. W., Westwick, J., Kasahara, K., and Kunkel, S. L. (1990) IL-4 inhibits the expression of IL-8 from stimulated human monocytes. *J. Immunol.* **145,** 1435–1439.
214. Cluitmans, F. H., Esendam, B. H., Landegent, J. E., Willemze, R., and Falkenburg, J. H. (1994) IL-4 down-regulates IL-2-, IL-3-, and GM-CSF-induced cytokine gene expression in peripheral blood monocytes. *Ann. Hematol.* **68,** 293–298.
215. Matsumoto, K., Taki, F., Miura, M., Matsuzaki, M., and Takagi, K. (1994) Serum levels of soluble IL-2R, IL-4, and soluble Fc epsilon RII in adult bronchial asthma. *Chest* **105,** 681–686.
216. de Waal Malefyt, R., Haanen, J., Spits, H., Roncarolo, M. G., te Velde, A., Figdor, C., et al. (1991) Interleukin 10 (IL-10) and viral IL-10 strongly reduce antigen-specific human T cell proliferation by diminishing the antigen-presenting capacity of monocytes via downregulation of class II major histocompatibility complex expression. *J. Exp. Med.* **174,** 915–924.
217. Yssel, H., De Waal Malefyt, R., Roncarolo, M. G., Abrams, J. S., Lahesmaa, R., Spits, H., and de Vries, J. E. (1992) IL-10 is produced by subsets of human CD4+ T cell clones and peripheral blood T cells. *J. Immunol.* **149,** 2378–2384.
218. de Waal Malefyt, R. (1998) IL-10, in *Cytokines* (Mire-Sluis, A. R. and Thorpe, R., eds.), Academic Press, London, pp. 151–168.
219. Wanidworanun, C. and Strober, W. (1993) Predominant role of tumor necrosis factor-alpha in human monocyte IL-10 synthesis. *J. Immunol.* **151,** 6853–6861.
220. van der Poll, T., Jansen, J., Levi, M., ten Cate, H., ten Cate, J. W., and van Deventer, S. J. (1994) Regulation of interleukin 10 release by tumor necrosis factor in humans and chimpanzees. *J. Exp. Med.* **180,** 1985–1988.
221. Chomarat, P., Rissoan, M. C., Banchereau, J., and Miossec, P. (1993) Interferon gamma inhibits interleukin 10 production by monocytes. *J. Exp. Med.* **177,** 523–527.
222. de Waal Malefyt, R., Yssel, H., and de Vries, J. E. (1993) Direct effects of IL-10 on subsets of human CD4+ T cell clones and resting T cells. Specific inhibition of IL-2 production and proliferation. *J. Immunol.* **150,** 4754–4765.
223. de Waal Malefyt, R., Abrams, J., Bennett, B., Figdor, C. G., and de Vries, J. E. (1991) Interleukin 10 (IL-10) inhibits cytokine synthesis by human monocytes: an autoregulatory role of IL-10 produced by monocytes. *J. Exp. Med.* **174,** 1209–1220.
224. Kim, J. M., Brannan, C. I., Copeland, N. G., Jenkins, N. A., Khan, T. A., and Moore, K. W. (1992) Structure of the mouse IL-10 gene and chromosomal localization of the mouse and human genes. *J. Immunol.* **148,** 3618–3623.
225. Turner, D. M., Williams, D. M., Sankaran, D., Lazarus, M., Sinnott, P. J., and Hutchinson, I. V. (1997) An investigation of polymorphism in the interleukin-10 gene promoter. *Eur. J. Immunogenet.* **24,** 1–8.

226. Go, N. F., Castle, B. E., Barrett, R., Kastelein, R., Dang, W., Mosmann, T. R., et al. (1990) Interleukin 10, a novel B cell stimulatory factor: unresponsiveness of X chromosome-linked immunodeficiency B cells. *J. Exp. Med.* **172,** 1625–1631.
227. Rousset, F., Garcia, E., Defrance, T., Peronne, C., Vezzio, N., Hsu, D. H., et al. (1992) Interleukin 10 is a potent growth and differentiation factor for activated human B lymphocytes. *Proc. Natl. Acad. Sci. USA* **89,** 1890–1893.
228. te Velde, A. A., de Waal Malefijt, R., Huijbens, R. J., de Vries, J. E., and Figdor, C. G. (1992) IL-10 stimulates monocyte Fc gamma R surface expression and cytotoxic activity. Distinct regulation of antibody-dependent cellular cytotoxicity by IFN-gamma, IL-4, and IL-10. *J. Immunol.* **149,** 4048–4052.
229. Defrance, T., Vanbervliet, B., Briere, F., Durand, I., Rousset, F., and Banchereau, J. (1992) Interleukin 10 and transforming growth factor beta cooperate to induce anti-CD40-activated naive human B cells to secrete immunoglobulin A. *J. Exp. Med.* **175,** 671–682.
230. Briere, F., Servet Delprat, C., Bridon, J. M., Saint-Remy, J. M., and Banchereau, J. (1994) Human interleukin 10 induces naive surface immunoglobulin D+ (sIgD+) B cells to secrete IgG1 and IgG3. *J. Exp. Med.* **179,** 757–762.
231. Briere, F., Bridon, J. M., Chevet, D., Souillet, G., Bienvenu, F., Guret, C., et al. (1994) Interleukin 10 induces B lymphocytes from IgA-deficient patients to secrete IgA. *J. Clin. Invest.* **94,** 97–104.
232. Fiorentino, D. F., Zlotnik, A., Vieira, P., Mosmann, T. R., Howard, M., Moore, K. W., and O'Garra, A. (1991) IL-10 acts on the antigen-presenting cell to inhibit cytokine production by Th1 cells. *J. Immunol.* **146,** 3444–3451.
233. Willems, F., Marchant, A., Delville, J. P., Gerard, C., Delvaux, A., Velu, T., et al. (1994) Interleukin-10 inhibits B7 and intercellular adhesion molecule-1 expression on human monocytes. *Eur. J. Immunol.* **24,** 1007–1009.
234. Ding, L., Linsley, P. S., Huang, L. Y., Germain, R. N., and Shevach, E. M. (1993) IL-10 inhibits macrophage costimulatory activity by selectively inhibiting the up-regulation of B7 expression. *J. Immunol.* **151,** 1224–1234.
235. D'Andrea, A., Aste-Amezaga, M., Valiante, N. M., Ma, X., Kubin, M., and Trinchieri, G. (1993) Interleukin 10 (IL-10) inhibits human lymphocyte interferon gamma- production by suppressing natural killer cell stimulatory factor/IL-12 synthesis in accessory cells. *J. Exp. Med.* **178,** 1041–1048.
236. Sher, A., Fiorentino, D., Caspar, P., Pearce, E., and Mosmann, T. (1991) Production of IL-10 by CD4+ T lymphocytes correlates with down- regulation of Th1 cytokine synthesis in helminth infection. *J. Immunol.* **147,** 2713–2716.
237. Taga, K. and Tosato, G. (1992) IL-10 inhibits human T cell proliferation and IL-2 production. *J. Immunol.* **148,** 1143–1148.
238. Katsikis, P. D., Cohen, S. B., Londei, M., and Feldmann, M. (1995) Are CD4+ Th1 cells pro-inflammatory or anti-inflammatory? The ratio of IL-10 to IFN-gamma or IL-2 determines their function. *Int. Immunol.* **7,** 1287–1294.
239. Yamamura, M., Uyemura, K., Deans, R. J., Weinberg, K., Rea, T. H., Bloom, B. R., and Modlin, R. L. (1991) Defining protective responses to pathogens: cytokine profiles in leprosy lesions. *Science* **254,** 277–279.

240. Caceres-Dittmar, G., Tapia, F. J., Sanchez, M. A., Yamamura, M., Uyemura, K., Modlin, R. L., et al. (1993) Determination of the cytokine profile in American cutaneous leishmaniasis using the polymerase chain reaction. *Clin. Exp. Immunol.* **91,** 500–505.
241. Barnes, P. F., Abrams, J. S., Lu, S., Sieling, P. A., Rea, T. H., and Modlin, R. L. (1993) Patterns of cytokine production by mycobacterium-reactive human T-cell clones. *Infect. Immun.* **61,** 197–203.
242. Sieling, P. A., Abrams, J. S., Yamamura, M., Salgame, P., Bloom, B. R., Rea, T. H., and Modlin, R. L. (1993) Immunosuppressive roles for IL-10 and IL-4 in human infection. In vitro modulation of T cell responses in leprosy. *J. Immunol.* **150,** 5501–5510.
243. Carvalho, E. M., Bacellar, O., Brownell, C., Regis, T., Coffman, R. L., and Reed, S. G. (1994) Restoration of IFN-gamma production and lymphocyte proliferation in visceral leishmaniasis. *J. Immunol.* **152,** 5949–5956.
244. King, C. L., Mahanty, S., Kumaraswami, V., Abrams, J. S., Regunathan, J., Jayaraman, K., et al. (1993) Cytokine control of parasite-specific anergy in human lymphatic filariasis. Preferential induction of a regulatory T helper type 2 lymphocyte subset. *J. Clin. Invest.* **92,** 1667–1673.
245. van der Poll, T., Jansen, P. M., Montegut, W. J., Braxton, C. C., Calvano, S. E., Stackpole, S. A., et al. (1997) Effects of IL-10 on systemic inflammatory responses during sublethal primate endotoxemia. *J. Immunol.* **158,** 1971–1975.
246. Riordan, F. A., Marzouk, O., Thomson, A. P., Sills, J. A., and Hart, C. A. (1996) Proinflammatory and anti-inflammatory cytokines in meningococcal disease. *Arch. Dis. Child.* **75,** 453–454.
247. Minty, A., Chalon, P., Derocq, J. M., Dumont, X., Guillemot, J. C., Kaghad, M., et al. (1993) Interleukin-13 is a new human lymphokine regulating inflammatory and immune responses. *Nature* **362,** 248–250.
248. Matthews, D. J. and Callard, R. E. (1998). IL-13, in *Cytokines* (Mire-Sluis, A. R. and Thorpe, R., eds.), Academic Press, London, pp. 205–216.
249. de Waal Malefyt, R., Abrams, J. S., Zurawski, S. M., Lecron, J. C., Mohan-Peterson, S., Sanjanwala, B., et al. (1995) Differential regulation of IL-13 and IL-4 production by human CD8+ and CD4+ Th0, Th1 and Th2 T cell clones and EBV-transformed B cells. *Int. Immunol.* **7,** 1405–1416.
250. Burd, P. R., Thompson, W. C., Max, E. E., and Mills, F. C. (1995) Activated mast cells produce interleukin 13. *J. Exp. Med.* **181,** 1373–1380.
251. McKenzie, A. N. and Zurawski, G. (1995) Interleukin-13: characterization and biologic properties. *Cancer Treat. Res.* **80,** 367–378.
252. Defrance, T., Carayon, P., Billian, G., Guillemot, J. C., Minty, A., Caput, D., and Ferrara, P. (1994) Interleukin 13 is a B cell stimulating factor. *J. Exp. Med.* **179,** 135–143.
253. Cocks, B. G., de Waal Malefyt, R., Galizzi, J. P., de Vries, J. E., and Aversa, G. (1993) IL-13 induces proliferation and differentiation of human B cells activated by the CD40 ligand. *Int. Immunol.* **5,** 657–663.
254. Punnonen, J., Aversa, G., Cocks, B. G., McKenzie, A. N., Menon, S., Zurawski, G., et al. (1993) Interleukin 13 induces interleukin 4-independent IgG4 and IgE

synthesis and CD23 expression by human B cells. *Proc. Natl. Acad. Sci. USA* **90,** 3730–3734.

255. de Waal Malefyt, R., Figdor, C. G., Huijbens, R., Mohan-Peterson, S., Bennett, B., Culpepper, J., et al. (1993) Effects of IL-13 on phenotype, cytokine production, and cytotoxic function of human monocytes. Comparison with IL-4 and modulation by IFN- gamma or IL-10. *J. Immunol.* **151,** 6370–6381.
256. Doyle, A. G., Herbein, G., Montaner, L. J., Minty, A. J., Caput, D., Ferrara, P., and Gordon, S. (1994) Interleukin-13 alters the activation state of murine macrophages in vitro: comparison with interleukin-4 and interferon-gamma. *Eur. J. Immunol.* **24,** 1441–1445.
257. Huang, S. K., Xiao, H. Q., Kleine-Tebbe, J., Paciotti, G., Marsh, D. G., Lichtenstein, L. M., and Liu, M. C. (1995) IL-13 expression at the sites of allergen challenge in patients with asthma. *J. Immunol.* **155,** 2688–2694.
258. Till, S., Durham, S., Dickason, R., Huston, D., Bungre, J., Walker, S., et al. (1997) IL-13 production by allergen-stimulated T cells is increased in allergic disease and associated with IL-5 but not IFN-gamma expression. *Immunology* **91,** 53–57.

25

Clinical Scoring Systems in Meningococcal Disease

Marino Festa and Bert Derkx

1. Introduction

Scoring systems used in meningococcal disease have been developed and validated to predict death or severity of illness in cohorts of patients, usually in the setting of intensive care. When using these scores, it is important to remember that any individual's score is only of limited value in prognosticating about that individual patient and can be misleading *(1)*. The accuracy of any score is determined by how well its estimated pattern of mortality compares with that observed in the score's developmental cohort, rather than in individual patients. Scores cannot be considered interchangeable; different scores, comprised of different sets of variables to arrive at the probability of mortality, may arrive at the same overall aggregate risk of mortality in a population of patients with meningococcal disease, despite individual estimates within this cohort of patients differing widely between scores. The ability of a score to predict death for patients who die and survival for those that live is best-described by the area under the receiver operator characteristic (ROC) curve *(2)*. This curve is a plot of sensitivity versus "(1-specificity)", i.e., the true-positive to false-positive fractions, at different decision thresholds. The greater the discriminative ability of a test, the closer the area under the curve comes towards 1.0, where the true-positive fraction is 1.0 or 100% (perfect specificity) and the false-positive fraction is 0 (perfect sensitivity). No score, however, has sufficient accuracy for individual prognostication and the use of scores in this way is inappropriate for clinical practice or research *(3)*.

Many scoring systems exist for use in pediatric intensive care (PICU), some of which have been designed and validated specifically for use in meningococcal disease. The aim of any score differs depending on the score's design. Most

From: *Methods in Molecular Medicine, vol. 67: Meningococcal Disease: Methods and Protocols*
Edited by: A. J. Pollard and M. C. J. Maiden © Humana Press Inc., Totowa, NJ

"generic" scores designed for general use in PICU attempt to allocate a risk of mortality to an individual and have been validated in the prediction of death in cohorts of patients in PICU. Allocation of mortality risk by mortality-prediction scores allows stratification of children by mortality-risk bands and comparison between bands as a marker of meningococcal disease severity rather than simply survivors vs nonsurvivors.

Other scores have been designed specifically for use in meningococcal disease or sepsis and are referred to as "meningococcal-specific" scores throughout this chapter. Most of these scores (e.g., Glasgow Meningococcal Septicaemia Prognostic Score [GMSPS], "MenOPP" bedside clinical score [MOC], Barcelona score, Neisseria Sepsis Index [NESI]) attempt to describe disease severity, rather than necessarily predict mortality, and in some cases are of more use in the prediction of survival rather than death.

1.1. The Ideal Scoring System

The ideal scoring system would need to be accurate enough to allow both prediction of mortality risk and also of serious morbidity, such as organ-system failure, in any individual child admitted to the PICU. Importantly, it should allocate the risk of subsequent morbidity or mortality early in the PICU admission using simple, easily available clinical and laboratory parameters to allow early scoring soon after admission in this clinically distinctive disease. Such a score could be used in a prospective fashion to allow consideration of new or experimental therapies in the most severe cases as well as being useful retrospectively to allow comparisons between centers and between treatment alternatives and pathophysiological markers of disease. Unfortunately, as already stated, no existing score is accurate enough to reliably prognosticate on an individual basis. Despite this, individual scoring of patients does allow children to be grouped in low- and high-risk groups and scores have been used to exclude low-risk groups from clinical trials designed to estimate treatment effects *(4)*. Stratification of children with meningococcal disease by mortality risk or severity scoring therefore allows early selection of "higher-risk" children and elimination of "low-risk" patients who will survive with current treatment strategies, for entry to clinical trials to assess novel therapies. Retrospective comparison of clinical and laboratory measures of disease pathophysiology is also facilitated by the use of scoring systems to bracket cases into severity groups for comparison and analysis.

1.2. Important Principles in the Application of Scoring Systems in Clinical Research

1. Analysis of research results should consider the group or "risk band" within which the patient falls, rather than considering any individual's score. Individuals in this group should be analyzed together and compared to other risk bands.

2. When applying any clinical score, it is important to compare like with like. Therefore children with meningococcal septicemia may need to be analyzed separately from those with meningococcal meningitis, because the clinical picture in these two distinct groups will differ sufficiently to impact on many scoring systems. An example of this is the prognostic significance of the C-reactive protein (CRP) level on admission in a series of patients with meningococcal purpura *(5)*. In children who were not shocked, the CRP had no prognostic value, whereas in children who were shocked, CRP was an accurate predictor of outcome.
3. Scores developed in one population should be used cautiously when applied to another population in a different setting or country where the score has not previously been validated. It has been shown that the performance of a score may differ depending on the clinical setting *(6)*. Unless a score has been validated in a multi-center study using a population similar to the one in which the score is to be applied, it cannot be assumed that the score will perform with the same degree of accuracy or discriminative ability in the study population *(7)*.
4. Because environmental, host, and bacterial factors may alter and as recognition and treatment of meningococcal disease improves, the validity of a score in this disease may also change *(8,9)*. Scoring systems in meningococcal disease therefore need revalidation after a period of time to mirror changes in mortality from this disease.

2. Methods

2.1. Generic Scoring Systems

Generic scoring systems are designed to predict mortality in all children admitted to PICU and are widespread and used routinely in most units. Commonly used scores in PICU include the Pediatric Risk of Mortality (PRISM) score developed in 1988 *(10)*, and the Paediatric Index of Mortality (PIM) score developed in 1997 *(11)*. PRISM III, an updated version of the PRISM score was published in 1996 *(12)* but is only available under license, and is not in widespread use outside the US and will not be described here. Generic scores have been designed and validated specifically for the prediction of mortality in children on PICU. The PRISM score has been used to assess severity of illness in children with meningococcal disease in a number of studies *(13–15)*; experience with PIM in meningococcal disease remains limited. Both scores have the advantage of being prospectively calculated and readily available in children admitted to most PICUs, but the disadvantage of poor accuracy in some studies *(6)*.

2.1.1. Pediatric Risk of Mortality (PRISM) Score

The original version of this score developed in 1988 by Pollack et al. *(10)* is in widespread clinical use in PICUs throughout the world. A number of important factors should be considered before using this score. Firstly, the score was developed and validated in units throughout the US, and doubts have been raised over its performance in other settings, particularly in developing countries *(6)*. Secondly, although Algren et al. showed the PRISM score to be an accurate predictor of mortality rate in meningococcal infection *(13)*, subsequent studies have shown the PRISM score may overpredict mortality in children in PICU with meningococcal disease *(11,15,16)*. Nevertheless, the PRISM score is accurate enough to allow stratification of children by mortality risk bands, and has been used in this way in a number of clinical studies *(17–19)*.

A practical difficulty with the use of this score is the number of parameters and the length of data collection required for the score. A total of 14 parameters over a 24-h period (minimum 8 h) are required prior to scoring (*see* **Table 1**). This delay in allocation of mortality risk leads to a methodological criticism of the PRISM and other "worst in 24-h" scores, namely that delay in scoring makes the score appear more accurate than it really is, with death being diagnosed rather than predicted in those that die. The delay in scoring also makes the PRISM score less useful for studies where early randomization for a planned intervention is required; for example, a prospective, randomized, controlled study to evaluate a novel treatment in the most unwell patients. Kanter et al. revalidated the PRISM score using hospital data from the 24 h prior to PICU admission *(20)*. This pre-ICU PRISM score can, therefore be scored on admission to PICU and may be suitable for the early stratification of children with meningococcal disease by mortality risk, although at present, there are no studies evaluating this score specifically in meningococcal disease. The number of variables and the dependence of this score on clinical and laboratory parameters are unchanged, however, and hence many of the practical difficulties with data collection with the PRISM score are also applicable to the pre-ICU PRISM.

2.1.2. Paediatric Index of Mortality (PIM) Score

Shann et al. introduced the PIM score in 1997 as an alternative mortality-prediction model for use in PICU *(11)*. It has the major advantage of being a quicker and simpler generic score, using only 8 explanatory variables to calculate a risk of mortality within 1 h of admission (*see* **Table 2**). Personal experience with this score in children with meningococcal disease in one tertiary PICU shows it performed as well as PRISM (ROC area 0.879 vs 0.880) *(16)*. However, experience in meningococcal disease with this score remains limited.

As previously stated, PIM has the advantage of being a simpler score using easily available test parameters. It is thus a quicker score to perform and may be a more useful generic score than PRISM where early stratification of children by mortality-risk bands is required. The PIM score may also be useful for comparison of survivors within and between institutions, in the same way as the PRISM score, as PIM becomes more widely used. Care, however, should be exercised when using either PRISM or PIM scores in settings outside those similar to the development and validation cohorts.

2.2 Disease-Specific Scores

A number of authors have published scoring systems designed specifically to predict morbidity and mortality in meningococcal disease. Many of these scores are based on the clinical criteria for prediction of outcome described by Stiehm and Damrosch in 1966 *(21)*. They developed a predictive model using the following criteria: Petechiae, shock, meningitis, blood leucocyte count, and erythrocyte sedimentation rate (ESR). A number of authors have subsequently published scores using various clinical and laboratory criteria. These severity scores vary in their dependence on laboratory measurements and this impacts on their speed of risk classification. Meningococcal specific scores do have the advantage of having been designed and validated specifically in cohorts of children, and in some cases adults, with meningococcal disease. Experience with individual scores varies greatly; one of the most commonly used scores is the Glasgow Meningococcal Septicaemia Prognostic Score (GMSPS). Thomson et al. published a 10-yr retrospective review of the performance of this score and found it was able to stratify children with meningococcal septicaemia by disease severity *(22)*. Other scores have been developed, mainly using easily available clinical parameters to attempt to classify patients early according to the expected course of the disease. Four factors should be considered when contemplating the use of such scores in clinical research:

1. Has the score been validated in a similar population to that in which the study is proposed?
2. Was the score developed specifically for use in meningococcal septicemia excluding cases of meningococcal meningitis, or for all meningococcal disease?
3. Was the score developed and validated in children and/or adults?
4. The age of the score. When was the score developed and validated; is it still valid?

Six meningococcal-specific scores are reviewed here:

2.2.1. Glasgow Meningococcal Septicaemia Prognostic Score (GMSPS)

The GMSPS is a simple clinical scoring system that can be performed rapidly at the bedside, allowing early risk allocation (*see* **Table 3**). The score was designed in the UK, as a dynamic system allowing for rescoring in the face of clinical deterioration; this use of rescoring is responsible for the high sensitivity

Table 1
Pediatric Risk of Mortality (PRISM) Score (Worst in 24-h values (minimum of 8 h) required for each parameter)

Variable	Age restrictions and ranges			Score
Systolic BP (mmHg)	Infants		Children	
	130–160		150–200	2
	55–65		65–75	
	>160		>200	6
	40–54		50–64	
	<40		<50	7
Diastolic BP (mmHg)		All ages		
		>110		6
Heart rate (beats/min)	Infants		Children	
	>160		>150	4
	<90		<80	
Resp rate (breaths/min)	Infants		Children	
	61–90		51–70	1
	>90		>70	5
	Apnea		Apnea	
PaO_2/FiO_2[a]		All ages		
		200–300		2
		<200		3
$PaCO_2$[b] (torr)		All ages		
		51–65		1
		>65		5
Glasgow Coma score[c]		All ages		
		<8		6
Pupillary reactions		All ages		
		unequal or dilated		4
		fixed and dilated		10
PT/PTT		All ages		
		>1.5 × control		2
Total bilirubin (mg/dl)		>1 mo		
		>3.5		6
Potassium (mEq/L)		All ages		
		3.0–3.5		1
		6.5–7.5		
		<3.0		5
		>7.5		

(continued)

Table 1 *(continued)*

Variable	Age restrictions and ranges	Score
Calcium (mg/dl)	All ages	
	7.0–8.0	2
	12.0–15.0	
	<7.0	6
	>15.0	
Glucose (mg/dl)	All ages	
	40–60	4
	250–400	
	<40	8
	>400	
Bicarbonate[d] (mEq/L)	All ages	
	<16	3
	>32	

[a]Cannot be assessed in patients with intracardiac shunts or chronic respiratory insufficiency; requires arterial blood sampling.

[b]May be assessed with capillary blood gases.

[c]Assessed only if there is known or suspected CNS dysfunction; cannot be assessed in patients during iatrogenic sedation, paralysis, anesthesia, etc. Scores <8 correspond to coma or deep stupor.

[d]Use measured values.

The total score (PRISM) is entered into the following equation to calculate r:

$$r = 0.207 \times \text{PRISM} - 0.005 \times \text{age (months)} - 0.433 \times \text{operative status} - 4.782$$

where operative status is defined as postoperative = 1, nonoperative = 0

The probability of death may then be calculated as follows:

$$p\text{ (ICU death)} = \exp r / (1 + \exp [R])$$

and specificity of the GMSPS in a published retrospective review of its performance over a 10-yr period in children with meningococcal septicemia ***(22)***. However, early scoring, for example on admission, significantly reduced the predictive accuracy of the GMSPS in this study. Prospective validation of this score has shown a score ≥8 to best identify children at risk of dying from meningococcal disease (odds ratio 0.87) ***(23)***. However, a retrospective review of cases between 1985 and 1991 in a tertiary referral PICU in London found a high rate of survival in children with a score of >8 (62%), and significant survival even with a GMSPS >10 ***(8)***. The improving survival rate in the higher-risk groups using this score emphasizes the need to revalidate scoring systems to bring the predictive capability of the score up

Table 2
Pediatric Index of Mortality (PIM)[a]

Booked or elective admission to PICU (no = 0, yes = 1)
Presence of one of the following underlying conditions (no = 0, yes = 1)
—Cardiac arrest out of hospital
—Severe combined immunodeficiency syndrome
—Leukemia/lymphoma after 1st induction
—Cerebral hemorrhage
—Cardiomyopathy or myocarditis
—Hypoplastic left heart syndrome
—HIV infection
—IQ probably <35, worse than Down's
—A neurodegenerative disorder
Response of pupils to bright light (both >3 mm and both fixed = 1, other = 0, unknown = 0)
Base excess in arterial or capillary blood, mmol/l (unknown = 0)
PaO_2, mmHg (unknown = 0)
FiO_2 at time of PaO_2 if oxygen via ETT or headbox (unknown = 0)
Systolic blood pressure, mmHg (unknown = 120)
Mechanical ventilation at any time during first hour in PICU (no = 0, yes = 1)

[a]Use the first value of each variable measured within the period from the time of first contact to 1 h after arrival in PICU. First contact is defined as the first face-to-face (not telephone) contact between the patient and a doctor from the PICU (or a doctor from a specialist pediatric transport team)

The information in table can be used to calculate the PIM logit:

PIM logit (e^{logit}) = (–1.552 × elective admission, y/n) + (1.826 × specified diagnosis, y/n) + (2.357 × pupillary reaction to light) + (0.071 × absolute base excess) + (0.415 × (100 × FiO_2/PaO_2)) + (0.021 × (absolute systolic BP-120)) + (1.342 × mechanical ventilation, y/n) – 4.873

The logit must be converted to the predicted probability of death using the following formula:

$$\text{Predicted probability of death} = e^{logit}/(1+ e^{logit})$$

to date with modern "conventional" management before using severity scores to select patients for entry into clinical trials designed to assess novel therapies. In 1996, in a comparison of eight severity scores in 125 children with meningococcal disease, Derkx et al. found the GMSPS to be a simple and reliable score for identification of low-risk patients, accurately identifying a subgroup of patients with no mortality ***(24)***. The GMSPS is a widely used score and has been used to identify and stratify children likely to benefit from a novel therapy in meningococcal disease in a large multi-center, international, randomized, controlled clinical trial ***(4)***.

Table 3
Glasgow Meningococcal Septicemia Prognostic Score (GMSPS)

Bedside parameter	Points
BP <75 mmHg systolic, age <4 yr <85 mmHg systolic, age >4 yr	3
Skin/rectal temperature difference >3°C	3
Modified coma scale score <8[a] or deterioration of ≥3 points in 1 h	3
Deterioration in hour before scoring	2
Absence of meningism	2
Extending purpuric rash or widespread ecchymoses	1
Base deficit (capillary or arterial) >8.0	1
Maximum score	15

[a]Modified coma scale

i. Eyes open	
Spontaneously	4
To speech	3
To pain	2
None	1
ii. Best verbal response	
Orientated	6
Words	4
Vocal sounds	3
Cries	2
None	1
iii. Best motor response	
Obeys commands	6
Localizes pain	4
Moves to pain	1
None	0

Add scores i, ii, and iii to give result.

Retrospective use of this score is potentially more difficult, as the score changes depending on the time of scoring during the admission in a deteriorating patient. Hence with repetitive scoring the GMSPS score tends to increase; the timing of scoring is therefore important when comparing patients and therapies. Use of the highest score during an admission will best describe an individual's disease severity, but it may be important to have a fixed time-point for scoring, because there is the potential for individuals to deteriorate because of a therapy rather than despite it. Another possible criticism of this score is its use of the modified Glasgow Coma Scale, which in young infants and children at highest risk of meningococcal disease may be difficult to assess.

Despite these concerns, the GMSPS remains a widely used and relatively simple score that enables easy identification of low-risk patients for exclusion

Table 4
MenOPP Bedside Clinical Score (MOC)

Bedside parameter	Points
Systolic BP: ≤100 mmHg (adult); ≤70 mmHg (child)	1
Cyanosis	1
Ecchymosis	1
Diarrhea before or at admission	1
Cold extremities	1
No nuchal or back rigidity	1
Temperature ≥40.0°C	1
Maximum score	7

from clinical trials evaluating the effectiveness of new treatment alternatives and comparison of patients by disease severity.

2.2.2. "MenOPP" Bedside Clinical Score (MOC)

The MOC was developed from the assessment of all hospital admissions with meningococcal disease in Norway over a 1-yr period ***(25)***. The main attraction of this score is its simplicity, and therefore its speed, as it includes only 7 easily available clinical parameters obtained at the bedside (*see* **Table 4**). In a combined prospective and retrospective study of 125 children, the MOC showed good accuracy (ROC area = 0.866) and compared well with other more complicated clinical-scoring systems ***(24)***. This study showed mortality increased markedly in patients with a MOC ≥3. Unlike some of the other scores described in this chapter, the MOC score has been developed for use in meningococcal disease in any hospital department and in ambulatory practice and is designed to allow early assignment of disease severity. This makes for a rapid, practical score, which may also be useful in the prehospital environment.

2.2.3. Tüysüz score

Tüysüz and colleagues have developed a simple bedside score using simple clinical parameters plus the initial leucocyte count and CSF analysis (*see* **Table 5**). This score was developed from a retrospective review of 140 patients with meningococcal disease in Turkey ***(26)***. The authors suggest that this score's 9-point scale is useful in identifying low-risk (0–5 points), medium-risk (6–7 points), and high-risk groups (8–9 points), with mortality rates in the developmental set of 1.7, 25.0, and 100% respectively. The Tüysüz score performed well in a comparative review of meningococcal severity scores in the Netherlands (ROC area = 0.825) ***(24)***. A major disadvantage of this score, however, is its dependence on cerbrospinal fluid (CSF) analysis. Lumbar puncture is not

Table 5
Tüysüz Score

Clinical parameter	Points
Hypotension (systolic <5th percentile for age)	3
Diffuse petechiae (uncountable) developed <12 h prior to hospital admission	2
Peripheral WBC count <10,000/mm^3	2
Disturbed consciousness (sensorial variability between somnolence and coma)	1
Absence of meningitis (clinical signs and >100 WBC in CSF or positive CSF culture)	1
Maximum score	9

routinely performed in children presenting with meningococcal disease and may be contraindicated in a large number cases owing to a significantly decreased conscious level or severe shock and hemodynamic instability *(27)*. Inability to analyze CSF in these children precludes the use of this scoring system in a significant number of cases.

2.2.4. The Barcelona Scale

This score was prospectively developed and validated in children and adults presenting with meningococcal disease in 24 hospitals in Barcelona in 1997 *(28)*. It is a simple scoring system based on 4 readily available bedside parameters (*see* **Table 6**) and therefore has the advantage of being rapidly calculated on admission to hospital. The authors of this score conclude that a Barcelona score ≥1 is associated with a significant mortality and should be used to prioritize patients for intensive-care management. Although the Barcelona score performed well in its validation set (area under ROC curve = 0.91), this may be expected as this population of patients was the same as the score's derivation set. It remains to be seen whether the discriminatory power of the Barcelona score remains high in populations outside of this.

2.2.5. Neisseria Sepsis Index (NESI)

The NESI was developed in Moscow and Düsseldorf and uses only four variables *(29)* (*see* **Table 7**). It avoids complicated laboratory parameters and is therefore a relatively simple and quick score to perform. The NESI generates a score from 0–8, with an increasing score indicating increasingly severe sepsis. The authors of this score only observed deaths in children with a NESI >4. A subsequent observational study using data collected from all German pediatric hospitals over a 1-yr period (1994–1995) suggested a cut-off NESI >5 may be appropriate for consideration of alternative adjunctive therapeutic strategies in children with meningococcal sepsis *(30)*. Experience with this score

Table 6
The Barcelona Score

Bedside parameter	Points
Pre-admission antibiotic (≥1 dose of an antibiotic active against *N. meningitidis* within 12 h of admission)	–1
Age	
0–59 yr	0
>60 yr	1
Focal neurological signs (sensory, motor, or cranial nerve disturbances of central origin not present before the episode of meningococcal disease)	1
Hemorrhagic diathesis	2
Maximum score	4

remains limited, however, and comparison with more established scoring systems is needed.

2.2.6. The Rotterdam Score

This score was developed retrospectively from the clinical and laboratory characteristics of 75 children with meningococcal septic shock ***(18)***. The Rotterdam score uses 4 laboratory parameters to predict a risk of mortality rather than attempting to grade severity of illness by a random scale. The estimated risk of mortality may then be used to group patients into mortality-risk bands as a marker of disease severity. Individual mortality risk predictions should not be used in the analysis of clinical research studies as, in keeping with generic mortality prediction scores described earlier (**Subheding 1.2.**), the score is not accurate enough to be used in this way.

A disadvantage of the score is that the assignment of mortality risk is not possible until these laboratory parameters are available following admission and initial management in the emergency department or PICU, making this score less useful if early assignment of mortality risk is the goal. The use of CRP as one of the score's parameters may preclude this score's use in some centers where CRP is unavailable. Other parameters identified by multiple regression analysis in the development set were base excess, serum potassium level, and platelet count. The values for each of these variables have been weighted and brought together in the following mathematical expression of the probability of death: $e^{RS}/1 + e^{RS}$, where RS = Rotterdam score, a value defined as 1.01 + (1.21 × serum potassium level) – (0.29 × base excess) – (0.024 × platelet count) – (3.75 × log serum CRP level). Comparison of this score with the PRISM score in the development set by the Rotterdam score's authors

Table 7
The Neisseria Sepsis Index (NESI)

	Points		
Physiological parameter	0	1	2
Heart rate (bts/min)			
<4 yr	≤140	>140 to <200	≥200
≥4 yr	≤120	>120 to <180	≥180
Mean arterial pressure (mmHg)			
<4 yr	≥45	<45 to >20	≤20
≥4 yr	≥60	< 60 to >30	≤30
Base Excess (mval/l)	≥–6	<–6 to >–12	≤–12
Newly developed subcutaneous bleeding and/or skin necrosis	No	—	Yes
(Maximum score = 8)			

showed correlation between the two scores (r = 0.58). However, experience with the Rotterdam score remains limited and a multi-center study is required to validate this score.

In conclusion, a number of scoring systems may be applied to children with meningococcal disease in order to describe severity and facilitate clinical research into this clinically distinctive disease. Scoring systems differ in their local availability, with generic scores used "routinely" in many PICUs, and in their ease of use and accuracy within any given clinical setting. Any score chosen should take into account the clinical setting in which it is to be applied and local experience with the score. Different types of studies require different performance characteristics from a score and this should be considered during the study design. For example a clinical trial of a new drug therapy to be given early in the management of meningococcal disease would require rapid, early risk stratification. Scores capable of doing this, e.g., Pre-ICU PRISM, PIM, MOC, Barcelona, NESI, and perhaps GMSPS scores may be most suitable for use in such a trial. In laboratory-based studies comparing pathophysiological markers of disease, however, it may be particularly important to differentiate between mild, moderate and severe disease. In such cases, the score's accuracy is of paramount importance. The GMSPS is often used in this setting, because experience has shown the GMSPS to be one of the more accurate scoring systems.

References

1. Marcin, J. P., Pollack, M. M., Patel, K. M., and Ruttimann, U. E. (1998) Decision support issues using a physiology based score. *Intensive Care Med.* **24,** 1299–1304.

2. Zweig, M. H. and Campbell, G. (1993) Receiver-operating characteristic (ROC) plots: a fundamental evaluation tool in clinical medicine [published erratum appears in Clin. Chem. 1993 Aug;39(8):1589]. *Clin. Chem.* **39,** 561–577.
3. Lemeshow, S., Klar, J., and Teres, D. (1995) Outcome prediction for individual intensive care patients: useful, misused, or abused? *Intensive Care Med.* **21,** 770–776.
4. Giroir, B. P., Quint, P. A., Barton, P., Kirsch, E. A., Kitchen, L., Goldstein, B., et al. (1997) Preliminary evaluation of recombinant amino-terminal fragment of human bactericidal/permeability-increasing protein in children with severe meningococcal sepsis. *Lancet* **350,** 1439–1443.
5. Leclerc, F., Hue, V., Martinot, A., and Delepoulle, F. (1991). Scoring systems for accurate prognosis of patients with meningococcal infections. *Am. J. Dis. Child* **145,** 1090–1091.
6. Wells, M., Riera-Fanego, J. F., Luyt, D. K., Dance, M., and Lipman, J. (1996) Poor discriminatory performance of the Pediatric Risk of Mortality (PRISM) score in a South African intensive care unit [see comments]. *Crit. Care Med.* **24,** 1507–1513.
7. Patel, P. A. and Grant, B. J. (1999). Application of mortality prediction systems to individual intensive care units. *Intensive Care Med.* **25,** 977–982.
8. Shah, A. and Matthew, D. J. (1992) Glasgow Meningococcal Septicemia Prognostic Score in meningococcal septicemia [letter; comment]. *Crit. Care Med.* **20,** 1495–1496.
9. Leclerc, F., Delepoulle, F., Diependaele, J. F., Martinot, A., Hue, V., Flurin, V., et al. (1995) Severity scores in meningococcal septicemia and severe infectious purpura with shock. *Intensive Care Med.* **21,** 264–265.
10. Pollack, M. M., Ruttimann, U. E., and Getson, P. R. (1988) Pediatric risk of mortality (PRISM) score. *Crit. Care Med.* **16,** 1110–1116.
11. Shann, F., Pearson, G., Slater, A., and Wilkinson, K. (1997) Paediatric index of mortality (PIM): a mortality prediction model for children in intensive care. *Intensive Care Med.* **23,** 201–207.
12. Pollack, M. M., Patel, K. M., and Ruttimann, U. E. (1996) PRISM III: an updated Pediatric Risk of Mortality score. *Crit. Care Med.* **24,** 743–752.
13. Algren, J. T., Lal, S., Cutliff, S. A., and Richman, B. J. (1993) Predictors of outcome in acute meningococcal infection in children. *Crit. Care Med.* **21,** 447–452.
14. Mok, Q. and Butt, W. (1996) The outcome of children admitted to intensive care with meningococcal septicaemia. *Intensive Care Med.* **22,** 259–263.
15. van Brakel, M. J., van Vught, A. J., and Gemke, R. J. (2000) Pediatric risk of mortality (PRISM) score in meningococcal disease. *Eur. J. Pediatr.* **159(4),** 232–236.
16. Festa, M., McDermott, W., Britto, J., Habibi, P., and Nadel, S. (1998) Validation and comparison of PRISM and PIM scores in prediction of mortality from meningococcal disease. *Intensive Care Med.* **24(S1),** S41(Abstract).
17. Goldman, A. P., Kerr, S. J., Butt, W., Marsh, M. J., Murdoch, I. A., Paul, T., et al. (1997) Extracorporeal support for intractable cardiorespiratory failure due to meningococcal disease. *Lancet* **349,** 466–469.
18. Kornelisse, R. F., Hazelzet, J. A., Hop, W. C., Spanjaard, L., Suur, M. H., van, d., V, and de Groot, R. (1997) Meningococcal septic shock in children: clinical and

laboratory features, outcome, and development of a prognostic score. *Clin. Infect. Dis.* **25,** 640–646.
19. Hazelzet, J. A., de Groot, R., van Mierlo, G., Joosten, K. F., van de Vort, E., Eerenberg, A., et al. (1998) Complement activation in relation to capillary leakage in children with septic shock and purpura. *Infect. Immun.* **66,** 5350–5356.
20. Kanter, R. K., Edge, W. E., Caldwell, C. R., Nocera, M. A., and Orr, R. A. (1997) Pediatric mortality probability estimated from pre-ICU severity of illness. *Pediatrics* **99,** 59–63.
21. Stiehm, E. R. and Damrosch, D. S. (1966) Factors in the prognosis of meningococcal infection. Review of 63 cases with emphasis on recognition and management of the severely ill patient. *J. Pediatr.* **68,** 457–467.
22. Thomson, A. P., Sills, J. A., and Hart, C. A. (1991) Validation of the Glasgow Meningococcal Septicemia Prognostic Score: a 10-year retrospective survey. *Crit. Care Med.* **19,** 26–30.
23. Marzouk, O., Thomson, A. P., and Sills, J. A. (1991) Clinical features and management of meningococcal disease. *Care Crit. Ill* **7,** 186–187 (Abstract).
24. Derkx, H. H., van den Hoek, J., Redekop, W. K., Bijlmer, R. P., van Deventer, S. J., and Bossuyt, P. M. (1996) Meningococcal disease: a comparison of eight severity scores in 125 children. *Intensive Care Med.* **22,** 1433–1441.
25. Gedde-Dahl, T. W., Bjark, P., Hoiby, E. A., Host, J. H., and Bruun, J. N. (1990) Severity of meningococcal disease: assessment by factors and scores and implications for patient management. *Rev. Infect. Dis.* **12,** 973–992.
26. Tuysuz, B., Ozlu, I., Aji, D. Y., and Erginel, A. (1993) Prognostic factors in meningococcal disease and a new scoring system. *Acta Paediatr.* **82,** 1053–1056.
27. Pollard, A. J., Britto, J., Nadel, S., DeMunter, C., Habibi, P., and Levin, M. (1999) Emergency management of meningococcal disease. *Arch. Dis. Child* **80,** 290–296.
28. Barquet, N., Domingo, P., Cayla, J. A., Gonzalez, J., Rodrigo, C., Fernandez-Viladrich, P., et al. (1997) Prognostic factors in meningococcal disease. Development of a bedside predictive model and scoring system. Barcelona Meningococcal Disease Surveillance Group. *JAMA* 278, 491–496.
29. Nurnberger, W., Platonov, A., Stannigel, H., Beloborodov, V. B., Michelmann, I., von Kries, R., et al. (1995) Definition of a new score for severity of generalized Neisseria meningitidis infection. *Eur. J. Pediatr.* **154,** 896–900.
30. Nurnberger, W., Kries, R., Bohm, O., and Gobel, U. (1999) Systemic meningococcal infection: which children may benefit from adjuvant haemostatic therapy? Results from an observational study. *Eur. J. Pediatr.* **158(Suppl. 3),** S192–S196.

26

Quantitative Detection of Bacterial Lipopolysaccharides in Clinical Specimens

Petter Brandtzaeg, Reidun Øvstebø, and Peter Kierulf

1. Introduction

Lipopolysaccharides (LPS) located to the outer leaflet of the outer membrane have been identified as the main common endotoxic component of Gram-negative bacteria *(1–3)*. Although other constituents of the bacterial cell wall, i.e., peptidoglycan, may contribute, LPS is considered to be the single most important constituent of *Neisseria meningitidis* that induces inflammation in the host *(4–12)*. Neisserial lipopolysaccharides are often referred to as lipooligosaccharides (LOS) owing to the short polysaccharide chains comprising approx 10 sugars or less that are attached to lipid A.

The ability of LPS to activate a variety of immune cells is primarily related to lipid A, which is considered to be the endotoxic center of bacterial LPS *(1–3)*. Lipid A in *N. meningitidis* LPS consists of two 1′–6 linked D-glucosamine molecules to which equimolar amounts of hydroxylaurate (3-OH-12:O), hydroxymyristate (3-OH-14:O), laurate (12:O), and phosphate are attached (**Fig. 1**). Lipid A in *N. meningitidis* differs from lipid A in *Neisseria gonorrhoae* in that both phosphate groups are largely substituted by 2-aminoethylphosphate *(13)*. The fatty acids hydroxylaurate, hydroxymyristate, and laurate are attached to each of the two D-glucosamine molecules of neisserial lipid A, making it a symmetrical molecule that differs from asymmetrical lipid A found in important disease-causing, Gram-negative rods, for example, *Escherichia coli* and Salmonella species *(1–3,13)*.

If meningococci gain access to the circulation, the subarachnoid space, or other normally sterile body compartments such as pericardium, joints, or eyes, they may activate a variety of cells directly or indirectly. During proliferation,

From: *Methods in Molecular Medicine, vol. 67: Meningococcal Disease: Methods and Protocols*
Edited by: A. J. Pollard and M. C. J. Maiden © Humana Press Inc., Totowa, NJ

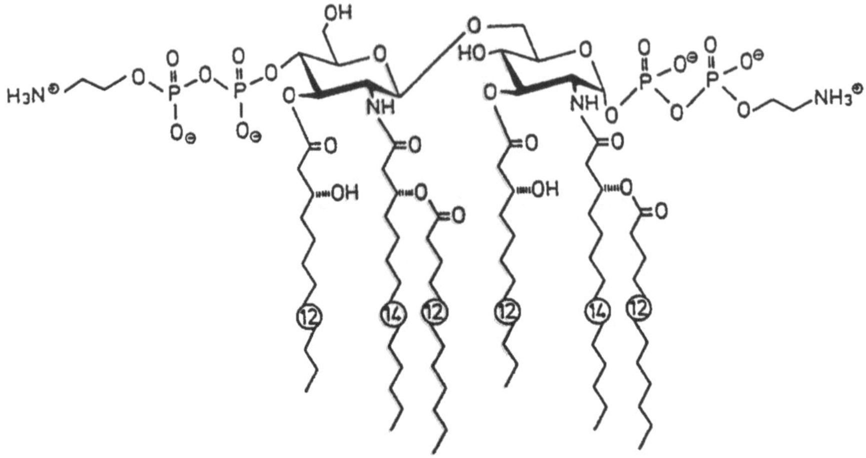

Fig. 1. Lipid A of pathogenic *Neisseria meningitidis*. Adapted with permission from **ref. *13***.

N. meningitidis tends to oversynthesize and shed outer-membrane vesicles (OMVs) containing LPS. In addition, meningococci readily undergo lysis, thereby releasing fragments of the outer membrane.

Host cells derived from the myeloid cell line and expressing CD14 on the surface, i.e., monocytes, macrophages, and neutrophils, play a key role in cellular inflammatory responses ***(14,15)***. How the LPS molecules, which normally are present in a lipid bilayer or as large aggregates in aqueous solution, induce cell activation in the host is presently only partly known. The LPS molecules are apparently detached from the bacterial outer membrane and form complexes with various plasma proteins, including LPS-binding protein (LBP), bactericidal permeability-increasing protein (BPI) derived from neutrophils, high-density lipoprotein (HDL), low-density lipoprotein (LDL), albumin, lactoferrin, serum amyeloid proteins (SAP), and others ***(16–21)***. LBP augments the CD14-mediated cellular reaction to lipid A whereas BPI, HDL, LDL, and lactoferrin reduce the cellular response to lipid A and function as a "buffer system" in the blood. SAP interferes with the LPS binding to HDL ***(21)***. Human hemoglobin binds LPS and enhances its toxicity ***(22)***. The latter observation may be of importance in meningococcal septicemia with coagulopathy, extensive hemorrhage, and disintegration of erythrocytes, particularly in the skin and the adrenals. The lipid A-LBP complex is recognized by CD14 and "guided" to the Toll-like receptor 4 expressed on the same cells. The Toll-like receptor 4 initiates transmembrane signaling activating the interleukin 1 (IL-1) intracellular signaling pathway, which finally induces DNA transcription in the nucleus ***(23,24)***.

1.1. The Role of Meningococcal LPS in Human Pathophysiology

Although endotoxin was suggested to play a central part in the pathogenesis of *N. meningitidis* at the beginning of the twentieth century, no direct proof was established before the 1980s and early 1990s *(5–7,25,26)*. At that time the Limulus amoebocyte lysate (LAL) assay using a chromogenic substrate was well-established as a reliable and reproducible method *(27–33)*. Systematic collection of patient samples revealed a consistent pattern that linked the levels of LPS to the clinical presentation of the meningococcal infection *(5–7,25,26,34–38)*. Patients developing fulminant meningococcal septicemia characterized by persistent septic shock, renal impairment, disseminated intravascular coagulation, and lack of significant pleocytosis were characterized by very high levels of LPS in the circulation and low levels in cerbebrospinal fluid (CSF) *(34–38)*. The circulating levels of LPS were quantitatively associated with the degree of activation of the plasma-cascade systems, i.e., the complement system, the coagulation system, and kallikrein-kinin system *(8,39–40)*. Plasminogen activator inhibitor 1 (PAI-1) was massively released in patients with the highest levels of circulating LPS, inducing a significant inhibition of the fibrinolysis *(41)*. The plasma levels of pro- and anti-inflammatory cytokines such as tumor necrosis factor-α (TNF-α), IL-1, interleukin 6 (IL-6), and interleukin 10 (IL-10) were associated with plasma levels of LPS *(42,43)*. The very high levels of LPS in plasma have been verified by quantifying hydroxylauric acid as a marker of neisserial LPS by gas-chromatography (GC) and mass-spectrometry (MS) *(7)*. The levels measured with the LAL assay, which is a bioassay and the chemical analysis employing GC-MS showed a close correlation *(7)*.

Patients presenting with distinct signs of meningitis without severe circulatory impairment revealed the opposite picture, i.e., low levels of LPS in plasma and high levels in CSF *(6,9,37)*. Patients presenting with both fulminant septicemia and distinct meningitis had LPS levels that were elevated in both compartments. A fourth group of patients is denoted "mild systemic meningococcal disease" or "mild meningococcemia" because they show no signs of severe circulatory impairment or clinically signs of distinct meningitis with marked pleocytosis (100×10^9 leukocytes/l CSF). These patients are characterized by low levels of LPS in both circulation and CSF *(11)*. The pathophysiological changes observed in our patients are in line with the pathophysiological responses observed in humans challenged with small doses of purified LPS intravenously *(44)*.

1.2. The LAL Assay

The levels of meningococcal LPS when detectable in plasma or CSF are in the order of few pg/mL to less than 1 μg/mL *(5–7,25,26,34–38)*. The only method presently available to quantify LPS in body fluids at these low levels is

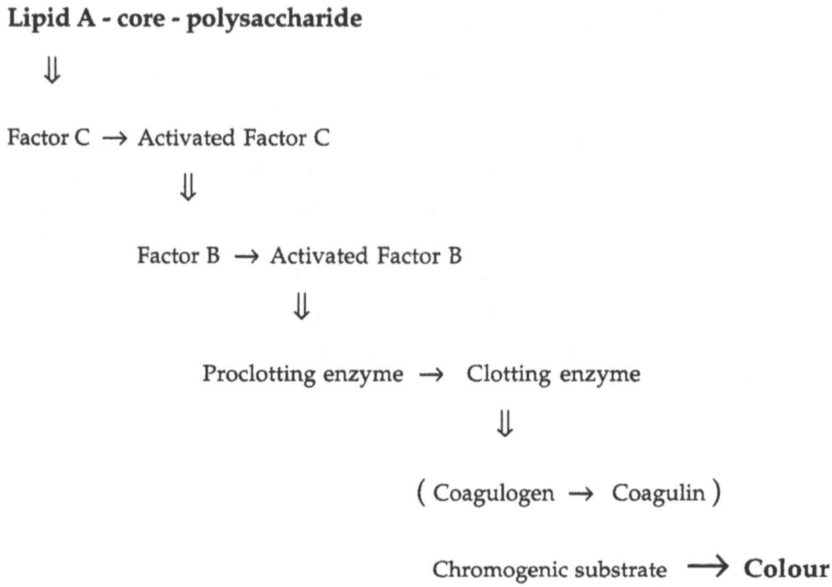

Fig. 2. The coagulation system of the *Limulus polyphemus* (horseshoe crab), which is used in the Limulus amoebocyte lysate, (LAL) assay. In assays using a chromogenic substrate, the coagulogen is removed so as not to interfere with the conversion of the chromogenic substrate.

the LAL assay. This assay makes use of purified components of the coagulation system of *Limulus polyphemus* (the horseshoe crab) (**Fig. 2**) ***(27,32)***. This primitive coagulation system is located within the amoebocytes, the only blood cell that circulates in the bluish hemolymph of the horseshoe crab ***(32)***. The coagulation system is activated by the lipid A moiety of the LPS molecule as a cascade of several enzymes: denoted factor C, factor B, proclotting enzyme, and coagulogen (**Fig. 2**). When proclotting enzyme is activated to clotting enzyme, it converts coagulogen to coagulin, transforming the hemolymph to a gel. Presently the final enzymatic step in this cascade is often read spectrophotometrically, substituting the terminal step, i.e., the conversion of coagulogen to coagulin (gel formation) with a chromogenic peptide substrate ***(25–33)*** (**Fig 2**).

1.3. Usefulness of the Method

Our experience with LPS measurements in 130 patients with documented meningococcal infections studied during a 16-yr period suggest that a persistent septic shock develops in patients with plasma LPS levels >700 ng/l (7 EU/mL). Persistent septic shock below this LPS level is rarely seen. When patients are grouped according to the admission level of plasma LPS, the case-fatality rate increases with increasing levels of LPS. Among our patients, a LPS content in plasma >15,000 ng/l has been associated with 100% fatality. Sequential measurements of LPS in plasma suggest that the LPS production in the circulation is immediately turned off after the first dose of antibiotic is injected. The rapidly declining levels of native LPS ($T_{1/2}$ = 1–3 h) are paralleled with declining levels of various inflammatory cytokines (TNF-α, IL-6, IL-10) and other mediators contributing to the vascular dysfunction (PAI-1, thrombin activation as measured by fibrinopeptide A). These observations provide a scientific base for early antibiotic treatment of these patients.

The quantitative measurements of LPS in plasma from patients with systemic meningococcal disease reveal a closer association with outcome and underlying pathophysiology than generally observed in other human infections caused by Gram-negative bacteria ***(45)***. The underlying causes of the bacterium's variable ability to proliferate and generate LPS-containing material in the circulation are still largely unknown.

2. Materials

1. Heparinized vacuum tubes. Endo Tube ET® (Chromogenix AB, Mölndal, Sweden). The tubes contain 30 IU heparin/mL blood and are guaranteed to be LPS-free. They collect 4 mL blood and have been developed specifically for LPS testing of blood.
2. Vials for storage of patient plasma and CFS. Cryotubes® 3-68632, (Nunc, Roskilde, Denmark) can be stored for more than 10 yr at –70°C.
3. Pooled heparinized normal plasma. Blood from 10 healthy blood donors is collected in Endo Tube ET®, centrifuged at 1,400*g* for 10 min, and the plasma pipetted off. Equal volumes from the 10 donors are mixed and stored in suitable volumes (for example, 2 mL).
4. Dilution fluid. Pooled heparinized plasma is thawed and diluted 1 + 9 with distilled H_2O to prepare a fluid of constant protein and ionic strength.
5. LAL (BioWhittaker, Inc, Walkersville, MD; Cat. no. N186).
6. Purified lipopolysaccharide. *E. coli* strain O55B5 LPS 7–10 endotoxin units (EU)/ng, (Cat. no. N185, BioWhittaker).
7. LPS samples for longitudinal controls. Divide a patient's plasma with high LPS concentration into single-use lots and store it deep-frozen (–70°C). Dilute one lot 1 + 9 with distilled H_2O; dilute further with dilution fluid to final concentrations of 7, 40, and 100 ng/L. Before each run, duplicate samples of 7, 40, and 100 ng/L are heat-inactivated (*see* **Subheading 3.4., step 2**) and used as longitudinal controls. Plot the results and estimate the mean and standard deviation (SD) of the measurements based on 30 observations.
8. Purified *E. coli* O55B5 LPS as alternative longitudinal controls. In lack of a patient plasma with high level of LPS, prepare pooled heparinized plasma enriched with *E. coli* O55B5 LPS to a concentration of 2,000 ng/L. Store deep

frozen in suitable small volumes (–70°C). For each run thaw a sample of the LPS-enriched control plasma and dilute to three different levels (7, 40, and 100 ng/L), heat inactivate (*see* above) and use as longitudinal controls.

9. Chromogenic peptide substrate. The chromogenic peptide substrate S-2423 (Chromogenix AB, Mölndal).
10. 0.5 *M* Tris-HCl, 0.2 *M* NaCl, ph 9.0.
11. Microtiter plates. The 96-well microtiter plates PS-Mikrotiterplatte® (Cat. no. 655101; Labortechnik, Nurtingen, Germany). Each new batch has to be tested for LPS contamination or nonspecific reactivity.
12. Microplate reader. The THERMOmax microplate reader equipped with SOFTware® version 2.01 (Molecular Devices Corporation, Menlo Park, CA).

3. Methods

3.1. Preparation of Patients' Plasma and Control Plasma

1. Collect blood in a Cryotube or a sterile vacuum tube containing 30 IU LPS-free heparin/mL blood. Centrifuge at 1,400*g* for 10 min at room temperature (+20°C). Pipet off the heparin plasma. Divide it into suitable volumes in Cryotubes and store at –70°C until the samples are analyzed. Thaw the samples at room temperature (+20°C). Mix the samples vigorously 3 min before the analysis.

3.2. Preparation of LAL

1. Reconstitute one vial of LAL (sensitivity varies from batch to batch, Cat. no. N186; BioWhittaker) with 6.0 mL of distilled H_2O. Aliquot the reconstituted LAL and store deep-frozen at –70°C in cryotubes. Owing to the varying sensitivity of the LAL-reagents, the reconstituted LAL solution of each new batch must be tested for possible further dilution with distilled H_2O to obtain the optimal working solution.
2. Determine the optimal incubation time of LAL reagents and LPS for each new batch of LAL by incubating different concentrations of the standard LPS (*see* **Subheading 3.8., step 3**) at varying times (usually between 30 and 45 min).
3. Thaw the solution before each run, invert three times, dilute with distilled H_2O to obtain the optimal working solution, keep on melting ice, and use within 10 min. Discard the surplus solution.

3.3. Preparation of LPS Standards

1. Prepare a stock solution by adding x mL of distilled H_2O to one freeze-dried vial containing *E. coli* strain O55B5 LPS 7–10 endotoxin units (EU)/ng (Cat. no. N185, BioWhittaker) to a concentration of 2 µg/L (2 ng/mL = 14–20 EU/mL).
2. Divide the solution in suitable volumes in cryotubes, keep it at +4°C for maximum 14 d, or store it at –70°C until use. Prepare standards (n = 7) by whirl-mixing a thawed aliquot for 3 min and dilute with dilution fluid (*see* **Subheading 2., item 4**)

to final LPS concentrations ranging from 2.5–500 ng/L. Dilution fluid without LPS serves as blank. Process the blank and the standards as diluted patients' plasma specimens and controls (*see* **Subheading 3.4.**).

3.4. Removal of Inhibitors of the LAL in Human Plasma, CSF Specimens and Controls

1. Dilute the samples 1 + 9 with distilled H_2O.
2. Heat to 75°C for 12 min.
3. Cool to room temperature (20°C).

3.5. Dilution of Samples

1. If further dilution than 1 + 9 is necessary (in case of high concentrations of LPS in the patient sample) use the dilution fluid (*see* **Subheading 2., item 4**) to keep a constant protein and ion strength. CSF is diluted in dilution fluid from the start.

3.6. Preparation of the Chromogenic Peptide Substrate

1. Reconstitute 25 mg of the chromogenic peptide substrate S-2423 with 3.4 mL of distilled H_2O and store at +4°C. Use the solution within 6 mo. The solution must be colorless.
2. Mix equal parts of prewarmed (37°C), reconstituted substrate S-2423 and prewarmed (37°C) Tris-HCl buffer, pH 9.0, immediately before use. Use the mixture without delay. Discard surplus solution.

3.7. Collection of CSF

1. Collect the CSF in sterile, LPS-free tubes, aliquot in plastic tubes (Cryotube 3-68632; Nunc) without centrifugation and store at –70°C.

3.8. Quantification of LPS in Patient Plasma with the LAL Assay (Detection Limit 25 ng/L).

1. Pipet 10 µL (duplicate analyses) of diluted and heat-inactivated samples (blank, standards, controls, and patient specimens) into the 96-well microtiter plate. The standards are placed in the center of the plate. The controls and samples are placed on each side of the standards.
2. Add 50 µL of reconstituted, diluted LAL in H_2O (*see* **Subheading 3.2., step 3**).
3. Incubate the plate at 37°C for 30–45 min with the optimal reaction time varying from batch to batch of LAL.
4. Add 50 UµL of prewarmed (37°C) S-2423/TRIS solution.
5. Monitor the reaction kinetically in a THERMOmax microplate reader at OD_{405}. All plates are accompanied by blank, a set of standards (n = 6), ranging from 2.5–500 ng of *E. coli* O55B5 LPS/l, and controls. Standard curves, based on duplicates, are drawn by the SOFTware® version 2.01. The detection limit for *E. coli* O55B5 LPS is 25 ng/L of heparinized plasma. Analyze all samples twice on separate days and cal-

culate the mean value. The day to day coefficient of variation (CV) is 16% based on 30 assays at 250 ng/L.

3.9. Sensitive LAL Assay (Detection Limit 4 ng/L)

1. Dilute all plasmas (patient samples, pooled heparinised plasma as blank, standards and controls) 1 + 3 with distilled H_2O.
2. Prepare six standards of *E. coli* O55B5 LPS ranging from 2.5–50 ng/L (*see* **Subheading 3.3.**).
3. Heat-inactivated the specimens for 12 min at 75°C, and cooled to room temperature (20°C).
4. Pipet 10 μL of the samples (duplicate analyses) into a 96-well microtiter plate.
5. Add 50 μL of LAL diluted with distilled H_2O.
6. Incubate the plate at 37°C for x (30–45) min.
7. Add 25 mg of chromogenic peptide substrate S-2423 to 7 mL of distilled H_2O.
8 Prewarm (37°C) equal parts of S-2423 and Tris-HCl buffer, pH 9.0 and mix.
9. Add 100 μL of the prewarmed S-2423 + Tris-HCl buffer to each well and incubate for 10 min at 37°C.
10. Terminate the reaction by adding 100 μL of 50% acetic acid.
11. Read the plate automatically at OD_{405} in a microtiter plate reader (THERMOmax). All plates are accompanied by blank, a set of standards (n = 6), ranging from 2.5–50 ng of *E. coli* O55B5 LPS/l, and controls. Analyze all samples twice on separate days and calculate the mean value. The longitudinal controls are essentially as described above.

3.10. Detection of LPS in the CFS

1. Thaw the CSF samples containing lysed leukocytes at room temperature (20°C).
2. Whirl mix vigorously for 3 min.
3. Dilute 1 + 9 with dilution fluid (*see* above). Further dilution are made with dilution fluid.
4. Heat-inactivate all samples at 75°C for 12 min and cool to room temperature (20°C).
5. Quantify the LPS content with the LAL assay as described above for plasma.

4. Notes

1. LPS-free equipment. All equipment and reagents should be tested to be LPS-free before use. The samples, i.e., patients' samples, blank and standards, can be prepared on an ordinary clean laboratory bench. The use of laminar flow cabinet for sample preparation is unnecessary.
2. Plasma vs serum. For optimal detection of circulating LPS, use heparinized plasma. The recovery of LPS in serum is much lower than in heparin plasma. LPS-containing material is apparently trapped during clot formation. Ex vivo experiments with whole blood suggest that less than 20% of the added purified meningococcal LPS is recovered in serum vs 75% in heparin plasma (**Fig. 3**).

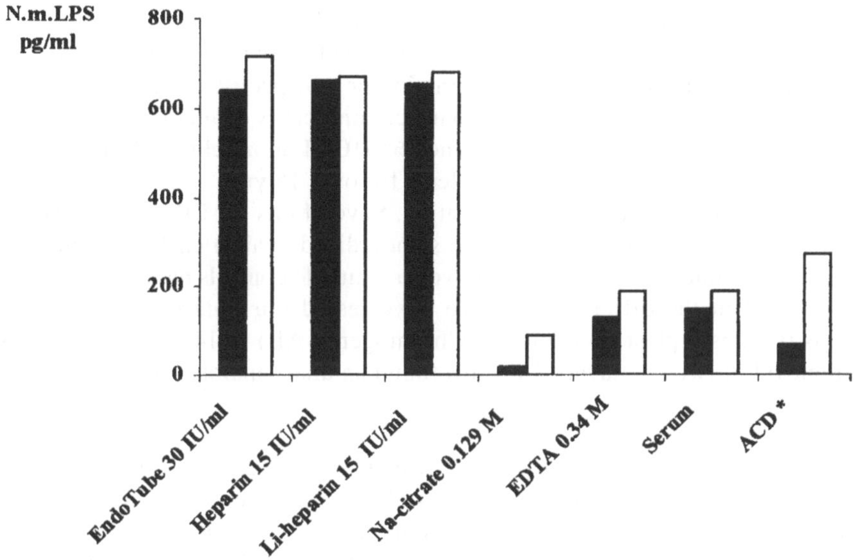

Fig. 3. Recovery of 1,000 pg/mL of purified *Neisseria meningitidis* LPS (N.m.LPS) extracted from the Norwegian strain 44/76 (B : 15 : P1.7,16,L3,7,9) *(7)* and added to whole blood from one healthy adult. Plasma and serum were prepared from blood collected in commercially available EndoTube® and vacuum tubes from Becton Dickinson. The vacuum tube containing heparin 15 IU/mL was prepared by injecting 60 IU/mL of concentrated heparin made for patient use in a 4-mL sterile vacuum tube. ACD denotes acid citrate dextrose. The black and white columns represent two separate experiments.

Studies of 10 paired serum and heparinized plasma samples collected simultaneously from patients with systemic meningococcal disease indicate that the mean LPS level in serum was 63% of that measured in plasma, ranging from 29–110%. Nine of 10 samples had higher LPS levels in plasma than in serum.

3. Heparinized vacuum tubes. In lack of commercially available, heparinized, LPS-free vacuum tubes, it is possible to prepare a sterile vacuum tube by injecting a small volume of concentrated heparin solution made for patient use (thus tested to be LPS-free). The final concentration of heparin should be 30 IU/mL blood. Do not use heparin contents >40 IU/mL blood. This high level of heparin may inhibit the LAL reaction. Perform pilot tests to ensure that the sterile vacuum tubes are not LPS contaminated. In our experience, sterile vacuum tubes without additive are usually LPS-free.
4. Heparin vs sodium citrate and EDTA as anticoagulants. The concentration of 0.129 *M* Na-citrate and 0.339 *M* EDTA used in commercially available vacuum tubes strongly inhibits the LAL-reaction in dilution 1 : 10 and 1 : 100 and are not suitable for LPS detection in human blood. When 1,000 pg/mL *N. meningitidis*

LPS is added to whole blood that is anticoagulated with either Na-citrate (0.129 *M*) or EDTA (0.339 *M*), <10% and <20%, respectively, are recovered (**Fig. 3**).

5. The microtiter plates. LPS contamination or nonspecific activation of the LAL cascade is a general problem with many commercially available microtiter plates. Using PS-Mikrotiterplatte® (Cat. no. 655101 Labortechnik, Nurtingen, Germany), we have avoided such problems for over 15 yr.
6. Commercial kits for LPS quantification. Several kits for LPS quantification are available. The various reagents are standardized against each other in order to reduce the interassay variation. However, suitable controls have, so far, not been included in the different kits. We have tested our controls in one of these kits (Coatest®-plasma endotoxin, Chromogenix AB) in 14 different runs. After removal of two "outlayers," we still found an unacceptably high CV (44%).

References

1. Rietschel, E. T., Brade, H., Brade, L., Brandenburg, K., Schade, U., Seydel, U., et al. (1987) Lipid A, the endotoxic center of bacterial lipopolysaccharides: relation of chemical structure to biological activity, in *Detection of Bacterial Endotoxins with the Limulus Amebocyte Lysate Test* (Watson, S. W., Levin, J., and Novitsky, T. J., eds.), Alan R. Liss, New York, 25–53.
2. Rietschel, E. T., Kirikae, T., Schade, F. U., Mamat U., Schmidt, G., Loppow, H., et al. (1994) Bacterial endotoxin: molecular relationships of structure to activity and function. *FASEB J.* **218,** 217–225.
3. Zähringer, U., Lindner, B., and Rietschel, E. T. (1999) Chemical structure of lipid A: recent advances in structural analysis of biologically active molecules, in *Endotoxin in Health and Disease* (Brade, H., Opal, S. M., Vogel, S. N., and Morrison, D. C., eds.), Marcel Dekker, New York, pp. 93–114.
4. De Voe, I. W. (1982) The meningococcus and mechanisms of pathogenicity. *Microb. Rev.* **46,** 162–190.
5. Brandtzaeg, P., Kierulf, P., Gaustad, P., Skulberg, A., Bruun, J. N., Halvorsen, S., and Sørensen, E. (1989) Plasma endotoxin as a predictor of multiple organ failure and death in systemic meningococcal disease. *J. Infect. Dis.* **159,** 195–204.
6. Brandtzaeg, P., Øvstebø, R., and Kierulf, P. (1992) Compartmentalization of lipopolysaccharide production correlates with clinical presentation in meningococcal disease. *J. Infect. Dis.* **166,** 650–652.
7. Brandtzaeg, P., Bryn, K., Kierulf, P., Øvstebø, R., Namork, E., Aase, B., and Jantzen, E. (1992) Meningococcal endotoxin in lethal septic shock plasma studied by gas-chromatography, mass-spectrometry, ultracentrifugation, and electron microscopy. *J. Clin. Invest.* **89,** 816–823.
8. Brandtzaeg, P. and Kierulf, P. (1992) Endotoxin and meningococcemia. Intravascular inflammation induced by native endotoxin in man, in *Bacterial Endotoxic Lipopolysaccharides. Immunopharmacology and Physiology*, vol. II (Ryan, J. L. and Morison, D. C., eds.), CRC Press, Boca Raton, FL, pp. 327–336.
9. Brandtzaeg, P., Halstensen, A., Kierulf, P., Espevik, T., and Waage, A. (1992) Molecular mechanism in the compartmentalized inflammatory response

presenting as meningococcal meningitis or septic shock. *Microb. Pathog.* **13,** 423–431.
10. Brandtzaeg, P. (1995) Pathogenesis of meningococcal infections, in *Meningococcal Disease* (Cartwright, K. A. V., ed.), John Wiley and Sons, Chichester, UK, pp. 71–114.
11. Brandtzaeg, P. (1996) Systemic meningococcal disease: Clinical pictures and pathophysiological background. *Rev. Med. Microbiol.* **7,** 63–72.
12. van Deuren, M., Brandtzaeg, P., and van der Meer, J. W. (2000) Update on meningococcal disease with emphasis on pathogenesis and clinical management. *Clin. Microbiol. Rev.* **13,** 144–166.
13. Kulshin, V. A., Zähringer, U., Lindner, B., Frasch, C. .E, Tsai, C. M., Dmiteiev, B. A., and Rietschel, E. T. (1992) Structural characterization of the lipid A component of pathogenic *Neisseria meningitidis. J. Bacteriol.* **174,** 1793–1800.
14. Wright, S. D., Ramos, R. A., Tobias, P. S., Ulevitch, R. J., and Mathison, J. C. (1990) CD14, a receptor for complexes of lipopolysaccharide (LPS) and LPS binding protein. *Science* **249,** 1431–1433.
15. Ulmer, A. J., El-Samalouti, V. T., Rietschel, E. T., Flad, H. D., and Dziarski, R. (1999) CD14, an innate immune receptor for various bacterial cell wall components, in *Endotoxin in Health and Disease* (Brade, H., Opal, S. M., Vogel, S. N., and Morrison, D. C., eds.), Marcel Dekker, New York, pp. 463–471.
16. Tobias, P. S. (1999) Lipopolysaccharide-binding protein, in *Endotoxin in Health and Disease* (Brade, H., Opal, S. M., Vogel, S. N., and Morrison, D. C., eds.), Marcel Dekker, New York, pp. 359–367.
17. Elsbach, P. (1999) Bactericidal/permeability-increasing protein, p15s and phospholipases A_2, endogenous antibiotics in host defence against bacterial infections, in *Endotoxin in Health and Disease* (Brade, H., Opal, S. M., Vogel, S. N., and Morrison, D. C., eds.), Marcel Dekker, New York, p. 369–377.
18. van Deventer, S. J. H. and Pajkrt, D. (1999) Interaction of lipopolysaccharides and lipoproteins, in *Endotoxin in Health and Disease* (Brade, H., Opal, S. M., Vogel, S. N., and Morrison, D. C., eds.), Marcel Dekker, New York, pp. 379–388.
19. David, S. A. (1999) The interaction of lipid A and lipopolysaccharides with human serum albumin, in *Endotoxin in Health and Disease* (Brade, H., Opal, S. M., Vogel, S. N., and Morrison D. C., eds.), Marcel Dekker, New York, pp. 413–422.
20. Appelmelk, B. J., An, Y. Q., Geerts, M., Thijs, B. G., de Boer, H. A., MacLaren, D. M., et al. (1994) Lactoferrin is a lipid A-binding protein. *Infect. Immun.* **62,** 2628–2632.
21. Gosselaar-de Haas, C. (1999) Serum Amyeloid Protein (SAP): A novel LPS-binding protein. PhD Thesis, University of Utrecht, the Netherlands.
22. Roth, R. J. and Levin, J. (1999) Effects of human hemoglobin on bacterial endotoxin in vitro and in vivo, in *Endotoxin in Health and Disease* (Brade, H., Opal, S. M., Vogel, S. N., and Morrison D. C., eds.), Marcel Dekker, New York, pp. 389–401.

23. Modlin R. L., Brightbill, H. D., and Godowski, P. J. (1999) The toll of innate immunity on microbial pathogens. *N. Engl. J. Med.* **340,** 1834–1835.
24. Zhang, F. X., Kirschning, J., Mancinella, R., Xu, X. P., Jin, Y., Faure, E., et al. (1999) Bacterial lipopolysaccharide activates nuclear factor-κB through interleukin-1 signaling mediators in cultured human dermal endothelial cells and mononuclear phagocytes. *J. Biol. Chem.* **274,** 7611–7614.
25. Harthug, S., Bjorvatn, B., and Østerud, B. (1983) Quantitation of endotoxin in blood from patients with meningococcal disease using a limulus lysate test in combination with chromogenic substrate. *Infection* **11,** 192–195.
26. Bjorvatn, B., Bjertnaes, L., Fadnes, H. O., Flaegstad, T., Gutteberg, T. J., Kristiansen, B. E., et al. (1984) Meningococcal septicaemia treated with combined plasmapheresis and leucapheresis or with blood exchange. *BMJ* **288,** 439–441.
27. Levin, J., Thomasulo, P. A., and Oser, R. S., (1970) Detection of endotoxin in human blood and demonstration of an inhibitor. *J. Lab. Clin. Med.* **75,** 903–911.
28. Iwanaga, S., Morita, T., Harada, T., Nakamura, S., Nina, M., Takada, K, et al. (1978) Chromogenic substrate for horseshoe crab clotting enzyme, its application for the assay of bacterial endotoxin. *Haemostasis* **7,** 183–188.
29. Thomas, L. L. M., Sturk, A., Kahlé, L. H., and ten Cate, J. W. (1981) Quantitative endotoxin determination in blood with a chromogenic substrate. *Clin. Chim. Acta.* **116,** 63–68.
30. Friberger, P., Knös, M., and Mellstam, L. (1982) A quantitative endotoxin assay utilising LAL and a chromogenic substrate, in *Endotoxin and Their Detection with the Limulus Amebocyte Lysate Test* (Watson, S. W., Levin, J., and Novitsky, T. J., eds.), Alan R. Liss, New York, pp. 195–205.
31. Sturk, A. and ten Cate, J. W. (1985) Endotoxin testing revisited. *Eur. J. Clin. Microbiol.* **4,** 382–385.
32. Levin, J. (1987) The Limulus amebocyte lysate test: perspectives and problems, in *Detection of Bacterial Endotoxins with the Limulus Amebocyte Lysate Test* (Watson, S. W., Levin, J., and Novitsky, T.J., eds.), Alan R. Liss, New York, pp. 1–24.
33. Sturk, A., Janssen, M. E., Muylaert, F. R., Joop, K., Thomas, L. L. M., and ten Cate, J. W. (1987) Endotoxin testing in blood, in *Detection of Bacterial Endotoxins with the Limulus Amebocyte Lysate Test* (Watson, S. W., Levin, J., and Novitsky, T. J. eds.), New York, Alan R. Liss, pp. 371–385.
34. Beloborodov V., Platonov A., and Troshansky D. (1994) Meningococcal disease as a problem of the special intensive care unit for patients with infectious disease, in *Proceedings of the Ninth International Pathogenic Neisseria Conference* (Evans, J. S., Yest, S. F., Maiden, M. L. N., and Fruers, J. M., eds.), pp. 400–401.
35. van Deuren, M., van der Ven-Jongekrijg, J., Bartelink, A. K. M., van Dalen, R., Sauerwein, R. W., and van der Meer, J. W. M. (1995) Correlation between proinflammatory cytokines and antiinflammatory mediators and the severity of disease in meningococcal infections. *J. Infect. Dis.* **172,** 433–439.

36. Gårdlund, B., Sjölin, J., Nilsson, A., Roll, R., Wickerts C. J., and Wretlind, B. (1995) Plasma levels of cytokines in primary septic shock in humans: correlation with disease severity. *J. Infect. Dis.* **172,** 296–301.
37. Brandtzaeg, P., Øvstebø, R., and Kierulf, P. (1995) Bacteremia and compartmentalization of LPS in meningococcal disease, in *Bacterial Endotoxins* (Levin, J., Alving, C. R., Munford, R. S., and Redl, H., eds.), Wiley-Liss, New York, pp. 219–233.
38. Derkx, B., Wittes, J., and McCloskey, R. Randomized, placebo-controlled trial of HA-1A in human monoclonal antibody to endotoxin, in children with meningococcal septic shock, European Pediatric Meningococcal Septic Shock Trial Study Group (1999) *Clin. Infect. Dis.* **28,** 770–777.
39. Brandtzaeg, P., Mollnes, T. E., and Kierulf, P. (1989) Complement activation and endotoxin levels in systemic meningococcal disease. *J. Infect. Dis.* **160,** 58–65.
40. Brandtzaeg, P., Sandset P. M., Joø, G. B., Øvstebø, R., Abildgaard, U., and Kierulf, P. (1989) The quantitative association of plasma endotoxin, antithrombin, protein C, extrinsic pathway inhibitor and fibrinopeptide A in systemic meningococcal disease. *Thromb. Res.* **55,** 459–470.
41. Brandtzaeg, P., Joø, G. B., Brusleto, B., and Kierulf, P. (1990) Plasminogen activator inhibitor 1 and 2, alpha-2-antiplasmin, plasminogen, and endotoxin levels in systemic meningococcal disease. *Thromb. Res.* **57,** 271–278.
42. Waage, A., Brandtzaeg, P., Halstensen, A., Kierulf, P., and Espevik, T. (1989) The complex pattern of cytokines in serum from patients with meningococcal septic shock. *J. Exp. Med.* **169,** 333–338.
43. Brandtzaeg, P., Osnes, L., Øvstebø, R., Joø, R., Westvik, Å. B., and Kierulf, P. (1996) Net inflammatory capacity of human septic shock plasma evaluated by a monocyte-based target cell assay: identification of interleukin-10 as a major functional deactivator of human monocytes. *J. Exp. Med.* **184,** 51–60.
44. Suffredini, A. F. and O'Grady, N. P. (1999) The pathophysiological responses to endotoxin in humans, in *Endotoxin in Health and Disease* (Brade, H., Opal, S. M., Vogel, S. N., and Morrison, D. C., eds.), Marcel Dekker, New York, pp. 817–830.
45. Hurley, J. and Levin, J. (1999) The relevance of endotoxin detection in sepsis, in *Endotoxin in Health and Disease* (Brade, H., Opal, S. M., Vogel, S. N., and Morrison, D. C., eds.), Marcel Dekker, New York, pp. 841–854.

27

Isolation and Analysis of Radiolabeled Meningococcal Endotoxin

Peter C. Giardina, Jerrold A. Weiss, Brad W. Gibson, and Michael A. Apicella

1. Introduction

The Gram-negative pathogen *Neisseria meningitidis*, is one of the leading causes of bacterial meningitis worldwide *(1)*. The host range for this organism is restricted to humans, where it colonizes the mucosal epithelium of the upper airway. It occasionally disseminates causing invasive disease (sepsis, disseminated intravascular coagulation [DIC], meningitis). Epidemic meningococcal meningitis is a major health problem, most notably in sub-Saharan Africa. In 1999, an outbreak of meningococcal disease spread across Guinea-Bissau, a region that is part of what is commonly called the African meningitis belt *(2)*. There were 2,169 reported cases and 404 deaths resulting from meningococcal disease in this outbreak from Jan. 1 to April 5, 1999. Also in 1999, there were reported outbreaks in Sudan (22,000 cases and 1,600 deaths) Rwanda (29 cases and 11 deaths), Angola (253 cases and 147 deaths), Ethiopia (126 cases and 4 deaths) and Senegal (2,709 cases and 372 deaths) *(2)*. According to the World Health Organization (WHO), each year approx 500,000 cases of meningitis and 50,000 deaths are attributable to *N. meningitidis* worldwide. In the United States, meningococcal disease is less common, although small outbreaks are reported each year *(3)*.

Meningococcal lipooligosaccharide (LOS; endotoxin) is a major virulence factor responsible for many of the symptoms associated with meningococcal disease, and is a primary focus of research *(4,5)*. Endotoxin is a pleiotropic effector molecule that promotes the production of pro-inflammatory mediators (i.e., interleukin [IL]-1, IL-6, IL-8, tumor necrosis factor [TNF] and arachi-

From: *Methods in Molecular Medicine, vol. 67: Meningococcal Disease: Methods and Protocols*
Edited by: A. J. Pollard and M. C. J. Maiden © Humana Press Inc., Totowa, NJ

donic acid) leading to shock syndrome with hypotension and DIC. Meningococci have been shown to shed LOS from the bacterial surface in culture and during disease, and free LOS has been detected in infected host tissues at concentrations sufficient to activate cultured host cells ***(6–9)***.

Various procedures for the purification of endotoxin have been published ***(10–16)***. These procedures generally involve organic extraction of bacterial lysates or culture supernatants. In **Subheading 1.2.** of this chapter, meningococcal LOS structure is reviewed, with an emphasis on LOS biosynthesized by meningococcal serogroup B strain, NMB (17). The role of LOS in pathogenesis is also discussed in **Subheading 1.2. Subheadings 2.**, **3.**, and **4.** outline a method by which meningococcal LOS has been radiolabeled to high specific radioactivity, and isolated for use in experiments involving small (physiological) amounts of LOS.

1.2. LOS Structure and Function

Meningococcal LOS is an amphipathic, phosphorylated glycolipid ($M_r \approx 4.8$ kDa), consisting of distinct and well-characterized lipid- and carbohydrate-containing regions ***(5)***. 3-hydroxy fatty acids (3-OH FA) (found only in endotoxin) are ligated to an *O*-phosphorylethanolamine substituted β(1′→6)-linked D-glucosamine disaccharide backbone (termed the lipid A backbone) to which charbohydrate moieties (core saccharides and variable terminal glycan structures) are attached ***(5,18)***. It has been well-established that the lipid A moiety is responsible for the host-cell activation and cytotoxicity. The variable terminal carbohydrate structures, anchored to lipid A through the core carbohydrate region and exposed to the outer environment, have been shown to mimic normal human glycoshingolipid blood-group antigens, and may be important for bacterial-host cell attachment and for pathogenesis. The implications of this antigenic mimicry have been described previously ***(4,19)*** and will be reviewed in brief in **Subheading 1.2.1.3.** of this chapter. Refer to Kahler and Stephens for a thorough review of meningococcal LOS structure and biosynthesis ***(20)***.

1.2.1. LOS Structure

1.2.1.1. Lipid A

The lipoidal portion of LOS, lipid A, anchors this molecule to the bacterial outer membrane and is the major lipid constituent of the outer leaflet of the Gram-negative outer envelope. The lipid A moiety of meningococcal LOS comprises a disaccharide backbone (1, 4′-bisphosphorylated β(1′→6)-linked D-glucosamine) with variable *O*-phosphorylethanolamine substitutions at positions 1 and 4′ ***(21)***. FA substitutions are present symmetrically at the disaccharide backbone 3 and 3′ positions (*O*-linked 3-hydroxydodecanoic acid) and at the 2 and 2′ positions (N-linked 3-(dodecanoyloxy)tetradecanoic acid). FA are also attached by ester linkage at the hydroxyl group of the 3-OH FA at positions 2 and 2′ (*O*-linked 3-hydroxydodecanoic acid). The symmetrical arrangement of FA in meningococcal LOS is one characteristic by which this molecule is distinguishable from LPS described in enteric Gram-negative bacteria ***(18,21)***.

1.2.1.2. Core

The conserved meningococcal LOS core saccharides ***(22)***, including L-glycero-D-manno-heptose (Hep), glucosamine (GlcNAc), and glucose (Glc), are attached to lipid A through Hep (HepI) by α(1→5) linkage to 2-keto-3-deoxyoctulosonic acid (Kdo). A second Hep (HepII) is attached to HepI via α(1→3) linkage and may contain phosphorylethanolamine and/or saccharide substituents (β-chain carbohydrates) at the HepI second carbon. A di-Kdo structure bridges the core saccharides and lipid A by α(2→6′) linkage to the 6′-hydroxyl group of the lipid A disaccharide backbone. This lipid A/KdoI linkage is susceptible to mild acid hydrolysis.

1.2.1.3. α-Chain Carbohydrates

The structurally variable α-chain carbohydrate moieties of meningococcal LOS ***(23–26)*** are assembled on HepI by Glcβ(1→4) linkage. These phase variable carbohydrate chains mimic mammalian blood-group antigens ***(4,19)***. As an example, the immunotypes L2 and L3, expressed by meningococcal strain NMB, consist of sialo- and asialo-lacto-*N*-neotetraose, [R-Galβ(1→4) GlcNAcβ(1→3)Galβ(1→4)Glc] (R= α(2→3)-linked sialic acid). These immunotypes mimic the human paragloboseries and sialoparagloboseries blood-group antigens, respectively.

1.2.2. LOS Function in Pathogenesis

The toxic properties of LOS and enteric LPS have been well-established and linked to the conserved lipid A moiety. LOS has also been shown to play a roll in bacterial attachment to host cells, and this function has been linked to the carbohydrate moiety. The terminal carbohydrates have also been implicated in evasion of the host immune response. In this section, the role of LOS in disease is described.

The mechanisms by which endotoxins activate mammalian cells are a subject of intense study. The Lipid A component of endotoxin is necessary and sufficient to activate mammalian cells, and this ability to activate host cells is related to the FA composition of lipid A ***(27)***. It has been established that host-cell activation is enhanced by LPS binding protein (LBP) ***(28)***, a 58 kDa mammalian serum glycoprotein that associates with lipid A, disaggregates LOS, and catalyzes the interaction of endotoxin with other host factors, including membrane-bound (glycosyl phosphatidylinositol-[GPI]-linked) and soluble CD14 (mCD14 or sCD14, respectively) ***(29)***. In general, the consequences of LOS interaction with these glycoproteins are: 1) clearance of LOS and 2) induction of host-cell activation leading to release of pro-inflammatory host factors. LOS uptake and host-cell activation have been shown to be separable events in cultured human neutrophils, in that LOS internalization may occur in the absence of the release of pro-inflammatory mediators, and cell activation may occur without LOS uptake by the host cells ***(30)***.

The β2 integrins, CD11a-c/CD18, have also been shown to bind endotoxin, and unlike mCD14, these adhesion molecules are transmembrane glycoproteins that could potentially participate directly in signal transduction ***(31)***. It has been proposed, however, that the β2 integrins interact (but may not require) a downstream signal transducer in response to LOS.

1.2.3. Clinical Aspects of Endotoxin

Over 3,300 cases of meningococcal disease in the US (1.24 cases per 100,000 population) were reported to the Centers for Disease Control and Prevention (CDC) in 1997, showing a slight overall increase in disease incidents from 1991 (0.84 cases per 100,000 population) ***(3)***. Most of these cases occured in young children and teenagers ***(32)***. Refer to Rosenstein et al. for a recent review of meningococcal disease in the US ***(33)***.

The mortality and serious morbidity caused by meningococcal infection are owing almost entirely to the LOS released by meningococcus ***(34–38)***. Although the outcome of meningococcal infection has improved greatly since the advent of antibiotics 50 years ago, the morbidity and mortality owing to this infection have changed very little during the last 25 years. This is due in large part to rapid onset of sepsis and the inability to control many of the consequences of the endotoxin-induced shock state.

Brandtzaeg and co-workers have made major contributions to our understanding of the physiologic effects of LOS during sepsis and meningitis caused by *N. meningitidis* ***(37–39)***. These investigators have demonstrated the ability to measure LOS in the plasma and cerbrospinal fluid (CSF) of infected patients and have shown that there is a close correlation between plasma LOS levels and prognosis. They have demonstrated that compartmentalization of LOS production correlates with the clinical presentation in meningococcal infection ***(38)***. LOS levels in patients defined as having septicemia showed high levels in plasma (median 3,500 ng) and low levels in CSF, whereas in patients with meningitis, LOS was detectable in the plasma of 3/19 patients and in the CSF in 18 of 19 patients with median levels of 2,500 ng. Physiologic studies of the meningococcal LOS in the plasma of infected patients revealed that it had a high sedimentation coefficient and assumed to be associated with a membrane-like structure. Bacterial outer-membrane fragments were found in the plasma of three patients. The plasma of one of these patients contained a bacterium covered with multiple, long membrane protrusions indicating that surplus outer membrane (blebbing) does occur in vivo ***(36)***. Mass spectrometric analysis of the endotoxin from patients with meningococcal sepsis indicated that it was of meningococcal origin rather than arising from the gastrointestinal tract owing to increased permeability during infection ***(39)***. Sedimentation analysis indicated that the majority of the LOS in these patients was not associated with high-density lipoproteins (HDLs) or low-density lipoproteins (LDLs).

Outer-membrane bleb formation by the group A meningococcus was first demonstrated by Cesarini and co-workers ***(40)***. DeVoe found that strains of meningococcal serogroup A, B, and C released membrane blebs in log phase of growth but not in the lag phase ***(41)***. The release of LOS from the surface of the meningococcus in the form of membrane blebs is now considered to be the principle factor associated with the high endotoxin levels in meningococcal sepsis.

1.2.4. Rationale

Our studies have shown that meningococcal (strain NMB) LOS exists as size-distinguishable aggregate forms that are separable by column chromatography ***(42)***. These aggregate forms are also distinguishable by their biological activities, as a measure of: 1) their ability to interact with the LPS-binding proteins LBP and CD14, and 2) their ability to activate host cells in vitro. These studies were accomplished using high specific radiolabeled LOS, achieved by disrupting the gene encoding the E1 subunit of pyruvate dehydrogenase (PDH) complex, *pdhA* ***(43)***, based on a method previously described ***(44)***. The PDH complex catalyzes the overall conversion of pyruvate to acetyl-CoA (the building block for lipid biosynthesis) and CO_2. Disruption of this gene in strain NMB resulted in the formation of an acetate auxotroph, NMBACE1, which was used to generate [^{14}C]-labeled LOS with specific activity from 500–700 cpm/ng.

The following sections describe the method by which meningococcal (NMB and NMBACE1) LOS was biosynthetically radiolabeled with [^{14}C]-acetate. This LOS isolation protocol is a modification of a method previously described for the isolation of LOS from the mucosal pathogen, *Haemophilus somnus* ***(13)***. In the method described here, [^{14}C]-radiolabeled meningococcal LOS is isolated from washed bacterial pellets by enzyme digestion, organic extraction, ethanol precipitation, and ultracentrifugation. Other methods, previously published, describe various organic extraction procedures for isolation of LOS from bacterial pellets as well as from spent culture supernatants, and in some instances utilize column chromatography in the purification ***(10–16)***.

Purified and desiccated LOS has the consistency of a fluffy white powder that is easily dispersed by static electricity and air currents. Therefore, necessary precautions must be taken to prevent radioactive contamination of equipment and personnel. We have attempted to minimize such problems in this procedure by minimizing the culture volume.

2. Materials

2.1. Medium Reagents

2.1.1. Bacto GC Agar Base Supplemented with Isovitalex

1. Bacto GC agar base: (Beckton Dickinson, Sparks, MD) 36g/L.
2. Isovitalex solution I (100 mL): 10 g L-glutamine, 1 g adenine, 0.03 g guanine HCl, 25.9 g L-cysteine HCl, 1.1 g L-cystine, 0.01 g vitamin B_{12}, 0.013 g p-aminobenzoic acid. Dissolve all ingredients in double-distilled water.
3. Isovitalex solution II (600 mL): 0.25 g β-NADH, 0.1 g thiamine pyrophosphate HCl (cocarboxylase), 2 g $Fe(NO_3)_3$, 0.03 g thiamine HCl, 100 g dextrose. Dissolve all ingredients in double-distilled water.
4. 100X Isovitalex stock solution (1 L): Combine all of Isovitalex solutions I and II, adjust the volume to 1L with double-distilled water, and filter-sterilize. Store 10 mL lots at –70°C. Cool autoclaved Bacto GC agar base to 60°C before addition of Isovitalex to a final concentration of 1X.

2.1.2. Morse's Defined Medium (MDM)

Modified from Morse and Barenstein ***(45)***.

1. MDM Solution I (1 L): 233.8 g NaCl, 40g K_2SO_4, 8.8 g NH_4Cl, 0.12 g EDTA·Na_2, 8.72 g $MgCl_2·6H_2O$. Dissolve in double-distilled water, autoclave, and store at –20°C.
2. MDM Solution II (1 L): 174.2g K_2HPO_4, 136.1 g KH_2PO_4. Dissolve in double-distilled water, autoclave, and store at –20°C.
3. MDM solution III (2 L): (*see* **Table 1**).
4. MDM Solution IV (100 mL): 0.02 g thiamine HCL, 0.005 g thiamine pyrophosphate HCl (cocarboxylase), 0.019 g Ca pantothenate (pantothenic acid), 0.03 g biotin. Dissolve in 50% ethanol, filter-sterilize, and store at –20°C.
5. MDM Solution V (500 mL): 100 g glucose. Dissolve in double-distilled water, autoclave, and store at –20°C.
6. MDM Solution VI (100 mL): 0.5 g hypoxanthine, 0.5 g uracil. Dissolve in 0.1 *M* NaOH, filter-sterilize, and store at –20°C.
7. 4X MDM stock medium (500 mL): (*see* **Table 2**).
8. 1 *M* $CaCl_2$ (50 mL): 7.35 g $CaCl_2$. Dissolve in double-distilled water, filter-sterilize, and store at room temperature.

Table 1
MDM Solution III (2 L)[a]

Reagent	Amount
L-aspartic acid	8 g
L-glutamic acid	20.8 g
L-arginine	2.4 g
Glycine	0.4 g
L-serine	0.8 g
L-leucine	1.44 g
L-isoleucine	0.48 g
L-valine	0.96 g
L-tyrosine	1.12 g
L-cystein $HCl \cdot H_2O$	0.88 g
L-cystine[b]	0.56 g
L-proline	0.8 g
L-tryptophan	1.28 g
L-threonine	0.8 g
L-phenylalanine	0.4 g
L-asparagine$\cdot H_2O$	0.4 g
L-glutamine	0.8 g
L-histadine $HCl \cdot H_2O$	0.4 g
L-methionine	0.24 g
L-alanine	1.6 g
L-lysine	0.8 g

[a]Heat gently to dissolve, filter-sterilize, and store at 4°C protected from light.

[b]First dissolve in 1 N HCl.

Table 2
4X MDM Stock Medium (500 mL)[a]

Reagent	Amount
MDM solution I	50 mL
MDM solution II	4 mL
MDM solution III	250 mL
MDM solution IV	20 mL
MDM solution V	50 mL
MDM solution VI	20 mL
Double-distilled water	86 mL
HEPES	20.0 g

[a]Adjust the pH to 7.4 with 10 N NaOH, adjust the volume to 500 mL with double-distilled water, and filter-sterilize. Store at 4°C protected from light.

9. 1 *M* $MgCl_2$ (50 mL): 10.17 g $MgCl_2$. Dissolve in double-distilled water, filter-sterilize, and store at room temperature.
10. 100 m*M* $Fe(NO_3)_3$ (50 mL): 2.02 g $Fe(NO_3)_3$. Dissolve in double-distilled water, adjust pH to 1.0 with 12 N HCl, and store at room temperature.
11. 1 *M* $NaHCO_3$ (50 mL): 4.2 g $NaHCO_3$. Dissolve in double-distilled water, filter-sterilize, and store at 4°C.
12. 1X MDM (500 mL): 125 mL 4X stock medium, 350 mL double-distilled water, 535 μL 1 *M* $MgCl_2$, 125 μL 1*M* $CaCl_2$. Add double-distilled water to a final volume of 500 mL, add 500 μL of 100 m*M* $Fe(NO_3)_3$, and filter-sterilize. Store at 4°C protected from light. Add sterile $NaHCO_3$ to the 1X MDM immediately prior to inoculation to a final concentration of 20 m*M*.

2.1.3. Sterile Plasticware and Glassware and [^{14}C]-Acetate

1. Dacron swabs.
2. 50-mL polypropylene conical tubes.
3. 100-mm plastic petri dishes.
4. Parafilm.
5. 0.2 micro filter units.
6. [1,2-^{14}C]-acetic acid, sodium salt (Moravek Biochemicals, Inc., Brea, CA) (1 mCi at 108 mCi/mmol) suspended in 1 mL of 1X MDM.

2.2. LOS Isolation Materials

1. 50 mL Oak Ridge centrifuge tubes (Nalge Nunc International, Rochester, NY).
2. 1.5 mL microcentrifuge tubes.
3. 13 × 51 mm thickwalled polyallomar ultracentrifuge tubes.
4. Parafilm.
5. 1 dram glass vials with screw caps.
6. 1-cm stir bars.
7. 13 × 100 mm disposable glass tubes with polypropylene screw caps.
8. 90% phenol in double-distilled water.
9. Chicken egg white lysozyme (Sigma, St. Louis, MO).
10. Micrococcal nuclease (from *Staphylococcus aureus* Foggi strain, Sigma).
11. Scintillation cocktail and vials.
12. TM buffer: 10 m*M* Tris-HCl, 50 m*M* $MgCl_2$, pH 8.0.

2.3. Sodium Dodecyl Sulfate Polyacrylamide Gel Electrophoresis (SDS-PAGE) Materials

1. 49.5% acrylamide stock solution (100 mL): 48.2 g acrylamide, 1.3 g bis-acrylamide. Dissolve in double-distilled water and store at 4°C protected from light (*see* **Note 1**).
2. SDS-PAGE gel buffer and reservoir buffer solutions: (*see* **Table 3**).
3. Sample dilution buffer base (500 mL): 3.63 g Tris base, 1.86 g EDTA·Na_2, 10 g SDS. Dissolve in double-distilled water, adjust pH to 6.8, and store at room temperature.

Table 3
SDS-PAGE Buffer Solutions

	Gel buffer	Anode (lower) buffer	Cathode (upper) buffer
Tris base	36.33 g	24.2 g	12.11 g
SDS	0.3 g	—	1 g
Glycine	—	—	—
Tricine	—	—	17.92 g
pH	8.45	8.9	8.25
Volume	100 mL	1000 mL	1000 mL

[a]Dissolve each solution in double distilled water to the volume indicated, and store at room temperature.

4. 2X sample dilution buffer: Add 0.8 mL β-mercaptoethanol, 4 mL glycerol, and 0.4 mL of saturated Bromophenyl Blue to 5.9 mL of the sample dilution buffer base, and store at 4°C.
5. Glycerol.
6. 10% ammonium persulfate (APS).
7. N,N,N′N′-tetra-methyl-ethylenediamine (TEMED).

2.4. Silver-Stain Reagents

1. SDS-PAGE gel fixing solution: 40% ethanol and 5% glacial acetic acid in double-distilled water.
2. Silver-stain solution A (30 mL): 2 mL conc. NH_4OH in 28 mL 0.1 *M* NaOH.
3. Silver-stain solution B (5 mL): 1 g $AgNO_3$ dissolved in 5 mL double-distilled water.
4. 1X silver-stain solution 150 mL: Slowly add silver-stain solution B to silver stain solution A with constant stirring. A brown precipitate will form briefly, but should quickly dissolve (add NH_4OH drops if necessary to dissolve). After the precipitate has dissolved, adjust the volume to 150 mL with double-distilled water.
5. Silver-stain developer (1L): 50 mg citric acid, 0.5 mL formaldehyde. Adjust the volume to 1 L with double distilled water.
6. Acid stop solution (1 L): 2 mL glacial acetic acid in double-distilled water.
7. Chromic-sulfuric acid cleaning solution.

2.5. FA Analysis Materials

1. Phosphate-buffered saline (PBS)
2. 12 *M* HCl.
3. 10 *M* NaOH.
4. Glacial acetic acid.
5. Chloroform : methanol (1 : 2 by volume).
6. 50 m*M* KCl, chloroform : methanol (2 : 1 by volume).
7. Acetonitrile : glacial acetic acid (1 : 1 by volume).

8. Reverse phase-(RP)-TLC plates (0.2 mm HPTLC RP-18; Merck Ltd., Dublin, Ireland).

3. Methods

3.1. Meningococcal Growth and Radiolabeling

3.1.1. Day 1

1. Inoculate a GC agar Petri dish with meningococci from freezer stock, and allow the culture to grow overnight (about 18 h) at 37°C in 5% CO_2/95% air atmosphere and 85% humidity. If a CO_2 incubator is not available, a candle jar can be used (*see* **Note 2**).

3.1.2. Day 2

1. Use a single bacterial colony from the overnight culture to inoculate a fresh GC agar plate, and allow the culture to grow, as in **Subheading 3.1.1.**
2. Prepare MDM and other sterile reagents for [^{14}C]-acetate labeling in continuous culture and for LOS isolation.

3.1.3. Day 3

1. Using a sterile Dacron swab, transfer meningococci from overnight culture to 5 mL of sterile, pre-warmed MDM in a sterile glass tube to an optical density (OD) of A_{600} = 0.24 (approx 2 × 10^8 cfu/mL) (*see* **Note 3**).
2. Dilute suspended bacteria in a total volume of 4.5 mL of pre-warmed MDM to an OD of A_{600} = 0.03 (approx 1 : 10 dilution) and transfer the inoculated medium to a sterile 50 mL polypropylene conical tube.
3. Add 0.75 mL of [^{14}C]-acetate (750 μCi) to the culture for a final volume of 5 mL and a final acetate concentration of 1.5 m*M* (*see* **Note 4**).
4. Secure the conical's cap tightly, and seal the cap with Parafilm.
5. Allow the culture to grow for 4–5 h (approximate final A_{600} = 0.8–1.0) at 37°C in a rotary shaking incubator (200 rpm).

   Henceforth, all manipulations of this [14C]-acetate labeled culture should be performed in a ventilated hood.
6. Chill the culture on ice, and sediment the bacteria by centrifugation at 3,200*g* for 10 min at 4°C.
7. Wash the bacterial pellet twice in sterile PBS follow by centrifugation, as in **Step 6**.
8. Suspend the bacteria in 1 mL of TM buffer containing 0.2% lysozyme and incubate overnight at room temperature with mild agitation.

3.2. LOS Isolation

Modified from Inzana et al., **ref. *13***.

3.2.1. Day 1

1. Add 5 μL (5U) of micrococcal nuclease to the 1 mL bacterial lysate, and incubate for 3–4 h at 37°C.

2. Transfer 500 µL of the bacterial lysate to 2 new 1 dram glass vials each containing a 1-cm magnetic stir bar, and add an equal volume of 90% phenol pre-warmed to 65°C.
3. Place the vials in a 65°C water bath on a heated magnetic stir plate, and incubate for 20 min with constant stirring.
4. Transfer the samples to 2 sterile 1.5-mL microcentrifuge tubes, and place the tubes on ice for 15 min.
5. Spin the samples in a refrigerated microcentrifuge at full speed (15,800*g*) for 10 min at 4°C.
6. Transfer the upper aqueous phase to a sterile 50-mL Oak Ridge tube.
7. Back extract the phenol phase twice with 500 µL each of sterile double-distilled water, spinning the samples and decanting the aqueous phase after each extraction, as in **steps 5** and **6**.
8. Measure the final volume of the pooled LOS-containing aqueous phases, and add 0.1 volume of 3 *M* sodium acetate and 2 volumes of 100% ethanol.
9. Mix the sample well, and incubate overnight at –20°C to precipitate the LOS.

3.2.2. Day 2

1. Sediment the precipitated LOS at 12,000*g* for 10 min.
2. Wash the LOS pellet twice with 100% ethanol followed by centrifugation, as in **step 8**, day 1.
3. Allow the pellet to dry at room temperature.
4. Suspend the LOS in 500 µL of endotoxin free sterile double-distilled water, and transfer the suspension to a sterile 1.5-mL microcentrifuge tube.
5. Seal the lid of the tube with Parafilm, and sonicate the sample for 15 min in a water-bath sonicator.
6. Transfer the sample to a 13 × 51 mm thickwalled polyallomar ultracentrifuge tube and sediment the LOS in a Beckman TL-100 ultracentrifuge at 100,000*g* for 90 min (*see* **Note 5**).
7. Suspend the LOS pellet in 500 µL of sterile endotoxin free double-distilled water, and sonicate, as in **step 5**, day 2.
8. Transfer 5 µL to scintillation cocktail, and count the sample.

A specific activity of approx 500–700 cpm/ng is achievable from the meningococcal (strain NMB) acetate auxotroph NMBACE1.

3.3. LOS Analysis

3.3.1. SDS-PAGE and Silver Staining

This procedure was modified from Lesse et al. ***(46)*** and Tsai and Frasch ***(47)***. The SDS-PAGE protocol was adjusted for use with the Hoefer SE600 SDS-PAGE Gel System and 1-mm spacers.

3.3.1.1. Day 1

1. Place two 12 × 16 cm glass SDS-PAGE plates in a 9 × 9 inch Pyrex dish, and add enough chromic-sulfuric acid cleaning solution to cover the plates.

Table 4
Resolving and Stacking Gel Solutions

Reagent	Resolving gel[a]	Stacking gel
Glycerol	5.2	—
H_2O	11.5	8.4
Gel buffer	16.6	3.1
Acrylamide:Bis	16.7	1.0
Final volume	50	12.5
10% APS[b]	0.1	0.15
TEMED[b]	0.01	0.015

[a]De-gas the resolving gel under vacuum for 10 min.
[b]Add APS and TEMED immediately prior to pouring the gel solutions.

2. After 15–30 min, wash the plates and the Pyrex dish with distilled H_20 (*see* **Note 6**).
3. Prepare the resolving and stacking gel solutions (*see* **Table 4**). Add the 10% APS and TEMED immediately prior to pouring the gel (*see* **Note 7**).
   This will provide enough gel solution to pour two 12 × 16 cm gels with 1-mm spacers (20 mL resolving gel solution is required for each gel).
4. Carefully add 1–2 mL of water saturated butanol to the top of the resolving gel, cover with plastic wrap, and allow to polymerize at least 4 h.
5. Pour the stacking gel no more than 1 h prior to loading the samples. It is not necessary to de-gas the stacking gel.
6. Assuming an LOS specific activity of 500 cpm/ng, prepare a range of LOS samples in loading buffer from 50–250 ng in 1.5 mL microcentrifuge tubes, and boil the samples for at least 10 min (*see* **Notes 8** and **9**).
7. Load the samples and run the gel at 105 volts until the dye front reaches the bottom of the gel (approx 18–20 h) (*see* **Note 10**).

3.3.1.2. Day 2

1. Separate the gel plates, discard the stacking gel, and submerge the resolving gel in 200–300 mL of gel fixing solution in the acid washed 9 × 9 Pyrex dish.
2. Agitate the gel for at least 4 h on a rotary platform with at least 2 changes of gel-fixing solution.
3. Incubate the gel in fixing solution containing 1.4 g periodic acid for 10 min with constant agitation.
4. Wash the gel for 30 minutes with at least 3 changes of 300–400 mL double-distilled water. During this washing step, make the silver-stain solution.
5. Incubate the gel in silver stain solution for 10 min with constant agitation.
6. Wash the gel as in **step 4**. During this step, make the silver-stain developing solution and the acid-stop solution.

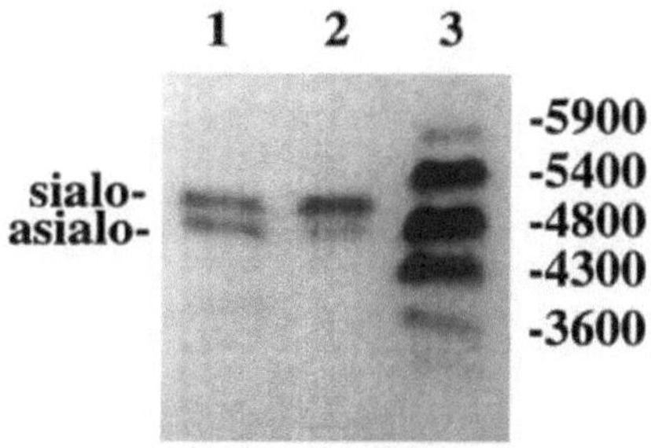

Fig. 1. SDS-PAGE and silver-staining analysis of meningococcal (NMB) LOS. [^{14}C]-LOS was analyzed by SDS-PAGE using gonococcal (PID2) and meningococcal (NMB) LOS standards for M_r and concentraion, respectively. Lane 1, (LOS conc. standard) 200 ng NMB LOS from large-scale isolation. Lane 2, ≈100,000 cpm [^{14}C]-LOS ≈500 cpm/ng. Lane 3, (LOS M_r standard) 800 ng gonococcal (PID2) LOS from large-scale isolation.

7. Add the developer solution to the gel, and allow 10–20 min for LOS bands to appear.
8. Replace the developer with acid stop solution, and agitate for 5 min (*see* **Note 11**). A typical silver-stained gel of NMB LOS is shown in **Fig. 1**.
9. Wash the gel, as in **step 4**, to remove the acetic acid.
10. Optional: If the gel is to be dried down under vacuum onto filter paper for radioautography, soak the gel overnight in a solution of 30% ethanol and 0.5% glycerol to prevent cracking.

3.3.2. FA Analysis

3.3.2.1. Day 1

1. Dry down 100,000–200,000 cpm (approx 200–400 ng) of [^{14}C]-LOS in a 13 × 100 mm screw cap disposable glass tube.
2. Suspend the [^{14}C]-LOS in 100 µL of saline.
3. Add 50 µL of 12 *N* HCl, and incubate for 90 min at 100°C.
4. Cool the sample in an ice/water bath.
5. Add 100 µL of 10 *N* NaOH, and incubate for 30 min at 100°C.
6. Add 110 µL of acetic acid. The pH of the hydrolyzed LOS solution should be between 4.0 and 5.0 with a final volume of 360 µL.
7. Add 2,160 µL of chloroform:methanol (1:2 by volume), and vortex 3 times at maximum speed for 3 min each with 1 min rest intervals.
8. Allow the phases to separate overnight at room temperature.

3.3.2.2. Day 2

1. Under a fume hood, equilibrate a TLC chamber with the mobile phase acetonitrile:glacial acetic acid (1:1 by volume).

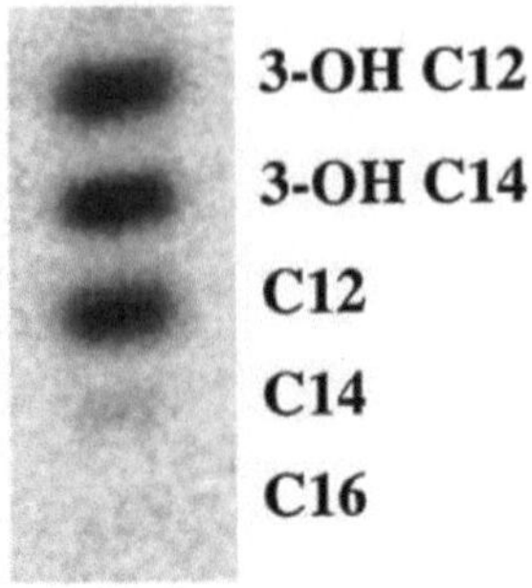

Fig. 2. Radioautography of RP-TLC analysis of hydrolyzed meningococcal (NMB) LOS. [^{14}C]-LOS was subjected to acid/base hydrolysis followed by organic extraction. Liberated FA were analyzed by RP-TLC. Mobile phase = acetonitrile:glacial acetic acid (1:1 by vol.). 3-OH FA are specific to endotoxin.

2. Add 1,080 µL of 50 m*M* KCl and 720 µL of chloroform to each sample, and vortex mix at maximum speed for 1 min.
3. Separate the chloroform (lower phase) and water/methanol (upper phase) by centrifugation at 1,800*g* for 5 min.
4. Prepare samples of the water/methanol phase (200 µL) and chloroform phase (50 µL) in scintillation fluid for counting (*see* **Note 12**).
5. Dry down 10,000–20,000 cpm of the chloroform phase under a stream of Nitrogen.
6. Using a 10 µL blunt Hamilton syringe, suspend the dried material in 10 µL of chloroform:methanol (2:1 by volume), and carefully and slowly load the material onto a HPTLC-RP18 plate (*see* **Note 13**).
7. Place the TLC plate into the equilibrated TLC chamber, and allow the mobile phase to migrate to the top of the plate.
8. Promptly remove the plate from the chamber for drying.
9. Expose the TLC plate to film for 24–48 h. A typical RP-TLC autoradiograph of hydrolyzed NMB LOS is shown in Fig. 2.

4. Notes

1. The stock acrylamide solution tends to precipitate at 4°C. If this happens, briefly warm the solution in a 37°C water bath with gentle mixing. Acrylamide is a potent neurotoxin, care should be taken to avoid exposure to skin and mucosal surfaces.
2. Growth of the NMB acetate auxotroph, NMBACE1, on GC agar requires addition of 3.5 m*M* sodium acetate to the medium for optimal growth.
3. Sterile Dacron-tipped swabs are used to pass meningococci to broth culture medium because meningococci seem to grow poorly upon passage with cotton-tipped swabs.
4. It is important to note that [^{14}C]-acetate is volatile below neutral pH.
5. The final step in this LOS purification procedure is ultracentrifugation at 100,000*g* to sediment the LOS while capsular polysaccharide and other trace soluble contaminants remain in the supernatant. It has been our experience that some LOS remains in

suspension following ultracentrifugation. Our most recent studies indicate that this LOS is biologically distinguishable from the LOS in the pellet ***(41)***.

6. The dish will be used to silver-stain the gel. Always handle the washed glassware and the polymerized acrylamide gel with powder-free gloves to prevent contamination that may interfere with silver-staining.
7. It is important to de-gas the resolving gel under vacuum for 10 min before pouring the gel.
8. LOS bands will resolve more clearly if the sample volume is kept to a minimum (e.g., 5–15 μL), and all of the wells contain either a LOS sample or sample buffer.
9. Known amounts of nonradiolabeled LOS (obtained from large-scale extraction in amounts large enough to accurately weight) can be used to calculate the amount of [^{14}C]-LOS in the stock suspension. Typically, densitometric analysis of silver-stained bands is used to generate a standard curve from which the concentration of [^{14}C]-LOS is calculated. The radiolabeled LOS should be compared only to large-scale LOS preparations from the same strain, as different LOS forms stain with different (LOS) to stain density ratios.
10. The dye front will move relatively quickly in the first few hours, but will slow considerably as the samples move through the gel.
11. It is a good idea to capture an image of the gel prior to adding the stop solution, as the acetic acid causes the bands to fade slightly.
12. Approximately 90–95% of the total radioactivity should partition to the chloroform phase. [^{14}C]-LOS samples containing capsular polysaccharide will generate a relatively large percentage of counts (30% or higher) in the water/methanol phase presumably resulting from [^{14}C]-labeled sialic acid liberated from the capsule during acid/base hydrolysis.
13. TLC samples should be loaded *slowly* onto the Rp-TLC plate approx 1 cm apart. Take care not to damage the surface of the plate while loading the sample. We have found that a blunt Hamilton syringe works well for loading these samples.

References

1. Apicella, M. A. (2000) *Neisseria meningitidis* in *Principles and Practice of Infectious Diseases* (Mandrell, G. L., Bennett, J. E., and Dolin, R., eds.), Churchill Livingstone, Philadelphia, pp. 2228–2241.
2. Anonymous (1999) Communicable Disease Surveillance and Response (CSR). World Health Organization, Geneva.
3. Anonymous (1997) Summary of Notifiable Diseases for 1997. *MMWR* **46,** 3.
4. Mandrell, R. E. and Apicella, M. A. (1993) Lipo-oligosaccharides (LOS) of mucosal pathoegns: molecular mimicry and host-modification of LOS. *Immunobiology* **187,** 382–402.
5. Verheul, A. F. M., Snippe, H., and Poolman, J. T. (1993) Meningococcal lipopolysaccharides: Virulence factor and potential vaccine component. *Microbiol. Rev.* **57,** 34–49.
6. Devoe, I. W. and Gilchrist, J. E. (1973) Release of endotoxin in the form of cell wall blebs during in vitro growth of *Neisseria meningitidis*. *J. Exp. Med.* **138,** 1156–1167.

7. Brandtzaeg, P., Oktedalen, O., Kierulf, P., and Opstad, P. K. (1989) Elevated VIP and endotoxin plasma levels in human gram-negative septic shock. *Regul. Peptides* **24,** 37–44.
8. Brandtzaeg, P., Kierulf, P., Gaustad, P., Skulberg, A., Bruun, J. N., Halvorsen, S., and Sorensen, E. (1989) Plasma endotoxin as a predictor of multiple organ failure and death in systemic meningococcal disease. *J. Infect. Dis.* **159,** 195–204.
9. Brandtzaeg, P., Bryn, K., Kierulf, P., Ovstebo, R., Namork, E., Aase, B., and Jantzen, E. (1992) Meningococcal endotoxin in lethal septic shock plasma studied by gas chromatography, mass-spectrometry, ultracentrifugation, and electron microscopy. *J. Clin. Invest.* **89,** 816–823.
10. Evans, J. S. and Maiden, M. C. (1996) Purification of meningococcal lipooligosaccharide by FPLC techniques. *Microbiology* **142,** 57–62.
11. Apicella, M. A., Griffiss, J. M., and Schneider, H. (1994) Isolation and characterization of lipopolysaccharides, lipooligosaccharides, and lipid A. *Methods Enzymol.* **235,** 242–252.
12. Gu, X. X. and Tsai, C. M. (1991) Purification of rough-type lipopolysaccharides of *Neisseria meningitidis* from cells and outer membrane vesicles in spent media. *Anal. Biochem.* **196,** 311–318.
13. Inzana, T. J., Iritani, B., Gogolewski, R. P., Kania, S. A., and Corbeil, L. B. (1988) Purification and characterization of lipooligosaccharides from four strains of *Haemophilus somnus. Infect. Immun.* **56,** 2830–2837.
14. Wu, L. H., Tsai, C. M., and Frasch, C. E. (1987) A method for purification of bacterial R-type lipopolysaccharides (lipooligosaccharides). *Anal. Biochem.* **160,** 281–289.
15. Johnson, K. G. and Perry, M. B. (1976) Improved techniques for the preparation of bacterial lipopolysaccharides. *Can. J. Microbiol.* **22,** 29–34.
16. Adams, G. A., Kates, M., Shaw, D. H., and Yaguchi, M. (1968) Studies of the chemical constituents of cell-wall lipopolysacchrides from *Neisseria perflava. Can. J. Biochem.* **46,** 1175–1184.
17. Rahman, M. M., Stephens, D. S., Kahler, C. M., Glushka, J., and Carlson, R. W. (1998) The lipooligosaccharide (LOS) of *Neisseria meningitidis* serogroup B strain NMB contains L2, L3 and novel oligosaccharides, and lacks the lipid-A 4′-phosphate substituent. *Carbohydrate Res.* **307,** 311–324.
18. Raetz, C. R. H. (1990) Biochemistry of endotoxin. *Ann. Rev. Biochem.* **59,** 129–170.
19. Giardina, P. C, Preston, A., Gibson, B., and Apicella, M. A. (1999) Antigenic mimicry in *Neisseria* species in *Endotoxin in Health and Disease* (Brade, H., Opal, S. M., Vogal, S. N., and Morrison, D. C., eds.), Marcel Dekker, New York, pp. 55–65.
20. Kahler, C. M. and Stephens, D. S. (1998) Genetic basis for biosynthesis, structure, and function of meningococcal lipooligosaccharide (endotoxin). *Crit. Rev. Microbiol.* **24,** 281–334.
21. Kulshin, V. A., Zahringer, U., Lindner, B., Frash, C. E., Tsai, C.-M., Dmitriev, B. A., and Rietschel, E. T. (1992) Structural characterization of the lipid A component of pathogenic *Neisseria meningitidis. J. Bacteriol.* **174,** 1793–1800.

22. Kahler, C. M., Carlson, R. W., Rahman, M. M., Martin, L. E., and Stephens, D. S. (1996) Inner core biosunthesis of lipooligosaccharide (LOS) in *Neisseria meningitidis* serogroup B: Identification and role in LOS assembly of the β 1,2 *N*-aetylglucosamine transferase (RfaK). *J. Bacteriol.* **178,** 1265–1273.
23. Lee, F. K., Stephens, D. S., Gibson, B. W., Engstrom, J. J., Zhou, D., and Apicella, M. A. (1995) Microheterogeneity of *Neisseria* lipooligosaccharide: analysis of the UDP-glucose 4 epimerase mutant of *Neisseria meningitidis* NMB. *Infect. Immun.* **63,** 2508–2515.
24. Jennings, M. P., Hood, D. W., Peak, I. R. A., Virji, M., and Moxon, E. R. (1995) Molecular analysis of a locus for the biosynthesis and phase-variable expression of the lacto-*N*-neotetraose terminal lipopolysaccharide structure in *Neisseria meningitidis. Mol. Microbiol.* **18,** 729–740.
25. Gamian, A., Beurret, M., Michon, F., Brisson, J.-R., and Jennings, H. J. (1992) Structure of the L2 Lipopolysaccharide core oligosaccharides of *Neisseria meningitidis. J. Biol. Chem.* **267,** 922–925.
26. Michon, F., Beurrett, M., Gamina, A., Brisson, J.-R., and Jennings, H. J. (1990) Structure of the L5 lipopolysacchardie core oligosaccharides of *Neisseria meningitidis. J. Biol. Chem.* **265,** 7243–7247.
27. Reitschel, E. T., Brade, H., Brade, L., Brandenburg, K., Schade, U., Seydel, U., et al. (1987) Lipid A, the endotoxic center of bacterial lipopolysaccharides: relation of chemical structure to biological activity. *Prog. Clin. Biol. Res.* **231,** 25–53.
28. Pugin, J., Schurer-Maly, C. C., Leturcq, D., Moriarty, D., Ulevich, R. J., and Tobias, P. S. (1993) Lipopolysaccharide activation of human endothelial and epithelial cells is mediated by lipopolysaccharide binding protein and soluble CD14. *Proc. Natl. Acad. Sci. USA* **90,** 2744–2748.
29. Wright, S. D., Ramos, R. A., Tobias, P. S., Ulevitch, R. J., and Mathison, J. C. (1990) CD14 is a receptor for complexes of lipopolysaccharide (LPS) and LPS binding proteins. *Science* **249,** 1431–1433.
30. Luchi, M. and Munford, R. S. (1993) Binding, internalization, and deacylation of bacterial lipopolysaccharide by human neutrophils. *J. Immunol.* **151,** 959–969.
31. Wright, S. D. and Jong, M. T. C. (1986) Adhesion-promoting receptors on human macrophages recognize *Escherichia coli* by binding to lipopolysaccharide. *J. Exp. Med.* **164,** 1876–1888.
32. Brandtzaeg, P., Sandset, P. M., Joo, G. B., Ovstebo, R., Abildgaard, U., and Kierulf, P. (1989) The quantitative association of plasma endotoxin, antithrombin, protein C, extrinsic pathway inhibitor and fibrinopeptide A in systemic meningococcal disease. *Thromb. Res.* **55,** 459–470.
33. Rosenstein, N. E., Perkins, B. A., Stephens, D. S., Lefkowitz, L., Cartter, M. L., Danila, R., et al. and the Active Bacterial Core Surveillance Team. (1999) The changing epidemiology of meningococcal disease in the United States, 1992–1996. *J. Infect. Dis.,* **180,** 1894–1901.

34. Girardin, E., Grau, G. E., Dayer, J. M., Roux-Lombard, P., and Lambert, P. H. (1988) Tumor necrosis factor and interleukin-1 in the serum of children with severe infectious purpura. *N. Engl. J. Med.* **319,** 397–400.
35. Brandtzaeg, P., Oktedalen, O., Kierulf, P., and Opstad, P. K. (1989) Elevated VIP and endotoxin plasma levels in human gram-negative septic shock. *Regul. Peptides* **24,** 37–44.
36. Brandtzaeg, P., Kierulf, P., Gaustad, P., Skulberg, A., Bruun, J. N., Halvorsen, S., and Sorensen, E. (1989) Plasma endotoxin as a predictor of multiple organ failure and death in systemic meningococcal disease. *J. Infect. Dis.* **159,** 195–204.
37. Brandtzaeg, P., Mollnes, T.E., and Kierulf, P. (1989) Complement activation and endotoxin levels in systemic meningococcal disease. *J. Infect. Dis.* **160,** 58–65.
38. Brandtzaeg, P., Ovsteboo, R., and Kierulf, P. (1992) Compartmentalization of lipopolysaccharide production correlates with clinical presentation in meningococcal disease. *J. Infect. Dis.* **166,** 650–652.
39. Brandtzaeg, P., Bryn, K., Kierulf, P., Ovstebo, R., Namork, E., Aase, B., and Jantzen, E. (1992) Meningococcal endotoxin in lethal septic shock plasma studied by gas chromatography, mass-spectrometry, ultracentrifugation, and electron microscopy. *J. Clin. Invest.* **89,** 816–823.
40. Cesarini, J. P., Vandekerkove, M., Faucon, M. R., and Nicoli, J. (1967) Ultrastructure of the wall of *Neisseria meningitidis. Ann. l'Institut Pasteur* **113,** 833–841.
41. Devoe, I. W. and Gilchrist, J. E. (1973) Release of endotoxin in the form of cell wall blebs during in vitro growth of *Neisseria meningitidis. J. Exp. Med.* **138,** 1156–1167.
42. Giardina, P. C., Gioannini, T., Buscher, B., Zaleski, A., Stoll, L, Zheng, D.-S., et al. (2000) Construction of acetate auxotrophs of *Neisseria meningitidis* to study host-meningococcal endotoxin interactions. *J. Biol. Chem.* [epub ahead of print].
43. Neveling, U., Bringer-Meyer, S., and Sahm, H. (1998) Gene and subunit organization of bacterial pyruvate dehydrogenase complexes. *Biochim. Biophys. Acta.* **1385,** 367–372.
44. Munford, R. S., DeVeaux, L. C., Cronan, J. E., and Rick, P. D. (1992) Biosynthetic radiolabeling of bacterial lipopolysaccharide to high specific activity. *J. Immunol. Meth.* **148,** 115–120.
45. Morse, S. A. and Barenstein, L. (1980) Purine metabolism in *Neisseria gonorrhoeae*: the requirement for hypoxanthine. *Can. J. Microbiol.* **26,** 13–20.
46. Lesse, A. J., Campagnari, A. A., Bittner, W. E., and Apicella, M. A. (1990) Increased resolution of lipopolysaccharides and lipooligosaccharides utilizing tricine-sodium dodecyl sulfate polyacrylamide gel electrophoresis. *J. Immunol. Methods* **126,** 109–117.
47. Tsai, C.M. and Frasch, C.E. (1982) A sensitive silver stain for detecting lipopolysaccharides in polyacrylamide gels. *Anal. Biochem.* **119,** 115–120.

28

Cytokine Measurement In Vivo and In Vitro

Marcel van Deuren and Petter Brandtzaeg

1. Introduction

1.1. Activation of the Cytokine Network In Vivo

1.1.1. Background

Cytokines play a pivotal role in both defense against meningococcal infection and the pathophysiology of invasive meningococcal disease. These chemical messengers are crucial cogwheels in the machinery of the innate immune system and are also powerful forces in the antigen-specific defense system.

In the mid 1980s, tumor necrosis factor α (TNF-α) was identified as a critical mediator in the genesis of Gram-negative or lipopolysaccharide (LPS)-induced septic shock *(1)*. It was demonstrated that infusion of Gram-negative bacteria or LPS induces a rise in the serum concentration of TNF-α, that antibodies against TNF-α abrogate the development of shock and that TNF-α infusion induces a clinical picture of fever, shock, disseminated intravascular coagulation (DIC), and multiple-organ failure (MOF) indistinguishable from that of Gram-negative septic shock. In 1987, Waage and co-workers reported that fatalities with meningococcal septic shock had extremely high serum TNF-α levels *(2)*, and from that moment meningococcal septic shock was labeled the "prototype, endotoxin-induced, cytokine-mediated, Gram-negative infection." Since then, approx 25 studies have reported on cytokine measurements in blood during meningococcal sepsis and more than 50 studies have described cytokine measurements in cerebrospinal fluid (CSF) during meningitis.

Still, our understanding of the role of cytokine activation in meningococcal disease is limited and skewed. The principal reason for this unbalanced view is that most studies have focused on the role of cytokines in the pathophysiology

From: *Methods in Molecular Medicine, vol. 67: Meningococcal Disease: Methods and Protocols*
Edited by: A. J. Pollard and M. C. J. Maiden © Humana Press Inc., Totowa, NJ

of meningococcal septic shock or meningitis and only a handful have discussed the role of cytokines in the processes that precede the condition of invasive disease. In brief, we know very little about the role of cytokines in the process of colonization of the nasal mucosa, the intracellular survival of meningococci in macrophages and mucosal cells, the trafficking of meningococci through mucosal cells, and the induction of the specific protective immune response.

Thus, although the information concerning cytokines in meningococcal disease reviewed in this chapter may seem substantial, it is important to note the complete picture is not yet known. It is likely that a majority of the missing pieces in the jigsaw cover areas that relate to defense against meningococcal disease rather than the extensively studied dramatic inflammatory response that occurs after invasion.

1.1.2. Cytokine Measurements In Vivo

In vivo, cytokines have a wide spectrum of autocrine, paracrine, and endocrine effects on the cells of origin, adjacent cells, or distant cells, respectively *(3)*. Cytokines are active intracellularly, bound to cellular membranes or in a released form in body fluids. Some cytokines may be present in a pro-form, some aggregate to bioactive multimeric aggregates. The activity of cytokines is further modulated by the presence of other cytokines, by the density of cytokine receptors on target cells, and by structures that interfere with the binding to cells such as soluble cytokine receptors.

A large variety of techniques have been developed for the immunochemical or functional assay of cytokines in body fluids. Significant differences exist between these techniques, which is not surprising given the multitude of factors that influence the concentration of free and bound cytokines and their activities ***(4–6)***. Even when a standardized kit is used, data from samples taken at different time-points during the course of the disease or values from plasma, serum or CSF may be not comparable. Thus, all available data should be regarded as reflecting relative and not absolute values.

The role of cytokines in CSF during bacterial meningitis of various etiologies has been reviewed recently by Täuber and Moser *(7)*. This chapter will focus primarily on cytokines in plasma or serum during meningococcal sepsis. Based on the more than 25 studies that measured in vivo cytokines in plasma or serum the following general picture can be deduced.

1.1.2.1. Pro-inflammatory Cytokines

Early in the disease, the serum concentrations of TNF-α and other proinflammatory cytokines like interleukin-1β (IL-1β), IL-6, IL-8, and interferon-γ (IFN-γ) correlate with degree of endotoxinemia and the severity of shock in meningococcal sepsis ***(2,8–21)***. Reportedly all these cytokines bring about a clinical picture characterized by fever, shock, DIC and MOF either alone or in synergy. Thus, the causal role of these pro-inflammatory cytokines in the genesis of meningococcal sepsis seems to be well established.

Recently, however, this concept has been disputed for a number of reasons. First, in vitro LPS-stimulation of blood cells from relatives of patients who died from meningococcal sepsis produce less pro-inflammatory TNF-α and more anti-inflammatory IL-10 than cells of family members of patients who survived ***(22)***. Second, in surgical sepsis where high TNF-α values are rarely encountered ***(23)***, serum TNF-α correlates with a good outcome ***(24–26)***, whereas serum IL-10 is associated with fatality ***(27,28)***. Third, blocking of TNF-α is detrimental in animal experiments that simulate abdominal sepsis or foreign-body infections ***(29–31)***. Together these observations suggest that in these types of infections TNF-α may be not as damaging as believed, but is essential for the appropriate antibacterial immune response.

However, meningococcal sepsis differs from these types of infections. In meningococcal sepsis, the overwhelming exposure to bacteria without preceding illness is clearly different from that during surgical sepsis or foreign-body infections. Therefore the pattern of cytokine activation in meningococcal sepsis differs from that in surgical sepsis ***(23)***. In addition, unlike the complement system, cytokines have no defined role in the restraint of the intravascular outgrowth of meningococci. Thus, we believe that in meningococcal sepsis high cytokine levels contribute clearly to tissue damage and clinical deterioration.

1.1.2.2. Compartmentalized Cytokine Production

Cytokine production in meningococcal infections is compartmentalized. This means that in septic shock, the cytokine network is activated in the plasma-compartment, whereas in meningitis, the major changes occur in the subarachnoid compartment ***(15,18,32–34)***.

The compartmentalized cytokine activation is a consequence of the site where meningococci multiplicate ***(35,36)***. In sepsis, the outgrowth in the bloodstream appears to occur exponentially. Within 12–18 h, plasma endotoxin concentration can reach very high levels, i.e., 7.5–1700 endotoxin units (EU) per mL equal to 0.75–170 ng/mL of *Escherichia coli* O55B5 LPS as measured by the *Limulus* amebocyte lysate (LAL) assay ***(11,37)***. This is equivalent to an estimated bacterial load of approx 7.5×10^5 to 1.7×10^8 cfu/mL (*see* **Subheading 1.2.4.**). However, much of the LPS is not present as live bacteria but presumably as outer membrane vesicles (OMV) or fragments of lysed bacteria ***(10)***. In patients with meningitis, the outgrowth in the bloodstream is restrained with plasma endotoxin concentrations less than (median) 250 pg/mL. On arrival in the subarachnoid space, meningococci proliferate in an uncontrolled fashion as a result of lesser immune suveillance in this compartment ***(38–41)***.

CSF endotoxin values during meningitis are as high as 2.5 ng/mL (median range 0.25–500 ng/mL) ***(40)***. Quantitative bacterial cultures in this condition reveal CSF-concentrations of 10^8 cfu/mL or more ***(42,43)***.

The experimental inoculation of meningococci in the subarachnoid space in rabbits elicits a pattern of cytokines similar to that in blood after the intravenous application ***(9)***. However, although both patterns appear similar, more detailed measurements of (for instance) the cytokine-soluble receptors, soluble TNF-receptor (sTNFR) and soluble IL-1-receptor type II (sIL-1RII), show that definite differences exist between the two compartments ***(18,34)***. The explanation for the dissimilarity lies in the differential cellular origin of the cytokines, different mechanisms of clearance, and in the different time-course of both infections ***(41)***. In addition, it should be kept in mind that meningococcal sepsis is primarily an intra-vascular infection with intra-vascular activation of the cytokine network, whereas meningococcal meningitis is a metastatic extra-vascular infection.

During sepsis, early complement activation, ignited immediately after invasion of meningococci into the bloodstream ***(11)***, influences the production of TNF-α, IL-1β, and IL-6 through C3a and C5a ***(44–47)***. Neutrophil activation stimulates cytokine production directly and also indirectly via damage to endothelial cells ***(48,49)***. Neutrophil activation in the blood compartment, reflected by upregulation of CD11b, shedding of L-selectin, and release of elastase starts within 15 min after contact with meningococci ***(50–52)***, while only after 90-min does cytokine production become detectable ***(51)***. In meningitis the sequence of these processes is the other way around. Here the cytokine activation precedes and induces the influx of activated neutrophils into the subarachnoid space by permeabilizing the blood liquor barrier ***(7,53,54)***.

In brief, the cytokine response in meningococcal sepsis in the blood compartment is modulated by the preceding and ongoing activation of the complement-system, coagulation-system, neutrophils, and endothelium. As all these factors are absent in the native subarachnoid space that is lined with meningothelial cells ***(7,38,39)***, cytokine activation in CSF will be differentially regulated.

1.1.2.3. Anti-inflammatory Cytokines

Early during the course of meningococcal infections, not only the pro-inflammatory cytokines such as TNF-α and IL-1β are produced and released, but also the anti-inflammatory cytokines like IL-1 receptor antagonist (IL-1Ra) and IL-10 ***(17,18,34,55)***. Similarly, the plasma concentrations of various soluble cytokine receptors are affected. Soluble TNFR-p55 and sTNFR-p75 are upregulated at an early stage ***(8,16,18,56,57)***. Soluble IL-1RII is increased in CSF at the onset of disease but unaffected in plasma during the early stage of sepsis where it increases gradually during recovery ***(34)***. In contrast, soluble IL-6 receptor (sIL-6R) is downregulated in blood during the acute stage of sepsis ***(20,21,58)***.

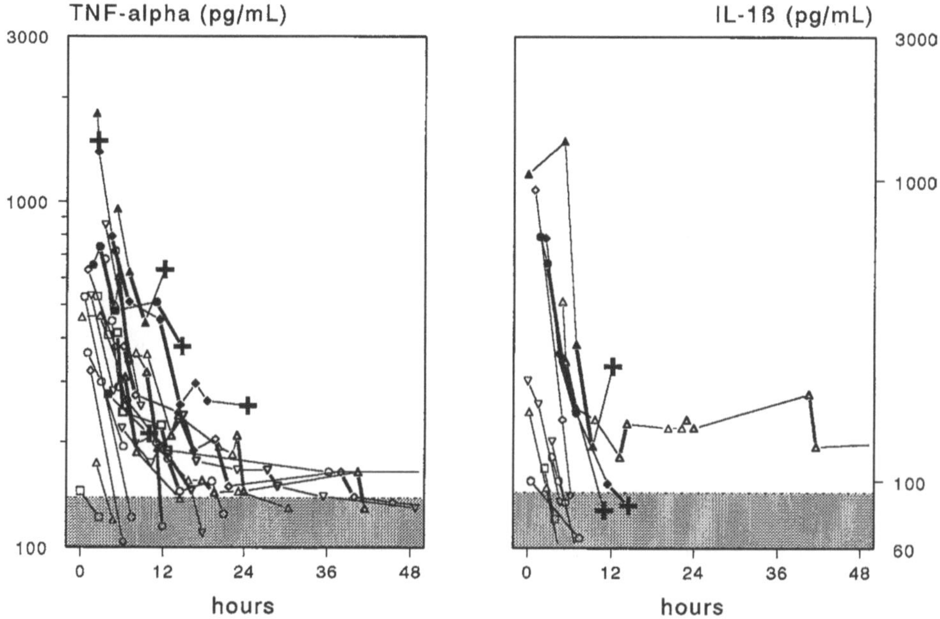

Fig. 1. Course of cytokines during first hours after admission. The individual plasma patterns of tumor necrosis factor α (TNF-α) and interleukin-1β (IL-1β) in patients with meningococcal sepsis during the first 2 d after admission. Open markers are survivors, closed markers nonsurvivors, crosses indicate moment of death. Thick lines indicate the cytokine pattern during a plasma exchange or whole-blood exchange session ***(162)***; thin lines represent data outside an exchange session. The shaded area indicates the normal cytokine value (mean ± SD); for the ease of survey, values within the normal range are not shown.

IL-10 is known to inhibit the production of pro-inflammatory cytokines like TNF-α. IL-1Ra blocks the effects of IL-1β. Soluble TNFRs and sIL-1RII restrain the effect of TNF-α and IL-1β in the early stage of the disease but may prolong the effects of both ligand cytokines by releasing them in a later stage. In contrast, sIL-6R is believed to potentiate the effect of IL-6. Thus, directly after onset of disease the cytokine network in meningococcal infections is regulated in a very complex fashion that makes it difficult to estimate the overall effect of its concerted action.

1.1.2.4. Kinetics of Cytokines

The plasma concentrations of most pro-inflammatory cytokines decrease promptly after admission and initiation of antibiotic therapy and normalize within 6–24 h even in patients with an ultimately fatal course (**Fig. 1**) ***(9,16,34,57,59)***. An increase in the plasma concentration of TNF-α and IL-1β

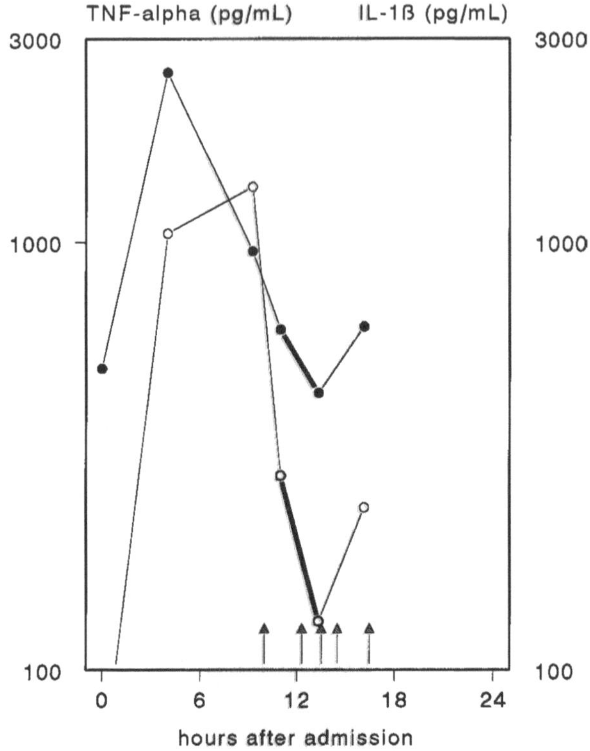

Fig. 2. Course of cytokines when antibiotics are delayed. The plasma pattern of tumor necrosis factor-α (TNF-α, closed dots) and interleukin-1β (IL-1β, open dots) in one nonsurviving patient who received, because of initial misdiagnosis, antibiotics only 5.5 h after admission. The patient died 19 h after admission. The thick lines indicate a plasma-exchange session ***(162)***. The arrows indicate resuscitation efforts.

after initiation of antibiotic treatment has never been observed. A rise of TNF-α and IL-1β after admission is only observed in those unfortunate patients from whom antibiotics are mistakenly withheld (**Fig. 2**); ***(60)***; (P. Brandtzaeg, personal observation).

Most anti-inflammatory cytokines and soluble receptors level off slowly after several days ***(9,14,16,17,34,59)***. This discrepancy in the kinetics of pro- and anti-inflammatory mediators implies that measurements of plasma concentrations at an arbitrary point in time are of limited value for the evaluation of the pro- or anti-inflammatory status of the cytokine network ***(12,18,27,57)***.

Some data exist on the time-course of cytokines in CSF during treatment of meningococcal meningitis ***(61–63)***. Cultures of CSF become sterile almost immediately ***(43)***. Although no data for meningococcal meningitis are available, sequential CSF-sampling in *Haemophilus influenzae* meningitis show a definite increase of TNF-α in the first 4 h after initiation of antibiotic therapy ***(64)***. Clinically this increase may coincide with the temporal deterioration during the first hours of treatment. This occurrence of a transient increase of TNF-α in CSF is in accordance with the finding that 18–30 h after start of therapy, TNF-α and IL-1β may still remain detectable in CSF in the majority of the patients ***(62)***. IL-6 remains increased for several days ***(63)***. There is some evidence that in meningococcal meningitis the inflammatory response in CSF extinguishes faster than in pneumococcal meningitis ***(65)***. This might be explained by the somewhat higher initial bacterial load in pneumococcal meningitis ***(43)***, the higher IFN-γ concentrations ***(66)*** or the different cytokine induction in CSF by the Gram-positive pneumococcus ***(67)***.

1.1.2.5. Endotoxin Responsiveness

Although conflicting data exist ***(22,68)***, in meningococcal sepsis the degree in rise of serum TNF-α is probably not explained by TNF-α polymorphism. However, in other infectious diseases, polymorphisms of the TNF-α promoter gene explain some of the clinical differences ***(69,70)***. In contrast, blood cells of patients or relatives of patients who die of meningococcal disease produce less TNF-α and more IL-10 after stimulation with LPS, compared to cells of patients who survive ***(71)***. Thus, the phenomenon of endotoxin responsiveness, i.e., the genetically determined trait to produce more or less cytokines after the exposure to LPS ***(72)***, is believed to be of minor importance for the degree of cytokine activation in meningococcal sepsis.

1.1.2.6. Regulation of Cytokine Production

Despite the rapid normalization of the TNF-α and IL-1β serum concentrations, mRNA for these cytokines in blood cells remains increased for several days. This suggests an early restraint of cytokine production in these cells by post-transcriptional regulatory mechanisms ***(73)***. The downregulation can also be observed when peripheral blood cells are stimulated ex vivo with LPS. Shortly after onset of disease these, cells have lost their capacity to produce and secrete TNF-α, IL-1β, or IL-6 after such stimulus ***(56,73)***. The duration and severity of the downregulated state correlates with the severity of disease and may be caused by IL-10 ***(74,75)*** and possibly transforming growth factor-β (TGF-β) ***(76–78)***. More detailed study of this phenomenon, that also occurs after experimental LPS-infusion, other types of sepsis, or severe trauma ***(79–81)***, shows that in meningococcal sepsis the TNF-α production is downregulated post-transcriptionally but IL-1β production is also regulated at the mRNA level ***(73)***. IFN-γ and granulocyte-macrophage colony stimulating factor (GM-CSF) can restore this state of monocyte deactivation ***(82–84)***.

It should be noted that the cellular source of cytokine production during meningococcal sepsis or meningitis is currently not known. Several candidate cells have been suggested, among them tissue macrophages, endothelial cells, microglial cells, and astrocytes *(7)*. Peripheral blood mononuclear cells (PBMCs) are assumed to play a minor role during the in vivo cytokine production in sepsis *(73,85)*. Therefore, studies on the regulation of cytokine production in monocytes may be less relevant for the in vivo regulation during invasive meningococcal disease and should be interpreted cautiously.

1.1.2. The In Vivo Data Summarized

From the above mentioned in vivo observations, we can conclude that the excessive pro-inflammatory cytokine production, which causes shock, DIC, and MOF (alone or in combination with other pro-inflammatory mediators), is not the result of an enhanced or dysregulated cytokine responsiveness, but rather the consequence of the explosive outgrowth of meningococci in the bloodstream. The production and activity of these pro-inflammatory cytokines is counter-regulated in a complex fashion. Early after onset of the disease, anti-inflammatory mediators appear in the circulation, pro-inflammatory cytokines disappear rapidly, and the production of pro-inflammatory cytokines in blood cells is downregulated. Cytokine activation in the CSF compartment during meningococcal meningitis shows both similarities and dissimilarities with that in blood during sepsis. Studies of the regulation of cytokine production in vivo are limited because the principal cellular sources of cytokine production during meningococcal sepsis and meningitis are still unknown.

1.2. Cytokine Production In Vitro

1.2.1. Background

In the in vivo situation during invasive meningococcal disease, cytokine production is induced after contact between growing meningococci and a plethora of immune-competent cells. For the in vitro study of this process, the in vivo situation has been curtailed and simplified.

The model that is most often used for these purposes evaluates cytokine induction by LPS in peripheral blood monocytes or cell-lines of macrophages. LPS, one of the outer-membrane components of Gram-negative micro-organisms, is considered the most potent cytokine inducing part of Gram-negative bacteria. LPS is an amphipatic molecule composed of a lipid-A part, a poly- or oligosaccharide part and one or more molecules of 2-keto-3-deoxy-octanate (KDO) connecting lipid-A with the saccharide tail *(86)*. Owing to its amphipatic structure, isolated LPS forms aggregates.

Studies with isolated LPS or parts of the LPS-molecule have broadened and deepened our insight in the mechanism of cytokine induction markedly. For a variety of reasons, the applicability of such knowledge to the in vivo situation during invasive meningococcal disease is limited.

First, we do not know which types of cells are responsible for cytokine production during invasive meningococcal disease. Second, the study of isolated cells requires removal of these cells from their possibly relevant physiologic environment. Third, the amount of LPS used in many of these studies considerably exceeds the LPS concentration during the onset of meningococcal infection. Because of these high concentrations, the LPS may engage LPS-receptors and cytokine inducing pathways other than those that would be active in vivo. Fourth, LPS from enterobacteriaceae generally evaluated in these types of studies differs in many aspects from that from *Neisseria meningitidis*. Lastly, meningococcal LPS is not the sole compound of *N. meningitidis* that is able to induce cytokine synthesis.

1.2.2. Cytokine Induction by LPS

LPS induces cytokine production when it ligates LPS-receptors (*see* next paragraph) on cytokine-producing cells and initiates a transfer of a stimulating signal to the nucleus. Here, by induction of the transcription factor, NF-κB, cytokine mRNA will be transcribed and cytokine synthesis follows after 60–90 min. TNF-α is the first cytokine to appear, followed by IL-β after 120 min and IL-6, IL-8, and IL-10 immediately thereafter. Notably, stimulation of monocytic cells with LPS induces only minute amounts of IFN-γ.

Several membrane-bound proteins are involved in the recognition of LPS. In higher LPS-concentrations, LPS may attach to the integrins CD11a,11b,11c/CD18, L-selectin, and the scavenger receptor. In lower LPS-concentrations the principal LPS-receptor is CD14 ***(87,88)***. CD14 is a 55-kDa membrane protein of cells belonging to the myeloid-cell lineage or mesangial cells. One of the functions of CD14 is a highly specific interaction with the lipid-A part and the KDO part of the LPS-molecule ***(88)***. There is evidence that the polysaccharide part of the LPS molecule also interacts with this binding but the exact role of the carbohydrate chain is still unsolved ***(89,90)***. Recently it was shown that variant types of LPS with a short carbohydrate chain tend to engage relatively more CD14-independent pathways ***(91)***.

Cells that do not bear membrane-bound CD14 (mCD14) on their surface, like endothelial cells and astrocytes, can react with LPS through a soluble form of CD14 (sCD14) ***(88,92–94)***, that is reported to increase slightly during sepsis and meningococcal infections ***(21,94,95)***. Because mCD14 is a glycosyl-phosphatidylinositol (GPI)-anchored membrane protein that lacks a cytoplasmatic signaling domain, a co-receptor is required to permit transfer of the signal across the plasma membrane ***(96)***. Recently a Toll-like receptor and possibly the so-called membrane-organizing extension spike receptor "moesin" have been demonstrated to be involved in this process ***(97–99)***.

Various serum proteins like LPS-binding protein (LBP) ***(100)***, serum amyloid-P (SAP) ***(101)***, apolipoproteins ***(101)***, and the synthetic peptide polymyxin B (PMB) ***(102,103)*** bind with high affinity to lipid-A. Many proteins derived from neutrophilic granules such as lactoferrin (LF) ***(104)***, bactericidal/permeability-increasing protein (BPI) ***(105)***, heparin-binding protein, and fucoidin ***(106)*** bind also to the lipid-A portion of LPS. Affinity of these peptides to LPS follows the electrostatic binding between a short cationic amino-acid sequence that is present in most of these peptides with the phosphorylated disaccharide portion of lipid-A and the stabilizing hydrophobic interaction between adjacent peptide loops with the fatty acid residues of lipid-A ***(101,107)***. BPI ***(105)***, SAP ***(101)***, lipoproteins ***(108)***, LF ***(104)***, and the synthetic peptide PMB ***(103,109)*** inhibit the binding of *E. coli* LPS to CD14, thereby decreasing the LPS-induced TNF-α production. This inhibitory action is believed to occur via stabilization of LPS-aggregates. In contrast, LBP catalyses the transfer of *E. coli* LPS to CD14 by dissociating LPS-monomers from LPS-aggregates ***(88)***. By doing so, LBP increases the affinity of LPS to CD14 100–1000 times ***(110)***. In vitro experiments show that in the presence of 5% serum or LBP, the threshold concentration of *E. coli* LPS that induces TNF-α or IL-1β production in cells of the monocytic cell-lineage is lowered from approx 10 ng/mL to 100 pg/mL ***(111)***.

It is of interest to note that in vivo during the early stage of infections the serum concentrations of LBP and BPI increase ***(112–114)***, that changes occur in the lipid metabolism ***(115)*** and that sCD14 increases slightly ***(21)***. Thus in the in vivo situation, several factors affect the binding of LPS to LPS-receptors. Also during in vitro experiments these serum factors and the presence of neutrophils that release various LPS-binding peptides modulate the LPS-induced cytokine production by monocytes. This may be one of the reasons why more LPS is required for the induction of cytokines in whole blood than is needed for the induction of cytokines in isolated mononuclear cells.

1.2.3. Cytokine Induction by Meningococcal LPS

Because meningococcemia is characterized by extremely high serum cytokine concentrations, which is not the case in other Gram-negative infections like gonococcemia or typhoid fever ***(116)***, several studies have tried to relate the observed degree of in vivo cytokine induction to the binding of the isolated type of LPS on monocytes and its cytokine inducing potency ***(89,117–127)***. From these studies, it can be concluded that for optimal induction of cytokines by meningococcal LPS, lipid-A, KDO, and saccharide are all required. Unfortunately, quantitative conclusions about the biological activity of meningococcal LPS compared to other types of LPS are difficult to draw, because most studies compare LPSs on a weight base without information about the molecular weight (MW), the number of LPS-molecules per bacterium, the efficacy of the extraction procedure, and the purity of the LPS-preparation. A recent study that dealt with this problem and evaluated various more uniformly extracted and calibrated types of LPS found only minor differences in the biological activity of these types of LPS ***(128)***. The qualitative picture based on the studies with meningococcal LPS is that that meningococcal LPS may be somewhat (but not much) more potent for induction of cytokines. The findings of Prins et al. that LPS from meningococcal strains isolated from patients with shock or isolated from patients with chronic meningococcemia induced equivalent amounts of TNF-α, support this view ***(127)***.

In recent experiments in our laboratory we compared, on a molar base, the potency of meningococcal serogroup B *H44/76* LPS (gift from Peter van der Ley, National Institute of Public Health and the Environment [RIVM], Bilthoven, the Netherlands) with that of a commercial *E. coli* 055:B5 LPS (L2880, Sigma Chemical Co, St. Louis, MO), both extracted with the same phenol-water method ***(129)***. The molar concentration of both preparations was estimated by assay of 2-keto-3-deoxy-octanate (KDO) ***(130)***, based on two KDO-molecules per molecule of meningococcal LPS and three KDO-molecules per molecule *E. coli* LPS. It appeared that the minimal concentration of meningococcal LPS that induces TNF-α or IL-1β release by human monocytes in the presence of serum, is 2 fmol/mL or 8 pg/mL (**Fig. 3**). For *E. coli* 055:B LPS, these values are 12 fmol/mL or 180 pg/mL. LPS from the meningococcal mutant strain *pB4* that lacks the oligosaccharide tail ***(131)*** was found to be less potent in the lower concentration ranges but induced more cytokines at concentrations > 1 nmol LPS/mL. As at this range non-CD14 mediated responses are assumed to become more important, our observations suggest a role for the saccharide tail in the binding to CD14 and are in accordance to the recent finding of Gangloff et al., who found that LPSs with a shorter carbohydrate chain induce stronger CD14-independent responses ***(91)***.

Despite the similarities between meningococcal LPS and other types of LPS, meningococcal LPS clearly differs from *E. coli* LPS with respect to the binding by polymyxin B (PMB) and the inhibitory effect of PMB on cytokine induction. PMB binds to *E. coli* LPS ***(102,103)*** and prevents attachment to CD14 by stabilising the LPS-aggregates ***(109)***. This stabilization results in a decrease of the cytokine-inducing potency with 50–100% ***(109,132)***. However, PMB binds only minimally to meningococcal LPS and, although results are somewhat conflicting ***(103,133)***, does not seem to interfere with the binding to LAL. Similarly, PMB has hardly any inhibitory effect on the cytokine-inducing potency of meningococcal LPS ***(123,132)***. The reason for the lack of a detoxifying effect of PMB on meningococcal LPS is currently unknown but it seems plausible to think of the structural differences between meningococcal LPS and *E. coli* LPS. PMB binds principally to the lipid-A part of LPS. In contrast to enterobacteriaceal

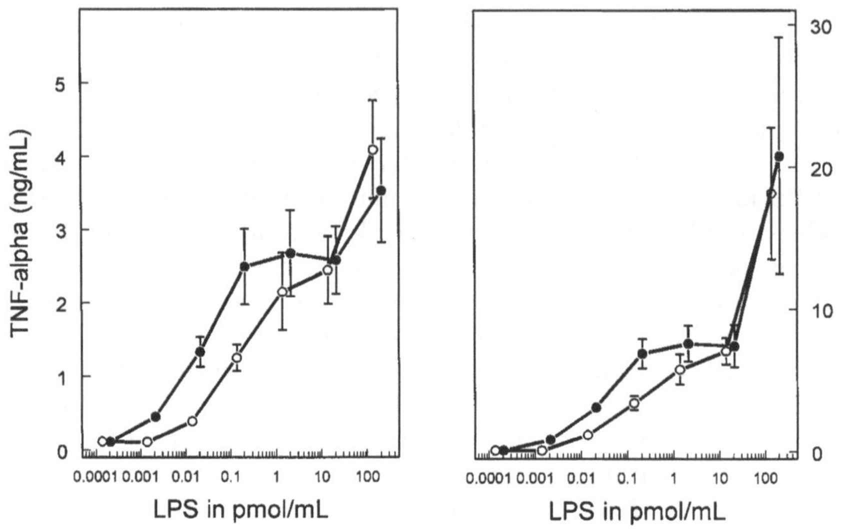

Fig. 3. Comparison of cytokine induction by meningococcal LPS and *E. coli* LPS. Concentrations of tumor necrosis factor α (TNF-α) and interleukin-1β (IL-1β) in the supernatant of human PBMCs stimulated 24 h with different concentrations of *N. meningitidis* serogroup B H44/76 lipo-oligosaccharide (closed dots) or *E. coli* 055:B5 lipopolysaccharide (LPS) (open dots). Meningococcal LPS and the commercially available *E. coli* LPS (L2880, Sigma) were isolated with phenol and water ***(129)***. The molar concentration was estimated based on 2-keto-3-deoxy-octanate (KDO) measurements in a 1 mg/mL LPS solution ***(130)***, and the composition of 2 KDO-molecules in one meningococcal serogroup B LPS molecule and 3 KDO-molecules in one *E. coli* LPS molecule ***(163)***. Data are mean ± SEM of 5 experiments.

lipid-A, meningococcal LPS contains 3-hydoxy lauric acid (3-OH-12:0), whereas the position of the fatty acids also differs ***(134,135)***. In addition, the core region of meningococcal LPS is formed by 2 KDO-molecules, whereas *E. coli* LPS contains 3 KDO-molecules. These or other differences may explain the poor binding of PMB to meningococcal LPS. Whether these structural differences will also influence the binding to LBP and other human LPS-binding proteins that play a role in the handling of LPS during invasive disease needs to be investigated further.

1.2.4. Cytokine Induction by Whole Meningococci

Cytokine induction in vivo during meningococcal infections occurs not after contact with isolated or purified LPS, but after contact with whole meningococci and outer-membrane structures designated as "blebs." The difference between these two types of stimulation is evident. During in vitro stimulation with LPS no IFN-γ is produced. However, after stimulation with whole meningococci, some IFN-γ is produced, which is in accordance with the in vivo observation that this cytokine is increased in serum during meningococcal sepsis and in CSF during meningitis ***(8,66)***.

From experiments with whole Gram-positive bacteria or isolated bacterial products, we know that many non-LPS components are able to elicit cytokine production ***(136)***. Identified potent cytokine inducers are lipopeptides ***(137)***, lipoteichoic acid ***(138)***, capsular polysaccharide ***(139)***, and peptidoglycan ***(140–142)***. Only a few studies assessed the cytokine inducing properties of non-LPS structures of meningococci. In 1992, Boutten et al. used muramyl-dipetide obtained from meningococci to induce cytokines ***(123)***. Recent studies identified IgA_1-proteases, outer-membrane proteins (OMPs) that accelerate the degradation of lysosomal proteins and facilitate the intracellular survival of the bacterium ***(143–145)***, as inducers of pro-inflammatory cytokine synthesis ***(146)***. Studies with whole meningococci show that pili have a synergistic effect on LPS-induced endothelial damage ***(147)*** and that the polysaccharide capsule influences LPS-induced expression of adhesion molecules ***(148,149)***. In these experiments, whole meningococci were more potent stimuli of some adhesion molecules than LPS ***(149)***. Other experiments with whole meningococci and isolated LPS showed that the threshold concentration of LPS that induces tissue factor (TF) on endothelial cells is approx 100 pg/mL, whereas whole meningococci induced TF-expression in a concentration as low as 10^4 CFU/mL ***(150)***.

The cytokine-inducing effect of whole meningococci in comparison to that of isolated LPS became more easily to assess with help of the recently engineered LPS-deficient serogroup B H44/76 mutant strain *pLAK33* by the National Institute of Public Health and the Environment (RIVM) in the Netherlands ***(134,151)***. With this strain, we and others showed that LPS is not the sole cytokine-inducing element of *N. meningitidis* (**151a,151b**). After estimation of the number of LPS molecules per bacterium of the wild-type strain by subtracting the amount of KDO in the LPS-free strain from that in the wild-type strain, a number of approx 150,000 LPS-molecules or 10^{-3} pg LPS per bacterium could be estimated, and the quantitative contribution of non-LPS structures to the cytokine induction could be assessed. It appeared that in concentrations $>2 \times 10^7$ bacteria or >2 ng LPS/mL, whole meningococci were more potent stimuli in vitro than isolated LPS. In addition it was shown meningococci free of LPS induce cytokines including some IFN-γ.

Further studies with these LPS-free meningococci revealed further that serum enhances the non-LPS induced cytokine production, comparable to the effect of serum on LPS-induced CD14 mediated cytokine production (**Fig. 4**). Which

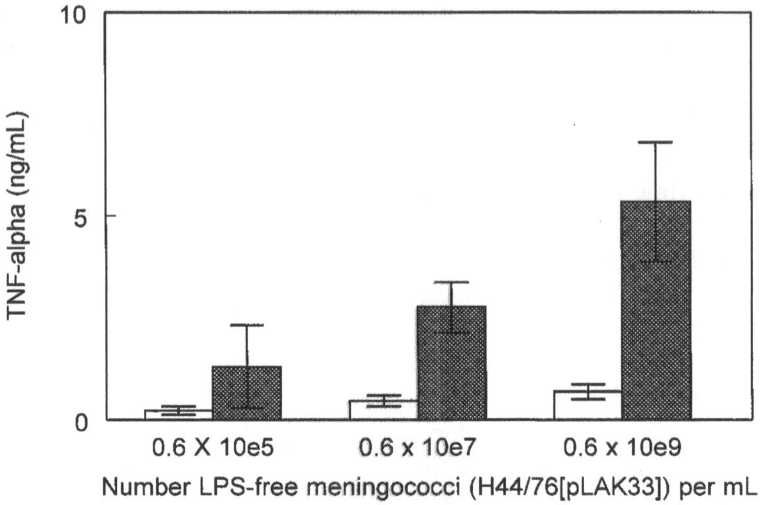

Fig. 4. Stimulatory effect of serum on cytokine induction by LPS-deficient meningococci. Concentrations of tumor necrosis factor α (TNF-α) and interleukin-1β (IL-1β) in the supernatants of human PBMCs stimulated 24 h with three different concentrations of heat-killed serogroup B *N. meningitidis* mutant *H44/76[pLAK33]* that is deficient of LPS. The white bars represent cytokine production in the absence of fresh-pooled serum, the gray bars show the result with 5% serum. Bars are mean values ± SEM, for n = 5 experiments with 0.6×10^5 cfu/mL, n = 9 with 0.6×10^7 cfu/mL and n = 11 with 0.6×10^9 cfu/mL.

particular component of the LPS-free meningococcus induces cytokine production, which serum factors are involved, and which receptors are engaged is currently subject to further study.

1.2.5. The In Vitro Data Summarized

LPS, an outer-membrane constituent of Gram-negative bacteria, is extensively studied for its cytokine-inducing properties. LPS stimulates cytokine production after binding to the CD14 receptor. Various serum peptides, which vary in vivo during different stages of the infection, influence the binding of LPS to CD14. LBP facilitates the binding of LPS to CD14; other peptides like BPI, LF, and the synthetic peptide PMB inhibit the binding to CD14.

The potency of meningococcal LPS in stimulating cytokine production is approximately similar to that of LPS from *E. coli*. However, clear differences exist with respect to the binding and detoxification by PMB. Whether this also reflects differential binding to the human LPS binding peptides warrants further research.

Because several undefined non-LPS structures of *N. meningitidis* are able to induce cytokines, whole meningococci induce more cytokines than isolated

LPS. Also the pattern of cytokines that is induced by whole meningococci is somewhat different. Thus, in spite of the generally accepted concept, invasive meningococcal disease is more than a "prototype endotoxin-induced, cytokine-mediated, Gram-negative infection."

1.3. Tip of the Iceberg

The only natural reservoir of *N. meningitidis* is the human nasal mucosa. Meningococci have found several ways to exploit human structures for their own benefit ***(152)***. The attachment of pili to the CD46 receptor and the class 5 Opa OMP to CD66a are examples of the tight relationship between these prokaryotes and humans ***(153,154)***. Binding of meningococci to human cells transduces a signal to the host ***(155)***. For gonococci, it has been shown that binding leads to activation of the transcription factor NF-κB and induction of a number of proinflammatory cytokines ***(156)***. IgA_1-proteases, that promote survival of meningococci in human cells by degrading some lysosomal constituents and promote trafficking trough epithelial cells ***(143–145,157)***, also induce pro-inflammatory cytokines ***(146)***.

During human evolution cytokines became pivotal elements of the immune system. In that same evolution, humans had intimate contacts with meningococci. The influences of meningococci on cytokines during invasive disease as described in this chapter are only the tip of an iceberg. The recently discovered interactions during binding to mucosal cells and survival in cells indicate that multiple relations will exist between these prokaryotes and the human cytokine network.

2. Materials

2.1. Collection of In Vivo Samples from Patients

1. Samples for plasma endotoxin are drawn in endotoxin-free tubes heparinized with pyrogen-free heparine. The tubes are centrifuged gently (1400*g* for 10 min) to obtain platelet-rich plasma. Aliquots are stored immediately at –70°C until assay. For CSF samples no heparine is required.
2. For circulating cytokines serum or plasma is needed, aprotinin 10,000 kallikrein inactivating U/mL (Bayer, Leverkusen, Germany) may be added to prevent proteolytic cleavage. Plasma samples are centrifuged immediately twice (at 2,250*g* for 10 min and 15,000*g* for 5 min) to eliminate ongoing cytokine production by blood cells or cytokine release from blood cells or platelets. Samples should be stored at –70°C. CSF samples are treated similarly.
3. For the measurement of cytokines bound to blood cells ***(158)***, the cell pellet of ethylene diammete tetracetic acid (EDTA)- or heparine-anticoagulated blood is resuspended in RPMI 1640 medium (Dutch modification, Flows Lab, Irvine, Scotland) and PBMCs are isolated by density-gradient centrifugation on Ficoll-Hypaque (Pharmacia Biotech AB, Uppsala, Sweden). Total cell-associated cytokines are measured after three cycles of freezing and thawing.

4. For the detection of cytokine mRNA in blood cells 0.5 mL EDTA-anticoagulated blood is mixed immediately with an equal amount 4 *M* guanidiumisothiocynate (GITC) freshly enriched with 7 μL mercaptoethanol and stored at –70°C until assay.

3. Methods

1. Endotoxin is measured by a commercially available chromogenic LAL assay (purchased from various companies). Higher concentrations (>10 ng/mL) can be measured chemically by employing gas chromatography and mass spectrophotometry (GC-MS) for the lauric acid part (3-OH-12:0) of lipid-A ***(37)***.
2. Cytokines are assessed by a bio-assays (*see* Chapter 29) or immuno-assays (suppliers including Pharmingen and R&D Systems).
3. Intracellular cytokines are assessed with immunohistochemical techniques or by flow cytometry ***(159,160)***.
4. Cytokine mRNA is assessed by a reverse transcriptase polymerase chain reaction (RT-PCR) ***(161)***.

4. Notes

1. Because the concentration of endotoxin and cytokines during the course of the disease changes rapidly, it is important to note exactly when sampels are taken, i.e., at what point in time with respect to the onset of disease and initiation of therapy.
2. Quantitative comparison between samples is only allowed for similar specimen measured with the same assay and measured in the same run ***(4)***.
3. Cytokine data obtained by immuno-assays do not allow conclusions about the biological activity of cytokines.
4. During meningococcal disease the cytokine network is extensively activated, i.e., various cytokines and their receptors with mutually interfering effects are modulated, produced, and released in different kinetic patterns. Thus the measurement of one selected member of the cytokine network does not allow conclusions about the effect and activity of cytokines during the course of meningococcal disease.

References

1. Beutler, B., Milsark, I. W., and Cerami, A. C. (1985) Passive immunization against cachectin/tumor necrosis factor protects mice from lethal effect of endotoxin. *Science* **229,** 869–871.
2. Waage, A., Halstensen, A., and Espevik, T. (1987) Association between tumour necrosis factor in serum and fatal outcome in patients with meningococcal disease. *Lancet* **i,** 355–357.
3. Van Deuren, M., Dofferhoff, A. S., and van der Meer, J. W. (1992) Cytokines and the response to infection. *J. Pathol.* **168,** 349–356.
4. Engelberts, I., Stephens, S., Francot, G. J., van der Linden, C. J., and Buurman, W. A. (1991) Evidence for different effects of soluble TNF-receptors on various TNF measurements in human biological fluids. *Lancet* **338,** 515–516.
5. Dinarello, C. A. and Cannon, J. G. (1993) Cytokine measurements in septic shock. *Ann. Intern. Med.* **119,** 853–854.

6. Cannon, J. G., Nerad, J. L., Poutsiaka, D. D., and Dinarello, C. A. (1993) Measuring circulating cytokines. *J. Appl. Physiol.* **75,** 1897–1902.
7. Täuber, M. G. and Moser, B. (1999) Cytokines and chemokines in meningeal inflammation: biology and clinical implications. *Clin. Infect. Dis.* **28,** 1–11.
8. Girardin, E., Grau, G. E., Dayer, J.-M., Roux-Lombard, P., The J5 Study Group, and Lambert, P. H. (1988) Tumor necrosis factor and interleukin-1 in the serum of children with severe infectious purpura. *N. Engl. J. Med.* **319,** 397–400.
9. Waage, A., Brandtzaeg, P., Halstensen, A., Kierulf, P., and Espevik, T. (1989) The complex pattern of cytokines in serum from patients with meningococcal septic shock. Association between interleukin 6, interleukin 1, and fatal outcome. *J. Exp. Med.* **169,** 333–338.
10. Brandtzaeg, P., Kierulf, P., Gaustad, P., Skulberg, A., Bruun, J. N., Halvorsen, S., and Sørensen, E. (1989) Plasma endotoxin as a predictor of multiple organ failure and death in systemic meningococcal disease. *J. Infect. Dis.* **159,** 195–204.
11. Brandtzaeg, P., Mollnes, T. E., and Kierulf, P. (1989) Complement activation and endotoxin levels in systemic meningococcal disease. *J. Infect. Dis.* **160,** 58–65.
12. Girardin, E., Roux-Lombard, P., Grau, G. E., Suter, P., Gallati, H., The J5 Study Group, and Dayer, J.-M. (1992) Imbalance between tumour necrosis factor-alpha and soluble TNF receptor concentrations in severe meningococcaemia. *Immunology* **76,** 20–23.
13. Van Deuren, M., van der Ven-Jongekrijg, J., and van der Meer, J. W. M. (1992) Interleukin-8 in acute meningococcal infections; correlation with severity of disease [abstract], in *Proceedings of the The 3rd International Symposium on Chemotactic Cytokines* (Lindley, I. J. D., Westwick, J., and Kunkel, S. L., eds.), Baden, Austria, p. 28.
14. Westendorp, R. G. J., Brand, A., Haanen, J., van Hinsbergh, V. W. M., Thompson, J., van Furth, R., and Meinders, E. A. (1992) Leukaplasmapheresis in meningococcal septic shock. *Am. J. Med.* **92,** 577–578.
15. Halstensen, A., Ceska, M., Brandtzaeg, P., Redl, H., Naess, A., and Waage, A. (1993) Interleukin-8 in serum and cerebrospinal fluid from patients with meningococcal disease. *J. Infect. Dis.* **167,** 471–475.
16. Gårdlund, B., Sjölin, J., Nilsson, A., Roll, M., Wickerts, C.-J., and Wretlind, B. (1995) Plasma levels of cytokines in primary septic shock in humans: correlation with disease severity. *J. Infect. Dis.* **172,** 296–301.
17. Lehmann, A. K., Halstensen, A., Sørnes, S., Røkke, O., and Waage, A. (1995) High levels of interleukin 10 in serum are associated with fatality in meningococcal disease. *Infect. Immun.* **63,** 2109–2112.
18. Van Deuren, M., van der Ven Jongekrijg, J., Bartelink, A. K. M., van Dalen, R., Sauerwein, R. W., and van der Meer, J. W. M. (1995) Correlation between proinflammatory cytokines and antiinflammatory mediators and the severity of disease in meningococcal infections. *J. Infect. Dis.* **172,** 433–439.
19. Kornelisse, R. F., Hazelzet, J. A., Savelkoul, H. F. J., Hop, W. C. J., Suur, M. H., Borsboom, A. N. J., et al. (1996) The relationship between plasminogen activator inhibitor-1 and proinflammatory and counterinflammatory mediators in children with meningococcal septic shock. *J. Infect. Dis.* **173,** 1148–1156.

20. Frieling, J. T. M., van Deuren, M., Wijdenes, J., van Dalen, R., Bartelink, A. K. M., van der Linden, C. J., and Sauerwein, R. W. (1996) Interleukin-6 and its soluble receptor during acute meningococcal infections: effect of plasma or whole blood exchange. *Crit. Care Med.* **24,** 1801–1805.
21. Arranz, E., Blanco-Quiros, A., Solis, P., and Garotte, J. A. (1997) Lack of correlation between soluble CD14 and IL-6 in meningococcal septic shock. *Pediatr. Allergy Immunol.* **8,** 194–199.
22. Westendorp, R. G., Langermans, J. A., Huizinga, T. W., Elouali, A. H., Verweij, C. L., Boomsma, D. I., and Vandenbroucke, J. P. (1997) Genetic influence on cytokine production and fatal meningococcal disease. *Lancet* **349,** 170–173.
23. Waage, A. and Aasen, A. O. (1992) Different role of cytokine mediators in septic shock related to meningococcal disease and surgery/polytrauma. *Immunol. Rev.* **127,** 221–230.
24. Hamilton, G., Hofbauer, S., and Hamilton, B. (1992) Endotoxin, TNF-alpha, interleukin-6 and parameters of the cellular immune system in patients with intraabdominal sepsis. *Scand. J. Infect. Dis.* **24,** 361–368.
25. Rigato, O., Ujvari, S., Castelo, A., and Salomao, R. (1996) Tumor necrosis factor alpha (TNF-alpha) and sepsis: evidence for a role in host defense. *Infection* **24,** 314–318.
26. Riche, F., Panis, Y., Laisne, M. J., Briard, C., Cholley, B., Bernard-Poenaru, O., et al. (1996) High tumor necrosis factor serum level is associated with increased survival in patients with abdominal septic shock: a prospective study in 59 patients. *Surgery* **120,** 801–807.
27. Van Dissel, J. T., van Langevelde, P., Westendorp, R. G., Kwappenberg, K., and Frolich, M. (1998) Anti-inflammatory cytokine profile and mortality in febrile patients. *Lancet* **351**, 950–953.
28. Gogos, C. A., Drosou, E., Bassaris, H. P., and Skoutelis, A. (2000) Pro- versus anti-inflammatory cytokine profile in patients with severe sepsis: a marker for prognosis and future therapeutic options. *J. Infect. Dis.* **181,** 176–180.
29. Echtenacher, B., Falk, W., Mannel, D. N., and Krammer, P. H. (1990) Requirement of endogenous tumor necrosis factor/cachectin for recovery from experimental peritonitis. *J. Immunol.* **145,** 3762–3766.
30. Vaudaux, P., Grau, G. E., Huggler, E., Schumacher-Perdreau, F., Fiedler, F., Waldvogel, F. A., and Lew, D. P. (1992) Contribution of tumor necrosis factor to host defense against staphylococci in a guinea pig model of foreign body infections. *J. Infect. Dis.* **166,** 58–64.
31. McMasters, K. M., Peyton, J. C., Hadjiminas, D. J., and Cheadle, W. G. (1994) Endotoxin and tumour necrosis factor do not cause mortality from caecal ligation and puncture. *Cytokine* **6,** 530–536.
32. Waage, A., Halstensen, A., Shalaby, R., Brandtzaeg, P., Kierulf, P., and Espevik, T. (1989) Local production of tumor necrosis factor alpha, interleukin 1, and interleukin 6 in meningococcal meningitis. Relation to the inflammatory response. *J. Exp. Med.* **170,** 1859–1867.

33. Waage, A., Halstensen, A., Espevik, T., and Brandtzaeg, P. (1993) Compartmentalization of TNF and IL-6 in meningitis and septic shock. *Mediators Inflamm.* **2,** 23–25.
34. Van Deuren, M., van der Ven-Jongekrijg, J., Vannier, E., van Dalen, R., Pesman, G., Bartelink, A. K. M., et al. The pattern of interleukin-1β (IL-1β) and its modulating agents IL-1 receptor antagonist and IL-1 soluble receptor type II in acute meningococcal infections. *Blood* **90,** 1101–1108.
35. Brandtzaeg, P., Halstensen, A., Kierulf, P., Espevik, T., and Waage, A. (1992) Molecular mechanisms in the compartmentalized inflammatory response presenting as meningococcal meningitis or septic shock. *Microb. Pathog.* **13,** 423–431.
36. Brandtzaeg, P., Ovstebo, R., and Kierulf, P. (1995) Bacteremia and compartmentalization of LPS in meningococcal disease. *Prog. Clin. Biol. Res.* **392,** 219–233.
37. Brandtzaeg, P., Bryn, K., Kierulf, P., Øvstebø, R., Namork, E., Aase, B., and Jantzen, E. (1992) Meningococcal endotoxin in lethal septic shock plasma studied by gas chromatography, mass-spectrometry, ultracentrifugation, and electron microscopy. *J. Clin. Invest.* **89,** 816–823.
38. Simberkoff, M. S., Moldover, N. H., and Rahal, J. J., Jr. (1980) Absence of detectable bactericidal and opsonic activities in normal and infected human cerebrospinal fluids. A regional host defense deficiency. *J. Lab. Clin. Med.* **95,** 362–372.
39. Zwahlen, A., Nydegger, U. E., Vaudaux, P., Lambert, P. H., and Waldvogel, F. A. (1982) Complement-mediated opsonic activity in normal and infected human cerebrospinal fluid: early response during bacterial meningitis. *J. Infect. Dis.* **145,** 635–646.
40. Brandtzaeg, P., Øvstebø, R., and Kierulf, P. (1992) Compartmentalization of lipopolysaccharide production correlates with clinical presentation in meningococcal disease. *J. Infect. Dis.* **166,** 650–652.
41. Van Deuren, M., Brandtzaeg, P., and van der Meer, J. W. M. (2000) Update on meningococcal disease with emphasis on pahogenesis and clinical management. *Clin. Micr. Rev.* **13,** 144–166.
42. Bingen, E., Lambert-Zechovsky, N., Mariani-Kurkdjian, P., Doit, C., Aujard, Y., Fournerie, F., and Mathieu, H. (1990) Bacterial counts in cerebrospinal fluid of children with meningitis. *Eur. J. Clin. Microbiol. Infect. Dis.* **9,** 278–281.
43. Mariani-Kurkdjian, P., Doit, C., Le Thomas, I., Aujard, Y., Bourrillon, A., and Bingen, E. (1999) Concentrations bacteriennes dans le liquide céphalo-rachidien au cours des méningites de l'enfant. *Presse Med.* **28,** 1227–1230.
44. Haeffner-Cavaillon, N., Cavaillon, J. M., Laude, M., and Kazatchkine, M. D. (1987) C3a(C3adesArg) induces production and release of interleukin 1 by cultured human monocytes. *J. Immunol.* **139,** 794–799.
45. Okusawa, S., Yancey, K. B., van der Meer, J. W., Endres, S., Lonnemann, G., Hefter, K., et al. (1988) C5a stimulates secretion of tumor necrosis factor from human mononuclear cells in vitro. Comparison with secretion of interleukin 1 beta and interleukin 1 alpha. *J. Exp. Med.* **168,** 443–448.
46. Takabayashi, T., Vannier, E., Clark, B. D., Margolis, N. H., Dinarello, C. A., Burke, J. F., and Gelfand, J. A. (1996) A new biologic role for C3a and C3a desArg: regulation of TNF-alpha and IL-1 beta synthesis. *J. Immunol.* **156,** 3455–3460.

47. Takabayashi, T., Vannier, E., Burke, J. F., Tompkins, R. G., Gelfand, J. A., and Clark, B. D. (1998) Both C3a and C3a(desArg) regulate interleukin-6 synthesis in human peripheral blood mononuclear cells. *J. Infect. Dis.* **177,** 1622–1628.
48. Walzog, B., Weinmann, P., Jeblonski, F., Scharffetter-Kochanek, K., Bommert, K., and Gaehtgens, P. (1999) A role for beta(2) integrins (CD11/CD18) in the regulation of cytokine gene expression of polymorphonuclear neutrophils during the inflammatory response. *FASEB J.* **13,** 1855–1865.
49. Yamaguchi, Y., Matsumura, F., Liang, J., Okabe, K., Ohshiro, H., Ishihara, K., et al. (1999) Neutrophil elastase and oxygen radicals enhance monocyte chemoattractant protein-expression after ischemia/reperfusion in rat liver. *Transplantation* **68,** 1459–1468.
50. Speer, C. P., Rethwilm, M., and Gahr, M. (1987) Elastase-alpha 1-proteinase inhibitor: an early indicator of septicemia and bacterial meningitis in children. *J. Pediatr.* **111,** 667–671.
51. Chan, B., Kalabalikis, P., Klein, N., Heyderman, R., and Levin, M. (1996) Assessment of the effect of candidate anti-inflammatory treatments on the interaction between meningococci and inflammatory cells *in vitro* in a whole blood model. *Biotherapy* **9,** 221–228.
52. Heyderman, R. S., Ison, C. A., Peakman, M., Levin, M., and Klein, N. J. (1999) Neutrophil response to *Neisseria meningitidis*: inhibition of adhesion molecule expression and phagocytosis by recombinant bactericidal/permeability-increasing protein (rBPI21). *J. Infect. Dis.* **179,** 1288–1292.
53. Quagliarello, V. J., Wispelwey, B., Long, W. J., Jr., and Scheld, W. M. (1991) Recombinant human interleukin-1 induces meningitis and blood-brain barrier injury in the rat. Characterization and comparison with tumor necrosis factor. *J. Clin. Invest.* **87,** 1360–1366.
54. Ramilo, O., Sáez-Llorens, X., Mertsola, J., Jafari, H., Olsen, K. D., Hansen, E. J., et al. (1990) Tumor necrosis factor α/cachectin and interleukin 1β initiate meningeal inflammation. *J. Exp. Med.* **172,** 497–507.
55. Derkx, B., Marchant, A., Goldman, M., Bijlmer, R., and van Deventer, S. (1995) High levels of interleukin-10 during the initial phase of fulminant meningococcal septic shock. *J. Infect. Dis.* **171,** 229–232.
56. Van Deuren, M., van der Ven-Jongekrijg, J., Demacker, P. N. M., Bartelink, A. K. M., van Dalen, R., Sauerwein, R. W., et al. (1994) Differential expression of proinflammatory cytokines and their inhibitors during the course of meningococcal infections. *J. Infect. Dis.* **169,** 157–161.
57. Van Deuren, M., Frieling, J. T. M., van der Ven-Jongekrijg, J., Neeleman, C., Russel, F. G. M., van Lier, H. J. J., et al. (1998) Plasma patterns of tumor necrosis factor-α (TNF) and TNF soluble receptors during acute meningococcal infections and the effect of plasma exchange. *Clin. Infect. Dis.* **26,** 918–923.
58. Bygbjerg, I. C., Hansen, M. B., Ronn, A. M., Bendtzen, K., and Jakobsen, P. H. (1997) Decreased plasma levels of factor II + VII + X correlate with increased levels of soluble cytokine receptors in patients with malaria and meningococcal infections. *APMIS* **105,** 150–156.

59. Van Deuren, M. and van der Meer, J. W. (1997) Extracorporal techniques to accelerate the clearance of TNF-α and IL-1β in septic patients, in *Yearbook of Intensive Care and Emergency Medicine* (Vincent, J. L., ed.), Springer-Verlag KG, Berlin, Germany, pp. 140–147.
60. Van Deuren, M. (1998) Acute meningococcal disease. A study of clinical management, cytokine activation and regulation. PhD thesis, University of Nijmegen, The Netherlands.
61. Kornelisse, R. F., Hoekman, K., Visser, J. J., Hop, W. C. J., Huijmans, J. G. M., van der Straaten, P. J. C., et al. (1996) The role of nitric oxide in bacterial meningitis in children. *J. Infect Dis.* **174,** 120–126.
62. Mustafa, M. M., Lebel, M. H., Ramilo, O., Olsen, K. D., Reisch, J. S., Beutler, B., and McCracken, G. H., Jr. (1989) Correlation of interleukin-1 beta and cachectin concentrations in cerebrospinal fluid and outcome from bacterial meningitis. *J. Pediatr.* **115,** 208–213.
63. Rusconi, F., Parizzi, F., Garlaschi, L., Assael, B. M., Sironi, M., Ghezzi, P., and Mantovani, A. (1991) Interleukin 6 activity in infants and children with bacterial meningitis. The Collaborative Study on Meningitis. *Pediatr. Infect. Dis. J.* **10,** 117–121.
64. Arditi, M., Manogue, K. R., Caplan, M., and Yogev, R. (1990) Cerebrospinal fluid cachectin/tumor necrosis factor-α and platelet-activating factor concentrations and severity of bacterial meningitis in children. *J. Infect. Dis.* **162,** 139–147.
65. Roine, I., Foncea, L. M., Ledermann, W., and Peltola, H. (1995) Slow recovery of cerebrospinal fluid glucose and protein concentrations distinguish pneumococcal from *Haemophilus influenzae* and meningococcal meningitis in children. *Pediatr. Infect. Dis. J.* **14,** 905–907.
66. Kornelisse, R. F., Hack, C. E., Savelkoul, H. F., van der Pouw Kraan, T. C., Hop, W. C., van Mierlo, G., et al. (1997) Intrathecal production of interleukin-12 and gamma interferon in patients with bacterial meningitis. *Infect. Immun.* **65,** 877–881.
67. Diab, A., Zhu, J., Lindquist, L., Wretlind, B., Bakhiet, M., and Link, H. (1997) *Haemophilus influenzae* and *Streptococcus pneumoniae* induce different intracerebral mRNA cytokine patterns during the course of experimental bacterial meningitis. *Clin. Exp. Immunol.* **109,** 233–241.
68. Nadel, S., Newport, M. J., Booy, R., and Levin, M. (1996) Variation in the tumor necrosis factor-α gene promoter region may be associated with death from meningococcal disease. *J. Infect. Dis.* **174,** 878–880.
69. McGuire, W., Hill, A. V., Allsopp, C. E., Greenwood, B. M., and Kwiatkowski, D. (1994) Variation in the TNF-alpha promoter region associated with susceptibility to cerebral malaria. *Nature* **371,** 508–510.
70. Stuber, F., Petersen, M., Bokelmann, F., and Schade, U. (1996) A genomic polymorphism within the tumor necrosis factor locus influences plasma tumor necrosis factor-alpha concentrations and outcome of patients with severe sepsis. *Crit. Care Med.* **24,** 381–384.
71. Westendorp, R. G. J., Langermans, J. A. M., de Bel, C. E., Meinders, A. E., Vandenbroucke, J. P., van Furth, R., and van Dissel, J. T. (1995) Release of tumor necrosis factor: an innate host characteristic that may contribute to the outcome of meningococcal disease. *J. Infect. Dis.* **171,** 1057–1060.

72. Bruin, K. F. (1994) Endotoxin responsiveness in humans. PhD thesis, University of Amsterdam.
73. Van Deuren, M., Netea, M. G., Hijmans, A., Demacker, P. N. M., Neeleman, C., Sauerwein, R. W., et al. (1998) Posttranscriptional down-regulation of tumor necrosis factor-α and interleukin-1β production in acute meningococcal infections. *J. Infect. Dis.* **177,** 1401–1405.
74. Brandtzaeg, P., Osnes, L., øvstebo, R., Joø, G. B., Westvik, Å.-B., and Kierulf, P. (1996) Net inflammatory capacity of human septic shock plasma evaluated by a monocyte-based target cell assay: identification of interleukin-10 as a major functional deactivator of human monocytes. *J. Exp. Med.* **184,** 51–60.
75. Marie, C., Fitting, C., Muret, J., Payen, D., and Cavaillon, J. M. (2000) Interleukin 8 production in whole blood assays: Is interleukin 10 responsible for the downregulation observed in sepsis? *Cytokine* **12,** 55–61.
76. Ayala, A., Meldrum, D. R., Perrin, M. M., and Chaudry, I. H. (1993) The release of transforming growth factor-beta following haemorrhage: its role as a mediator of host immunosuppression. *Immunology* **79,** 479–484.
77. Ayala, A., Knotts, J. B., Ertel, W., Perrin, M. M., Morrison, M. H., and Chaudry, I. H. (1993) Role of interleukin 6 and transforming growth factor-beta in the induction of depressed splenocyte responses following sepsis. *Arch. Surg.* **128,** 89–94.
78. Randow, F., Syrbe, U., Meisel, C., Krausch, D., Zuckermann, H., Platzer, C., and Volk, H. D. (1995) Mechanism of endotoxin desensitization: involvement of interleukin 10 and transforming growth factor beta. *J. Exp. Med.* **181,** 1887–1892.
79. Granowitz, E. V., Porat, R., Mier, J. W., Orencole, S. F., Kaplanski, G., Lynch, E. A., et al. (1993) Intravenous endotoxin suppresses the cytokine response of peripheral blood mononuclear cells of healthy humans. *J. Immunol.* **151,** 1637–1645.
80. Ertel, W., Kremer, J. P., Kenney, J., Steckholzer, U., Jarrar, D., Trentz, O., and Schildberg, F. W. (1995) Downregulation of proinflammatory cytokine release in whole blood from septic patients. *Blood* **85,** 1341–1347.
81. Van Deuren, M., Twickler, T. B., de Waal Malefyt, M. C., Van Beem, H., van der Ven-Jongekrijg, J., Verschueren, C. M. M., and van der Meer, J. W. M. (1998) Elective orthopedic surgery, a model for the study of cytokine activation and regulation. *Cytokine* **10,** 897–903.
82. Frankenberger, M., Pechumer, H., and Ziegler-Heitbrock, H. W. (1995) Interleukin-10 is upregulated in LPS tolerance. *J. Inflamm.* **45,** 56–63.
83. Döcke, W. D., Randow, F., Syrbe, U., Krausch, D., Asadullah, K., Reinke, P., et al. (1997) Monocyte deactivation in septic patients: restoration by IFN-gamma treatment. *Nature Med.* **3,** 678–681.
84. Williams, M. A., Withington, S., Newland, A. C., and Kelsey, S. M. (1998) Monocyte anergy in septic shock is associated with a predilection to apoptosis and is reversed by granulocyte-macrophage colony-stimulating factor ex vivo. *J. Infect. Dis.* **178,** 1421–1433.
85. Munoz, C., Carlet, J., Fitting, C., Misset, B., Bleriot, J. P., and Cavaillon, J. M. (1991) Dysregulation of in vitro cytokine production by monocytes during sepsis. *J. Clin. Invest.* **88,** 1747–1754.

86. Luderitz, O., Tanamoto, K., Galanos, C., McKenzie, G. R., Brade, H., Zahringer, U., et al. (1984) Lipopolysaccharides: structural principles and biologic activities. *Rev. Infect. Dis.* **6,** 428–431.
87. Antal-Szalmás, P. (2000) Evaluation of CD14 in host defence. *Eur. J. Clin. Invest.* **30,** 167–179.
88. Tobias, P. S., Tapping, R. I., and Gegner, J. A. (1999) Endotoxin interactions with lipopolysaccharide-responsive cells. *Clin. Infect. Dis.* **28,** 476–481.
89. Cavaillon, J. M., Fitting, C., Caroff, M., and Haeffner-Cavaillon, N. (1989) Dissociation of cell-associated interleukin-1 (IL-1) and IL-1 release induced by lipopolysaccharide and lipid A. *Infect. Immun.* **57,** 791–797.
90. Otterlei, M., Sundan, A., Skjak-Braek, G., Ryan, L., Smidsrod, O., and Espevik, T. (1993) Similar mechanisms of action of defined polysaccharides and lipopolysaccharides: characterization of binding and tumor necrosis factor alpha induction. *Infect. Immun.* **61,** 1917–1925.
91. Gangloff, S. C., Hijiya, N., Haziot, A., and Goyert, S. M. (1999) Lipopolysaccharide structure influences the macrophage response via CD14-independent and CD14-dependent pathways. *Clin. Infect. Dis.* **28,** 491–496.
92. Arditi, M., Zhou, J., Dorio, R., Rong, G. W., Goyert, S. M., and Kim, K. S. (1993) Endotoxin-mediated endothelial cell injury and activation: role of soluble CD14. *Infect. Immun.* **61,** 3149–3156.
93. Loppnow, H., Stelter, F., Schonbeck, U., Schluter, C., Ernst, M., Schutt, C., and Flad, H. D. (1995) Endotoxin activates human vascular smooth muscle cells despite lack of expression of CD14 mRNA or endogenous membrane CD14. *Infect. Immun.* **63,** 1020–1026.
94. Landmann, R., Reber, A. M., Sansano, S., and Zimmerli, W. (1996) Function of soluble CD14 in serum from patients with septic shock. *J. Infect. Dis.* **173,** 661–668.
95. Landmann, R., Zimmerli, W., Sansano, S., Link, S., Hahn, A., Glauser, M. P., and Calandra, T. (1995) Increased circulating soluble CD14 is associated with high mortality in gram-negative septic shock. *J. Infect. Dis.* **171,** 639–644.
96. Ulevitch, R. J. and Tobias, P. S. (1995) Receptor-dependent mechanisms of cell stimulation by bacterial endotoxin. *Ann. Rev. Immunol.* **13,** 437–457.
97. Kirschning, C. J., Wesche, H., Merrill Ayres, T., and Rothe, M. (1998) Human toll-like receptor 2 confers responsiveness to bacterial lipopolysaccharide. *J. Exp. Med.* **188,** 2091–2097.
98. Modlin, R. L., Brightbill, H. D., and Godowski, P. J. (1999) The toll of innate immunity on microbial pathogens. *N. Engl. J. Med.* **340,** 1834–1835.
99. Tohme, Z. N., Amar, S., and Van Dyke, T. E. (1999) Moesin functions as a lipopolysaccharide receptor on human monocytes. *Infect. Immun.* **67,** 3215–3220.
100. Tobias, P. S., Soldau, K., Gegner, J. A., Mintz, D., and Ulevitch, R. J. (1995) Lipopolysaccharide binding protein-mediated complexation of lipopolysaccharide with soluble CD14. *J. Biol. Chem.* **270,** 10,482–10,488.
101. De Haas, C. J., Van der Zee, R., Benaissa-Trouw, B., Van Kessel, K. P., Verhoef, J., and Van Strijp, J. A. (1999) Lipopolysaccharide (LPS)-binding synthetic pep-

tides derived from serum amyloid P component neutralize LPS. *Infect. Immun.* **67,** 2790–2796.

102. Morrison, D. C. and Jacobs, D. M. (1976) Binding of polymyxin B to the lipid A portion of bacterial lipopolysaccharides. *Immunochemistry* **13,** 813–818.
103. Rustici, A., Velucchi, M., Faggioni, R., Sironi, M., Ghezzi, P., Quataert, S., Green, B., and Porro, M. (1993) Molecular mapping and detoxification of the lipid A binding site by synthetic peptides. *Science* **259,** 361–365.
104. Appelmelk, B. J., An, Y. Q., Geerts, M., Thijs, B. G., de Boer, H. A., MacLaren, D. M., et al. (1994) Lactoferrin is a lipid A-binding protein. *Infect. Immun.* **62,** 2628–2632.
105. Weiss, J., Elsbach, P., Shu, C., Castillo, J., Grinna, L., Horwitz, A., and Theofan, G. (1992) Human bactericidal/permeability-increasing protein and a recombinant NH2-terminal fragment cause killing of serum-resistant gram-negative bacteria in whole blood and inhibit tumor necrosis factor release induced by the bacteria. *J. Clin. Invest.* **90,** 1122–1130.
106. Heinzelmann, M., Polk, H. C., Jr., and Miller, F. N. (1998) Modulation of lipopolysaccharide-induced monocyte activation by heparin-binding protein and fucoidan. *Infect. Immun.* **66,** 5842–5847.
107. Porro, M. (1994) Structural basis of endotoxin recognition by natural polypeptides. *Trends Microbiol.* **2,** 65–66.
108. Cavaillon, J. M., Fitting, C., Haeffner Cavaillon, N., Kirsch, S. J., and Warren, H. S. (1990) Cytokine response by monocytes and macrophages to free and lipoprotein-bound lipopolysaccharide. *Infect. Immun.* **58,** 2375–2382.
109. Iwagaki, A., Porro, M., and Pollack, M. (2000) Influence of synthetic antiendotoxin peptides on lipopolysaccharide (LPS) recognition and LPS-induced proinflammatory cytokine responses by cells expressing membrane-bound CD14. *Infect. Immun.* **68,** 1655–1663.
110. Hailman, E., Lichenstein, H. S., Wurfel, M. M., Miller, D. S., Johnson, D. A., Kelley, M., et al. (1994) Lipopolysaccharide (LPS)-binding protein accelerates the binding of LPS to CD14. *J. Exp. Med.* **179,** 269–277.
111. Schumann, R. R., Leong, S. R., Flaggs, G. W., Gray, P. W., Wright, S. D., Mathison, J. C., et al. (1990) Structure and function of lipopolysaccharide binding protein. *Science* **249,** 1429–1431.
112. Opal, S. M., Palardy, J. E., Marra, M. N., Fisher, C. J., Jr., McKelligon, B. M., and Scott, R. W. (1994) Relative concentrations of endotoxin-binding proteins in body fluids during infection. *Lancet* **344,** 429–431.
113. Froon, A. H., Dentener, M. A., Greve, J. W., Ramsay, G., and Buurman, W. A. (1995) Lipopolysaccharide toxicity-regulating proteins in bacteremia. *J. Infect. Dis.* **171,** 1250–1257.
114. Opal, S. M., Scannon, P. J., Vincent, J. L., White, M., Carroll, S. F., Palardy, J. E., et al. (1999) Relationship between plasma levels of lipopolysaccharide (LPS) and LPS-binding protein in patients with severe sepsis and septic shock. *J. Infect. Dis.* **180,** 1584–1589.

115. Henter, J. I., Carlson, L. A., Hansson, M., Nilsson-Ehle, P., and Ortqvist, E. (1993) Lipoprotein alterations in children with bacterial meningitis. *Acta Paediatr.* **82,** 694–698.
116. Keuter, M., Dharmana, E., Gasem, M. H., van der Ven Jongekrijg, J., Djokomoeljanto, R., Dolmans, W. M., et al. (1994) Patterns of proinflammatory cytokines and inhibitors during typhoid fever. *J. Infect. Dis.* **169,** 1306–1311.
117. Haeffner-Cavaillon, N., Cavaillon, J. M., Etievant, M., Lebbar, S., and Szabo, L. (1985) Specific binding of endotoxin to human monocytes and mouse macrophages: serum requirement. *Cell. Immunol.* **91,** 119–131.
118. Lebbar, S., Cavaillon, J. M., Caroff, M., Ledur, A., Brade, H., Sarfati, R., and Haeffner-Cavaillon, N. (1986) Molecular requirement for interleukin 1 induction by lipopolysaccharide-stimulated human monocytes: involvement of the heptosyl-2-keto-3-deoxyoctulosonate region. *Eur. J. Immunol.* **16,** 87–91.
119. Haeffner-Cavaillon, N. and Cavaillon, J. M. (1987) Involvement of the LPS receptor in the induction of interleukin-1 in human monocytes stimulated with endotoxins. *Ann. Inst. Pasteur Immunol.* **138,** 473–477.
120. Haeffner-Cavaillon, N., Caroff, M., and Cavaillon, J. M. (1989) Interleukin-1 induction by lipopolysaccharides: structural requirements of the 3-deoxy-D-manno-2-octulosonic acid (KDO). *Mol. Immunol.* **26,** 485–494.
121. Laude-Sharp, M., Haeffner-Cavaillon, N., Caroff, M., Lantreibecq, F., Pusineri, C., and Kazatchkine, M. D. (1990) Dissociation between the interleukin 1-inducing capacity and Limulus reactivity of lipopolysaccharides from gram-negative bacteria. *Cytokine* **2,** 253–258.
122. Couturier, C., Haeffner-Cavaillon, N., Caroff, M., and Kazatchkine, M. D. (1991) Binding sites for endotoxins (lipopolysaccharides) on human monocytes. *J. Immunol.* **147,** 1899–1904.
123. Boutten, A., Dehoux, M., Deschenes, M., Rouzeau, J. D., Bories, P. N., and Durand, G. (1992) Alpha 1-acid glycoprotein potentiates lipopolysaccharide-induced secretion of interleukin-1 beta, interleukin-6 and tumor necrosis factor-alpha by human monocytes and alveolar and peritoneal macrophages. *Eur. J. Immunol.* **22,** 2687–2695.
124. Muller-Alouf, H., Alouf, J. E., Gerlach, D., Ozegowski, J. H., Fitting, C., and Cavaillon, J. M. (1994) Comparative study of cytokine release by human peripheral blood mononuclear cells stimulated with *Streptococcus pyogenes* superantigenic erythrogenic toxins, heat-killed streptococci, and lipopolysaccharide. *Infect. Immun.* **62,** 4915–4921.
125. Blondiau, C., Lagadec, P., Lejeune, P., Onier, N., Cavaillon, J. M., and Jeannin, J. F. (1994) Correlation between the capacity to activate macrophages in vitro and the antitumor activity in vivo of lipopolysaccharides from different bacterial species. *Immunobiology* **190,** 243–254.
126. Blondin, C., Le Dur, A., Cholley, B., Caroff, M., and Haeffner-Cavaillon, N. (1997) Lipopolysaccharide complexed with soluble CD14 binds to normal human monocytes. *Eur. J. Immunol.* **27,** 3303–3309.

127. Prins, J. M., Lauw, F. N., Derkx, B. H. F., Speelman, P., Kuijper, E. J., Dankert, J., and van Deventer, S. J. H. (1998) Endotoxin release and cytokine production in acute and chronic meningococcaemia. *Clin. Exp. Immunol.* **114,** 215–219.
128. Luchi, M. and Morrison, D. C. (2000) Comparable endotoxic properties of lipopolysaccharides are manifest in diverse clinical isolates of gram-negative bacteria. *Infect. Immun.* **68,** 1899–1904.
129. Westphal, O. and Jann, J. K. (1965) Bacterial lipopolysacharide extraction with phenol- water and further application of the procedure. *Methods Carbohydr. Chem.* **5,** 83–91.
130. Weissbach, A. and Hurwitz, B. (1959) The formation of 2-keto-3-deoxyheptonic acid in extracts of *Escherichia coli* B. *J. Biol. Chem.* **234,** 705–709.
131. Van der Ley, P., Kramer, M., Martin, A., Richards, J. C., and Poolman, J. T. (1997) Analysis of the icsBA locus required for biosynthesis of the inner core region from *Neisseria meningitidis* lipopolysaccharide. *FEMS Microbiol. Lett.* **146,** 247–253.
132. Cavaillon, J. M., and Haeffner-Cavaillon, N. (1986) Polymyxin-B inhibition of LPS-induced interleukin-1 secretion by human monocytes is dependent upon the LPS origin. *Mol. Immunol.* **23,** 965–969.
133. Baldwin, G., Alpert, G., Caputo, G. L., Baskin, M., Parsonnet, J., Gillis, Z. A., et al. (1991) Effect of polymyxin B on experimental shock from meningococcal and *Escherichia coli* endotoxins. *J. Infect. Dis.* **164,** 542–549.
134. Steeghs, L., Jennings, M. P., Poolman, J. T., and van der Ley, P. (1997) Isolation and characterization of the *Neisseria meningitidis* lpxD-fabZ-lpxA gene cluster involved in lipid A biosynthesis. *Gene* **190,** 263–270.
135. Odegaard, T. J., Kaltashov, I. A., Cotter, R. J., Steeghs, L., van der Ley, P., Khan, S., et al. (1997) Shortened hydroxyacyl chains on lipid A of *Escherichia coli* cells expressing a foreign UDP-N-acetylglucosamine O-acyltransferase. *J. Biol. Chem.* **272,** 19,688–19,696.
136. Henderson, B., Poole, S., and Wilson, M. (1996) Bacterial modulins: a novel class of virulence factors which cause host tissue pathology by inducing cytokine synthesis. *Microbiol. Rev.* **60,** 316–341.
137. Kreutz, M., Ackermann, U., Hauschildt, S., Krause, S. W., Riedel, D., Bessler, W., and Andreesen, R. (1997) A comparative analysis of cytokine production and tolerance induction by bacterial lipopeptides, lipopolysaccharides and *Staphylococcus aureus* in human monocytes. *Immunology* **92,** 396–401.
138. Bhakdi, S., Klonisch, T., Nuber, P., and Fischer, W. (1991) Stimulation of monokine production by lipoteichoic acids. *Infect. Immun.* **59,** 4614–4620.
139. Soell, M., Diab, M., Haan-Archipoff, G., Beretz, A., Herbelin, C., Poutrel, B., and Klein, J. P. (1995) Capsular polysaccharide types 5 and 8 of *Staphylococcus aureus* bind specifically to human epithelial (KB) cells, endothelial cells, and monocytes and induce release of cytokines. *Infect. Immun.* **63,** 1380–1386.
140. Schrijver, I. A., Melief, M. J., Eulderink, F., Hazenberg, M. P., and Laman, J. D. (1999) Bacterial peptidoglycan polysaccharides in sterile human spleen induce proinflammatory cytokine production by human blood cells. *J. Infect. Dis.* **179,** 1459–1468.

141. Kengatharan, K. M., De Kimpe, S., Robson, C., Foster, S. J., and Thiemermann, C. (1998) Mechanism of gram-positive shock: identification of peptidoglycan and lipoteichoic acid moieties essential in the induction of nitric oxide synthase, shock, and multiple organ failure. *J. Exp. Med.* **188,** 305–315.
142. Mattsson, E., Rollof, J., Verhoef, J., Van Dijk, H., and Fleer, A. (1994) Serum-induced potentiation of tumor necrosis factor alpha production by human monocytes in response to staphylococcal peptidoglycan: involvement of different serum factors. *Infect. Immun.* **62,** 3837–3843.
143. Ayala, P., Lin, L., Hopper, S., Fukuda, M., and So, M. (1998) Infection of epithelial cells by pathogenic neisseriae reduces the levels of multiple lysosomal constituents. *Infect. Immun.* **66,** 5001–5007.
144. Lin, L., Ayala, P., Larson, J., Mulks, M., Fukuda, M., Carlsson, S. R., Enns, C., and So, M. (1997) The Neisseria type 2 IgA1 protease cleaves LAMP1 and promotes survival of bacteria within epithelial cells. *Mol. Microbiol.* **24,** 1083–1094.
145. Vitovski, S., Read, R. C., and Sayers, J. R. (1999) Invasive isolates of *Neisseria meningitidis* possess enhanced immunoglobulin A1 protease activity compared to colonizing strains. *FASEB J.* **13,** 331–337.
146. Lorenzen, D. R., Dux, F., Wolk, U., Tsirpouchtsidis, A., Haas, G., and Meyer, T. F. (1999) Immunoglobulin A1 protease, an exoenzyme of pathogenic Neisseriae, is a potent inducer of proinflammatory cytokines. *J. Exp. Med.* **190,** 1049–1058.
147. Dunn, K. L., Virji, M., and Moxon, E. R. (1995) Investigations into the molecular basis of meningococcal toxicity for human endothelial and epithelial cells: the synergistic effect of LPS and pili. *Microb. Pathog.* **18,** 81–96.
148. Klein, N. J., Ison, C. A., Peakman, M., Levin, M., Hammerschmidt, S., Frosch, M., and Heyderman, R. S. (1996) The influence of capsulation and lipooligosaccharide structure on neutrophil adhesion molecule expression and endothelial injury by *Neisseria meningitidis. J. Infect. Dis.* **173,** 172–179.
149. Dixon, G. L., Heyderman, R. S., Kotovicz, K., Jack, D. L., Andersen, S. R., Vogel, U., et al. (1999) Endothelial adhesion molecule expression and its inhibition by recombinant bactericidal/permeability-increasing protein are influenced by the capsulation and lipooligosaccharide structure of *Neisseria meningitidis. Infect. Immun.* **67,** 5626–5633.
150. Heyderman, R. S., Klein, N. J., Shennan, G. I., and Levin, M. (1991) Deficiency of prostacyclin production in meningococcal shock. *Arch. Dis. Child.* **66,** 1296–1299.
151. Steeghs, L., den Hartog, R., den Boer, A., Zomer, B., Roholl, P., and van der Ley, P. (1998) Meningitis bacterium is viable without endotoxin. *Nature* **392,** 449–450.
151a. Uronen, H., Williams, A. J., Dixon, G., Anderson, S. R., van der Ley, P., van Deuren, et al. (2000) Gram-negative bacteria induce pro-inflammatory cytokine production by monocytes in the absence of lipopolysaccharide (LPS). *Clinical Exp. Immunol.* **122,** 312–315.
151b. Sprong, T., Stikkelbroeck, N., van der Ley, P., Steeghs, L., van Alphen, L., Klein, N., et al. (2001) Cytokine induction by *N. meningitidis* LPS and non-LPS. *J. Leukocyte Biol.*, in press.

152. Meyer, T. F. (1999) Pathogenic neisseriae: complexity of pathogen-host cell interplay. *Clin. Infect. Dis.* **28,** 433–441.
153. Kallstrom, H., Liszewski, M. K., Atkinson, J. P., and Jonsson, A. B. (1997) Membrane cofactor protein (MCP or CD46) is a cellular pilus receptor for pathogenic Neisseria. *Mol. Microbiol.* **25,** 639–647.
154. Virji, M., Watt, S. M., Barker, S., Makepeace, and K., Doyonnas, R. (1996) The N-domain of the human CD66a adhesion molecule is a target for Opa proteins of *Neisseria meningitidis* and *Neisseria gonorrhoeae*. *Mol. Microbiol.* **22,** 929–939.
155. Kallstrom, H., Islam, M. S., Berggren, P. O., and Jonsson, A. B. (1998) Cell signaling by the type IV pili of pathogenic Neisseria. *J. Biol. Chem.* **273,** 21,777–21,782.
156. Naumann, M., Wessler, S., Bartsch, C., Wieland, B., and Meyer, T. F. (1997) *Neisseria gonorrhoeae* epithelial cell interaction leads to the activation of the transcription factors nuclear factor kappaB and activator protein 1 and the induction of inflammatory cytokines. *J. Exp. Med.* **186,** 247–258.
157. Hopper, S., Vasquez, B., Merz, A., Clary, S., Wilbur, J. S., and So, M. (2000) Effects of the immunoglobulin A1 protease on *Neisseria gonorrhoeae* trafficking across polarized T84 epithelial monolayers. *Infect. Immun.* **68,** 906–911.
158. Munoz, C., Misset, B., Fitting, C., Bleriot, J. P., Carlet, J., and Cavaillon, J. M. (1991) Dissociation between plasma and monocyte-associated cytokines during sepsis. *Eur. J. Immunol.* **21,** 2177–2184.
159. Björk, L., Fehniger, T. E., Andersson, U., Andersson, J. (1996) Computerized assessment of production of multiple human cytokines at the single-cell level using image analysis. *J. Leukoc. Biol.* **59,** 287–295.
160. Tayebi, H., Lienard, A., Billot, M., Tiberghien, P., Herve, P., and Robinet, E. (1999) Detection of intracellular cytokines in citrated whole blood or marrow samples by flow cytometry. *J. Immunol. Methods* **229,** 121–130.
161. Netea, M. G., Drenth, J. P., De Bont, N., Hijmans, A., Keuter, M., Dharmana, E., et al. (1996) A semi-quantitative reverse transcriptase polymerase chain reaction method for measurement of MRNA for TNF-alpha and IL-1 beta in whole blood cultures: its application in typhoid fever and exentric exercise. *Cytokine* **8,** 739–744.
162. Van Deuren, M., Santman, F. W., van Dalen, R., Sauerwein, R. W., Span, L. F., and van der Meer, J. W. (1992) Plasma and whole blood exchange in meningococcal sepsis. *Clin. Infect. Dis.* **15,** 424–430.
163. Pavliak, V., Brisson, J. R., Michon, F., Uhrin, D., Jennings, H. J. (1993) Structure of the sialylated L3 lipopolysaccharide of *Neisseria meningitidis*. *J. Biol. Chem.* **268,** 14,146–14,152.

29

Cytokine Bioassays

Nina-Beate Liabakk, Anders Waage, Egil Lien, Jørgen Stenvik, and Terje Espevik

1. Introduction

Cytokines are important mediators in inflammation, and play a key role in inflammation induced by Gram-negative bacteria. Cytokines are released into serum during different pathological conditions, such as meningococcal disease, and the cytokine levels in serum seem to correlate with fatal outcome of septic shock *(1–3)*. Consequently, detection of cytokines in serum samples from patients with pathological diseases may be of prognostic and clinical value. Cytokines can be detected using bioassays and immunoassays, and this chapter focuses on description of bioassays for detection of tumor necrosis factor-α (TNF-α), interleukin-1 (IL-1), and IL-6 in serum samples.

Cytokine bioassays are based on specific biological activities of cytokines on various cell lines, such as proliferation *(4,5)*, induction of surface molecules, secretion of other cytokines *(6)*, inhibition of cytokine secretion and activity, and cytotoxicity *(7,8)*. The TNF bioassay is a cytotoxic bioassay and the TNF bioactivity is determined by its cytotoxic effect on the murine fibrosarcoma cell line WEHI 164 clone 13 *(8)*. The principle behind the cytotoxic TNF bioassay involves binding of TNF to membrane-bound cell surface TNF receptors, which results in killing of the TNF-sensitive cell line. The IL-1 bioassay uses two T-cell lines, the EL-4-NOB-1 *(6)* and HT-2 *(4)*, and is based on both secretion of other cytokines and proliferation. IL-1 stimulation of the EL-4-NOB-1 cell line results in secretion of IL-2 and IL-2 has growth-stimulatory effect on the the HT-2 cells. The IL-6 bioassay uses the IL-6 dependent B-cell line B13.29 clone B9 *(5)* and is also classified as a proliferation bioassay.

From: *Methods in Molecular Medicine, vol. 67: Meningococcal Disease: Methods and Protocols*
Edited by: A. J. Pollard and M. C. J. Maiden © Humana Press Inc., Totowa, NJ

Furthermore, the cytokines are measured by a colorimetric method for growth and survival by use of a tetrazolium salt (MTT) as described by Mosmann *(9)*. The salt binds to mitochondrial dehydrogenase enzymes, which catalyzes the formation of blue-colored formazan crystals in metabolizing cells. Subsequently, these crystals can be dissolved in detergents and the color of the resulting solution measured automatically using a microtiter plate reader. The absorbance at 570 nm correlates with the number of living cells and with the cytokine concentration in the samples.

The other strategy to quantiate cytokines are immunoassays. The choice of assay type may be difficult, because each type has its own particular quality. In contrast to bioassays, immunoassays measure immunoactive cytokines, which include both degraded cytokines and neutralized cytokines, i.e., cytokines in complexes with cytokine receptors. **Figure 1** illustrates detection of TNF-α in supernatants from monocytes stimulated with Lipid A, which is a part of the endotoxin lipopolysaccharide (LPS), in the cytotoxic TNF bioassay and in an immunoassay. Analysis of the supernatants with the TNF bioassay and immunoassay demonstrates a bell shaped TNF production curve peaking at 8 h *(10)*. After this peak, the bioactivity of TNF is lost faster than the immunoactivity. Further on, in sera from sepsis patients, Stenvik et al. *(10)* found moderate to high levels of immunoactive TNF, but considerably less bioactive TNF. This discrepancy between the assay types indicates that bio-inactive forms of TNF, recognized by the immunoassay, and not by the bioassay, were present. Formation of complexes between TNF and soluble TNF receptors or degradation of the bioactive TNF trimer may be explanations of differences in detection of immunoactive vs bioactive TNF.

This chapter describes in detail the bioassays for TNF-α, IL-1, and IL-6, with focus on the TNF-α bioassay.

2. Materials

2.1. Preparation of Medium

1. RPMI 1640 (Gibco, Paisley, UK).
2. L-glutamine (Gibco). Make a stock solution of 20 mg/mL by dissolving 2 g in 100 mL sterile water. Sterile-filtrate, make aliquots of 5 mL, and store at –20°C.
3. Garamycin, 40 mg/mL (Schering-Plough, Labo n.v., Belgium).
4. Fetal calf serum (FCS) (HyClone, Logan, UK). Heat-inactivate the serum at 56°C for 30 min before use. Make aliquots of 5 mL and store at –20°C (*see* **Note 1**).
5. 2-Mercaptoethanol (Sigma). Make a stock solution of 2.5×10^{-2} *M* by adding 53 µL of concentrated 2-mercaptoethanol to 30 mL RPMI 1640. Store in the fridge at 4°C.
6. Actinomycin D (Sigma). Make a stock solution of 250 µg/mL by dissolving 5 mg in 20 mL sterile water. Make aliquots and store at –20°C. Actinomycin D is a mutagen. It should be handled with gloves only and should be kept contained.

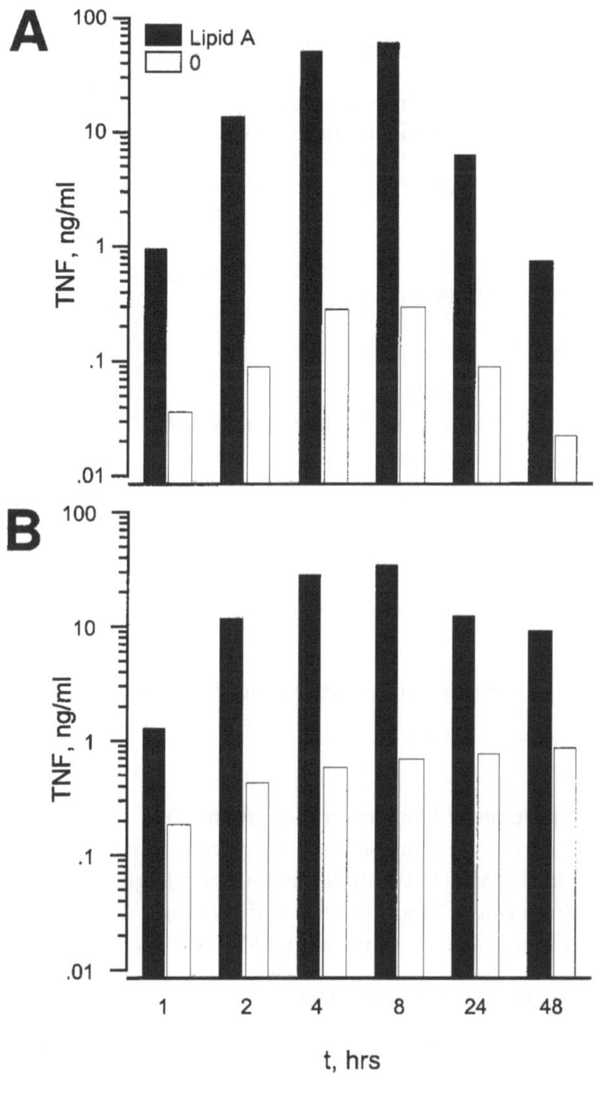

Fig. 1. Time course of TNF release from freshly isolated adherent primary monocytes, analysed by cytotoxicity WEHI 164 clone 13 bioassay **(A)** or 6H11 TNF immunoassay **(B)**, both developed in our laboratory. The cells are exposed to medium only (0, open bars) or 125 ng/mL of lipid A (filled bars) from *Salmonella minnesota* (Sigma). Medium used was AIM (Gibco) containing 10% FCS. Cell-free supernatants are harvested at the indicated time points, and analyzed simultaneously in the two assays.

Table 1
Description of the Medium Used in the Bioassays

Type of bioassay	Cell line	Growth medium: basic medium added	Dilution medium: basic medium added
TNF-α	WEHI 164 clone 13	5% FCS	5% FCS[a] 0.5 μg/mL Actinomycin D
IL-1	EL-4-NOB-1[b]	10% FCS	10% FCS 2.5×10^{-5} *M* 2-Mercaptoethanol
	HT-2	10% FCS, 2.5×10^{-5} *M* 2-Mercaptoethanol, 2-Mercaptoethanol, 25U/ml IL-2	10% FCS, 2.5×10^{-5} *M* 2-Mercaptoethanol
IL-6	B13.29 clone B9	10% FCS 5×10^{-5} *M* 2-Mercaptoethanol IL-6[c]	5% FCS 5×10^{-5} *M* 2-Mercaptoethanol,

[a]*See* **Note 2**.
[b]*See* **Note 3**.
[c]Preparation of IL-6 for addition in the growth medium is described in **Subheading 3.7., step 1**.

7. IL-2 (can be purchased from several companies).
8. IL-6 (can be purchased from several companies, *see* **Subheading 3.7., step 1**).
9. Basic medium (RPMI 1640 supplemented with L-glutamine and garamycin).
10. Growth medium (basic medium with additives; *see* **Table 1**).
11. Dilution medium (basic medium with additives; *see* **Table 1**).

2.2. Maintenance of Cell Culture

1. The cell lines used in the cytokine bioassays are listed in **Table 1**.
2. Trypsin (Gibco).
3. Growth medium (basic medium with additives; *see* **Table 1**).
4. 75 cm^2 tissue culture flasks (Nunc).
5. Incubator (Forma Scientific, OH).

2.3. Preparation of Standards and Samples

1. r (recombinant) hu (human) TNF-α.
2. rIL-1.
3. rIL-2.

4. rIL-6. (The cytokines can be purchased from several companies.)
5. Dilution medium (basic medium with additives; *see* **Table 1**).

2.4. TNF-α Bioassay

1. Dilution medium (basic medium with additives; *see* **Table 1**).
2. Neutralizing TNF-α antibodies. Monoclonal anti-TNF-α called 6H11 ***(11)*** or polyclonal anti-TNF-α rabbit serum. Neutralizing TNF-α antibodies can also be purchased from many companies. If a polyclonal rabbit serum is used as a neutralizing antibody, this serum should also be heat-inactivated (56°C, 30 min) before use.
3. 96-well microtiterplates (Costar).
4. MTT (3-(4,5-dimethylthiazol-2-yl)-2,5-diphenyltetrazolium bromid (Sigma). Make a stock solution of 5 mg/mL by dissolving 500 mg in 100 mL phosphate buffered saline (PBS) (Dulbecco 'A' Tablets). Sterile-filtrate and store in the fridge at 4°C. MTT is a mutagen. It should be handled with gloves only and should be kept contained.
5. Acidic sodium dodecyl sulfate (SDS) solution: 10% (w/v) SDS (Bio-Rad Laboratories) dissolved in 0.01 *M* HCl (Merck).
6. Isopropanol-0.04 *M* HCl. Prepare the solution by adding 3.3 mL HCl to 1 L isopropanol (Merck). Should be made at least 1 d before use.
7. Shaker (Titertek, Flow Laboratories).
8. Microplate reader (Bio-Rad, model 3550-UV, Richmond, CA).

2.5. IL-1 Bioassay

1. *See* **Subheading 2.4.**
2. HBSS (Hank's Balanced Salt Solution) (Gibco).
3. Neutralizing IL-1 antibodies (can be purchased from several companies).

2.6. IL-6 Bioassay

1. *See* **Subheading 2.4.**
2. PBMC were isolated from human A+ blood buffy coats (The Blood Bank, University Hospital, Trondheim, Norway) as described by Bøyum et al. ***(12)***.
3. LPS (Sigma L-8274). Make a stock solution of 10 mg/mL by dissolving 100 mg in 10 mL NaCl. Make working stocks of 50 μL and store at –20°C.
4. Neutralizing IL-6 antibodies (can be purchased from several companies).

3. Methods

3.1. Preparation of Medium

1. Make basic medium by adding 5 mL L-glutamine and 0.5 mL garamycin to 1 L of RPMI 1640.
2. Make the growth medium required by the cell lines by adding heat-inactivated FCS and additional substances (*see* **Table 1**).

3. Make the dilution medium required by the bioassays by adding heat-inactivated FCS and additional substances (*see* **Table 1**).
4. Store media in the fridge at 4°C for a maximum of 2 wk.

3.2. Maintenance of Cell Culture

1. The cell lines should be replaced with freshly thawed cells regularly, because the cells lose their sensitivity to the cytokines after some months in culture. For instance, the WEHI 164 clone 13 cell line should be replaced after a couple of months of cultivation, while the B13.29 clone B9 should be replaced three times a year.
2. Stock cells are usually subcultured when they reach a cell density of 5×10^5 cells/mL, usually twice a week; for instance, every Monday and Friday. However, the growth of cell lines varies and have to be optimized for each cell line (*see* **Note 4**).
3. When subculturing the cells, dilute the cells in fresh growth medium in a new culture flask. Use 15 mL of medium per flask, and add 10 mL extra growth medium the day before the bioassay is performed.
4. Incubate the culture flask at 37°C in a humidified 5% CO_2 incubator.

3.3. Preparation of Standards

1. When the standards are initially purchased, high-concentration stocks are prepared (500 μg/mL in PBS for the rhuTNF-α standard). These are divided (100 μL lots) and stored at –70°C. From these, working stocks (50 μg/mL, diluted in bacic medium with 5% heat-inactivated FCS) are prepared and stored in the fridge at 4°C for several months without losing activity.
2. Standards are carried out in triplicates in 96-well microtiter plates. Dilute the standards in dilution medium, dependent on what cytokine bioassay is carried out (*see* **Table 1**).
3. Typically, make twofold dilutions of the standards 15 times (making standard curves). The final volume of standard per well should be 100 μL.
4. Make the standard curves by first adding 50 μL dilution medium to the first 6 rows of the microtiter plate. Then, add 50 μL of the titrated cytokine standard in the first well of the first three rows. Mix the solutions by pipetting, withdraw 50 μL, and pipet into the adjacent wells along the row. When reaching the end of the three rows, continue the dilution curve in the three next rows. After 15 dilutions, discard the final 50 μL, leaving 50 μL in the end wells.
5. Add only dilution medium (50 μL/well) in the three last wells as a negative control.
6. In order to confirm the specificity of the cytokine bioassay, a neutralizing antibody against the cytokine should be added in order to inhibit the specific effect of the cytokine on the target cell line. Fifty μL of the neutralizing cytokine antibody (10 μg/mL) is therefore added to 50 μL of each standard dilution in one of the three parallels. In the two other parallels, add only 50 μL dilution medium. The total volume per well is now 100 μL.

1	2	3	4	5	6	7	8	9	10	11	12
S1	S1	S1+	S9	S9	S9+	A1	A1	A1+	C1	C1	C1+
S2	S2	S2+	S10	S10	S10+	A2	A2	A2+	C2	C2	C2+
S3	S3	S3+	S11	S11	S11+	A3	A3	A3+	C3	C3	C3+
S4	S4	S4+	S12	S12	S12+	A4	A4	A4+	C4	C4	C4+
S5	S5	S5+	S13	S13	S13+	B1	B1	B1+	IS1	IS1	IS1+
S6	S6	S6+	S14	S14	S14+	B2	B2	B2+	IS2	IS2	IS2+
S7	S7	S7+	S15	S15	S15+	B3	B3	B3+	IS3	IS3	IS3+
S8	S8	S8+	M	M	M+	B4	B4	B4+	IS4	IS4	IS4+

Fig. 2. Typical experimental design of a microtiter plate for a cytokine bioassay with standard curve, internal standard, and three samples with and without a neutralizing antibody.

Key:

S1-S15: 15 dilutions of cytokine standard, where S1 represent the start concentration, S2 represent 1;2 dilution, S3 1;4 dilution and further on.

S2+–S15+: 15 dilution of the cytokine standard added a neutralising antibody.

M: medium control

A1–A4: 4 dilutions of a serum sample, where A1 represent the start dilution 1;10, A2 the second dilution 1;50, A3 the third dilution 1;250 and A4 the fourth dilution 1;1250.

A1+–A4+: 4 dilutions of serum sample A added a neutralizing antibody. B and C: 2 other serum samples, diluted in the same way as sample A.

IS1–IS4: 4 dilutions of an internal standard, diluted in the same way as serum samples A, B and C.

IS1+–IS4+: 4 dilutions of the internal standard added a neutralising antibody.

3.4. Preparation of Samples

1. Serum samples are divided into working stocks and stored at –70°C before analysis. Working stocks should not be repeatedly frozen and thawed.
2. If serum samples are tested, it is important to first inactivate the samples by heating at 56°C for 30 min (*see* **Note 5**).
3. Make serially dilutions of the samples in dilution medium, dependent on what cytokine bioassay is done (*see* **Table 1**).
4. Typically, start the dilution of the serum sample at 1:10 and thereafter do 1:5 dilutions. The final volume of sample per well should be 100 μL.
5. Make the sample dilution curves by first adding 50 μL dilution medium to the first wells of three rows. Add 12.5 μL serum sample to the first well, mix by pipetting and transfer 12.5 μL into the adjacent wells along the row, 4 times in total.
6. In order to confirm the specificity, a neutralizing antibody against the cytokine should be added to the serum samples in order to inhibit the specific effect of the cytokine on the target cell line. 50 μL of a neutralizing cytokine antibody (10 μg/mL)

is therefore added to 50 μL of each serum dilution in one of the three parallels. In the two other parallels, add only 50 μL dilution medium. The total volume per well is now 100 μL. **Figure 2** illustrates a typical experimental design of a microtiter plate for a cytokine bioassay, with the standard curve and four samples, with and without a neutralizing antibody (*see* **Note 6**).

7. An internal standard (IS) should be included every time the bioassays are run, in order to control inter-assay variations. The IS could for instance be a serum sample or a cell-culture supernatant known to contain high amounts of the actual cytokine. Make a serially dilution curve of the IS in the same way as the sample dilution curve.

3.5. TNF-α Bioassay

1. Make dilution medium as described (*see* **Subheading 3.1.**).
2. Prepare standards and samples as described (*see* **Subheadings 3.2.** and **3.3.**). Start the TNF-α standard curve at 200 pg/mL.
3. After preparation of standards and samples, place the microtiter plates in the incubator at 37°C and 5% CO_2 atmosphere while the cells are prepared.
4. Dilute the WEHI 164 clone 13 cells to 6 × 10^4 cells/ml in dilution medium (*see* **Table 1**). Add 100 μL cell suspension to the samples (6 × 10^3 cells/well). The final volume of the well should be 200 μL.
5. Incubate the plate over night in the incubator.
6. Add 20 μL MTT to each well.
7. Incubate the plate for 4 h in the incubator.
8. Remove 100 μL supernatant from each well (*see* **Note 7**). Do not touch the cells in the bottom of the well.
9. Add 100 μL 10% SDS-0.01M HCl and incubate over night in the incubator.
10. Read the absorbance at 570 nm on a microplate reader.
11. The detection limit of the TNF-α bioassay is 1 pg/mL.

3.6. IL-1 Bioassay

1. Make dilution medium as described (*see* **Subheading 3.1.**).
2. Prepare standards and samples as described (*see* **Subheadings 3.2.** and **3.3.**). Start the IL-1 standard curve at 250 pg/mL.
3. After preparation of standards and samples, place the microtiter plates in the incubator at 37°C and 5% CO_2 atmosphere while the cells are prepared.
4. Dilute the EL-4-NOB-1 (*see* **Note 2**) cells to 2 × 10^6 cells/mL in dilution medium (*see* **Table 1**). Add 100 μL EL-4-NOB-1 cells to the samples (2 × 10^5 cells/well). The total volume of the well is now 200 μL.
5. Incubate the plate over night in the incubator.
6. Centrifuge the plate (1500 rpm, 8 min).
7. Transfer 75 μL supernatant to a new plate, avoid transfering the cells.
8. Add 125 μL HT-2 cells per well to the new plate. The HT-2 cells are first centrifuged (1500 rpm, 8 min), washed 3 times with HBSS, and seeded at a concentration of 3.2 × 10^4 cells/mL or 4 × 10^3 cells/well in dilution medium (*see* **Table 1**). The final volume of the well is now 200 μL (*see* **Note 8**).

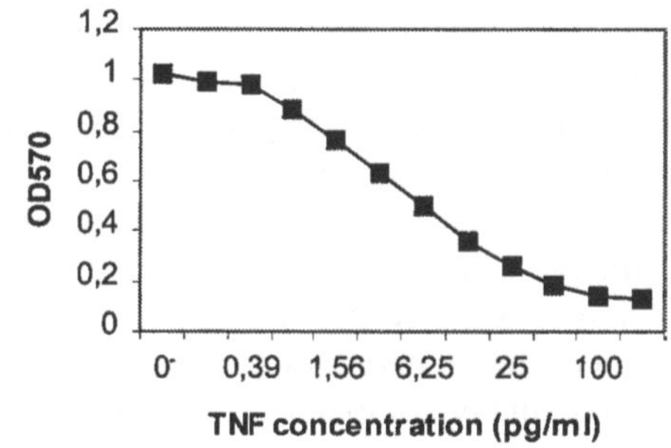

Fig. 3. Typical standard curve for the cytotoxic TNF-α bioassay.

9. Incubate the plate for 2 d in the incubator.
10. Continue the same procedure as the TNF-α bioassay (*see* **Subheading 3.5., steps 6–10**).
11. The detection limit of the IL-1 bioassay is 5 pg/mL.

3.7. IL-6 Bioassay

1. Preparation of IL-6 added in the growth medium for the B13.29 clone B9 cells is made as follows: Isolate PBMC as described *(12)*, wash 2 times in HBSS, and resuspend in IL-6 assay medium (*see* **Table 1**) supplemented with 0.1 μg/mL LPS. Seed the PBMC at a cell concentration of 2×10^6 cells/mL in cell-culture flasks and incubate for 24 h. Harvest the supernatant and store by freezing at –20°C. The IL-6 concentration in the supernatant is decided by comparison with the rIL-6 standard. The concentration of IL-6 added to the medium should be about 500 μg/mL.
2. Make dilution medium as described (*see* **Subheading 3.1.**).
3. Prepare standards and samples as described (*see* **Subheadings 3.2.** and **3.3.**). Start the IL-6 standard curve at 125 pg/mL.
4. After preparation of standards and samples, place the microtiter plates in the incubator at 37°C and 5% CO_2 atmosphere while the cells are prepared.
5. Centrifuge the B13.29 clone B9-cells and wash 3 times in HBSS. Resuspend the cells to 5×10^4 cells/mL and add 100 μL cell suspension to the samples or 5×10^3 cells per well. The total volume per well should now be 200 μL.
6. Incubate the plates for 3 d.
7. Continue the same procedure as the TNF-α bioassay (*see* **Subheading 3.5., steps 6–10**).
8. The detection limit of the IL-6 bioassay is 3 pg/mL.

3.8. Calculations

1. Plot a standard curve of absorbance vs concentration of the cytokine. Use a logarithmic scale on the x-axis for the concentration of the cytokine, and a linear scale on the y-axis for the absorbance. **Figure 3** illustrates a typical standard curve for the TNF-α bioassay. Generally, for cytotoxic bioassays (the TNF-α

bioassay), the greater the cytokine concentration, the lower the assay response. In contrast, for proliferation assays (like the IL-1 and the IL-6 bioassays), the greater the cytokine concentration, the larger the assay response.

2. Plot dose-response curve of the samples.
3. Compare the sample dilution curves with the standard curve. The linear range of the curves is used for the calculations. Samples and standards should produce parallel straight sections of dose-response curves. The distance between the two curves is an indication of the relative biological activity of the cytokine between the two samples. Today, many computer programs are available that automatically calculate the cytokine concentrations (*see* **Note 9**).

4. Notes

1. It is important to screen different FCS batches and types before use, because FCS batch and type may influence the cell lines with regard to growth, assay specificity, and assay sensitivity. This can be achieved by: 1) testing cell growth of different cell lines; 2) carrying out different bioassays; 3) cloning of hybridoma cells, and 4) quantitation of endotoxin content.
2. When the WEHI 164 clone 13 cells are thawed and split the first time, use 10% FCS and then change to 5% at the second splitting.
3. The T-cell line LBRM-33-1A5 ***(13)*** can be used instead of EL-4-NOB-1 cells in the IL-1 bioassay.
4. Culturing of the cell lines used in the different bioassays have to be optimized for each cell line. However, it is supposed that the cell lines used in the bioassays are subcultured like this every Monday (and Friday): WEHI 164 clone 13 cell line is diluted 1:30 and (1:20), the EL-4-NOB-1 is diluted 1:40 and (1:40), the HT-2 is diluted 1:80 and (1:40), and the B13.29 clone B9 is diluted about 1:10 and (1:10).
5. If cell supernatants are tested instead of serum samples, it is not necessary to first heat inactivate the samples. Typically, the cell-culture supernatants are serially diluted 1:5.
6. It is not necessary to include the standard curve on each plate, if many samples and plates are going to be analyzed.
7. If the samples to be tested are cell supernatants, etc. (not serum samples), it is not necessary to add 10% SDS-0.01 *M* HCl. Instead, remove 150 μL (instead of 100 μL) supernatant from each well, add 100 μL isopropanol-0.04 *M* HCl, and incubate for 1 h at room temperature with shaking before reading the absorbance. Adding isopropanol to serum samples may result in precipitation, which in turn gives higher optical density (OD) values than expected. The strategy using isopropanol-0.04N HCl instead of 10% SDS-0.01 *M* HCl reduces the total assay time by 1 d.
8. To control that the proliferation of HT-2 cells is not caused by IL-2 present in the test samples, add positive samples to cultures of HT-2 without prior conditioning by EL-4-NOB-1 cells. Start the IL-2 standard curve at 100 U/mL.

9. One disadvantage with bioassays compared to immunoassays is the great variability between the runs. This is mainly owing to the cells, which differ with regard to both growth and sensitivity and result in high-variation coefficients.

References

1. Waage, A., Halstensen, A., and Espevik, T. (1987) Association between tumour necrosis factor in serum and fatal outcome in patients with meningococcal disease. *Lancet* **i,** 355–357.
2. Girardin, E., Grau, G. E., Dayer, J. M., Roux-Lombard, P., and Lambert, P. H. (1988) Tumor necrosis factor and interleukin-1 in the serum of children with severe infection purpura. *N. Engl. J. Med.* **319,** 397–400.
3. Waage, A., Brandtzaeg, P., Halstensen, A., Kierulf, P., and Espevik, T. (1989) The complex pattern of cytokines in serum from patients with meningococcal septic shock. *J. Exp. Med.* **169,** 333–338.
4. Mosmann, T. R., Cherwinski, H., Bond, M. W., Giedlin, M. A., and Coffman, R.L. (1986) Two types of murine helper T cell clone. I. Definition according to profiles of lymphokine activities and secreted proteins. *J. Immunol.* **136,** 2348–2357.
5. Aarden, L. A., De Groot, E. R., Schaap, O. L., and Lansdorp, P. M. (1987) Production of hybridoma growth factor by human monocytes. *Eur. J. Immunol.* **17,** 1411–1416.
6. Gearing, A. J. H., Bird, C. R., Bristow, A., Poole, S., and Thorpe, R. (1987) A simple sensitive bioassay for interleukin-1 which is unresponsive to 103 U/ml of interleukin-2. *J. Immunol. Methods* **99,** 7–11.
7. Kramer, S. M. and Carver, M. E. (1986) Serum-free in vitro bioassay for the detection of tumor necrosis factor. *J. Immunol. Meth.* **93,** 201–206.
8. Espevik, T. and Nissen-Meyer, J. (1986) A highly sensitive cell line, WEHI 164 clone 13, for measuring cytotoxic factor/tumor necrosis factor from human monocytes. *J. Immunol. Meth.* **24,** 739–743.
9. Mosmann, T. (1983) Rapid colorimetric assay for cellular growth and survival: Application to proliferation and cytotoxicity assays. *J. Immunol. Methods* **65,** 55–63.
10. Stenvik, J., Lien, E., Jahr, T. G., Halstensen, A., and Espevik, T. Detection of TNF in monocyte cultures and in sepsis sera with bio- and immunoassays-differences related to TNF and TNF-soluble TNF receptor complexes. *In press.*
11. Liabakk, N. B., Nustad, K., and Espevik, T. (1990) A rapid and sensitive immunoassay based on magnetic monodisperse particles for the detection of Tumor Necrosis Factor. *J. Immunol. Methods* **134,** 253–259.
12. Bøyum, A. M. (1976) Separation of Monocytes and Lymphocytes. *Scand. J. Immunol.* **5,** 9–15.
13. Conlon, P.J. (1983) A rapid biological assay for the detection of interleukin 1. *J. Immunol.* **131,** 1280.

30

Molecular Analysis of Gene-Polymorphisms Affecting the Host Response to Infection

Rudi G. J. Westendorp and Tom W. J. Huizinga

1. Introduction

The genetic regulation of the host response to infection is crucial for understanding susceptibility to and outcome of meningococcal disease. The initial host response depends on the innate immune system, after which specific immunity is attained when antibodies from the adaptive immune system appear. The comparison of genetic markers in patients who have suffered from the disease, their families, and appropriate control populations thus identifies components of the host response that are key to combat meningococcal infection. A similar reasoning can be followed when studying susceptibility to or when studying outcome of meningococcal disease. A better understanding of the host response at a molecular level also allows for estimating individual risk. This accumulating knowledge can be used to develop new preventive and therapeutic interventions and to vary these strategies dependent on risk profiles.

1.1. Strengths and Weaknesses of Genetic Analyses

The importance of studying gene-polymorphisms to unravel the pathogenesis of meningococcal disease in humans cannot be emphasized enough. Conclusive arguments for a causal relation generally come up from experimental studies. In humans, experimental studies to understand susceptibility and outcome of meningococcal disease are not feasible apart from testing efficacy of vaccines to prevent infection. Note that meningococcal infection is already at a late phase when the efficacy of therapeutic interventions is studied. For that reason these studies do not add much to our basic understanding of the disease. Our insight into the host response to infection is thus based on the earliest

From: *Methods in Molecular Medicine, vol. 67: Meningococcal Disease: Methods and Protocols*
Edited by: A. J. Pollard and M. C. J. Maiden © Humana Press Inc., Totowa, NJ

clinical observations in patients who contracted the disease. The major caveat is that the observed signs and symptoms may just reflect the "natural course" of meningococcal infection instead of being part of a causal pathway (*see* **ref. *1***, pp. 67–78). This implies that most of the circulating factors that associate with outcome are merely risk-indicators and not risk-factors. The strength of a genetic analysis is that the genes under study are not distorted by the course of the disease, as genomic DNA is invariable since conception. When patients with meningococcal disease are thus characterized by a particular genotype, this observation certainly indicates a causal mechanism that is related to susceptibility or outcome of the disease. Although this logic has been known for a long time, genetic research has been held up by the absence of the molecular tools to prove it.

Cytokines have been identified as key players in the host response to infection ***(2)***. Their significance has been shown in various experimental models. However, the contribution of the various cytokines to, among others, meningoccal infection is less clear. The reason is that the conclusions from experimental models seem to contradict the observations in humans. High levels of circulating, pro-inflammatory cytokines were reported in patients who suffered from meningoccocal sepsis ***(3)***. The high circulating levels were also related to an adverse outcome and replicated in patients with other types of (Gram-negative) sepsis. These observations led to the general conclusion that production of pro-inflammatory cytokines in humans contributed to the development of sepsis syndrome ***(4)***. The idea initiated a major development into specific antibodies that were capable of blocking the various pro-inflammatory cytokines, or to block their biologic propensities. The initiative lasted for nearly a decade before it became apparent that this approach was unsuccessful ***(5)***. Some of the large randomized controlled trials that were instigated showed even a higher mortality in patients who were treated with these antibodies ***(6)***. What went wrong?

There is a lively discussion whether the observations from the various experimental models can be extrapolated to humans ***(7)***. This discussion acknowledges our general caution to equate mice and humans. The quintessential fault, however, was that the presence of circulating, pro-inflammatory cytokines in patients was not properly understood. Instead of playing a causal role in the development of sepsis, the circulating cytokines in patients with meningococcal disease only reflect the disease course and indicate an adverse outcome ***(8)***. A recent and more likely interpretation of the data is that a pro-inflammatory response is necessary to combat infection and to prevent adverse outcome ***(9–11)***.

An analysis of gene-polymorphisms that affect cytokine responses could have shed another light on the topic ***(12)***. The reason being that gene-polymorphisms of patients with meningococcal disease do not change during the course of the disease. This would in principle have prevented the misinterpretation of a risk-indicator for a risk-factor. So far, the studies using polymorphisms in genes encoding for pro-inflammatory cytokines are not conclusive (see the discrepancy between **refs.** ***8*** and ***13*** for meningococcal disease, and between **refs.** ***12*** and ***14*** for sepsis syndrome in general). The reason is that these polymorphisms have not unequivocally been shown to be functional ***(15,16)***. Functional polymorphisms associate with variation of the gene-product in in vitro studies, affect the phenotype of transgene-animal models, and relate to human biology in vivo.

Conclusive arguments for causality could be obtained when the role of fibrinolysis in complicated meningococcal disease was studied using a functional polymorphism. First, high circulating levels of inhibitors of fibrinolysis had been observed in patients with adverse outcome ***(17)***. These observations were difficult to interpret, as it could only be a reflection of the disease course. Later studies, however, showed that a polymorphism that associates with increased transcription of the plasminogen-activator-inhibitor (PAI) gene in vitro as well as in vivo was enriched in patients with adverse outcome ***(18,19)***. From these data, it was concluded that inhibition of fibrinolysis is not only a marker of complicated meningococcal disease but also contributes to an adverse outcome.

There is yet another rationale for contending that the analysis of gene-polymorphisms is especially suitable for studying pathogenesis of meningoccocal disease. The incidence of meningococcal disease in the general population is low. Hence, prospective follow-up studies of nonaffected persons are unrealistic, whereas case-control studies that gather consecutive series of patients are possible. Case-control studies that use genetic markers do not suffer from the various biases and confounders that are generally associated with this type of study. For instance, it is not relevant that the determinant under study is assessed after disease has occurred, as the genetic code is invariable. Moreover, it is not likely that the genetic analysis is confounded by other determinants of disease, as these risk factors tend to segregate independently. As a rule of thumb, the presence of a genetic polymorphism is independent of other genetic risk factors (e.g., complement deficiencies), and environmental (e.g., crowding) risk factors and adjustment is not indicated (how to deal with more complicated situations, *see* **ref.** ***20***, pp. 82–123).

1.2. Different Types of Genetic Studies

The study of gene-polymorphisms affecting immune responses can principally be divided into three types (for review see **ref.** ***21***). The first type is the analysis of a gene-polymorphism that is functional (*see* **Table 1**). This analysis is the most intuitive and most powerful. The gene-polymorphism leads to different levels of the gene-product in vitro and in vivo and/or is associated with outcome of other diseases. Depletion or enrichment of such a gene-polymorphism in patients who have had meningococcal disease directly allow

Table 1
Characteristics of Various Studies Analyzing Genetically Determined Immune Responses

	Study makes use of		
Characteristic	Gene-polymorphism that is functional	Polymorphism of candidate gene	Inherited functional polymorphism
Prior knowledge on	Gene-expression	Location on genome	Biological mechanism
Presumed regulation	Simple	Simple	Complex
Family approach	Not necessary	Increases sensitivity	Necessary
Input	Relatively easy	Genetically complicated	Labor intensive
Causal inference	Good	Poor	Good

for causal inference. A clear example is the study of a polymorphism in the gene encoding for plasminogen-activator-inhibitor type I (PAI-1) inhibiting fibrinolysis as described earlier.

The second type of genetic studies is the analysis of a gene polymorphism for which functional data are not yet available (*see* **Table 1**). With the genetic code for *Homo sapiens* (nearly) finished, the number of single nucleotide polymorphic markers is rapidly increasing. Markers in all genes that are involved in the host response to meningococcal disease will become available, and it can be tested whether the frequencies are different in patients from control persons. When it becomes apparent that meningococcal disease associates with a marker in an unknown gene, a search into the function of that gene is indicated. The location of the marker in (the proximity) of a gene does not necessarily imply that the gene in which the marker is located is causally related to the disease. The explanation is that most of the markers are nonfunctional. This implies that the marker may be linked to another polymorphism in a nearby gene that is causing the association.

A word of caution is necessary to interpret data from forthcoming genome screens with a large number of nonfunctional single nucleotide polymorphisms at fixed intervals. The reason is that linkage between these nonfunctional single nucleotide polymorphisms and the causal gene cannot always be assumed to be present. An example is the identification of Factor V Leiden mutation as a risk factor for venous thrombosis. This association could not have been identified with the CA-dinucleotide repeat closest to the factor V Leiden mutation *(22)*. Thus even when the frequency of these nonfunctional polymorphisms is similar in patients and control persons, it cannot be excluded that a gene that is located in the proximity of the marker is involved in the pathogenesis of meningococcal infection. When searching for genes involved in the pathogenesis of meningococcal infection that are not yet known (i.e., candidate genes), the sensitivity of the analysis can be improved when using haplotypes *(23)*. Haplotypes are combinations of polymorphic markers that are inherited as one. This necessitates the inclusion of family members. The techniques are beyond the scope of this chapter and the reader is referred to other textbooks.

The third type of genetic analysis is that of an inherited functional polymorphism and actually combines the strengths of the first two types of analyses (*see* **Table 1**). Some of the immune responses have already been shown to be under genetic control by heritability testing in families and twin pairs. The loci on the genome that encode for these responses, however, are not yet known. Identification may be difficult because several interacting genes are involved. Although the genomic loci are not yet known, patients and control persons can be characterized for this inherited trait by functional testing. A clear example is the innate responsiveness of cytokine production upon incubation of whole blood samples ex-vivo *(8)*. Similar as assessing the frequencies of a gene polymorphism that is functional, the comparison of inherited functional polymorphism between patients and control persons directly allows for causal inference.

A modification of the third type of study is when first-degree relatives of patients are enrolled. There are three indications for this modified approach; (1) the patient is deceased, (2) the patient is using medication that interacts with the functional assay (e.g., corticosteroids), or (3) the disease activity interacts with the functional assay. Under these circumstances, the patient cannot be characterized for the functional polymorphism. Instead, first-degree relatives can be studied because the functional polymorphism is inherited. **Figure 1** shows the results of such an analysis *(8)*. Each dot represents the mean of all first-degree relatives of the person under study. These family means reflect the best estimate of the polymorphism for ill or deceased patients. The data depicted in the figure strongly suggest that patients with an adverse outcome of meningococcal disease were characterized by low production of tumor necrosis factor-α (TNF-α) and high production of interleukin-10 (IL-10). The data can be alternately stated. Patients with an adverse outcome of meningococcal disease stem from families with low production of TNF-α and high production of IL-10. This emphasizes the heritable character of the increased susceptibility for adverse outcome. Using a similar approach, heritable differences in production of TNF-α and IL-10 could be linked with susceptibility of systemic lupus erythematodes (SLE) and multiple sclerosis (MS) *(24,25)*.

The drawback of using a family approach is that the difference between family means is expected to be lower than would be obtained when patients and control persons were characterized directly. The difference is less because the patients and control persons and their respective first-degree relatives only

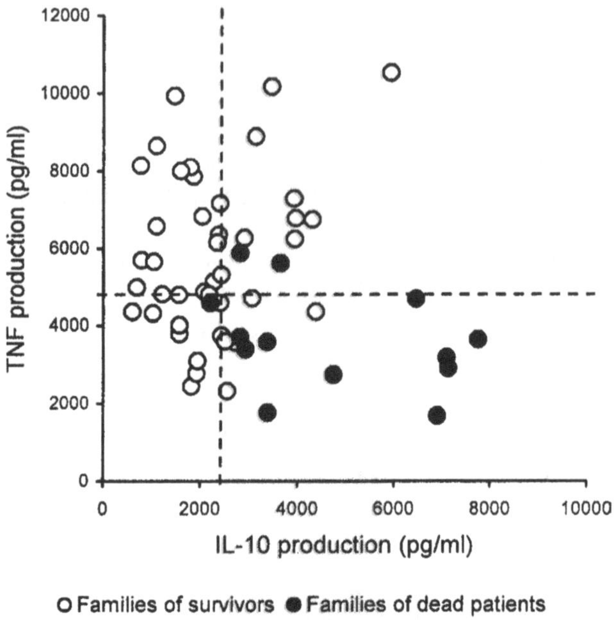

Fig. 1. Production of TNF and IL-10 in whole-blood samples incubated with 1000 ng/mL endotoxin. Symbols represent the family means of TNF production and IL-10 production. Open circles represent cytokine production in 42 families of patients who survived (121 first-degree relatives), and closed circles represent production of cytokines in 13 families of patients who died from meningococcal infection (43 first-degree relatives). Dotted lines indicate medians of the family estimates for both cytokines. Adapted with permission from **ref.** ***8***.

share 50% of their genome. The risk estimates are thus deflated to the null value. Causal inference is, however, unaffected. Again, the force of persuasion may even be larger as it appears that families of patients who suffered from meningococcal disease have specific innate characteristics.

1.3. Aim of the Chapter

The aim of this chapter is to provide sufficient detail to perform three variants of genetic studies to unravel the host response to meningococcal infection.

2. Materials

2.1. Isolation of Genomic DNA from Peripheral Blood Mononuclear Cells (PBMCs)

1. PBS: 140 m*M* NaCl, 9.2 m*M* Na_2HPO_4, 1.3 m*M* Na H_2PO_4.
2. Ficoll with specific gravity 1.076 g/mL.

3. Isotonic NH_4Cl.
4. 25 m*M* Tris-HCl, 100 m*M* NaCl, 10 m*M* EDTA, pH 8.0.
5. Proteinase K: 100 ug/ml.
6. Phenol/chloroform/isoamylalcohol (25:24:1).
7. Chloroform/isoamylalcohol (24:1).
8. Sodiumacetate, pH 5.5.
9. Ethanol 100%.

2.2. Polymerase Chain Reaction

1. Oligonucleotide primers for studying the TNF promoter polymorphism –238 G to A are 5′-AAACAGACCACAGACCTGGTC-3′ and 5′-AAGGATACCCC TCACACTCCCCATCCTCCCGGATA-3′. For the –308 G to A polymorphism the primers are 5′-GAGGCAATAGGTTTTGAGGGCCAT-3′ and 5′-GGGAC ACACAAGCATCAAG-3′.
2. Restriction enzymes *Bam*HI and *Nco*I.
3. Biotin labeled primers for studying the IL-10 promoter polymorphism –1082 G to A are 5′-TTCTTTGGGAGGGGGAAG-3′ for –1082G and 5′-ACTTCCCC TTCCCAAAGAA-3′ for –1082A.

2.3. Whole-Blood Stimulation Assay

1. Vacutainer® blood collecting system and sterile endotoxin-free blood collection tubes (Chromogenix Endotube®, Mölndal, Sweden) containing 120 IU sodium heparin.
2. RPMI 1640 (Cat. no. 041-02400, Gibco Life Technologies, Paisley, UK).
3. A single batch of a 5 mg/mL stock solution of lipopolysaccharide (LPS, *Escherichia coli* 0111;B4, Boivin method, Difco Laboratories, Detroit, MI) is prepared and stored in 250 μL aliquots at –70°C, undiluted aliquots were taken once a week and stored at 4°C.
4. Antibodies against cytokines (for instance, Central Laboratory of the Blood Transfusion Service, Amsterdam, The Netherlands, and BioSource, Fleurus, Belgium).
5. Standard cytokines calibrated against WHO International Standard (National Institute for Biological Standards and Control, Potters Bar, UK).

3. Methods

3.1. Isolation of Genomic DNA from PBMCs (*see* Notes 1–3)

1. Collect blood into heparinized tubes and dilute 1:1 with PBS.
2. Carefully pipet the diluted blood on Ficoll and centrifuge at 1000*g* for 20 min.
3. Lyse the remaining erytrocytes with isotonic NH_4Cl at 4°C.
4. Wash the cells with PBS and dilute the cell pellet in 1 mL of isolation buffer consisting of Tris-HCl pH 8.0, 100 μg/mL proteinase K and 0.6% sodium dodecyl sulfate (SDS). From this step onwards the pellet can be kept at –20°C.
5. Incubate the cell pellet for at least for 4 h at 37°C. Extract with an equal volume of phenol/chloroform/isoamylalcohol (25:24:1). Harvest the upperlayer.

Repeat until the interphase has disappeared. Wash last time with chloroform/isoamylalcohol.

6. Add sodium acetate, pH 5.5, till a final concentration of 0.3 *M*. Precipitate DNA with two volumes of 100% ethanol.
7. Centrifuge the DNA at 4000 rpm (2000*g*) for 5 min and wash the pellet once with 70% ethanol. Incubate DNA in 500 µL TE.

3.2. Polymerase Chain Reaction (PCR) (*see* Notes 4 and 5)

1. Design primers from the sequence data base using the websites (*see* **Note 6**). As an example to study the TNF promoter polymorphism for the –238 G to A or –308 G to A polymorphism, PCR fragments are generated using the primer combinations mentioned in **Subheading 2.2.1.**
2. Type the –238 G to A polymorphism by using the restriction enzyme *Bam*HI yielding a fragment for the GG genotype of 123 bp and 42 bp, for the AA genotype of 165 bp and for the GA genotype all three fragments. For the –308 G to A polymorphism the use of the restriction enzyme *Nco*I yields fragments of 126 bp and 21 bp for the GG, 147 bp for the AA and all three fragments for the GA (for a detailed description *see* **ref. *26***).
3. Use biotin-labeled primers to hybridize the PCR fragment by dotblot. The advantage of this technique is that one PCR fragment can be generated for a large part of the promoter. As an example use IL-10 promoter fragments by PCR using primer combinations as described in **Subheading 2.2.3.**
4. Blot to PCR fragments to nitrocellulose. Hybridize with biotin labeled primers described in **Subheading 2.2.3.** This technique necessitates binding of the blotted PCR product at a specific temperatures (for a detailed description *see* **ref. *27***).

3.3. Whole-Blood Stimulation Assay (*see* Note 7)

1. Collect whole blood samples of 4.5 mL using a Vacutainer® blood collecting system in sterile endotoxin-free blood collection tubes (Chromogenix Endotube®, Mölndal, Sweden) containing 120 IU sodium heparin. Perform venepuncture and transportation uniformly in all experiments without agitating the samples. Time from sampling to incubation must be synchronized.
2. Dilute samples 1:1 with RPMI and divide into 1.0 mL volumes in polystyrene microtiter plates.
3. Prepare serial 10-fold dilutions using 10 µL of the 250 µL aliquots and adding these to the RPMI-diluted whole-blood aliquots to obtain LPS final concentrations of 0, 10, 100, and 1000 ng/mL.
4. Incubate blood aliquots for 4 or 24 h at 37°C under a 5% CO_2 atmosphere depending on the cytokine studied. Centrifuge microtiter plates twice at 600*g* and store the supernatants at –70°C.
5. Perform ELISAs for cytokine measurements by coating polystyrene microtiter wells overnight at room temperature with specific monoclonal human antibodies followed by washing and blocking steps (*see* **Note 8**).

6. Incubate freshly thawed samples and a human standard followed by washing steps and the separate addition of biotinylated second specific antibody, streptavidin-HRP antibody, and enzyme substrate.

3.4. Identification of Patient and Control Populations

1. Enroll a consecutive series of patients with meningococcal disease (*see* **Note 9**). Diagnosis of patients should be based on: (1) the typical clinical presentation, and (2) bacterial confirmation by positive cultures from blood and cerebrospinal fluid (CSF) or positive antigen testing. Viable meningococci can be detected in the thrombotic skin lesions of most patients with sepsis even after the start of antimicrobial treatment and allows for increasing the yield of culture-positive patients *(28)*.
2. Classify patients as suffering from septic shock if blood pressure is persistently low (systolic pressure <100 mm Hg in those older than 14 yr, and systolic pressure <70 mm Hg in children younger than 14 yr) after volume replacement (10 mL/kg), and signs of end-organ failure. Nuchal rigidity is absent. The number of white blood cells in CSF is below 100/mL. All patients with septic shock have widespread purpura, skin necrosis, and consumption coagulopathy.
3. Classify patient as suffering from meningitis when pleiocytosis in CSF is present (white blood cell count >1000/mL) without hemodynamic deterioration. Patients with meningitis have petechiae only, without signs of disseminated intravascular coagulation.
4. Classify patients as exhibiting a mixed clinical picture when both signs of septic shock and meningitis are present (*see* **Subheadings 3.4.2.** and **3.4.3.**).
5. Sample control subjects who have not suffered from meningococcal disease from the similar population as where the patients originate (*see* **Note 10**). Comparison of patients with this control group enables to study susceptibility to meningococcal disease.
6. Sample control subjects embedded within the same consecutive series of patients, i.e., those who survived from meningococcal disease. Comparison of the patients who died from meningococcal disease with this control group enables to study outcome of meningococcal disease. A similar contrast can be created when sampling patients who suffered from septic shock vs those who suffered from meningitis only within the same consecutive series of patients.
7. Enroll as many first-degree relatives of a series of patients and control persons when taking a family approach. Parents, siblings, as well as children can be recruited as they all share 50% of their genome with the patient and control persons.

3.5. Calculation of Risks

1. Compare distributions of alleles and genotypes between the groups with a Chi-square test of significance. Comparison of a functional polymorphism is assessed by applying the Mann-Whitney test, which avoids any distributional assumption. As a rule, results from a functional assay are not normally distributed.
2. Estimate the risk of susceptibility for contracting the disease or developing an adverse outcome with the exposure odds ratio by simple cross-tabulation (*see*

ref. *1*, pp. 241–245). When a functional polymorphism is studied, risks can be estimated when the patients and the control persons are reclassified for the polymorphism as present/absent when dichotomized around the median of the *total* group of subjects under study.

3. Obtain a representative estimate of a functional polymorphism for patients based on their first-degree relatives. This estimate is calculated as the mean of all first-degree relatives of the patient per family. The patient is thus not included in the analysis. The estimate of the functional polymorphism for control families is calculated as the mean of all family members.
4. Adjust risk estimates for potential confounders using logistic regression. In general, there is no indication for adjustment when there are differences in demographics such as age and sex. The prevalence of a genetic polymorphism is not dependent on age and sex. Adjustment for confouding may be indicated when studying two genetic polymorphisms that are in linkage desequilibrium (*see* **Note 11**). When adjusting for confounding in a family approach, the family means are imputed in the regression models as best estimates of the patients and the control persons.

4. Notes

1. The isolation method described is a classical way giving high yields of highly purified genomic DNA suitable for almost all PCRs. Alternatively, DNA can be purified using an almost one step procedure using the QIAamp blood kit (QIAGEN, Hilden, Germany). This method with small columns is much more efficient but the DNA obtained is less pure which may result in problems when the DNA is used for PCR.
2. If it is unfeasible to sample blood for DNA, other sources that containing cellular material can be used as for instance mouth swabs ***(29)***. DNA can be isolated from this material using the aforementioned method. Instead of adding to the cell pellet, the isolation-buffer is added to the cellular material.
3. Genomic DNA can also be isolated from tissue obtained from biopsies during life as well as from material obtained from post-mortal examinations ***(30)***. This may be particularly valuable to complement a series of consecutive patients. Some of them have deceased before admitted to hospital.
4. A critical problem when performing large-scale genetic studies is contamination of the genomic DNA samples. If in the same laboratory-room PCR products and plasmids encoding a cytokine promoter are being produced it is likely that minute amounts will contaminate the genomic DNA samples. This results in the detection of the polymorphic allele of the contaminating PCR product or plasmid instead of the genotype of the patient. It is therefore essential to physically separate the rooms in which PCR products are being produced from rooms in which isolation of DNA from patient samples is being performed.
5. The design of primers is dependent on the technique that is being used. To identify alleles two ways can be chosen. First a PCR fragment is generated that contains differences in restriction sites in the allelic variant and in the wild-type. The

advantage is the simplicity of the technique, the disadvantage is incomplete digestions that may cause interpretation problems. The other way is to make PCR fragments of the whole promoter and subsequently design labeled primers that bind specifically to one of the two alleles. The advantage of the latter procedure is that a large number of patients can be tested simultaneously, but the disadvantage is that the hybridization temperatures are critical. However, the method is more time-consuming and is not applicable for fragments larger than about 2000 bp. When using highly purified genomic DNA especially the larger PCR fragments give more accurate readings of the dotblots.

6. Cytokine polymorphisms can be found on: http://www.pam.bris.ac.uk/services/GAI/cytokine4.htm. Human cytokine gene nucleotide sequence alignments can be found on: http://www.pam.bris.ac.uk/services/cytokine2.htm.
7. Different from working with genomic DNA the standardization of a functional polymorphism is decisive. We have experienced that considerable variation is introduced when procedures are only slightly changed ***(31)***. For instance, different heparin tubes, batches of endotoxin, or time-intervals between blood sampling and stimulation are all able to introduce systematic variation in the functional assays. The worst-case scenario is that the whole patient series is sampled and/or stimulated within a different time-frame than the control series. Such a practice offers the greatest chance that small differences in procedures introduce differences between the patient and the control series. Once the data are obtained, this systematic error can not be distinguished from different biological characteristics between the groups. This type of error can easily be avoided when patients and control persons are simultaneously enrolled using identical procedures.
8. The quantification of the concentration of a soluble protein is hindered by variation. All independent, noncommercial working parties on studies of concentration of cytokines (e.g., the European League against Rheumatism Study Party or **ref.** ***32***) have failed to identify a specific method that yields similar results in different laboratories of aliquots of one sample shipped to all different laboratories. We have studied the sources of variation by always including samples of pools of plasma that should give identical results. By doing this we found considerable variation over time. The best way to prevent this source of variation is to do all measurements of one particular study in one enzyme-linked immunosorbent assay (ELISA) batch within a limited time frame. In line with **Note 7**, samples of patients and control persons should be randomly distributed over the various plates.
9. A consecutive series of all patients with meningococcal disease who are admitted to a particular center should be studied. When only patients admitted to the general wards are taken into account, the series will predominantly include patients with meningitis. Series will predominantly include sepsis when only patients admitted to intensive care units are enrolled. Moreover, some patients have died before admitted to hospital. Because the polymorphism under study may well be associated with outcome, it is clear that the prevalence of the polymorphism is strongly dependent on how the patients for the study are identified. Series of patients with meningococcal disease are also different between hospitals.

Patients with meningococcal meningitis are over represented in series from district hospitals whereas patients with sepsis are over represented in series of tertiary centers. Most suitable is a consecutive series of patients that are identified within a geographical region, for instance via an obligatory notification system.
10. There is strong heterogeneity among control groups. Frequencies of gene polymorphisms are dependent on geographical and ethnic variation. Therefore it is crucial that the control series have the same distribution of geographical regions and ethnic groups. When this basic principle is neglected, spurious false-positive and false-negative associations will occur (for further reading, *see* **ref. *33***).
11. An alternative approach is to restrict the series of patients and control persons to a particular allele or genotype of the first polymorphism to study the effect of the second polymorphism ***(34)***.

References

1. Rothman, K. J. and Greenland, S. (1999) *Modern Epidemiology.* Lippincott-Raven, Philadelphia.
2. Van der Poll, T. and van Deventer, S. J. (1999) Cytokines and anticytokines in the pathogenesis of sepsis. *Infect. Dis. Clin. North Am.* **13,** 413–426.
3. Girardin, E ., Grau, G. E., Dayer, J. M., Roux-Lombard, P., J5 Study Group, and Lambert, P. H. (1988) Tumor necrosis factor and interleukin-1 in the serum of children with severe infectious purpura. *N. Engl. J. Med.* **319,** 397–400.
4. Parillo, J. E. (1993) Pathogenetic mechanisms of septic shock. *N. Engl. J. Med.* **328,** 1471–1477.
5. Wheeler, A. P. and Bernard, G. R. (1999) Treating patients with severe sepsis. *N. Engl. J. Med.* **340,** 207–214.
6. Fisher, C. J., Agosti, J. M., Opal, S. M., Lowry, S. F., Balk, R. A., Sadoff, J. C., et al. (1996) Treatment of septic shock with the tumor necrosis factor receptor: Fc fusion protein. *N. Engl. J. Med.* **334,** 1697–1702.
7. Bone, R. C. (1996) Why sepsis trials fail. *JAMA* **276,** 565–566.
8. Westendorp, R. G. J., Langermans, J. A. M., Huizinga, T. W. J., Elouali, A. H., Verweij, C. L., Boomsma, D. I., and Vandenbroucke, J. P. (1997) Genetic influence on cytokine production and fatal meningococcal disease. *Lancet* **349,** 170–173.
9. Alexander, H. R., Sheppard, B. C., Jensen, J. C., Langstein, H. N., Buresh, C. M., Venzon, D., et al. (1991) Treatment with recombinant human tumor necrosis factor-alpha protects rats against the lethality, hypotension, and hypothermia of gram-negative sepsis. *J. Clin. Invest.* **88,** 34–39.
10. Rothe, J., Lesslauer, W., Lotscher, H., Lang, Y., Koebel, P., Kontgen, F., et al. (1993) Mice lacking the tumour necrosis factor receptor 1 are resistant to TNF-mediated toxicity but highly susceptible to infection by Listeria monocytogenes. *Nature* **364,** 798–802.

11. Van Dissel, J. T., van Langevelde, P., Westendorp, R. G. J., Kwappenberg, K., and Frolich, M. (1998) Anti-inflammatory cytokine profile and mortality in febrile patients. *Lancet* **351,** 950–953.
12. Mira, J-P., Cariou, A., Grall, F., Delclaux, C., Losser, M-R., Heshmati, F., et al. (1999) Association of TNF2, a TNF-α promoter polymorphism, with septic shock susceptibility and mortality. *JAMA* **282,** 561–568.
13. Nadel, S., Newport, M. J., Booy, R., and Levin, M. (1996) Variation in the tumor necrosis factor-α gene promoter region may be associated with death from meningococcal disease. *J. Infect. Dis.* **174,** 878–880.
14. Stüber, F., Udalova, I. A., Book, M., Drutskaya, L. N., Kuprash, D. V., Turetskaya, R. L., et al. (1995) –308 tumor necrosis factor (TNF) polymorfism is not associated with survival in severe sepsis and is unrelated to lipopolysaccharide inducibility of the human promoter. *J. Inflamm.* **46,** 42–50.
15. Brinkman, B. M. N., Zuydgeest, D., Kayzel, L., Breedveld, F. C., and Verwey, C. C. (1996) Relevance of the TNF -308 promotor polymorphism in the TNF gene regulation. *J. Inflamm.* **46,** 32–41.
16. Kroeger K. M., Steer, J. H., Joyce, D. A., and Abraham, L. J. (2000) Effects of stimulus and cell type on the expression of the –308 tumor necrosis factor promoter polymorphism. *Cytokine* **12,** 110–119.
17. Kornelisse, R. F., Hazelzet, J. A., Savelkoul, H. F. J., Hop, W. C. J., Suur, M. H., Borsboom, A. N. J., et al. (1996) The relationship between plasminogen activator inhibitor-1 and proinflammatory and counterinflammatory mediators in children with meningococcal septic shock. *J. Infect. Dis.* **173,** 1148–1156.
18. Hermans P. W. M., Hibberd, M. L., Booy, R., Daramola, O., Hazelzet, J. A., de Groot, R., Levin, M., and the Meningococcal Research Group (1999) 4G/5G promoter polymorphism in the plasminogen-activator-inhibitor-1 gene and outcome of meningococcal disease. *Lancet* **354,** 556–560.
19. Westendorp, R. G. J., Hottenga, J.-J., and Slagboom, P. E. (1999) Variation in the plasminogen activator inhibitor-1 gene and risk of meningococcal septic shock. *Lancet* **354,** 561–563.
20. Khoury, M. J., Beaty, T. H., and Cohen, B. H. (1993) *Fundamentals of Genetic Epidemiology*. Oxford University Press, New York.
21. Clerget-Darpoux, F., Bonaïti-Pellié, E. (1992) Strategies based on marker information for the study of human diseases. *Ann. Hum. Genet.* **56,** 145–153.
22. Koeleman B. P., Reitsma, P. H., Bakker, E., and Bertina, R. M. (1997) Location on the human genetic linkage map of 26 genes involved in blood coagulation. *Thromb. Haemost.* **77,** 873–878.
23. Eskdale, J., Gallagher, G., Verweij, C. L., Keijsers, V., Westendorp, R. G. J., and Huizinga, T. W. J. (1998) Interleukin-10 secretion in relation to human Il-10 locus haplotypes. *Proc. Natl. Acad. Sci. USA* **95,** 94,565–94,570.
24. Van der Linden, M. W., Westendorp, R. G. J., Sturk, A., Bergman, W., and Huizinga, T. W. J. (2000) Interleukin-10 production in first degree relatives of

patients with generalized, but not cutaneous lupus erythemathodes. *J. Invest. Med.* **48,** 327–334.

25. De Jong, B. A., Schrijver, H. M., Huizinga, T. W. J., Bollen, E. L. E. M., Polman, C. H., Uitdehaag, B. M. J., et al. (2000) Innate production of IL-10 and TNF affects the risk of multiple sclerosis. *Ann. Neurol.* **48,** 641–646.
26. Brinkman, B. M. H., Huizinga, T. W. J., Breedveld, F. C., and Verwey, C. C. (1996) Allele specific quantification of TNF-α transcripts in rheumatoid arthritis. *Human Genet.* **97,** 813–818.
27. Verduyn, W., Doxiadis, I. I. N., Aholts, J., Drabbels, J. J. M., Naipal, A., D'Amaro, J., et al. (1993) Biotinylated DRB sequence-specific oligonucleotides. Comparison to serological HLA-DR typing of organdonors in Europdonor. *Human Immunol.* **37,** 59–66.
28. Van Deuren, M., van Dijke, B. J., Koopman, R. J. J., Horrevorts, A. M., Meis, J. F. G. M., Santman, F. W., and van der Meer, J. W. M. (1993) Rapid diagnosis of acute meningococcal infections by needle aspiration or biosy of skin lesions. *BMJ* **306,** 1229–1232.
29. Meulenbelt, I., Droog, S., Trommelen, G. J. M., Boomsma, D. I., and Slagboom, P. E. (1995) High yield noninvasive human genomic DNA isolation method for genetic studies in geographically dispersed families and populations. *Am. J. Hum. Genet.* **57,** 1252–1254.
30. Vandenbroucke, J. P., Bertina, R. M., Holmes, Z. R., Spaargaren, C., van Krieken, J. H., Manten, B., and Reitsma, P. H. (1998) Factor V Leiden and fatal pulmonary embolism. *Thromb. Haemost.* **79,** 511–516.
31. Van der Linden, M. W., Huizinga, T. W. J., Stoeken, D.-J., Sturk, A., and Westendorp, R. G. J. (1998) Determination of tumour necrosis factor and IL-10 in a whole blood stimulation system: assessment of laboratory error and individual variation. *J. Immunol. Methods* **218,** 63–71.
32. De Kossodo, S., Houba, V., Grau, G. E., and the WHO Collaborative Study Group. Assaying Tumor Necrosis Factor concentrations in human serum. A WHO international collaborative study (1995). *J. Immunol. Methods* **182,** 107–114.
33. Izaks, G. J., Remarque, E. J., Schreuder, G. M. T, Westendorp, R. G. J., and Ligthart, G. J. (2000) The effect of geographic origin on the frequency of HLA antigens and their association with aging. *Eur. J. Immunogen.* **27,** 107–114.
34. Rood, M. J., van Krugten, M. V., Zanelli, E., van der Linden, M. W., Keijsers, V., Schreuder, G. M. T., et al. (2000) TNF -308A and HLA-DR3 alleles contribute independently to susceptibility to systemic lupus erythematosus. *Arthritis Rheum.* **43,** 129–134.

31

Coagulation Studies

Jan A. Hazelzet, C. Erik Hack, and Ronald de Groot

1. Introduction

Disseminated intravascular coagulation (DIC) is a complex acquired, coagulopathy resulting from excessive thrombin formation. Abnormal tissue factor (TF) expression is a major mechanism initiating DIC in many disorders, including obstetric complications, sepsis, cancer, and trauma. Numerous laboratory tests are available to monitor DIC, but most patients can be adequately managed using only routine hemostasis screening tests, and assays for fibrinogen and D-dimers. Treatment of DIC should focus on reversing the underlying disorder that initiated the coagulopathy. Novel treatments are being investigated for the treatment of DIC; many of these experimental modalities target the excessive TF activity that characterizes DIC.

1.1. Activation of the Coagulation System

In severe infections, activation of coagulation can be mediated by toxins, cytokines, and several other mediators of inflammation. An important part of current insights into these pathogenic pathways has been gained from experimental studies in humans and primates. Until recently, activation of coagulation was believed to be divided into an intrinsic (contact-dependent) and an extrinsic (tissue factor-dependent) pathway both leading to the formation of thrombin and subsequently fibrin. Primary physiological importance was given to the intrinsic pathway. Although the intrinsic pathway is activated during sepsis *(1)*, it is probably not of major importance in the initiation of DIC *(2)*. More knowledge of tissue factor and the rediscovery of its inhibitor (TFPI), have led to a reappraisal of the of the coagulation system *(3)*. In this revised hypothesis, factor 7a/tissue factor complex is responsible for the initiation of

From: *Methods in Molecular Medicine, vol. 67: Meningococcal Disease: Methods and Protocols*
Edited by: A. J. Pollard and M. C. J. Maiden © Humana Press Inc., Totowa, NJ

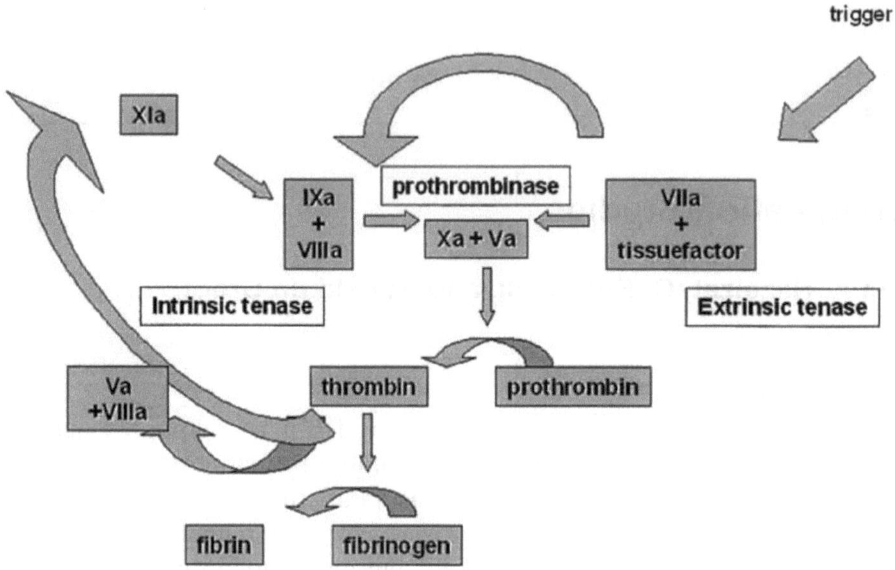

Fig. 1. Activation of coagulation.

coagulation but, owing to TFPI-mediated feedback inhibition, amplification of the procoagulant response through the actions of factor 8, 9, and 11 is required for sustained hemostasis *(3,4)*. It is now assumed that thrombin plays a crucial role in the further activation of systemic activation (**Fig. 1**). Not only may thrombin affect the aforementioned positive feedback loops, but also stimulate further platelet activation. Endotoxin-stimulated coagulation activation seems to be mediated by proinflammatory cytokines like tumor necrosis factor (TNF-α), interleukin (IL)-1, and IL-6. Experimental studies in primates suggest that IL-6 is mainly involved in the activation of coagulation, and TNF-α in the subsequent inhibition of fibrinolysis. The specific role of IL-1 is not clear.

1.2. Disseminated Intravascular Coagulation in Sepsis

1.2.1. Definition

DIC is an acquired syndrome characterized by the activation of intravascular coagulation resulting in intravascular fibrin formation. The process may be accompanied by secondary fibrinolysis or inhibition of fibrinolysis. This definition implies that clot formation in the microcirculation and consequent organ failure and/or a hemorrhagic diathesis may occur *(5)*.

1.2.2. Pathophysiology

Activation of coagulation and fibrinolysis is a normal component of the acute inflammatory response. Inflammatory cytokines initiate coagulation events locally at sites of inflammation by converting the endothelium from an antithrombotic surface to a prothrombotic surface; by stimulating tissue-factor production, which activates the extrinsic pathway of coagulation; and by stimulating production of platelet-activating factors. The fibrinolytic system is initially activated but is subsequently inhibited. This results in a marked imbalance in coagulation and fibrinolysis resulting in a net procoagulant state. When thrombin generation and platelet activation exceed the body's capacity to inactivate or remove these factors, DIC results. DIC directly contributes to multiple organ failure and death associated with sepsis.

1.2.3. Diagnosis

According to the definition of DIC, the presence of soluble fibrin is crucial for the diagnosis. There is no reliable test available for quantitatively measuring soluble fibrin at the moment, nor is there a test that is sensitive or specific enough to allow a definitive diagnosis *(5)*. However, several tests are used; *see* **Table 1** for a list of tests. To assess the presence and severity of DIC in individual patients, several diagnostic pathways have been proposed. The working group on DIC of the International Society for Thrombosis and Haemostasis is currently developing a standardized definition, a scoring system not only to establish overt DIC, but also non-overt DIC and to follow the progress of this syndrome. This scoring system is based on the score described in **Table 2**. Six points means probable DIC, 7 or more means definitive DIC. This DIC score was based on that established by the Japanese Ministry of Health and Welfare *(6)*. A simplified score is that in **Table 3**; the presence of 3 or more points is considered a positive result for presence of DIC. Another approach is to grade the clinical situation into phase of DIC as is depicted in **Table 4**.

1.3. Coagulation Disorders in Meningococcal Disease

Levels of natural inhibitors of coagulation are markedly altered during meningococcal sepsis. Several studies confirmed that antithrombin III (AT-III) levels *(7–11)*, protein S, and notably protein C *(7–9,11–14)*, are decreased in meningococcal septic shock possibly as a result of leakage of these proteins from the circulation and also as a result of consumption, inactivation, and decreased liver function. The decline in protein C levels is more pronounced than the decrease in ATIII and protein S levels. The decrease in ATIII, protein C, and protein S levels is associated with the presence of DIC and poor out-

Table 1
Laboratory Tests

Parameter	Test character	Commercially available	Behavior in sepsis	Reference in SMD
Functional				
APTT	A	Y	↑	*(15,27)*
PT	A	Y	↑	
TT	A	Y	↑	
Reptilase time	A	Y	↑	
Protamine sulfate test		Y	+	
Coagulation factors				
Fibrinogen	C	Y	↓	***(15,27–30)***
Prothrombin	A,C	Y	↓	***(8,14,15,29)***
F5	A,C	Y	↓	***(8,14,15,29)***
F7	A,C	Y	↓	***(8,14,15,29)***
F8	A,C	Y	↓	***(14)***
von Willebrand factor	C	Y	↑	***(15)***
VWF/F8			↑	***(15)***
F9	A,C	Y	↓	***(15)***
F10	A,C	Y	↓	***(15)***
F11	A,C	Y	↓	***(31)***
F12	A,B,C	Y	↓	***(31)***
Prekallikrein	A,B,C	Y	↓	***(15,31)***
Plasminogen	B,C	Y	↓	***(14–16,32)***
α1-antiplasmin	B,C	Y	↓	***(14–16,32)***
t-PA	C	Y	↑	***(15)***
PAI-1	C	Y	↑↑	***(16,17,21,32)***
Activation markers				
F1+2	C	Y	↑	
Fp A+B	C	Y	↑	
TAT	C	Y	↑	***(15,31)***
PAP	C	Y	↑	***(15)***
s-fibrin	A		↑	
FDP		Y	↑	***(16)***
D-dimers	C	Y	↑	
s-TF	C	Y	↑	
s-Protein C R	C	N	↑	
s-Thrombomodulin	C	N	↑	

(continued)

Table 1 *(continued)*

Parameter	Test character	Commercially available	Behavior in sepsis	Reference in SMD
Anticoagulant pathways				
Protein C antigen	C	Y	↓↓	*(7,8,11,12,33)*
Protein C activity	B	Y		
Protein S total	C	Y	↓	*(7,8,11,12,33)*
Antithrombin	B,C	Y	↓	*(7,8,11,33)*
TFPI	C	N	↑	*(7)*
C4BP	C	N	↓	*(15)*
Fibronectin	C	Y	↓	*(34)*

Tests
A. Clotting assay.
B. Chromogenic assay.
C. Immunoassay.

come. The higher mortality of infants with meningococcal septic shock is probably related to immaturity of the protein C system ***(13,15)***. Elevated initial levels of the extrinsic pathway inhibitor (EPI), another inhibitor of coagulation, were found in patients with fulminant meningococcemia ***(7)***. This is in contrast to the levels of ATIII and protein C. The levels of EPI were significantly higher in nonsurvivors in comparison to survivors. Furthermore, levels of EPI increased during the course of disease ***(7)***. The fibrinolytic system becomes activated by tissue plasminogen activator (TPA) during the early course of meningococcal sepsis. Subsequently, fibrinolysis is inhibited by increased levels of plasminogen activator inhibitor (PAI-1) ***(15–17)***. In patients with sepsis and septic shock TPA levels are increased and related to outcome and severity of disease ***(18,19)***. However, we could not detect significant differences in the initial levels of t-PA in survivors and nonsurvivors with meningococcal septic shock ***(15,17)***. In adult patients with nonmeningococcal septic shock, levels of plasminogen and alpha-2-antiplasmin are low in septic shock but not related to outcome ***(18,20)***. In contrast in children with meningococcal septic shock, alpha-2-antiplasmin levels as well as the ratio PAI-1/tPA were related to outcome ***(14–16)***. These changes in fibrinolytic parameters result in an ineffective fibrinolysis. Of interest, a genetic polymorphism in the promoter of the PAI-1 gene has been proposed as the explanation for higher PAI-1 levels in nonsurvivors following a similar TNF stimulus ***(17,21)***.

The massive consumption coagulopathy is characterized by low levels of coagulation factors VII, X, V, prothrombin, fibrinogen, and platelets. Because

Table 2
Extensive DIC score[a]

Diagnostic criteria for DIC	Value	DIC Score (points)
PT ratio	1.25–1.66	1
	>1.67	2
Fibrinogen (g/L)	1.00–1.50	1
	<1.00	2
FDP (μg/mL)	10–20	1
	20–40	2
	>40	3
Platelet count ($\times 10^3/\mu L$)	80–120	1
	50–80	2
	<50	3
Symptoms of bleeding	+	1
Organ failure owing to thrombosis	+	1

[a]Adapted from **ref. *6***.

Table 3
Simple DIC Score

Platelet count (10^9/L)	<150
Fibrinogen (g/L)	<2
Factor 5 (% of normal)	<60
FDP (μg/mL)	>10

of the massive demand of anticoagulation factors owing to widespread activation of the anticoagulant pathway, the host's endogenous anticoagulants are depleted causing purpura fulminans ***(13)***. This depletion is possibly age-dependent ***(13,15)***.

1.4. Relation Coagulation and Inflammation

The coagulation system can no longer be seen as an independent process in the defensive host response during inflammation. Many studies have shown several connecting points, which makes the coagulation system an integral part of the inflammatory response to all kinds of trauma (hypoxia, tissue destruction, and infectious stimuli). The endothelium can be considered as the first link between inflammation and coagulation, because damaged endothelium represents a surface where proteins involved in both coagulation and inflammation are expressed. Cytokines modulate the coagulation system by

Table 4
Phases and Laboratory Data of Acute DIC

Phases	Laboratory data
Phase 1 compensated activation	
Clinical findings:	
No symptoms	
Lab:	
• No measurable consumption of hemostasis components	• PT, aPTT, TT: within normal limits
• ↑ Activation markers	• Platelets: normal, F_{1+2}, TAT: ↑
• ↑ Enzyme-inhibitor complexes	• ATIII, Prot C: ↓
	• Soluble fibrin: present
Phase 2 decompensated activation	
Clinical findings:	
Bleeding from injuries and puncture sites, decreased organ function	
Lab:	
• Continuous ↓ platelets and coagulation factors	• PT, aPTT prolonged
• Continuous ↑ activation markers	• Platelets, fibrinogen, coagulation factor activities, ATIII, Prot C: ↓
• Continuous ↑ enzyme-inhibitor complexes	• F_{1+2}, TAT, FDP's: ↑
	• Soluble fibrin: increased
Phase 3 full-blown DIC	
Clinical findings:	
Skin bleeding of different sites, multi-organ failure	
Lab:	
Clearly expressed consumption of hemostasis components	• PT, aPTT: extremely ↑ or unclottable
	• Platelets, fibrinogen, coagulation factors, ATIII, Prot C: ↓↓
	• F_{1+2}, TAT, FDP's: ↑↑
	• Soluble fibrin: increased

Adapted from ***ref. 5***.

downregulating the expression of thrombomodulin and the activation of protein C pattern, and they induce the expression of tissue factor. At the same time, at the site of tissue injury, platelets become activated and release several mediators that further modify the balance between procoagulant and anticoagulant activities. Thrombin, formed following activation of the coagulation cascade, will promote fibrin formation, but also induces several immunological

Table 5
List of Abbrevations

APTT	Activated partial thromboplastin time
C4bp	Complement C4b binding protein
F	Factor
F1+2	Prothrombin fragment 1 + 2
FDP	Fibrin/fibrinogen degradation product
FPA	Fibrinopeptide A
MAb P	Monoclonal antibody against a proteinase
PAI-1	Plasminogen activator inhibitor-1
PAP	Plasmin-antiplasmin complex
PBS	Phosphate-buffered saline
PBST	PBS containing 0.2% (w/v) Tween 20
Poly HRP	Polymerized horseradish peroxidase
PT	Prothrombin time
SMD	Severe meningococcal disease
s-TF	Soluble tissue factor
TAT	Thrombin antithrombin complex
TFPI	Tissue-factor pathway inhibitor
TMB	Tetra-methyl-benzidin
t-PA	Tissue plasminogen activator
TT	Thrombin time

cell functions, including chemotaxis and mitogenesis *(22–25)*. Therefore, in the study of inflammation, and certainly in meningococcal disease, the involvement of the coagulation pathway has to be taken into account.

1.5. Therapeutic Options

Therapies directed towards modulating the coagulation system, have so far shown little benefit in clinical practice. Heparin, antithrombin, fresh frozen plasma, protein C concentrate (human), and recombinant TPA have all been studied, but all published therapeutic trials were descriptive studies, or used historical controls. In the beginning of 2000, a small (n = 40 pts) dose-finding, placebo-controlled study using human protein C concentrate, was concluded, but the results are not yet available (de Klein, 2001, in press). From a theoretical point of view, protein C is the most promising candidate for a phase 3 study.

- The protein C plasma levels are dramatically decreased in patients, the levels are related to outcome and severity of disease, more than any other anticoagulant.
- Treatment in septic baboons improved outcome and coagulation disturbances.
- Protein C complexes with PAI-1 and in this way decreases the inactivation of the fibrinolytic system.

However, before protein C can be an anticoagulant, it needs to be activated. During sepsis this activation might be downregulated, and it is uncertain whether supranormal levels of protein C, which were used during this study, can overcome this downregulation; in other words, can we use (human) protein C concentrate or do we need (recombinant) activated protein C. The dose-finding study should give answers to these questions. Recent experimental studies in septic animals have suggested an encouraging effect on outcome following treatment with antithrombin and TFPI *(26)*.

1.6. General Method for the Determination of Activated Clotting Proteins Bound to Inhibitors

Coagulation factors circulate in the blood as inactive precursor molecules. Hence, the coagulation factors, which upon activation are active serine proteinases, circulate as zymogens. Activation of precursor molecules occur via limited proteolysis. For example, prothrombin is converted into thrombin by activated factor X (factor Xa), which cleaves prothrombin at two sites. This reaction is much accelerated in the presence of the cofactor, factor Va. The activity of serine proteinases in plasma is tightly regulated by a set of inhibitors, including antithrombin III, α2-antiplasmin, and others. Hence, to measure activation of coagulation in plasma, measurement of the activity of coagulation factors with for example chromogenic substrates, is not a good option because most activated proteinases of the clotting system will be bound to an inhibitor at the time of testing. As complexes between most inhibitors and activated clotting proteinases are very stable, measurement of the levels of these complexes in plasma may provide an alternative to measure activation of coagulation in vivo. Indeed measurement of, for example, thrombin-antithrombin III complexes has been done in a number of studies.

Complexes between activated clotting proteinases and inhibitors can be sensitively measured with enzyme-linked immunosorbent assay (ELISA) systems, in particular with monoclonal antibodies (MAbs) against neoepitopes expressed on the complex. If such antibodies are not available, the complexes can be measured with a so-called double-antibody sandwich ELISA, in which an antibody against one moiety of the complex (f/e thrombin) is used to catch the complexes, and a labeled antibody against the other moiety to detect bound complexes. The disadvantage of the latter system is that the catching antibody will bind both the activated factor (as a complex with an inhibitor) as well as the nonactivated zymogen (prothrombin). Hence, at too low dilutions of the samples, the zymogen will compete with the complex for binding to the catching antibody, and negatively influence the detection of the latter. This problem can be overcome by testing higher dilutions, but this has the disadvantage that the assay becomes less sensitive. In practice, levels of most clotting proteinases in plasma are within a range that, considering the sensitivity of the assay, dilutions can be tested at which the catching antibody is able to capture all zymogen and activated proteinases form a sample. A general procedure to measure such complexes is given in **Subheading 3.** Such a procedure applies to various complexes. The authors have experience with measuring factor XIIa-C1-inhibitor, kallikrein-C1-inhibitor, factor XIa-complexes (C1-inhibitor, antithrombin III, α2-antiplasmin, α1-antitrypsin), thrombin-antithrombin III, plasmin-α2-antiplasmin, TPA/PAI-1, and UPA/PAI-1 complexes. In the procedure presented here, a MAb against a clotting proteinase (MAb P) is used for coating, and a biotinylated MAb against the inhibitor (biot-MAb I) is used for the detection of bound complexes. P can be thrombin, factor XIa etc, I can be antithrombin III or other inhibitors. Many suitable antibodies can be purchased from companies. Results obtained are measured and related with those obtained with a standard, whereafter the concentration of the complex in the sample to be tested can be calculated.

2. Materials

1. 96-well ELISA plates (for example Maxisorb Nunc).
2. 0.1 *M* sodium-carbonate-bicarbonate buffer, pH 9.6 (coating buffer).
3. Distilled water.
4. Phosphate-buffered saline (PBS), pH 7.4.
5. PBS containing 0.2% (w/v), Tween 20 (PBST).
6. PBS containing 2% (v/v), cow milk (blocking buffer).
7. High-performance ELISA (HPE) buffer (CLB, Amsterdam, the Netherlands).
8. Polymerized horseradish peroxidase coupled to streptavidin (poly HRP; CLB).
9. Tetra-methyl-benzidin 0.1 mg/mL in 0.11 *M* sodium acetate, pH 5.5, containing 3% (v/v), H_2O_2 (TMB solution).
10. 2 *M* H_2SO_4.

3. Methods

1. Dilute MAb P appropriately (usually 1–5 μg/mL) in coating buffer.
2. Add 100 μL of diluted MAb P to each well of the ELISA plate.
3. Incubate plates for overnight at room temperature.
4. Wash plates 3 times with distilled water.
5. Add 100 μL of blocking buffer to each well.
6. Incubate the plates with for one hour at 37°C.
7. Wash plates 5 times with PBST.
8. Dilute samples to be tested: for example, EDTA (10 m*M*), plasma appropriately in HPE buffer.
9. Add 100 μL of the diluted samples per well of the ELISA plate (*see* **Note 1**).
10. Incubate the plates for 1 h at 37°C.
11. Wash plates 5 times with PBST.

12. Dilute biotinylated MAb I appropriately diluted HPE-buffer (1 mg/mL solution usually has to be diluted about 1 : 1000).
13. Add 100 µL of diluted biotinylated MAb I to each well.
14. Incubate plates for 1 h at 37°C.
15. Wash plates 5 times with PBST.
16. Dilute poly-HRP appropriately (1 mg/mL solution usually 1 : 10,000) in blocking buffer.
17. Add 100 µL of diluted poly-HRP to each well of the ELISA plate.
18. Incubate the plates for 1 h at 37°C.
19. Wash plates 5 times with PBST.
20. Add 100 µL of TMB solution to each well.
21. Incubate the plates for an appropriate time (usually 10–30 min) at room temperature.
22. Add 100 µL of 2 *M* H_2SO_4 to each well to block further conversion of the substrate.
23. Measure the absorption of the wells at 450 nm (*see* **Note 2**).

Most active serine proteinases are inactivated in plasma by proteinase inhibitors. Among the inhibitors, those belonging to the superfamily of serine proteinase inhibitors ("serpins") are important. They inhibit their target proteinases by forming covalent complexes in which the active site serine of the proteinase is covalently linked to the amino acid residue at the so-called P1-position of the reactive site loop of the serpin. These complexes are only formed between serpin and active proteinase and not between serpin and zymogen. Hence, the level of proteinase-serpin complexes in biological fluids is a parameter for the amount of active proteinase generated. Generally, these complexes form within seconds to minutes after the formation of an active proteinase, so direct measurement of the active proteinase, for example with chromogenic substrates should occur within seconds to minutes after that formation, which is for practical reasons not feasible. Proteinase-serpin complexes are cleared from the circulation with a half-life time of 15–120 min by specific receptors in the liver. In the liver, complexes are digested and degraded, and in this way the proteinase is removed. Hence, the presence of increased levels of proteinase-serpin complexes points to enhanced formation of the active serine proteinase, and in case the proteinase is a member of the coagulation system, to activation of the coagulation system. The absence of complexes in a plasma sample itself does argue against the formation of an active proteinase in vivo, and in case of a clotting proteinase, against activation of the coagulation system, because the activation process has proceeded more slowly and over a longer period of time, which, considering the relatively rapid clearance of the complexes in vivo, may only induce a moderate increase of complex levels in the circulation.

Alternatively, serine proteinases bound to biological compounds may be protected against the inactivation by serpins. In such a situation, complexes between the active proteinase and the serpins are not formed. For example, thrombin bound to fibrin is protected against inactivation by antithrombin III. In such a situation, concentrations of so-called activation peptides, for example, the F1+2-fragment that is cleaved from prothombin upon activation by the prothrombinase complex, may better reflect the activation of the serine proteinase.

4. Notes

1. Each plate should contain a dose-response curve (that is, different dilutions) of a standard that is used to derive concentrations from the measured absorption at 450 nm. In addition, each plate should contain negative and positive control samples (preferably plasma samples from patients with high and normal levels of the parameter tested. Increased responses of negative controls or decreased responses of positive controls point to errors in the assay or problems with reagents, and in generally are a reason for repeated testing of samples in the hope that a mistake during the initial testing has been made. If the abnormal responses of negative and/or positive controls are repeatedly found, the various reagents used in the ELISA should be tested. For example, upon storage, MAbs used in the assay may become aggregated, leading to worse performance of the assay. Reproducibility of the assay can be assessed by establishing the variation coefficient for samples with high or low values, and should for this type of assay be below 20%, preferably below 10%.
2. To correct for aspecific background of the plates (opalescence) absorption at 450 nm can be corrected by measuring absorbance at 540 nm as well.

References

1. Wuillemin, W. (1997) Activation of the contact system in patients with sepsis and with septic. *Blood* **89(10),** 3893.
2. Pixley, R., Cadena, R. D. L., Page, J., Kaufman, N., Wyshock, E., Chang, A., Taylor, F., and Colman, R. (1993) The contact system contributes to hypotension but not disseminated intravascular coagulation in lethal bacteremia. *J. Clin. Invest.* **91,** 61–68.
3. Broze, G. J., Jr. (1995) Tissue factor pathway inhibitor and the revised theory of coagulation. *Annu. Rev. Med.* ***46,*** *103–112.*
4. Luchtman-Jones, L. and Broze, G. J. Jr. (1995) The current status of coagulation. *Ann. Med.* **27(1),** 47–52.
5. Muller-Berghaus, G., ten Cate, H., and Levi, M. (1999) Disseminated intravascular coagulation: clinical spectrum and established as well as new diagnostic approaches. *Thromb. Haemost.* **82(2),** 706–712.
6. Wada, H., Wakita, Y., Nakase, T., Shimura, M., Hiyoyama, K., Nagaya, S., Mori, Y., and Shiku, H. (1995) Outcome of disseminated intravascular coagulation in relation to the score when treatment was begun. Mie DIC Study Group. *Thromb. Haemost.* **74(3),** 848–852.

7. Brandtzaeg, P., Sandset, P. M., Joo, G. B., Ovstebo, R., Abildgaard, U., and Kierulf, P. (1989) The quantitative association of plasma endotoxin, antithrombin, protein C, extrinsic pathway inhibitor and fibrinopeptide A in systemic meningococcal disease. *Thromb. Res.* **55(4),** 459–470.
8. Fourrier, F., Lestavel, P., Chopin, C., Marey, A., Goudemand, J., Rime, A., and Mangalaboyi, J. (1990) Meningococcemia and purpura fulminans in adults: acute deficiencies of proteins C and S and early treatment with antithrombin III concentrates. *Intensive Care Med.* **16(2),** 121–124.
9. Fourrier, F., Chopin, C., Goudemand, J., Hendrycx, S., Caron, C., Rime, A., et al. (1992) Septic shock, multiple organ failure, and disseminated intravascular coagulation. Compared patterns of antithrombin III, protein C, and protein S deficiencies. *Chest* **101(3),** 816–823.
10. Fourrier, F., Chopin, C., Huart, J., Runge, I., Caron, C., and Goudemand, J. (1993) Double-blind, placebo-controlled trial of antithrombin III concentrates in septic shock with disseminated intravascular coagulation. *Chest* **104,** 882–888.
11. Leclerc, F., Hazelzet, J. A., Jude, B., Hofhuis, W., Hue, V., Martinot, A., and van der Voort, E. (1992) Protein C and S deficiency in severe infectious purpura of children: a collaborative study of 40 cases. *Intensive Care Med.* **18(4),** 202–205.
12. Powars, D. R., Rogers, Z. R., Patch, M. J., McGehee, W. G., and Francis, R. B. (1987) Purpura fulminans in meningococcemia: association with acquired deficiencies of protein C and S. *N. Engl. J. Med.* **317(9),** 571–572.
13. Powars, D., Larsen, R., Johnson, J., Hulbert, T. Sun, T., Patch, M. J., Francis, R., and Chan, L. (1993) Epidemic meningococcemia and purpura fulminans with induced protein C deficiency. *Clin. Infect. Dis.* **17,** 254–261.
14. Fijnvandraat, K., Derkx, B., Peters, M., Bijlmer, R., Sturk, A., Prins, M. H., et al. (1995) Coagulation activation and tissue necrosis in meningococcal septic shock: severely reduced protein C levels predict a high mortality. *Thromb. Haemost.* **73,** 15–20.
15. Hazelzet, J. A., Risseeuw-Appel, I. M., Kornelisse, R. F., Hop, W. C. G., Dekker, I., Joosten, K. F. M., de Groot, R., and Hack, C. E. (1996) Age-related differences in outcome and severity of DIC in children with septic shock and purpura. *Thromb. Haemost.* **76(6),** 932–938.
16. Brandtzaeg, P., Joo, G. B., Brusletto, B., and Kierulf, P. (1990) Plasminogen activator inhibitor 1 and 2, alpha-2-antiplasmin, plasminogen, and endotoxin levels in systemic meningococcal disease. *Thromb. Res.* **57(2),** 271–278.
17. Kornelisse, R. F., Hazelzet, J. A., Savelkoul, H. F. J., Hop, W. C. J., Suur, M. H., Borsboom, A. N. J., Risseeuw-Appel, I. M., v. d. Voort E., and d. Groot, R. (1996) The relationship between plasminogen activator inhibitor-1 and proinflammatory and counterinflammatory mediators in children with meningococcal septic shock. *J. Infect. Dis.* **173,** 1148–1156.
18. Voss, R., Matthias, R. R., Borkowski, G., and Reitz, D. (1990) Activation and inhibition of fibrinolysis in septic patients in an internal intensive care unit. *Br. J. Haematol.* **75,** 99–105.

19. Philippé, J., Offner, F., Declerck, P. J., Leroux-Roels, G., Vogelaers, D., Baele, G., and Collen, D. (1991) Fibrinolysis and coagulation in patients with infectious disease and sepsis. *Thromb. Haemost.* **65(3),** 291–295.
20. Hesselvik, J. F., Blombäck, M., Brodin, B., and Maller, R. (1989) Coagulation, fibrinolysis, and kallikrein systems in sepsis: relation to outcome. *Crit. Care Med.* **17(8),** 724–733.
21. Hermans, P. W., Hibberd, M. L., Booy, R., Daramola, O., Hazelzet, J. A., de R., Groot, and Levin M. (1999) 4G/5G promoter polymorphism in the plasminogen-activator-inhibitor-1 gene and outcome of meningococcal disease. Meningococcal Research Group. *Lancet* **354(9178),** 556–560.
22. Taylor, F. (1994) The inflammatory-coagulant axis in the host response to gram-negative sepsis: regulatory roles of proteins and inhibitors of tissue factor. *N. Horizons* **2,** 555–565.
23. Esmon, C. T., Fukudome, K., Mather, T., Bode, W., Regan, L. M., Stearns-Kurosawa, D. J., and Kurosawa, S. (1999) Inflammation, sepsis, and coagulation. *Haematologica* **84(3),** 254–259.
24. Cicala, C. and G. Cirino (1998) Linkage between inflammation and coagulation: an update on the molecular basis of the crosstalk. *Life Sci.* **62(20),** 1817–1824.
25. de Jonge, E., Levi, M., Stoutenbeek, C. P., and van Deventer, S. J. (1998) Current drug treatment strategies for disseminated intravascular coagulation. *Drugs* **55(6),** 767–777.
26. de Jonge, E., Dekkers, P. E., Creasey, A. A., Hack, C. E., Paulson, S. K., Karim, A., et al. (2000) Tissue factor pathway inhibitor dose-dependently inhibits coagulation activation without influencing the fibrinolytic and cytokine response during human endotoxemia. *Blood* **95(4),** 1124–1129.
27. McManus, M. L. and Churchwell, K. B. (1993) Coagulopathy as a predictor of outcome in meningococcal sepsis and the systemic inflammatory response syndrome with purpura. *Crit. Care Med.* **21,** 706–711.
28. Vik-Mo, H., Lote, K., and Nordoy, A. (1978) Disseminated intravascular coagulation in patients with meningococcal infection: laboratory diagnosis and prognostic factors. *Scand. J. Infect. Dis.* **10(3),** 187–191.
29. Giraud, T., Dhainaut, J. F., Schremmer, B., Regnier, B., Desjars, P., Loirat, P., et al. (1991) Adult overwhelming meningococcal purpura. A study of 35 cases, 1977–1989. *Arch. Intern. Med.* **151(2),** 310–316.
30. Leclerc, F., Beuscart, R., Guillois, B., Diependaele, J. F., Krim, G., Devictor, D., Bompard, Y., and van-Albada, T. (1985) Prognostic factors of severe infectious purpura in children. *Intensive Care Med.* **11(3),** 140–143.
31. Wuillemin, W. A., Fijnvandraat, K., Derkx, B. H. F., Peters, M., Vreede, W., Cate, H. T., and Hack, C. (1995) Activation of the intrinsic pathway of coagulation in children with meningococcal septic shock. *Thromb. Haemost.* **74,** 1436–1441.
32. Engebretsen, L., Kierulf, P., and Brandtzaeg, P. (1986) Extreme plasminogen activator inhibitor and endotoxin values in patients with meningococcal disease. *Thromb. Res.* **42,** 713–716.

33. Fijnvandraat, K., Peters, M., Derkx, B., van Deventer, S., and ten Cate, J. W. (1994) Endotoxin induced coagulation activation and protein C reduction in meningococcal septic shock. *Prog. Clin. Biol. Res.* **388,** 247–254.
34. Blanco, A., Guisasola, J. A., Solis, P., Bachiller, R., and Gonzalez, H. (1990) Fibronectin in meningococcal sepsis. Correlation with antithrombin III and protein C. *Acta Paediatr. Scand.* **79(1),** 73–76.

32

Complement Pathways and Meningococcal Disease

Diagnostic Aspects

Anders G Sjöholm, Lennart Truedsson, and Jens C. Jensenius

1. Introduction

1.1. Description of the Complement System

Complement is an immunological effector system that bridges innate and acquired immunity in several ways. There is a striking association between susceptibility to meningococcal disease and various forms of complement deficiency *(1,2)*. In defense against bacterial infection, the most important function of complement is probably to serve as a mediator of antibody-dependent immunity. Specific antibodies can trigger activation of the classical and the alternative pathways of complement activation *(3–5)*. It is well known that antibody-independent mechanisms interfere with alternative pathway activation on the bacterial surface *(6,7)*. The newly discovered mannan-binding lectin (MBL) pathway of complement activation appears to be protective against many types of infection *(8)* and adds previously unsuspected aspects of innate immunity to complement-mediated defense. Interestingly, immune responses are influenced by complement *(9)*, and it could be that acquisition of protective antibodies is impaired in some types of complement deficiency. A further aspect of interactions between *Neisseria* and complement is the potential role of membrane-bound complement regulators as cellular receptors for the microbes *(7)*.

The complement system consists of more than 30 proteins, including soluble complement proteins, membrane-bound regulators, and cellular complement receptors *(3)*. The soluble complement proteins may be divided into different functional units: the classical activation pathway, the alternative activation pathway, the MBL activation pathway, and the membrane attack pathway con-

From: *Methods in Molecular Medicine, vol. 67: Meningococcal Disease: Methods and Protocols*
Edited by: A. J. Pollard and M. C. J. Maiden © Humana Press Inc., Totowa, NJ

sisting of the late complement components that assemble to form the membrane attack complex (MAC, C5b-C9n). C3, the major complement protein in plasma, has several functions and participates in recruitment of MAC through the three activation pathways.

The classical pathway comprises $C1qr_2s_2$, C4, C2, and C3 is usually triggered by specific antibodies forming immune complexes with antigens on the surface of target cells or in the fluid phase *(3)*. The $C1qr_2s_2$ complex binds through the C1q subcomponent to the Fc portion of IgM and IgG antibodies. Binding results in activation of zymogen C1r, which in turn activates C1s. C1s cleaves C4 and C2 with formation of classical pathway C3 convertase (C4b2a). When activated C3 (C3b) is generated, the convertase acquires C5-cleaving activity, and can then recruit cytotoxic C5b-C9n. C3 and C4 contain an internal thiol ester bond, which is exposed as a result of activation. The carbonyl group of the thiol ester is reactive with hydroxyl and amino groups, whereby C3b and C4b bind covalently to polysaccharides and proteins with formation of ester and amide bonds, respectively. The classical pathway is controlled by C1 inhibitor (C1 INH), which dissociates activated $C1qr_2s_2$ complexes with formation of complexes containing C1 INH, C1r, and C1s ***(10)***, and by C4-binding protein, which together with factor I contributes to downregulation of classical pathway C3 convertase *(7)*.

The MBL pathway is antibody-independent, and includes MBL and the MBL-associated serine proteases 1 and 2 (MASP-1 and MASP-2), C4, C2, and C3 ***(8,11)***. MBL recognizes sugars such as mannose and N-acetylglucosamine on microbial and other surfaces. MBL resembles C1q, and MBL/MASP complexes are partly analogous to the $C1qr_2s_2$ complex. Activation leads to recruitment of classical pathway C3 convertase. MASP-1 reportedly cleaves C3 directly ***(12)***. C1 INH contributes to the control of MBL/MASP complexes ***(13)***.

The alternative pathway consists of C3, factor B, factor D, and properdin. The control proteins factor H and factor I may be described as integral parts of the pathway ***(3)***. The alternative pathway lacks a distinct recognition molecule analogous to C1q or MBL. Activation of the pathway depends on continuous formation of a C3b-like molecule, $C3(H_2O)$, by hydrolysis of the internal thiol ester of C3. $C3(H_2O)$ binds factor B allowing factor D to cleave factor B. This gives rise to limited amounts of a fluid-phase C3-cleaving enzyme $C3(H_2O)Bb$. Part of the C3b generated by the action of the initial enzyme will fix covalently to microbial or other target surfaces with hydroxyl or amino groups. Some surfaces allow the deposited C3b to form alternative pathway C3 convertase (C3bBb), while other surfaces allow the control proteins factor H and factor I to abolish alternative pathway activation by dissociation of C3bBb and degradation of C3b to iC3b. Further degradation leads to the release of C3c from C3dg fragments that remain covalently bound to the antigen. The C3dg fragment (39 kD) is a likely physiological end-product of C3 breakdown, but can be further degraded into C3d (34 kD) and C3g (5 kD) by proteolytic enzymes such as trypsin. Properdin stabilizes the C3bBb complex and sometimes appears to be of critical importance for alternative pathway activation. Deficiencies of factor I or factor H lead to secondary C3 deficiency through uncontrolled activation and breakdown of C3 in the circulation.

The surface properties that distinguish between activators and nonactivators of the alternative pathway are not altogether well-defined. Sialylated structures and other polyanions are often found on the surface of non-activators and are known to promote factor H function *(6)*. Specific uptake of factor H and C4-binding protein by microbial surface proteins probably protects microorganisms against complement *(7)*.

The immunological importance of the alternative pathway in antibody-mediated defense may not be fully appreciated. In complement-sufficient persons, the alternative pathway is considered to serve as a powerful amplification mechanism for complement activation initiated through the classical pathway by small amounts of antibody. Complement activation initiated through the MBL pathway may be amplified in a similar fashion. Antibodies can also activate the alternative pathway independent of classical pathway C3 convertase, which is most clearly important in classical pathway-deficiency states *(14)*. Antibodies binding to appropriate targets provide sites for C3b deposition that are protected from factors I and H *(4)*. Evidence suggests that specific IgA and IgG2 antibodies that bind to antigens with high epitope density are efficient activators of the alternative pathway *(5)*.

C3 convertases (C4b2a and C3bBb) combined with C3b cleave C5 into C5a and C5b. The smaller C5a fragment has anaphylatoxic and chemotactic activity, while the larger C5b fragment combines with C6 and initiates assembly of MAC, the cytotoxic complex of C5b, C6, C7, C8, and C9 that inserts into cell membranes *(3)*. MAC formation is controlled by S protein and clusterin in the fluid phase and by the membrane-bound regulators HRF and CD 59.

1.2. Complement-Mediated Defense

Complement supports several functions that contribute to protection against disease as well as to expression of disease manifestations *(1,2,15)*. With regard to protection against bacterial infection, deposition of opsonic C3 fragments (C3b and iC3b) on the bacterial surface, and assembly of MAC resulting in serum bactericidal activity, are probably the principal effector mechanisms. Phagocytes have receptors that recognize the C3b (complement receptor 1,

CR1) and iC3b (complement receptor 3, CR3) ligands on the bacterial surface. Gram-positive bacteria such as *Streptococcus pneumoniae* can be eliminated by opsonophagocytosis, but are completely resistant to the bactericidal action of MAC. By contrast, both mechanisms are functional in defence against Gram-negative bacteria such as *Neisseria meningitidis* and *Hemophilus influenzae* type b. Phagocytic killing probably predominates in defence against *N. meningitidis* serogroup B, while other meningococci such as serogroup Y may preferentially be eliminated by direct killing in serum ***(16)***. Perhaps surprisingly, the consequences of C5 deficiency appear to be similar to those of other late complement component deficiencies indicating that the chemotactic C5a fragment is not of critical importance in this context.

1.3. Complement and Meningococcal Disease

1.3.1. Complement Deficiencies Associated with Meningococcal Disease

Deficiencies of the late complement components C5-C9 and of the alternative pathway component properdin demonstrate a very clear association with susceptibility to meningococcal disease. The incidence of meningococcal disease is probably about 50% in both groups, but may be lower in properdin deficiency ***(1,2,15)***. Recurrent disease is typical in patients with deficiencies of C5-C8. Although some patients with deficiencies of C5-C8 have severe disease, the survival rate is higher than in complement-sufficient patients. C9-deficiency is fairly common in the Japanese population with an approximate prevalence of 0.1%. C9 deficiency appars to have milder consequences than deficiencies of the other late complement components. Meningococcal disease in properdin deficiency is associated with high mortality, at least in some families. As in complement-sufficient patients, properdin-deficient survivors of meningococcal infections do not show recurrent disease.

Meningococccal disease has been reported in almost every form of complement deficiency. Patients with rare genetic defects of C3 are susceptible to infections caused by encapsulated bacteria such as meningococci and are also susceptible to other infections. C2 deficiency is fairly common in Western populations with an estimated prevalence of 0.01–0.0025%. Invasive infections with encapsulated bacteria have been documented in about 25% of reported C2-deficient patients. Deficiencies of classical pathway components are also associated with development of systemic lupus erythematosus (SLE).

While MBL has been firmly established as a component of the complement system, the issue of MBL deficiency and disease is partly distinct from that of the other complement deficiency states. MBL deficiency is found in about 10% of the general population ***(17)***, and one must assume that for yet unknown reasons a balanced polymorphism must be of some biological advantage. On the other hand, an increased prevalence of MBL deficiency has been reported in many types of infection *(8,18,19)*. Recent evidence also suggests that MBL deficiency may be an important predisposing factor for meningococcal disease *(20)*, even if this question is still controversial. Interestingly, the MBL pathway has been shown to be activated by *N. meningitidis* mutants with unsialylated lipooligosaccharides *(21)*.

Properdin deficiency is X-linked, which implies that many males in affected families may be at risk of developing meningococcal disease. Other complement deficiencies show an autosomal-recessive mode of inheritance, which implies that the risk of more than one case of homozygous deficiency in a family is usually limited to first-degree relatives. The genetics of MBL deficiency are fairly complex. The deficiency phenotype is determined by mutations of structural genes as well as by promoter region alleles *(22)*. Thus, MBL deficiency can occur in persons with heterozygous defects of MBL structural genes as well as in persons with homozygous defects, and even in persons homozygous for the wild type structural allele *(23)*.

Autoantibodies to alternative pathway convertases, C3 nephritic factors (C3NeF), block the action of factors H and I and produce C3 hypercatabolism and persistently low C3 concentrations *(24)*. This condition is the most common form of C3 deficiency, and may present with meningococcal disease. Other conditions with acquired complement deficiency are not usually associated with meningococcal disease.

For unknown reasons, meningococcal disease in complement deficiency is mostly caused by the *N. meningitidis* serogroups W-135 and Y, even if the serogroups B and C have also been observed *(1,2,15)*.

1.3.2. Complement Activation in Meningococcal Disease

In patients with meningococcal disease, complement activation leading to manifest hypocomplementaemia has long been known to be associated with a poor prognosis *(25)*. Later studies have shown that endotoxin levels in meningococcal disease are correlated with fatal outcome and with the degree of complement activation as assessed by measurement of C3 fragments and SC5b-C9 complexes in the circulation *(26)*.

1.4. Prophylactic Treatment in Complement Deficiency

Vaccination responses to tetravalent meningococcal vaccine covering the serogroups A, C, W-135, and Y have been documented in terminal component deficiencies, properdin deficiency, and in a few patients with C3 deficiency *(27,28)*. In addition, bactericidal and opsonic vaccination responses have recently been reported in C2 deficiency *(14)*. Experience of vaccination in complement deficiency is still limited. Considering the risk of fulminant infection in X-linked properdin deficiency, identification and vaccination of properdin-deficient relatives of index cases is strongly recommended. Long-term prophylaxis with antibiotics has been tried in patients with recurrent meningococcal disease *(2)*. It is likely that a new generation of protein-polysaccharide conjugate vaccines against A, C Y, and W135 meningococci, and perhaps other vaccines currently under development, will be used in this context in the future.

1.5. Detection of Complement Deficiency

Ordinary immunochemical measurements of C3 and C4 will often reveal acquired hypocomplementemia and form an important part of basic complement analysis. However, given the large number of complement proteins in serum, complement analysis must include screening procedures for assessment of whole complement function in order to detect the various complement deficiencies. Hemolytic titration of the classical pathway and the alternative pathway by CH50 procedures *(29)* is often considered the gold standard for the purpose. On the other hand, these techniques are time-consuming and not altogether well suited for analysis of clinical samples. In this chapter, we have chosen to describe three simplified procedures for assessment of whole complement function. Qualitative hemolytic gel *(30)* and quantitative hemolytic approaches *(31)* were chosen. The third assay system is an enzyme-linked immunosorbent assay (ELISA) based on detection of complement deposition *(32)*. As yet there are no validated methods for functional assessment of the MBL pathway. Instead, we describe specific measurements of MBL *(17,33)*. For measurement of other individual complement proteins, we refer to the literature *(29,34)*.

In our opinion, all patients with an invasive infection caused by *N. meningitidis*, or other encapsulated bacteria, should be screened for complement function with the main purpose of excluding complement deficiency in individual patients and families. Quite clearly, the identification of various complement deficiency states provides a basis for clinical guidance and for prophylactic treatment policies. Complement investigation should be mandatory in some patient groups: 1) Patients with a family history of meningococcal disease occurring in accordance with an X-linked pattern (properdin deficiency), 2) patients with recurrent meningococcal disease (deficiencies of C5-C9), 3) patients with meningococcal disease caused by serogroups Y and W-135 and by very rare serogroups, and 4) patients with severe infections caused by different encapsulated bacteria (deficiencies of the classical pathway and C3). Investigations may be performed in convalescence a few weeks following infection. When available, sera from patients with fulminant infection should be analyzed with regard to the possible importance of subsequent family investigation, particularly in properdin deficiency. With regard to the MBL pathway, it is important to stress that this complement activation pathway was only recently discovered and that our understanding of the clinical manifestations of MBL deficiency is still poorly developed.

Widespread application of the assays for MBL measurement described here will undoubtedly promote our understanding of the significance of this phylogenetically ancient defense mechanism.

2. Materials

2.1. Qualitative Hemolytic Gel Assays

1. Blood-collection tubes with no anticoagulant.
2. Ethylene diamine tetraacetic acid (EDTA) blood collection tubes with enough EDTA for 10 mmol/L final concentration.
3. Serum and EDTA plasma: collect blood specimens by venepuncture into tubes without anticoagulant and with EDTA. Allow coagulation to proceed for about 1 h at room temperature. Keep the blood at 4°C for another hour before centrifugation (2000*g* for 5 min). The EDTA blood can be centrifuged immediately. Concerning handling and transportation of samples, *see* **Note 1**.
4. Veronal-buffered saline (VBS): 2.5 m*M* 5,5 diethyl barbituric acid, 4.5 m*M* sodium 5,5 diethyl barbiturate, pH 7.4, 145 m*M* NaCl. Prepare a stock VBS solution that is five times the concentration of the isotonic VBS used in the assays. For preparation of the stock VBS, dissolve 85.0 g NaCl and 3.75 g Na-5,5 diethyl barbiturate in 1400 mL of distilled water and 5.75 g 5,5 diethyl barbituric acid in 500 mL hot distilled water. Mix the two solutions and cool to room temperature. Adjust the volume to 2000 mL. The stock VBS is stable for at least 1 mo at 4°C.
5. Make stock solutions containing 0.3M $CaCl_2$, 1M $MgCl_2$, 0.2 M sodium EDTA (pH 7.5), and 0.2 M ethylene glycol tetraacetate EGTA for addition to VBS as required. The EGTA (Sigma Chemical Co, St. Louis, MO) is most easily dissolved at alkaline pH.
6. For the classical pathway assay, VBS with 0.15 m*M* Ca^{2+} and 0.5 m*M* Mg^{2+} (VBS^{++}) is used. For comments on divalent cations and complement function, *see* **Note 2**.
7. For the alternative pathway assay, VBS containing EGTA and Mg^{2+} is used (VBS-MgEGTA). VBS-MgEGTA with 10 m*M* EGTA and 5 m*M* Mg^{2+} is suitable for the hemolytic gel assay. For further comment, *see* **Note 2**.
8. Target erythrocytes: Sheep and guinea-pig erythrocytes (E) stored in Alsever's solution at 4°C for a few days before use. Cells from sheep, guinea pigs, and rabbits for hemolytic assays are commercially available from many sources (National Health or Veterinary Institutes of several countries; Bradsure Biologicals Ltd, UK) and remain stable for up to 4 wk. Antibody-sensitized sheep E ($_{sh}$EA) are used for the classical pathway assay. The cells (10^9 E/mL, 5% packed E [v/v]) are thoroughly washed in VBS containing 10 m*M* EDTA (VBS-EDTA) until no hemoglobin is visible in the supernatant.

9. Rabbit anti-sheep hemolysin containing IgM and IgG antibodies is commercially available from several sources (Sigma; Dade-Behring, Deerfield, IL). For further comment, *see* **Note 3**. The lowest dose of hemolysin that does not limit lysis of $_{sh}$EA by guinea-pig serum is used ***(35)***. Alternatively, a subagglutinating dose of hemolysin can be determined ***(29)***. For determination of a subagglutinating dose, serial dilutions of hemolysin in VBS-EDTA (0.05 mL) are mixed in microtiter plate wells with equal volumes of E (10^9/mL). The highest antibody dose that does not cause agglutination is chosen.
10. For hemolytic assays, $_{sh}$E (10^9/mL) and the selected dose of hemolysin are mixed in equal volumes and incubated for 15–30 min at room temperature or at 37°C before use. The $_{sh}$EA are stable at 4°C for about a week.
11. Unsensitized guinea-pig E ($_{gp}$E) are used for the alternative pathway assay.
12. Preparation of hemolytic gels: For the classical pathway assay, agarose (Agarose ME, SeaKem, FMC Bioproducts, Rockland, ME) at 0.6% (w/v) is suspended in VBS^{++} and is then dissolved by heating. The agarose is allowed to cool to about 50°C and is then rapidly mixed with $_{sh}$EA. Before mixing, the required amount of $_{sh}$EA is pelleted by centrifugation (2000*g*, 5 min). The pelleted $_{sh}$EA are resuspended in VBS^{++} at 5×10^8 cells/mL and the suspension is prewarmed to 37°C before mixing with the agarose. The final cell concentration in the gel should be 0.5–1.0%. The gel, 1-mm thick, is cast between glass plates held apart by a plastic U-frame and assembled with paper clips. The gel is allowed to set, and one of the glass plates is then removed by carefully sliding it across the base of the plastic frame. Preferably, the gel can be cast onto the hydrophilic surface of a Gel-bond film (FMC Bioproducts) placed between the U-frame and one of the glass plates. The procedure for preparation of gels for the alternative pathway assay is the same apart from the use of VBS-MgEGTA buffer and of unsensitized $_{gp}$E as target cells. After preparation, the hemolytic gels are stored in moist chambers at 4°C and can be used for at least 1 wk.

2.2. Simplified Quantitative Hemolytic Assays

1. Serum samples: *see* **Subheading 2.1.1.** EDTA plasma is not recommended for this assay.
2. Buffers: *see* **Subheading 2.1., items 4–7**. In these assays, gelatin (Sigma) is added at 0.1% (w/v) to VBS^{++} and VBS-MgEGTA in order to minimize spontaneous hemolysis of target cells. The gelatin is dissolved in the buffers by brief heating during agitation.
3. Target erythrocytes: For preparation of $_{sh}$EA for the classical pathway assay, *see* **Subheading 2.1., items 8–10**. Unsensitized rabbit E ($_{ra}$E) (for source, *see* **Subheading 2.1.8.**) suspended in VBS-MgEGTA containing 4 m*M* Mg^{++} and at 16 m*M* EGTA are used as target cells in the quantitative alternative pathway assay.

2.3. Complement Deposition ELISA

1. Serum samples: *see* **Subheading 2.1.1.** EDTA plasma is not recommended for this assay.
2. Microtiter plates: Falcon cat. no. 3915, Becton Dickinson (Lincoln Park, NJ).

3. Coating buffer: 50 m*M* carbonate buffer, pH 9.5.
4. Complement activators: Purified polyclonal IgM (IgMκ PHP 003, Serotec, Oxford, UK) and lipopolysaccharide (LPS) from *Salmonella typhosa* (Sigma).
5. Blocking agents: human serum albumin (HSA; Sigma, Cat. no. A-9511), Tween 20 (Sigma).
6. Assay buffers: phosphate-buffered saline (PBS), 10 m*M* sodium phosphate, pH 7.2, 100 m*M* NaCl; PBS containing 0.05% Tween 20 (PBS-T); VBS^{++} (*see* **Subheading 2.1.6.**) containing 1% HSA; VBS-EGTA (*see* **Subheading 2.1.7.**) containing 1% HSA.
7. Microtiter plate incubation: thermoblock (Dri.block, DB-IM, Techne, Cambridge; UK).
8. Conjugated antibodies: monoclonal mouse antihuman $C5b\text{-}C9_n$ IgG (Code no. M 777, Dakopatts, Glostrup, Denmark) and polyclonal rabbit antihuman properdin IgG. We have used properdin antibodies prepared in the laboratory. Commercial preparations are available from several sources (Sigma; Binding Site Ltd, Birmingham, UK). The antibodies were conjugated with alkaline phosphatase (P 6774, Sigma)
9. Substrate: disodium-*p*-nitrophenyl phosphate (Sigma) 1 mg/mL dissolved in 10% (w/v) diethanolamine, pH 9.8, with 101 mg $MgCl_2$ and 200 mg NaN_3 added per L (Sigma).

2.4. Specific Measurement of MBL

2.4.1. Sandwich ELISA for the Estimation of MBL as Antigen

1. Serum or EDTA plasma samples (*see* **Subheading 2.1.3.**). MBL is very stable (*see* **Note 1**).
2. Calibration: standard curves are constructed using dilutions of an in-house serum or plasma pool (2–3 μg MBL/mL), which is calibrated against the World Health Organization (WHO) standard serum obtainable from Statens Serum Institut, Copenhagen, Denmark. In our laboratory the WHO standard was estimated to contain MBL at 2.8 μg/mL when compared with purified MBL (quantified by amino acid analysis).
3. Quality controls: in order to cover the range of MBL encountered, four internal controls are included in each assay. Serum or plasma with MBL concentrations at about 10, 50, 250, and 1250 ng/mL are suitable.
4. Microtiter plates: for ELISA we use conventional microtiter plates (Maxisorb, Nunc, Kamstrup, Denmark).
5. Coating buffer: PBS, 10 m*M* phosphate, pH 7.4, 140 m*M* NaCl (*see* **Note 10**).
6. Monoclonal antibodies (MAbs) for coating: anti-MBL (MAb 131-1, Statens Serum Institut). MAb 131-10 (Statens Serum Institut) also works well.
7. Assay and washing buffer: Tris-buffered saline (TBS) with Tween 20 (TBS/Tween), 10 m*M* Tris/HCl, pH 7.4, 140 m*M* NaCl, 7.5 m*M* NaN_3, with or without 0.05% (v/v) Tween 20 (Sigma).
8. Biotin-labeled anti-MBL: biotinylate MAb 131-1 with biotin-N-hydroxysuccinimide (BNHS, Sigma). Thirty μL of a 1 mg BNHS/mL DMSO and 1 mg antibody in 1 mL PBS/bicarbonate, pH 8.5, are mixed and incubated for 2 h at

room temperature followed by dialysis against TBS in the cold. For storage at 4°C the biotinylated antibody is diluted with an equal volume of TBS containing 2% (w/v) HSA (Sigma).
9. Alkaline phosphatase-labeled avidine (Sigma, A2527).
10. Substrate: 0.12 m*M* bromochloroindolyl phosphate, 0.12 m*M* nitroblue tetrazolium, 4 m*M* $MgCl_2$, 0.1 *M* ethanolamine, pH 9.0.

2.4.2. Time-Resolved Immunofluorometric Assay (TRIFMA)

1. Materials for TRIFMA are largely the same as those used for the ELISA (**steps 1–7**).
2. Microtiter plates: Another type of plate is used for TRIFMA (Fluoroplates, Nunc). Conventional ELISA plates can be used for TRIFMA, but may vary considerably in background reading from batch to batch.
3. Europium-labeling is carried out similarly to biotinylation using 0.2 mg Eu-chelate of diethylene-triamine-tetraacetic acid (DTTA) phenylisothiocyanate (Wallac Oy, Turku, Finland) and 1 mg antibody at pH 8.5 for 20 h at room temperature, followed by dialysis against TBS. The labeled antibody, diluted with 10 mL TBS containing 1% (w/v) HSA, is stable for years at 4°C.

2.4.3. Lectin ELISA for Determination of MBL

1. Materials are largely the same as those used for the sandwich ELISA for estimation of MBL as antigen.
2. Coating: mannan (Sigma) in carbonate buffer (*see* **Subheading 2.3.3.**) is used.

3. Methods

3.1. Qualitative Hemolytic Gel Assays

3.1.1. Sample Application and Diffusion

1. Apply undiluted serum or EDTA plasma samples to 3-mm wide wells punched in the $_{sh}$EA and $_{gp}$E gels. The wells should be fairly closely spaced (10–12 mm) so as to allow partial interaction between adjacent samples (**Fig. 1**). Keep gels cool during application.
2. Allow diffusion in a moist chamber to proceed at 4°C for 18 h.
3. Transfer the gels to a moist chamber at 37°C for development of hemolytic reactions for about 2 h.
4. Inspect the gels directly and then dry them to preserve indefinitely.

3.2.2. Drying of Gels

1. Cover gels with a filter paper soaked in physiological saline and a 10 mm thick wad of soft absorbent paper.
2. Place a weight (2.5–10 g/cm^2) on top of the absorbent paper to exert a gentle pressure over the gel surface for 15 min.
3. The filter paper is removed and the gel is dried in the air or in front of a hot air fan.

3.2.3. Evaluation of Results

1. The hemolytic gel assays should be strictly regarded as a qualitative means to detect complement deficiencies. Measurement of zone diameters may be very misleading, particularly when pathological sera are concerned.
2. Concerning controls including pooled normal serum and complement-deficient sera, *see* **Notes 1** and **4**.
3. Three patterns should lead to suspicion of complement deficiency: absent hemolysis, partial hemolysis within the entire hemolytic area, and extremely small hemolytic zones. The presence of hemolytic crescents produced when adjacent wells provide a missing complement protein very strongly suggests complement deficiency (**Fig. 1**). The finding of full hemolysis virtually always excludes the presence of complement deficiency. Various inhibitory ring patterns are owing to antibodies interfering with the sensitized cells or immune complexes and are not associated with complement deficiency. Inhibitory antibodies include antibodies to $_{sh}E$ and rheumatoid factors.
4. Occasional properdin-deficient sera may produce normal patterns of hemolysis.
5. Examples of results obtained with complement-deficient sera are shown in **Fig. 1.**

3.2. Simplified Quantitative Hemolytic Assays

3.2.1. Classical Pathway

1. Mix serum (0.1 mL) diluted 1/5 in VBS^{++} with 0.1 mL of a 50% suspension of $_{sh}EA$ (10^9 cells/mL).
2. Incubate the mixture at 37°C for 20 min during agitation.
3. Stop the reaction by addition of ice-cold VBS-EDTA (3 mL).
4. Centrifuge (2000*g* for 10 min) and then read the optical density (OD) of the supernatant at 541 nm.
5. Correct the OD for background (cells incubated in buffer). The proportion of hemolysed cells is obtained by dividing the corrected OD with the OD obtained with cells completely lysed with 0.1% Na_2CO_3.
6. Express classical pathway activity in a test serum as a percentage of the activity in a reference serum, usually pooled normal human serum.

3.2.2. Alternative Pathway

1. Mix undiluted serum (0.05 mL) with 0.1 mL of a 50% suspension of $_{ra}E$ (10^9 cells/mL) in VBS-MgEGTA (*see* **Note 7**).
2. **Steps 2–6** are identical to those described for the classical pathway (**Subheading 3.2.1.**).

3.2.3. Evaluation of Results

1. Reference values should be established in each laboratory. Normal sera are expected to yield values in the approximate range between 50 and 150% of that obtained with pooled normal serum.

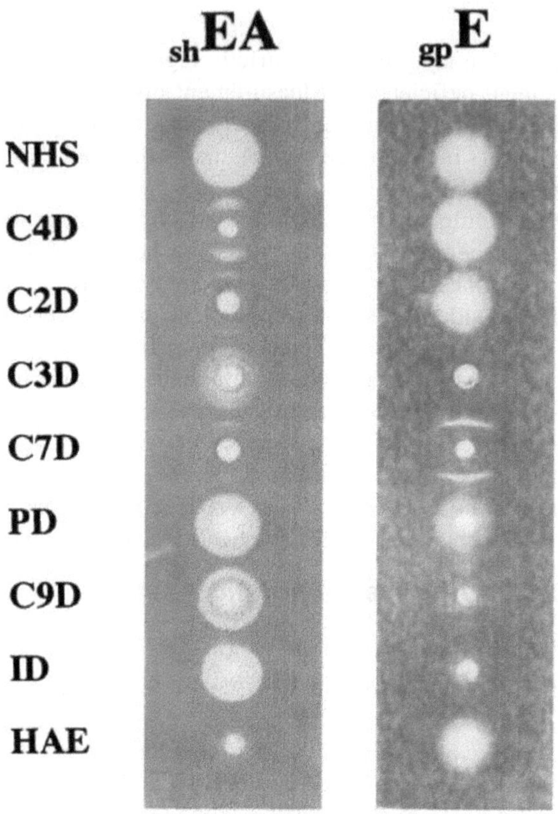

Fig. 1. Hemolytic gels for detection of complement deficiency. Classical pathway-mediated lysis of antibody-coated sheep erythrocytes ($_{sh}$EA) and alternative pathway-mediated lysis of guinea-pig erythrocytes ($_{gp}$E). Normal human serum (NHS) produces full lysis in both assays. Sera deficient in classical pathway proteins, exemplified with C4- and C2-deficient sera (C4D, C2D), and hereditary angioedema serum (HAE), show impaired lysis of $_{sh}$EA and normal lysis of $_{gp}$E. Sera with defects of the alternative pathway such as properdin- and factor I-deficient sera (PD and ID) show impaired lysis of $_{gp}$E and normal lysis of $_{sh}$EA. C3- and C7-deficient sera show impaired lysis of both target cell types. C9-deficient serum (C9D) masquerades as a defect of the alternative pathway. "Hemolytic crescents" in conjunction with absence of lysis is caused by a missing factor diffusing in from neighboring wells. Ring patterns as seen with C9D and $_{sh}$EA may occur and do not indicate complement deficiency.

2. Concerning controls including pooled normal serum and complement-deficient sera (*see* **Notes 1** and **4**).
3. Detection of subtotal properdin deficiency (*see* **Note 7**).

3.3. Complement Deposition ELISA

3.3.1. Coating Procedure

1. Coat microtiter plates with IgM for the classical pathway and with LPS for the alternative pathway. The coating dose is 1 μg/well in 0.05 mL of carbonate buffer with incubation overnight at 4°C.
2. Use two coated wells and one uncoated background control well for each serum sample.
3. Wash the wells twice with PBS after coating, and then block all wells with HSA (1% [w/v] 0.15 mL/well) for 2 h at room temperature.

3.3.2. Complement Deposition, Classical Pathway

1. Incubate IgM-coated wells and control wells for 15 min at 37°C with 0.05 mL serum diluted 1/4 in VBS^{++} containing 1% HSA. Incubations are preferably carried out in a thermoblock.
2. Stop the reaction by washing 3 times with PBS-T.
3. Add conjugated antihuman C5b-$C9_n$ (0.05 mL) in VBS^{++} with 1% HSA. After 2 h at room temperature the plates are washed 3 times with PBS-T.
4. Add substrate (0.05 mL) to the microtiter plate wells.
5. Measure the absorbance at 405 nm after 1 h at room temperature. A corrected absorbance value is obtained as the difference between the mean value with coated wells and the background well.

3.3.3. Complement Deposition, Alternative Pathway

1. Incubate LPS-coated wells and control wells for 30 min at 37°C with 0.05 mL serum diluted 1/4 in VBS-EGTA containing 1% HSA. Incubations are preferably carried out in a thermoblock.
2. Stop the reaction by washing 3 times with PBS-T.
3. Add anti-properdin conjugate (0.05 mL) in VBS^{++} with 1% HSA. After 2 h at room temperature the plates are washed 3 times with PBS-T.
4. **Steps 4** and **5** are identical to those described for the classical pathway assay.

3.3.4. Evaluation of Results

1. The combination of the classical and the alternative pathway complement deposition assays will probably reveal all known types of complement deficiency. Pooled normal serum is a suitable reference (*see* **Notes 1** and **4**). The results should be regarded as semiquantitative: complement deficiency is expected to result in absent or markedly reduced complement deposition in either or both of the assays.

2. An additional IgM-ELISA with detection of properdin deposition could be used for differentiation between terminal component deficiencies and defects of the classical activation pathway *(32)*.

3.4. Specific Measurement of MBL

3.4.1. Sandwich ELISA for the Estimation of MBL as Antigen

1. Coat wells by incubation overnight at 4°C with anti-MBL (300 ng MAb 131-1 or 100 ng MAb 131-10).
2. Wash the wells with TBS/Tween. The plates may then be kept with the wells filled with TBS at 4°C for months until use.
3. Empty the wells of the microtiter plate and add the test samples, internal controls, and calibrator after 20-fold dilution in TBS/Tween with 1 m*M* EDTA. Further twofold dilutions of the calibrator for the standard curve are made with the same buffer.
4. Incubate the plate overnight at 4°C (if a faster test is deemed desirable, shorter incubations may be used, e.g., 1 or 2 h at room temperature).
5. Wash with TBS/Tween, and then incubate for 2 h with 100 ng biotinylated anti-MBL antibody in 100 µL TBS/Tween.
6. Wash with TBS/Tween, and then add 100 µL of AP-labeled avidine diluted 2500-fold in TBS/Tween.
7. Incubate for 1 h at room temperature, wash.
8. Add enzyme substrate, and incubate at room temperature or at 37°C until satisfactory color development has occurred (*see* **Note 11**).
9. Read the OD at 405 nm on an ELISA reader.

3.4.2. TRIFMA for the Estimation of MBL as Antigen

1. General considerations: *see* **Note 12**.
2. The assay is carried out essentially as the ELISA.
3. One alternative is to add Eu-labeled streptavidin (Wallac, diluted 1000 fold in TBS/Tween with 25 µ*M* EDTA) instead of the enzyme-labeled avidin.
4. Incubate 1 h, wash, and then add 200 µL of enhancement reagent (Wallac).
5. Shake for 5 min, and read in the time resolved fluorometer (Wallac) whenever convenient (cover the plate or keep moist to prevent evaporation if the reading is delayed).
6. For routine analyses, we use a secondary antibody directly labeled with Eu (**Subheading 2.4.2., item 3**). Thus, instead of biotinylated MAb 131-1 add 20 ng Eu-labeled 131-1, incubate for 2 h, wash, add enhancement reagent and continue as above.

3.4.3. Assay for MBL as Lectin

1. Except for coating the plates with mannan instead of primary antibody, and the use of calcium-containing buffers *(17)*, this assay is carried out as described for the antigen ELISA or TRIFMA (*see* **Note 13**).

2. Microtiter wells are coated with 100 μL of mannan at 10 μg/mL in bicarbonate buffer (**Subheading 2.3.3.**) as described above.
3. It is important to remember that MBL is a calcium-dependent lectin. Thus all buffers for dilution and for wash should contain calcium (we use 5 m*M* $CaCl_2$), until the addition of substrate or enhancement solution (the only exception being the buffer for diluting the Eu-labeled reagent, when the assay is carried out as TRIFMA, which must be 25 μ*M* in EDTA).

4. Notes

1. For most purposes, including the functional complement assays described in this chapter, it is quite satisfactory if serum and EDTA plasma samples are kept at 4°C and are frozen at –80°C the same day that the blood samples are obtained. Generation of complement activation products such as C3dg fragments and SC5b-C9 is negligable in EDTA plasma stored at 4°C overnight ***(36)***. Transportation of frozen samples should preferably be in boxes with dry ice. A practical advantage with the qualitative hemolytic gel assays is that complement deficiencies can usually be discerned or excluded in unfrozen samples that are 2–3 d old. MBL and most of the other complement proteins are very stable as antigens for detection by immunochemical assays. Thus, samples conserved with merthiolate or sodium azide may be sent by ordinary mail and can be stored at –20°C for prolonged periods.
2. During complement activation, Ca^{2+} is required for complex formation between C1q, C1r, and C1s, while Mg^{2+} is required for complex formation between C4b and C2 and between C3b and factor B, i.e., for generation of the C3 convertases. Ca^{2+} is also required for binding of MBL to sugar structures, but does not appear to influence the integrity of MBL/MASP complexes. In alternative pathway assays, the Ca^{2+}-dependent $C1qr_2s_2$ complex is dissociated by the chelator EGTA, which binds Ca^{2+} with high affinity and blocks classical-pathway and MBL-pathway activation. Mg^{2+} is added to the system to ensure efficient generation of C3 convertase. The chelator EDTA blocks complement activation altogether through binding of Ca^{2+} and Mg^{2+}.
3. IgM antibodies usually predominate in commercial hemolysins; isolated IgM antibodies are preferable and can be obtained by gel filtration on Sephacryl S300 (Pharmacia, Uppsala, Sweden) or other suitable media.
4. Pooled normal serum is useful as a reference in screening tests for detection of complement deficiency. Sera from healthy donors are obtained as described above (*see* **Note 1**). The sera are pooled and subdivided and the individual lots then frozen at –80°C. With regard to other controls, it is wise to include complement-deficient sera in the assays, at least at regular intervals. Sera representing deficiencies of different functional units, e.g., C2-deficent serum, properdin-deficent serum, and serum from persons with C5, C6, C7, or C8 deficiency are recommended.
5. In hemolytic assays, C2 deficiency can be overlooked if the concentrations of rabbit antibody to sheep erythrocytes are too high.

6. In the quantitative hemolytic assays, target erythrocytes are added in such an excess that normal sera will be able to lyse about 25% of the cells. This implies that hemolysis within a very wide range can be measured with a single dose of serum. It has been shown that the number of cells lysed by a certain amount of serum is unchanged even in a large excess of target cells ***(31)***. With particular regard to alternative pathway function, we believe that the option to use a high serum concentration (>30%) in the assay is an important advantage.
7. Detection of subtotal properdin deficiency by quantitative hemolysis may require kinetic studies ***(37)***.
8. Commercial kits for assessment of complement function do not usually include tests for the alternative pathway.
9. Hemolytic gels for assessment of the classical and the alternative pathways are available (Binding Site).
10. For coating of plates in MBL assays, do NOT use the traditional bicarbonate coating buffer, which is detrimental to many specific antibodies during the coating procedure.
11. Obviously, peroxidase-labeled avidin or streptavidin with a suitable substrate may be used instead of phosphatase. In our experience, phosphatase is superior owing to ease of handling, e.g., no stop reagent is needed, and the sensitivity of the assay is easily increased by prolonged incubation with substrate.
12. TRIFMA takes advantage of the long fluorescence of the rare earth metal, europium (Eu). The costs of the the time-resolved fluorometer (Wallac) is not much above that of an ELISA reader. We find TRIFMA to be superior to ELISA on several accounts: the detection range is substantially larger, typically covering five orders of magnitude, the signal to noise ratio is about one thousand, and the sensitivity and reproducibility is better.
13. The quantitative results of the assay for MBL as a lectin ***(17)*** correlated closely (>97%) with the results of the TRIFMA, when the same monoclonal developing antibody (MAb 131-1) was used.

References

1. Sjöholm, A. G. (1990) Inherited complement deficiency states: implications for immunity and immunological disease. *APMIS* **98,** 861–874.
2. Figueroa, J. E. and Densen, P. (1991) Infectious diseases associated with complement deficiencies. *Clin. Microbiol. Rev.* **4,** 359–395.
3. Law, S. K. A and Reid, K. B. M. (1995) *Complement* (Male, D., ed.), In Focus, IRL Press, Oxford, UK, pp. 1–88.
4. Fries, L. F., Gaither, T. A., Hammer, C. H., and Frank, M. M. (1984) C3b covalently bound to IgG demonstrates a reduced rate of inactivation by factors H and I. *J. Exp. Med.* **160,** 1640–1655.
5. Valim, Y. M. L. and Lachmann, P. J. (1991) The effect of antibody isotype and antigenic density on the complement-fixing activity of human immune complexes: a system study using chimaeric anti-NIP antibodies with human Fc regions. *Clin. Exp. Immunol.* **84,** 1–8.

6. Vogel, U. and Frosch, M. (1999) Mechanisms of neisserial serum resistance. *Mol. Microbiol.* **32,** 1133–1139.
7. Lindahl, G., Sjöbring, U., and Johnsson, E. (2000) Human complement regulators: a major target for pathogenic microorganisms. *Curr. Opin. Immunol.* **12,** 44–51.
8. Turner, M. W. (1996) Mannose-binding lectin: the pluripotent molecule of the innate immune system. *Immunol. Today* **17,** 532–540.
9. Fearon, D. T. and Locksley, R. M. (1996) The instructive role of innate immunity in the acquired immune response. *Science* **272,** 50–54.
10. Laurell, A.-B., Mårtensson, U., and Sjöholm, A. G. (1987) C1 dissociation: the spontaneous generation in human serum of a trimer complex containing C1 inactivator, activated C1r and zymogen C1s. *J. Immunol.* **139,** 4145–4151.
11. Thiel, S., Vorup-Jensen, T., Stover, C. M., Schwaeble, W., Laursen, K., Poulsen, K., et al. (1997) A second serine protease associated with mannan-binding lectin that activates complement. *Nature* **386,** 506–510.
12. Matsushita, M. and Fujita, T. (1995) Cleavage of the third component of complement (C3) by mannose-binding protein-associated serine protease (MASP) with subsequent complement activation. *Immunobiology* **194,** 443–451.
13. Wong, N. K. H., Kojima, M., Dobó, J., Ambrus, G., and Sim, R. B. (1999) Activities of the MBL-associated serine proteases (MASPs) and their regulation by natural inhibitors. *Mol. Immunol.* **36,** 853–861.
14. Selander, B., Käyhty, H., Wedege, E., Holmström, E., Truedsson, L., Söderström, C., and Sjöholm, A. G. (2000) Vaccination responses to capsular polysaccharides of *Neisseria meningitidis* and *Haemophilus influenzae* type b in two C2-deficient sisters: alternative pathway-mediated bacterial killing, and evidence for a novel type of blocking IgG. *J. Clin. Immunol.* **20,** 138–149.
15. Sullivan, K. E. and Winkelstein, J. A. (1999) Genetically determined deficiencies of the complement system, in *Primary Immunodeficiency Diseases* (Ochs, H. D., Smith, C. I. E., and Puck, J. M., eds.), Oxford University Press, New York, pp. 397–416.
16. Ross, S. C., Rosenthal, P. J., Berberich, H. M., and Densen, P. (1987) Killing of *Neisseria meningitidis* by human neutrophils: implications for normal and complement-deficient individuals. *J. Infect. Dis.* **155,** 1266–1275.
17. Christiansen, O. B., Kilpatrick, D. C., Souter, V., Varming, K., Thiel, S., and Jensenius, J. C. (1999) Mannan-binding lectin deficiency is associated with unexplained recurrent miscarriage. *Scand. J. Immunol.* **49,** 193–196.
18. Summerfield, J. A., Sumiya, M., Levin, M., and Turner, M. W. (1997) Association of mutations in mannose binding protein gene with childhood infection in consecutive hospital series. *BMJ* **314,** 1229–1232.
19. Nielsen, S. L., Andersen, P. L., Koch, C., Jensenius, J. C., and Thiel, S. (1995) The level of the serum opsonin, mannan-binding protein in HIV-1 antibody-positive patients. *Clin. Exp. Immunol.* **100,** 219–222.
20. Hibberd, M. L., Sumijya, M., Summerfield, J. A., Booy, R., Levin, M., and the Meningococcal Research Group. (1999) Association of variants of the gene for mannose-binding lectin with susceptibility to meningococcal disease. *Lancet* **353,** 1049–1053.

21. Jack, D. L., Dodds, A. W., Anwar, N., Ison, C. A., Law, A., Frosch, M., et al. (1998) Activation of complement by mannose-binding lectin in isogenic mutants of *Neisseria meningitidis* serogroup B. *J. Immunol.* **160,** 1346–1353.
22. Madsen, H. O., Garred, P., Thiel, S., Kurtzhals, J. A., Lamm, L. U., Ryder, L. P., and Svejgaard, A. (1995) Interplay between promoter and structural gene variants control basal serum level of mannan-binding protein. *J. Immunol.* **155,** 3013–3020.
23. Steffensen, R., Thiel, S., Varming, K., Jersild, C., and Jensenius, J. C. (2000) Detection of structural gene mutations and promoter polymorphisms in the mannan-binding lectin (MBL) gene by polymerase chain reaction with sequence-specific primers. *J. Immunol. Methods* **241,** 33–42.
24. Spitzer, R. E., Stitzel, A. E., and Tsokos, G. C. (1996) Nephritic factor autoantibodies, in *Autoantibodies* (Peter, J. B. and Shoenfeld, Y., eds.), Elsevier Science B. V., Amsterdam, pp. 540–545.
25. Greenwood, B. M., Onyewotu, I. I., and Whittle, H. C. (1976) Complement and meningococcal infection. *BMJ* **1,** 797–799.
26. Brandtzaeg, P., Mollnes, T. E., and Kierulf, P. (1989) Complement activation and endotoxin levels in systemic meningococcal disease. *J. Infect. Dis.* **160,** 58–65.
27. Söderström, C., Braconier, J. H., Käyhty, H., Sjöholm, A.G., and Thuresson, B. (1989) Immune response to tetravalent meningococcal vaccine: opsonic and bactericidal functions of normal and properdin deficient sera. *Eur. J. Clin. Microbiol. Infect. Dis.* **8,** 220–224.
28. Fijen, C. A. P., Kuijper, E. J., Drogari-Apiranthitou, M., van Leeuwen, Y., and Daha, M. R. (1998) Protection against meningococcal serogroup ACYW disease in complement-deficient individuals vaccinated with the tetravalent meningococcal capsular polysaccharide vaccine. *Clin. Exp. Immunol.* **114,** 362–369.
29. Whaley, K. and North, J. (1997) Haemolytic assays for whole complement activity and indivual components, in *Complement: A Practical Approach* (Dodds, A. W. and Sim, R. B., eds.), Oxford University Press, Oxford, UK, pp. 19–47.
30. Truedsson, L., Sjöholm, A. G., and Laurell, A.-B. (1981) Screening for deficiences of the classical and alternative pathways of complement by hemolysis in gel. *Acta Pathol. Microbiol. Scand. (C)* **89,** 161–166.
31. Nilsson, U. R. and Nilsson, B. (1984) Simplified assays of hemolytic activity of the classical and alternative complement pathways. *J. Immunol. Methods* **72,** 49–59.
32. Nordin Fredrikson, G., Truedsson, L., and Sjöholm, A. G. (1993) New procedure for the detection of complement deficiency by ELISA. Analysis of activation pathways and circumvention of rheumatoid factor influence. *J. Immunol. Methods* **166,** 263–270.
33. Fischer, P. B., Ellermann-Eriksen, S., Thiel, S., Jensenius, J. C., and Mogensen, S. C. (1994) Mannan-binding protein and bovine conglutinin mediate enhancement of herpes simplex virus type 2 infection in mice. *Scand. J. Immunol.* **39,** 439–445.
34. Svehag, S.-E. and Leslie, R. G. Q. (1997) Immunochemical methods for the detection of complement components and complement activation, in *Complement:*

A Practical Approach (Dodds, A. W. and Sim, R. B., eds.), Oxford University Press, Oxford, UK, pp. 19–47.
35. Mayer, M. M. (1961) Complement and Complement fixation in *Experimental Immunochemistry* (Kabat, E. A. and Mayer, M. M., eds.), Thomas, Springfield, IL, pp. 133–240.
36. Mollnes, T. E. (1985) Early- and late-phase activation of complement evaluated by plasma levels of C3d,g and the terminal complement complex. *Complement* **2,** 156–164.
37. Sjöholm, A. G., Söderström, C., and Nilsson, L.-Å. (1988) A second variant of properdin deficiency: the detection of properdin protein at low concentration in affected males. *Complement* **5,** 130–140.

33

Evaluation of New Treatments for Meningococcal Disease

Simon Nadel, Iain Macintosh, and Michael Levin

1. Introduction

It is recognized that improvement in the practice of clinical medicine, including confirmation of the safety and efficacy of some current interventions, depends greatly on the pursuit of appropriate research. It therefore follows that improved clinical care of children depends on their participation in pediatric research. Furthermore, in the absence of relevant research, harm to children may result. Thus formal studies of therapeutic modalities in children is seen as a moral imperative to ensure that children have equal and safe access to existing and new agents *(1)*.

1.1. Meningococcal Disease

Meningococcal disease is now the most common infectious disease cause of death in children in the UK *(2)*. Recent years have seen an explosion in our understanding of the pathophysiology of meningococcal disease and other forms of sepsis and septic shock. Along with this increased understanding has come improved recognition of the complexity of the humoral and cellular immune responses, unraveling of the dynamic interaction between host and pathogen, and huge advances in the understanding of the genetic regulation of the host response to infection. The complexity of these factors ensures that significant improvements in treatment of meningococcal disease will not come about solely by simple approaches to therapy, but by improved understanding of the increasingly complex pathophysiology that occurs following invasion of *Neisseria meningitidis* into the bloodstream.

From: *Methods in Molecular Medicine, vol. 67: Meningococcal Disease: Methods and Protocols*
Edited by: A. J. Pollard and M. C. J. Maiden © Humana Press Inc., Totowa, NJ

1.2. A Model of Sepsis

Several features regarding meningococcal disease make it an ideal model to investigate potential new therapies.

Meningococcal disease:

1. Is a severe illness in which outcome can be accurately predicted and its morbidity readily documented;
2. Is readily recognized and confirmed;
3. Is relatively common;
4. Occurs in previously healthy children;
5. Has well defined pathophysiology;
6. Has standard treatment protocols; and
7. Is well-characterized for disease classification.

Meningococcal infection causes a spectrum of disease from meningitis, with a case-fatality rate of less than 3%, to septicemia and fulminant shock, with a case-fatality rate of up to 50%. Most cases occur in children under 5 yr of age. The overall case-fatality rate for children with meningococcal disease is about 10%. Up to 50% of children with meningococcal disease have features of septicemia with evidence of systemic sepsis or septic shock *(3)*.

Several scoring systems have been validated for use in children with meningococcal disease, in order to more accurately predict those who have more severe illness who would benefit from admission to intensive care units, and also those with a high risk of death who may benefit from the use of potentially beneficial but unproven experimental therapies.

Because of these factors, it would appear that meningococcal disease would be an ideal disease model for the assessment and evaluation of new therapies. Unfortunately, there have been disappointingly few well conducted studies of potentially useful treatments for patients with meningococcal disease. There are many reasons why this is the case, including the failure of many adult sepsis studies, the lack of a good animal model for meningococcal disease, and the fact that most cases of meningococcal disease occur in children.

1.3. Adult Sepsis Studies

There are many examples of failed clinical trials in the field of sepsis and septic shock in adult patients. These studies have enrolled many thousands of patients in multi-center, placebo-controlled, double-blind studies to evaluate new treatment strategies *(4)*. Most of these studies have failed in their aim of demonstrating a reduction in mortality owing to the use of an experimental anti-inflammatory treatment. Unfortunately, studies on improving the treatment of meningococcal disease have suffered because of the failure of these trials. Only by understanding the reasons for these failures will we be able to learn how to conduct more successful trials in the future.

Meningococcal disease is a remarkable illness in that it most commonly affects previously healthy children and adolescents. Adult sepsis studies have often failed because of the heterogeneous nature of the patients recruited. Usually, patients recruited in trials of adult sepsis treatments are critically ill for a variety of reasons. They may be elderly, and have several underlying illnesses that precipitated their admission to intensive care units, including cancer, trauma, cardiovascular disease, and post-surgery.

Sepsis and the systemic inflammatory response syndrome (SIRS) (*see* Appendix for definitions) is the final common pathway that occurs in many critically ill patients for a variety of reasons and secondary to a variety of pathogens. Many of the failed sepsis studies have evaluated a single therapeutic agent determined by a variety of in vitro and in vivo experiments. Expecting this agent to act as a magic bullet that uniformly benefits adult septic shock is a major challenge.

1.4. Animal Studies

Meningococcal infection is a human disease. Unfortunately, there is no natural animal host for *N. meningitidis*. Expecting to extrapolate useful information from animal models of septic shock can give misleading and overly optimistic estimates of the efficacy of new treatment regimens. Apart from the fact that clinically the time of onset of infection is impossible to evaluate, animal models use uniform subjects with known nutritional and genetic makeup, with a specified onset of infection and a timed treatment intervention in relation to the insult. Many human studies of new therapies follow their successful evaluation in animal models.

In addition, many of the anti-cytokine studies in human sepsis follow animal experiments in which pro-inflammatory cytokines are demonstrated to be centrally implicated in the pathophysiology of sepsis. In these animal studies, blocking the pro-inflammatory cytokine under investigation leads to improved survival. Unfortunately, the situation in human septic shock is much more complex. At the time of presentation, patients may have variable levels of endotoxin or other bacterial-derived inflammatory factors in their bloodstream, together with a bewildering array of pro- and anti-inflammatory cytokines and other factors in their blood and tissues. The relation between blood levels of these factors and tissue levels, which are likely to be much more relevant, has yet to be determined. Also, some adult studies have shown a worsening of outcome following blockade of pro-inflammatory cytokines in patients with septic shock. This suggests that timing of intervention is critical, as there is a delicate balance between pro- and anti-inflammatory host response, which may be vital for survival.

2. Methods

As alluded to earlier, adult sepsis studies include a heterogeneous mix of patients with different underlying diseases, different microbiological causes, and a variety of hemodynamic parameters. These factors and the appropriateness of anti-microbial therapy are major determinants of outcome. It may be difficult or impossible to control for these variables in large multi-center studies. Because of this, the trial agent must be highly effective for its effects to be recognized. Unfortunately, most studies of new therapies for sepsis have been underpowered to detect positive effects of the agent being studied. In addition, failure to reach the primary endpoint for the study, which is usually mortality, leads to rejection of specific agents that may be clinically useful in certain designated groups of patients. These agents may not be as effective as isolated modes of therapy, but in combination with other agents they may provide a significant survival advantage.

2.1. The Need to Study Drugs in Children

Drug studies carried out using adult subjects may not provide adequate information about relevant effects (either positive or negative) and toxicity in children. Apart from concerns with respect to toxicity, various other factors have contributed to a reluctance to carry out drug studies in children. These include a heightened sensitivity to risks entailed, especially since the thalidomide disaster, and a limited market potential. The result has been that children of all ages have been rendered "therapeutic orphans." For example, in the developed world approx 80% of the drugs listed are not licensed for children or are limited in their use to defined age groups *(5)*. There is, therefore, as a matter of justice and of concern for their well-being, a crucial need to develop appropriate drug research in children.

When designing a study in meningococcal infection, several factors need to be taken into account, as described in the following sections.

2.2. Disease Onset

Despite meningococcal disease being relatively easy to recognize by the appearance of fever and a hemorrhagic rash, this is confounded by the presence of nonspecific features in a sizeable proportion of patients. These nonspecific features include flu-like symptoms such as myalgia, sore throat, headache, vomiting, and rigors, together with a nonspecific rash or no rash in up to 25% of patients *(3)*. These factors make strict definition of the time of onset of illness difficult to define accurately. This becomes important in the evaluation of agents that are designed to halt disease progression by inhibiting the actions of endotoxin. The half-life of meningococcal endotoxin is 3–6 h following appropriate antibiotic therapy, suggesting that, even if an effective anti-endotoxin treatment existed, if it was evaluated more than 6 h after antibiotics were administered, it would be difficult to prove its efficacy ***(6)***.

2.3. Disease Classification

Meningococcal disease has a well-documented natural history, with clearly defined adverse prognostic factors. Several scoring systems exist to identify severe disease. Many trials in sepsis are designed with entry criteria that must be present before the patient is able to be entered into a trial of adjunctive therapy. The promptness of appropriate antibiotic and resuscitation therapy may make the entry criteria for these trials difficult to meet, despite the presence of severe disease. This is particularly the case in previously healthy children who are able to compensate for the loss of large volumes of intravascular fluid before suffering hypotension. It is possible that these children are therefore much more seriously ill before satisfying entry criteria for interventional studies, and therefore the beneficial effects of a study agent may not be so clearly apparent. However, relaxation of entry criteria to allow less sick children to be enrolled in the study would lead to enrolment of large numbers of children who have less risk of an adverse outcome, and therefore are more likely to survive. This dilutes the beneficial effects of the study agent as most children in the study would be likely to survive whether they received the investigational agent or not.

2.4. Experience of the Disease

Apart from in sub-Saharan Africa, meningococcal disease is a relatively uncommon disease, affecting about 6/100,000 of the population in the UK. Therefore, single institutions are unlikely to treat more than a few tens of patients each year. The recruitment of large numbers of patients into a properly conducted, randomized, placebo-controlled, double-blind phase III study of new treatments for sepsis needs several hundred patients to be studied to demonstrate a significant reduction in mortality. Therefore such studies need to be carried out at several centers. This causes further confounding of the treatment effect of the study drug owing to possible differences in clinical regimens in each center. While this may be compensated for by statistical stratification by center, if one center enrolls a sizeable proportion of patients, this may significantly affect the overall result.

2.5. Improvement in Outcome with Experience

The experience of St. Mary's Hospital, London has demonstrated that improvement in outcomes may occur during the period of a clinical study, not owing to the study agent, but owing to improvement in the management of patients with meningococcal disease because of familiarity with the disease and better knowledge of the natural history and appropriate pre-emptive intervention. The improved management of the disease at St. Mary's Hospital has lead to a dramatic reduction in mortality over the last 5 yr, despite disease severity remaining relatively constant *(7)*, and has been mirrored to some extent in other pediatric intensive care units in the UK. Centralization of pediatric intensive care in tertiary centers is an effective method of improving outcome in all critically ill children, but is a relatively recent phenomenon not mirrored in adult practice *(8)*. This may be one reason why the mortality rate for patients >/= 16 yr in the UK has not changed significantly for the last 5 yr *(7)*.

2.6. Statistical Power

A large sample size in a randomized trial provides the maximum chance of reliably detecting an overall treatment effect. However, particularly for a relatively rare disease, and for expensive interventions, large trials are extremely costly in both financial and logistical terms. Attempts to reduce the numbers required to demonstrate a significant treatment effect are made by enrolling only those most seriously ill, in whom the primary endpoint (usually significant reduction in mortality in septic shock studies) is most likely. Studies of new therapies for sepsis are usually powered on the assumption that there will be a 30–50% mortality in the control arm and the investigational agent would be effective if there was a 50% reduction in mortality in the treatment arm.

In the study of the monoclonal antibody (MAb) against endotoxin (HA-1A) in children with meningococcal septic shock, the study was powered assuming a 30% mortality in the control arm and a 15% mortality in the HA-1A arm *(9)*. It was calculated that 270 children would need to be enrolled to demonstrate this with 80% power. If the mortality in the control arm of the study were lower than predicted, then larger numbers of patients would be required to reach the primary endpoint.

For multi-center studies of expensive treatments in rare diseases, significant increases in numbers of patients required to be enrolled may be prohibitively expensive and logistically impossible.

2.7. Clinical Efficacy

Because of the difficulty in demonstrating significant differences in large clinical trials of experimental agents in adults with sepsis, researchers have attempted to carry out sub-group analyses to demonstrate patient groups in whom the treatment may be beneficial, although the treatment may show no overall benefit. In addition, attempts may be made to make sense of smaller studies by the use of meta-analyses. However, attempts to use meta-analyses of multiple small trials as a substitute for well-conducted large studies has proven to be a flawed concept from the clinician's viewpoint. A meta-analysis may suggest a potential benefit of a certain treatment, which should then be confirmed by a sufficiently powered randomized controlled trial.

When an investigational agent has been demonstrated to show a significant treatment benefit, it is important to focus on whether the agent is important for clinical practice. Clinical trials may show that treatments work, but there is increasing doubt whether they show if and how these treatments should be introduced into widespread clinical practice. In addition, financial implications of potential new therapies should become a routine part of clinical trial design. That is, a cost-effectiveness analysis and health economic modeling should be a part of all randomized, controlled clinical trials.

2.8. Ethics

Obviously, there is a need for properly conducted studies to evaluate fully prospective new therapies. The need for placebo control is clear in the absence of anything other than conventional therapy. However, owing to technical advances, conventional therapy may differ according to the intensive care unit where the patient is admitted. For example, in one unit conventional treatment of shock may consist of high-dose epinephrine and fluid loading to maintain a central venous pressure of 15 mmHg. In another unit, conventional therapy may include a pulmonary artery catheter, a vasoconstrictor agent such as norepinephrine, and an inotropic agent such as dobutamine. Both are standard therapies for the units concerned because evidence does not exist to value one therapeutic maneuver over the other. Add to this a placebo-controlled trial of a new therapy and at once the trial is confounded by center.

Another issue concerns whether consent to participate in a trial of a potentially life-saving therapy is really a coercive offer. The meaning of informed consent becomes a real concern in all clinical trials in critically ill patients. The attempt to obtain informed consent from parents or relatives of patients who are, by definition, close to death, may lead investigators to be exploitative in their efforts to recruit subjects to the trial. Some preliminary data from our own unit suggests that parents in this most stressful of times do not really understand the issues of a placebo group. They remember that the only prospect of being offered a potentially life-saving therapy is being enrolled in the trial, but often do not recall the meaning of the control group being offered just standard therapy and placebo.

A recent study performed in Australia revealed that of 64 parents questioned after their child had taken part in a clinical trial, only a small minority realized that the trial was meant to assess safety as well as efficacy. Of more concern was the fact that most parents believed that drug trials performed in hospitals were of low or no risk. Also, many regarded the informed consent as being unnecessary because parents would routinely do what the doctor advised ***(10)***.

2.9. Financial Considerations

In this era of extremely costly new therapies, it is now extremely unlikely that studies will be fully funded by charity or governmental bodies; usually an industrial sponsor is involved. The sponsor will usually offer financial inducements to the investigators to recruit patients. This money is usually spent by the investigator to enable the study to be carried out at that center, i.e., to recruit research personnel in order to carry out the study. This alliance between industry and research makes the role of the Data and Safety Monitoring Committee (DSMC) even more important. The DSMC is a committee independent of both the steering committee and any sponsor. Its primary objective is to assure safety for the patients in the trial. Legal requirements to report serious adverse events to the regulating authorities (e.g., the Food and Drug Administration), which is usually the task of the sponsor (drug company), may be taken over by the DSMC, which should be the only body that has access to unblinded data until the trial is completed.

The DSMC, which usually consists of 1–2 clinicians knowledgeable in the field, 1–2 statisticians, and an epidemiologist, monitors negative as well as positive results of the trial. Rules for interim analyses should be decided before the trial starts. In addition, the DSMC must be sure that the overall quality of the data is adequate for monitoring purposes.

The DSMC is the body that conducts interim analyses on unblinded data and may recommend early termination of the study, either for strongly positive treatment effects, or an increased incidence of adverse events in the treatment group. The DSMC is less likely to recommend discontinuation of a study for positive effects than for negative effects. It must be certain that early discontinuation does not lead to statistical uncertainty, inasmuch as it may be clear that the study will never reach a positive result, but in order to achieve a reliable result, the DSMC will often recommend continuation until the numbers recommended by the initial power calculation are achieved.

The sponsor usually covers the costs of the drug during the study. However, should the drug prove efficacious, the question arises as to who should cover future provision and costs of widespread drug usage. The role of bodies such as the National Institute for Clinical Excellence in the UK may prove to be instrumental in the decision of whether to allow a drug to be prescribed by the National Health Service, dependent on a cost-benefit analysis.

2.10. Conclusion

Because of all these aforementioned factors, large, well-conducted, double-blind, randomized, controlled trials in children with meningococcal disease have proved difficult to carry out. There have been very few properly conducted studies of anti-inflammatory or other novel interventions in meningococcal disease. Until the last 5 yr, no pharmaceutical company or grant-funding body has been likely to fund a study in children of an agent that has failed to meet its primary endpoint in a large adult study.

Recently it has become clear that therapeutic trials in children with meningococcal disease could provide a much clearer picture of sepsis treatments than trials in adults with a multitude of critical illnesses, in order to determine agents that may be beneficial in adults with SIRS and septic shock.

3. Evaluation of New Therapies

Understanding the pathophysiology of meningococcal disease has offered us hope of interrupting the pathways leading to the disordered physiology characterizing meningococcal disease.

The mortality from meningococcal disease has remained unacceptably high despite major advances in conventional management (i.e., the development of powerful antibiotics to counteract the emergence of drug-resistant bacteria and the improvement of organ-support techniques in intensive care). This has lead to research into novel methods of therapy aimed at decreasing or neutralizing the effects of endotoxin, inflammatory mediators, and coagulation abnormalities, or improving organ function.

3.1. Summary of Pathophysiology

It is now clear that meningococci invading the bloodstream from the nasopharynx may proliferate in the bloodstream, releasing endotoxin. This causes a host response characterized by release of inflammatory mediators and activation of the complement and coagulation cascades. These processes, if not interrupted, lead to effects on end organs and eventually multiple-organ failure and death. In the case of meningococcal meningitis without sepsis, these processes occur in the relatively closed system of the meninges leading to cerebral edema, vascular thrombosis, and eventually raised intracranial pressure, and possibly cerebral herniation and brain death *(11)*.

3.2. Anti-Endotoxin Therapy (*see* Table 1)

Endotoxin is probably one of the most important bacterial components contributing to the inflammatory process. Levels of endotoxin directly correlate with severity of disease and with elaboration and release of inflammatory mediators, including the cytokines tumore necrosis factor (TNF-α) and interleukin (IL-1) and IL-6 and the complement and coagulation components.

The assumption that these processes are related to the presence of endotoxin in the bloodstream is based on the findings that much of the pathophysiology

Table 1
Anti-Endotoxins

Agent	Study	Outcome	Comments	Reference
HA-1A	2199 adults with sepsis (Phase III).	No effect on 14-d mortality.		*(18)*
HA-1A	269 children with meningococcal sepsis (Phase III).	No significant difference from placebo.		*(9)*
$rBPI_{21}$	26 patients 1–18 yr (Phase I/II).	Safe to administer.	Incidental finding of reduction in expected mortality.	*(23)*
$rBPI_{21}$	393 children with severe meningococcal sepsis (Phase III)	No significant difference in 60 mortality.	Improvement in all primary and secondary endpoints. Suggestion that efficacy would be enhanced by earlier administration	*(24)*
E5	550 adults (Phase III).	No significant difference in 14- or 28-d mortality.	Slight reduction in mortality. May need to be given earlier to make a significant difference. No increase in adverse events.	*(105)*
E5531	Rabbits: *E. coli* endotoxin exposure.	Reduction in fever.		*(106)*
HDL (High density lipoprotein)	8 Adult volunteers. Randomized, double-blind, cross-over.	Reduced TNF, IL-6, IL-8.		*(27)*
LALF (Limulus Anti-lipopolysaccharide factor)	Mice: endotoxin exposure.	Reduced amount of biologically active LPS and reduced lethality of endotoxin.		*(30)*

of Gram-negative sepsis can be reproduced by the administration of purified endotoxin or a variety of endotoxin-free inflammatory mediators released by endotoxin. In addition, most of these effects can be blocked in vitro and in vivo by agents that neutralize the effects of endotoxin or the inflammatory mediators.

A variety of anti-endotoxin strategies have been proposed, including agents that bind and neutralize endotoxin, efforts to enhance endotoxin clearance, or agents that inhibit the interaction of endotoxin with its receptors.

3.2.1. Anti-Endotoxin Antibodies

Since the 1960s, investigators have attempted to produce neutralizing antibodies to the highly conserved elements in the core regions of endotoxin (such as Lipid A). This is a particularly attractive strategy as it would enable a single product, if effective, to be useful in all forms of Gram-negative sepsis. Early studies indicated that passively administered antisera raised to vaccines generated from rough mutant bacteria (such as *Escherichia coli* J5) protected against challenge from heterologous Gram-negative bacteria ***(12–15)***. These rough mutants expose core elements of endotoxin on their surface. Based on the assumption that the antisera contained immunoglobulin that bound and neutralized endotoxin, or by anti-Lipid A antibodies, researchers attempted to develop cross-protective IgM MAbs apparently directed against Lipid A. Two antibodies went into mass production that were found to bind weakly, but not to neutralize endotoxin ***(16)***. Neither of these antibodies was found consistently to neutralize endotoxin in vitro and in animal models. Each antibody has been subjected to clinical trials. Despite encouraging results in initial studies, both antibodies were subjected to further, better-controlled studies. In particular, HA-1A was studied in a randomized, double-blind, placebo-controlled trial in children with meningococcal septic shock ***(9)***. This trial demonstrated a 33% absolute reduction in mortality in the treatment group. However, this did not reach statistical significance. The authors concluded that there may be several reasons for these findings:

1. There may have been a genuine beneficial effect of HA-1A that was dampened by nonoptimal timing of intervention (i.e., treatment with an effective anti-endotoxin therapy is likely to be more effective if given earlier in the disease course). The median time from initiation of antibiotic therapy to administration of study medication in this study was 6.4 h with 25% of patients receiving study medication >9.7 h following antibiotic therapy.
2. The improvement in mortality may have been a chance finding. Since this study started, in vitro data have suggested that HA-1A is not efficient in binding and neutralizing meningococcal endotoxin. The antibody has low affinity for endotoxin and no activity against some species of endotoxin ***(17)***. It may be that HA-1A was not the best anti-endotoxin agent to study in clinical trials.

Other studies in adults with septic shock have failed to demonstrate any benefit from monoclonal anti-endotoxin antibodies *(18,19)* (**Table 1**).

Despite the disappointment of the HA-1A study in children with meningococcal septic shock, what was demonstrated was that a collaborative effort to determine effective treatment interventions could be efficiently performed in children with meningococcal disease, and this model could serve as a template for future studies.

3.2.2. Other Anti-Endotoxin Therapies

There are several promising anti-endotoxin therapies currently under development. These are derived from the existence of peptides and proteins in insects and animal species that have evolved for the purpose of binding and neutralizing endotoxin.

Endotoxin, which is present in the circulation, forms complexes with circulating proteins and lipoproteins, such as the acute-phase reactant lipopolysaccharide binding protein (LBP), which facilitates the transfer of endotoxin to its receptor CD14 and other lipoproteins *(20)*. Endotoxin is also bound and neutralized by several neutrophil granule proteins, including the bactericidal/permeability-increasing protein (BPI) and the cationic antibacterial protein hCAP-18 (a cathelicidin) *(21,22)*.

Only one of these compounds has been the subject of clinical trials in meningococcal disease: a recombinant form of BPI ($rBPI_{21}$) that consists of 21 amino acids of the N-terminal fragment of naturally occurring BPI, which has been shown to kill meningococci and bind to and neutralize endotoxin. This recombinant protein was the subject of an uncontrolled clinical study in children with severe meningococcal septicemia *(23)*.

The study evaluated 26 children (1–18 yr) with meningococcal septicemia (GMSPS>8) within 8 h of receiving antibiotics. The study noted a significant reduction in mortality in the treated patients (only 1 death) compared with historical controls (expected 4–8 deaths). The results of this study prompted a phase III randomized, double-blind, placebo-controlled study of $rBPI_{21}$ *(24)*. This study enrolled 393 patients with meningococcal septic shock. There was a nonsignificant trend towards reduced mortality in the $rBPI_{21}$ group (7.4 vs 9.9%, $p = 0.48$). Assessment of all the outcome measures together (both primary and secondary endpoints) revealed there was a statistically significant improvement in outcome in the rBPI group compared to placebo. Unfortunately, the study was underpowered to detect a statistically significant improvement in the primary endpoint (mortality) suggesting that a further, larger, study is required, possibly designed to allow earlier administration of $rBPI_{21}$ or placebo. It is likely that any anti-endotoxin therapy will be more effective if given earlier on in the disease course. In the meantime, there is much more pre-clinical and clinical evidence of efficacy of $rBPI_{21}$ to suggest that further clinical studies of $rBPI_{21}$ will take place.

Endotoxin is known to bind to lipid-containing particles such as high-density lipoprotein (HDL), low-density lipoprotein (LDL), and very low-density lipoprotein (VLDL). These particles appear to be involved in detoxification and clearance of circulating endotoxin through the reticulo-endothelium ***(25)***. Preparations of HDL that are reconstituted from plasma are able to neutralize endotoxin more potently than natural lipoproteins ***(26)***. These have shown promising results in adult volunteers challenged with endotoxin in that the volunteers showed reduction in symptoms, pro-inflammatory cytokines, and endotoxin-induced changes in leukocyte counts ***(27)***. A dose-finding study of reconstituted HDL has just started in children with meningococcal septic shock.

At present, conflicting data regarding the use of recombinant soluble CD14, LBP, and hCAP18 exist from in vitro and in vivo studies, making it unlikely that these agents will be studied in clinical trials in the near future.

Several nonhuman anti-endotoxin agents are known to exist. Of these, Limulus anti-LPS factor (LALF), which is present in amoebocytes of the horseshoe crab, has been shown to bind to endotoxin with high affinity and neutralize the toxic effects of Lipid A ***(28)***. A recombinant version of LALF has been formulated (endotoxin-neutralizing protein, ENP) which, like its original form, protects animals against endotoxin and Gram-negative bacterial challenge ***(29)***. A recently reported study demonstrated that LALF protected mice from mortality owing to endotoxin challenge even if given up to 24 h following the insult ***(30)***. However, both the toxicity and immunogenicity of LALF and ENP may prevent their use in humans.

3.2.3. Endotoxin Removal

Enhancement of the clearance of endotoxin to reduce plasma levels has been proposed as a mechanism behind the anecdotal use of extracorporeal methods of endotoxin removal. These methods include plasmapheresis, exchange transfusion, hemofiltration, and adsorption to charcoal or Polymyxin B-containing membranes. Despite many anecdotal reports of the use of these methods (particularly plasmapheresis or blood exchange) in meningococcal disease and other forms of sepsis, there have been no well-controlled studies of their use, and only a small number of patients have been recruited to these studies ***(31–34)***. Despite the impression of clinical improvement following initiation of therapy in many reports, properly conducted studies are required to prove clinical efficacy. However, there is little doubt that whatever the mechanism, there is clinical benefit following high-volume hemofiltration in critically ill adults. A recent study comparing volumes of filtration per hour in acute renal failure patients (only about 10% of which had sepsis) treated with veno-venous hemofiltration demonstrated a significantly higher survival rate in those patients treated with at least 35 mL/kg/h of filtration *(35)*. However, another study of 30 patients (including 8 children) with septic shock, 14 of which were randomized to treatment by plasma exchange showed no difference between the two groups *(36)*.

A study of plasma or whole-blood exchange in meningococcal septicemia showed transient reduction in soluble TNF-α receptors that rebounded following exchange. There was no influence on mortality *(37)*.

Although removal of endotoxin and other inflammatory mediators would appear to be theoretically beneficial in patients with septic shock, there is no properly derived data to prove it.

3.2.4. Analogs of Lipid A

These are compounds that are structurally similar to lipid A but have absent or reduced toxicity. They compete with lipid A for binding to LBP and other endotoxin receptors, thereby inhibiting host inflammatory-cell activation. Several analogs have been produced that have demonstrated promising in vitro and animal data.

E5531 is a synthetic lipid A analog-based on the structure of *Rhodobacter capsulatus* lipid A. It is a potent antagonist of lipid A without obvious toxic activity in mice *(38)*. Monophosphoryl lipid A is a nontoxic lipid A derivative that is not a potent lipid A antagonist. It induces tolerance to endotoxin if used prophylactically in human volunteers, and may become a useful adjunct in critically ill patients, but is not likely to be useful in the treatment of meningococcal disease *(39)*.

Although large, well-controlled studies have so far failed to prove the beneficial effects of anti-endotoxin therapy, there is much experimental data to support the further development of anti-endotoxin agents as adjuncts in therapy of meningococcal disease.

3.3. Anti-Cytokine Therapy (see **Table 2***)*

Sepsis is a clinical syndrome resulting from the host's response to an invading pathogen. Activation of the cytokine network triggered by endotoxin is thought to play a major role in the pathophysiology of meningococcal disease.

Clinical trials with anti-inflammatory therapy in patients with sepsis have been based on the assumption that excessive pro-inflammatory activity may be harmful to the host. Numerous studies have been published that demonstrate increased levels of cytokines in patients with sepsis, including meningococcal disease *(40,41)*. However, pro-inflammatory cytokines may only be detected

Table 2
Anti-Cytokines

Agent	Patient Group	Outcome	Comments	Reference
Corticosteroids	Meta-analysis of 9. Randomized, controlled trials	No benefit and potential risk patients	Higher mortality in sickest patients and in the most rigorous trials.	*(102)*
Ibuprofen	455 adults with sepsis (phase III).	No change in outcome.	Improvement in temperature but nothing else.	*(107)*
IL-1 Receptor Antagonist	696 patients with severe sepsis or septic shock (phase III).	Small but insignificant reduction in mortality.		*(108)*
TNF Antibody	553 patients with sepsis (phase III).	No change in 28-d mortality.	Faster reversal of shock.	*(109)*
Platelet-Activating Factor Inhibitor	609 patients with presumed gram-negative sepsis (phase III).	No significant effect on mortality.		*(110)*
Soluble TNF receptor: Fc fusion protein	141 patients (phase III).	No reduction in mortality.	Higher doses may increase mortality.	*(47)*
Interferon-γ	9 septic patients. No controls.	All patients showed recovery of monocyte function and production of TNF-α.		*(46)*
Beta Glucan	Mice: endotoxin exposure.	Suppression of TNF-α and reduced mortality.		*(111)*
IL-10	16 adult volunteers exposed to placebo and endotoxin.	Inhibition of release of Macrophage inflammatory protein (MIP)- 1 alpha, -1 β and Monocyte Chemoattractant Protein (MCP)-1.		*(112)*
IL-11	Rats: Pseudomonal Aeruginosa sepsis.	Reduced endotoxin levels. Reduced mucosal necrosis. Improved survival.		*(113)*
Lisophylline	Rats	Reduced TNF-α. Aspirin-induced mucosal damage ameliorated.		*(114)*

in a subset of all patients with sepsis, whereas anti-inflammatory cytokines and soluble cytokine inhibitors are detected in most and are also found in healthy individuals. It has been argued that those patients who fulfill the clinical criteria for SIRS (*see* Appendix) do not have detectable levels of pro-inflammatory cytokines in their circulation because they are studied late in the septic process ***(42)***. This may explain why the cytokines TNF-α, IL-1β, IL-12, and interferon (IFN-γ), which according to animal models play a central role in the pathogenesis of septic shock, are not consistently correlated with disease severity or outcome in patients with septic shock. In comparison with other cytokines, IL-6 (a mixed pro and anti-inflammatory cytokine) has been reported most consistently in patients with sepsis, although actual levels of IL-6 show considerable variation ***(43)***.

Induction of anti-inflammatory pathways to inhibit excessive pro-inflammatory activity can be demonstrated in most patients with sepsis. This has lead to the concept of "compensatory anti-inflammatory response" (CARS), following SIRS in time-course ***(43)***. For example, the plasma levels of soluble TNF-α receptors and the IL-1β inhibitors, soluble IL-1 receptor II and IL-1 receptor antagonist, increase substantially during the septic process, probably reflecting an attempt by the host to limit inflammation caused by TNF-α and IL-1β. Similarly, severe sepsis is associated with detectable serum IL-10 levels in 80–100% of patients ***(44)***. In addition, shortly after the onset of a septic event, a "refractory state" develops that is characterized by a relative inability of host inflammatory cells to respond to usually pro-inflammatory stimuli (such as endotoxin challenge) ***(45)***. The mechanisms for this state remain to be elucidated, but it is likely to be a purposeful adaptation of the host rather than a generalized hyporesponsiveness.

It is also important to realize that measuring cytokine levels in the circulation may not accurately reflect the situation at the tissue level. Particularly in generalized infections such as meningococcal septicemia, plasma levels of cytokines may not reflect the interactions occurring on the endothelial surface.

Clinical trials with anti-inflammatory strategies in patients with severe bacterial infection are based on agents that have been studied in animal models where bacteria or their products are administered as a systemic bolus. In such circumstances, overwhelming pro-inflammatory cytokine activation occurs leading to SIRS. In patients with sepsis who are involved in clinical trials, it is likely that a state of immunological refractoriness is already present by the time they are entered into the study. This has even led to the performance of one uncontrolled study in which an attempt was made to stimulate the immune status of patients with sepsis by the use of IFN-γ ***(46)***.

Unfortunately, most of the clinical trials of anti-inflammatory agents in adult sepsis have proven to be of no overall benefit with regard to a significant reduction in mortality, and in some cases (such as treatment with a soluble TNF-α receptor-Fc fusion protein) have proven to be deleterious *(47)*.

Despite much evidence regarding the presence of pro-inflammatory cytokines and their influence in meningococcal disease, there have been no published studies of the use of anti-cytokine agents in this group of patients.

3.4. Neutrophil/Endothelial Cell Interactions

Many of the pro-inflammatory mediators discussed earlier stimulate adhesion molecule expression on leukocytes, platelets, and endothelial cells. There is much evidence to implicate the adhesion of neutrophils to endothelial cells in the tissue injury and multiple-organ dysfunction that occurs during sepsis *(48)*. However, patients with inherited abnormalities of adhesion molecules have recurrent, severe infections typically characterized by a marked leucocytosis and may develop systemic sepsis and septic shock *(49)*. This highlights the important role these molecules have in host defense during infection. Although there is in vitro data suggesting the importance of these interactions in meningococcal disease, the inhibition of adhesion molecules in animal and human studies show results that are consistent with their important role in host defense; that is, inhibition of adhesion molecules results in either no benefit or a worse outcome in the treatment groups *(50,51)*.

3.5. Nitric Oxide (*see* Table 3)

Activation of the inflammatory response results in elaboration of a number of mediators with direct effects on vasomotor tone. Nitric oxide (NO), bradykinin, histamine, and prostacyclin (PGI2) can all decrease vascular tone and cause hypotension. Hypotension in shock also results from myocardial dysfunction, and decreased cardiac preload, which may occur owing to increased capillary permeability *(11)*.

NO is formed by the enzymatic action of NO synthase (NOS) on the guanidino group of the amino acid L-arginine *(52)*. The inducible isoform of NOS (iNOS) is produced in response to endotoxin, platelet-activating factor (PAF), IL-1, and TNF-α. Glucocorticoids, IL-1ra, PAF antagonists, TNF-α, tyrosine kinase inhibitors, and dihydropyridine calcium-channel blockers inhibit iNOS induction *(53)*.

NO is a highly diffusible compound that activates soluble guanylate cyclase in smooth-muscle cells. This converts GTP to cGMP, which relaxes the smooth-muscle cell via a protein kinase by promoting calcium entry into the sarcoplasmic reticulum *(54)*. It appears that iNOS is the predominant source of the excessive NO production responsible for the hypotension and profound and refractory vasodilation frequently observed in septic shock.

Table 3
NO Antagonists

Agent	Study	Outcome	Comments	Reference
N(G)-methyl-L-arginine hydrochloride(L-NMMA)	Multicenter, open-label, uncontrolled, dose range finding. 32 adults with sepsis.	Reduced requirement for Norepinephrine therapy.	No major adverse events.	***(115)***
N(G)-methyl-L-arginine hydrochloride(L-NMMA)	Multicenter, randomized, placebo-controlled, double blind. 797 patients with septic shock.	Increased mortality in treatment group.	Trial stopped early. Excess deaths mainly attributed to cardiovascular causes.	***(68)***
S-methyl-isothiourea (SMT)	Rats: endotoxin exposure.	Maintenance of CO and BP and also less organ dysfunction and lactic acidosis.		***(69)***
Transforming Growth Factor-β1(TGF-β1)	Rats: Salmonella Typhosa endotoxin exposure.	Inhibition of iNOS after endotoxin exposure. BP maintained and reduced mortality.		***(70)***

Normally, vasomotor tone is tightly regulated through the generation of NO by vascular endothelial cells being rapidly inhibited by binding to circulating hemoglobin in red blood cells. NO is highly soluble in water and may react with the superoxide ion to form peroxynitrite, which is highly toxic and relatively stable. This moiety then reacts with water to form nitrites and nitrates, which can be measured as a surrogate indicator of NO production ***(53,54)***.

Other molecules are also highly active in controlling vascular tone. These include the vasoconstrictors:

- Endothelin 1
- Angiotensin II
- Vasopressin
- Thromboxane A2
- Prostaglandin H2
- Superoxide

and the vasodilators:

- Prostacyclin (PGI2)
- Hydroxyeicosatetraenoic acid (HETE)
- Bradykinin
- Histamine

Endothelin 1 (ET1) is a potent vasoconstrictor that has been implicated in the vasomotor nephropathy of acute renal failure. ET1 production is inhibited by NO ***(55)***.

Although a variety of factors with opposing actions on the vasculature have been detected in sepsis and septic shock, NO has been implicated as one of the most potent and most important that contributes to the production of vasodilatation and unresponsiveness to exogenous vasopressors. High levels of nitrates and nitrites have been detected in sepsis models and patients with septic shock, including meningococcal disease ***(56)***.

The inflammatory response in sepsis, including increased NO production by iNOS, may result in endothelial cell dysfunction affecting vascular smooth muscle. The resulting affects on organ perfusion may be instrumental in the pathogenesis of the multiple organ dysfunction syndrome seen in sepsis and septic shock, which is associated with increased morbidity and mortality.

The role of iNOS and cGMP in the vasculopathy of septic shock have been supported by the finding that competitive NOS inhibitors such as L-N monomethyl arginine (L-NMMA) and N(G)-nitro-L-arginine methyl ester (L-NAME), act as vasopressors when administered to patients with septic shock ***(55,57)***.

In addition to the vasculopathy of sepsis, sepsis induces a state of reversible biventricular myocardial depression ***(53)***. The cause of this is probably multifactorial, including impaired coronary perfusion, inflammatory cell infiltration of the myocardium and myocardial edema, a direct effect of endotoxin and inflammatory mediators, and a poorly defined "myocardial depressant factor" ***(58)***.

The increased NO resulting from iNOS induction may contribute to the myocardial depression and β-adrenergic hyporesponsiveness associated with sepsis. The NO-induced production of cGMP in cardiac myocytes inhibits the β-adrenergic-stimulated increase in the slow calcium channel and decreases the affinity of calcium for the contractile apparatus. This results in negative inotropism and increases the relaxation phase of the cardiac cycle ***(59)***. NO has been highly implicated in the myocardial depression of sepsis. L-NMMA has been shown to block the cardiac myocyte depression induced by human septic serum, TNF-α and IL-1 ***(60,61)***.

The implication of NO in the vascular hyporesponsiveness and cardiac depression of sepsis supports the hypothesis that blockage or reduction of NO production will produce clinical benefit in patients with sepsis.

There are many animal models of sepsis in which various inhibitors of NO production have demonstrated potential benefit as well as potentially harmful effects. It has become clear, however, that nonspecific NOS inhibitors cause detrimental effects secondary to reduced organ perfusion and elevation of pulmonary artery pressures and renal vascular resistance ***(62,63)***. This is probably owing to inhibition of baseline NO production, which is essential for control of organ perfusion under normal circumstances. In addition, there are reports of increased capillary permeability and intestinal damage associated with L-NMMA after endotoxin challenge, together with a decrease in cardiac index and tissue oxygen delivery ***(53)***. This leads to an increase in lactic acidosis and hepatic toxicity. From animal studies it appeared that reduction of NO activity is associated with the potential benefit of treatment of hypotension and vasodilatation at the expense of reduction of cardiac output and tissue oxygen delivery, with an increase in pulmonary vascular resistance and increased mortality ***(63,64)***.

Despite these concerns, human studies have been carried out. All of these have shown similar effects to those demonstrated in animal models ***(57,65)***. In addition, concerns have been raised over increased activation of intravascular coagulation ***(66)***.

Despite some positive reports in small groups of patients ***(57,67)***, a phase III multicenter study of L-NMMA in adults with septic shock was halted prematurely owing to increased mortality in the L-NMMA group ***(68)***.

The use of L-NMMA and other nonselective iNOS inhibitors is associated with indiscriminate vasoconstriction of vital vascular beds, including those of the brain, kidney, liver, and lung, which result in compromised organ function. It therefore appears that clinical application of such agents is limited.

The recent development of selective iNOS inhibitors such as S-methylisothiourea (SMT) and transforming growth factor-β (TGF-β), which inhibit iNOS mRNA, and their application in animal models of septic shock suggest that these agents may offer the benefits of reduced NO production owing to iNOS inhibition, without the adverse effects of nonselective NOS inhibition ***(69,70)***.

3.6. Manipulation of Coagulation in Meningococcal Disease (see Table 4*)*

One of the hallmark features of meningococcal septicemia is disseminated intravascular coagulation and purpura, ischaemia, and gangrene of digits and sometimes limbs, leading to amputation in up to 10% of patients ***(11)***. Increased understanding of the pathological processes leading to the coagulopathy has allowed several potentially beneficial treatments to be introduced into clinical practice.

Patients with severe disease have all measurable aspects of coagulation disturbed early in the illness. In addition, reduction in the coagulation inhibitors antithrombin III, protein C, and protein S as well as tissue factor pathway inhibitor have been described ***(71)***. Severe depression of the levels of these inhibitors is associated with severe disease. Defective fibrinolysis has also been documented with low levels of plasminogen and alpha 2 antiplasmin and high levels of plasminogen activator inhibitor-1 (PAI-1). The finding of the latter has recently been associated with a polymorphism in the PAI-1 gene which, is associated with increased mortality ***(72)***.

The mechanisms responsible for the coagulopathy are incompletely understood. Endotoxin is a potent inducer of tissue factor expression on endothelial cells and on circulating monocytes, and the degree of coagulopathy has been correlated with levels of endotoxin. Congenital deficiencies of protein C and S are associated with purpuric lesions similar to those found in meningococcal disease, suggesting that depletion of these inhibitors may be involved in the pathogenesis of the purpuric lesions of meningococcal infection ***(73,74)***. More recent studies have suggested that loss of the anticoagulant glycosaminoglycans heparan sulphate and dermatan sulphate from the endothelial surface may result in defective thromboresistance owing to a failure to bind and activate antithrombin III and Heparin cofactor II ***(75)***. In addition, preliminary data suggests that the mechanism to convert protein C to its active form (the endothelial protein C receptor) may be lacking in patients with meningococcal disease (S. Faust, personal communication). A defect in endothelial thromboresistance may therefore coexist with upregulation of endothelial procoagulant activities and reduction of intrinsic fibrinolytic mechanisms. Microvascular thrombosis owing to these defects leads to impaired organ perfusion and func-

Table 4
Anti-Coagulants/Fibrinolytics

Agent	Patient group	Outcome	Comments	Reference
Anti-thrombin III	120 adults with sepsis.	No overall effect.	Septic shock subgroup showed nonsignificant reduction in mortality.	*(84)*
Anti-thrombin III	42 adults with severe sepsis (phase II study).	Safe to use and nonsignificant reduction in 30 d all cause mortality.	Meta-analysis of three other trials confirms trend towards reduced mortality.	*(116)*
Protein C	3 Meningococcal patients. Case series.	Improvement in global markers of hemostasis. No adverse events. Increase in Protein C.	Uncontrolled.	*(80)*
Protein C	12 pediatric Meningococcal patients. Case series.	Improvement in Protein C levels. No adverse events. Better than predicted mortality.	Uncontrolled.	*(79)*
Activated Protein C	1690 adults with sepsis. Randomized, placebo-controlled, Phase III	Significant improvement in all-cause mortality.	Increased serious bleeding events in treatment group	*(82)*
Heparin	30 healthy volunteers. Randomized, double-blind, controlled trial.	Significantly inhibited activation of coagulation after exposure to endotoxin.		*(117)*
Tissue-factor pathway inhibitor	12 TFPI pigs, 20 controls. Peritonitis-induced bacteremia.	TFPI attenuated cytokine response.	No survival benefit.	*(87)*
Tissue-factor pathway inhibitor	16 Adult Volunteers. Randomized, double-blind, placebo cross-over.	TFPI inhibits coagulation.	No effect on cytokines or fibrinolysis.	*(118)*
PAI-1 inhibitor	Mice: endotoxin exposure.	Attenuated increase in PAI-1 and decrease in Anti-thrombin III.	Effect observed after PAI-1 inhibitor given orally for 8 d prior to endotoxin.	*(90)*

tion, and eventually to multiple-organ failure and death. These findings have led investigators to examine the role of replacement of the natural inhibitors of coagulation (heparin, protein C, antithrombin III) and the use of fibrinolytic agents.

Heparin has been advocated for many years in the treatment of Disseminated Intravascular Coagulation (DIC). Several small studies were carried out in meningococcal disease and other forms of sepsis, but there was no convincing evidence of benefit, and some patients experienced hemorrhagic complications *(76,77)*.

Protein C in its inactive form was found to be effective in reducing inflammation and mortality in a baboon model of septic shock *(78)*. Following these findings, it has been anecdotally used in human sepsis, including meningococcal disease, with promising results *(79–81)*. However, as mentioned earlier, the mechanism for converting protein C to its active form may be defective in clinical sepsis. In addition, this product is extremely expensive and should not be introduced into widespread clinical use without properly derived evidence of its effectiveness.

The activated form of protein C (aPC) has recently been developed and has been evaluated in a phase III adult sepsis study, and a phase II pediatric sepsis study. The adult study was stopped by the DSMC following an interim analysis following the enrollment of 1690 patients (840 in the placebo group and 850 in the treatment group) *(82)*. There was a highly significant reduction in all cause mortality at 28 days in the treatment group (30.8% in the placebo group vs 24.7% in the aPC group P = 0.005). This reduction in mortality rate was consistent regardless of age, diagnosis, organism and severity of illness and presence of protein C deficiency. However, this study excluded patients at significant risk of bleeding (severe thrombocytopenia or other conditions that increased the risk of bleeding). There was nearly double the number of serious bleeding adverse events in the aPC group (3.5%) when compared to the placebo group (2%). This is not surprising considering that aPC is an anticoagulant that inhibits factors Va and VIIIa, and a pro-fibrinolytic agent that inhibits PAI-1 activity. There is a phase IIIb open-label study in both adults and children planned. One major concern regarding the use of aPC in children with meningococcal disease is the risk of hemorrhagic complications. There is a clear risk of intracranial hemorrhage in meningoccal disease without the use of anticoagulant agents. It is possible that this will be made greater by the use of aPC. Close monitoring of patients being treated with aPC is required before it is widely used in the treatment of meningococcal disease.

There have been several phase II studies and one phase III study of antithrombin III in adult sepsis *(83,84)*. These have suggested a reduction in mortality in patients with septic shock and reduced antithrombin III levels when treated with antithrombin III replacement. A further phase III study of this agent in adult septic shock is nearing completion. The tissue-factor pathway is thought to be important in the pathogenesis of the coagulopathy of sepsis. There have been several studies of anti-tissue-factor antibodies and tissue-factor pathway inhibitor itself, with encouraging results in animal models of sepsis ***(85–87)***.

The finding of a direct relationship between PAI-1 levels and mortality in meningococcal disease has lead to the proposal of the use of fibrinolytic therapy for meningococcal disease. There have been some anecdotal reports of the successful use of tissue plasminogen activator (tPA) in children with meningococcal disease ***(88,89)***. Understandably there are concerns regarding the potential for catastrophic bleeding in patients with a hemorrhagic diathesis. At present there are no plans for further studies of this agent in meningococcal disease.

A recent study has demonstrated beneficial effects in mice treated with an inhibitor of PAI-1. This may be a future direction for research as it is likely not to be associated with the hemorrhagic complications of fibrinolytic therapy ***(90)***.

Because of the recognized interactions between inflammation and coagulation, manipulation of the coagulation cascade would appear to be an attractive target for new therapies.

3.7. Miscellaneous New Therapies (*see* Table 5)

Despite the huge advances in our understanding of the pathophysiology of sepsis and an explosion in potential new therapies, the treatment of septic shock remains: eradication of the invading organism and support of organ dysfunction.

3.7.1. Volume Resuscitation

The most important therapeutic maneuver to correct hypovolemia and organ hypoperfusion in meningococcal sepsis remains volume resuscitation. A recent meta-analysis of fluid resuscitation in various clinical states has suggested that the use of Human Albumin Solution (HAS) may be associated with increased mortality ***(91)***. We have demonstrated a huge leak of albumin and other proteins from the circulation in children with severe meningococcal septicemia, which suggests that replacement with a colloidal solution would be optimal ***(92)***. In our practice, 4.5% HAS has been the primary fluid used to restore circulating volume, with no obvious adverse effects on mortality. In fact, using this regimen we have been able to reduce our pediatric intensive care unit (PICU) mortality to the lowest reported in children with meningococcal septic shock ***(7)***. However, the doubts raised regarding the use of HAS have increased the need for artificial colloid solutions in the resuscitation of children with septic shock. Unfortunately, there has never been an adequate study of artificial colloid solutions in patients with sepsis, although the development

Table 5
Miscellaneous

Agent	Patient Group	Outcome	Comments	Reference
Bradykinin Antagonists	504 adults with sepsis (phase II).	No significant overall benefit.	Gram-negative sepsis group showed improvement in 28-d mortality.	*(119)*
Polymyxin B Hemoperfusion	Prospective,controlled trial. 37 adult patients with sepsis.	Significant improvement in survival.	Endotoxin levels lowered in treatment group and improvement in cardiovascular parameters.	*(120)*
Plasmapheresis	Multicenter, prospective, randomized, controlled trial. 30 patients (22 adults, 8 children).	Reduction in acute phase reactants.	No difference in mortality. Trend towards less organ failure.	*(36)*
GCSF	Prospective, randomized, placebo-controlled. 42 neonates with presumed bacterial sepsis.	Significant increase in neutrophil concentration.		*(121)*
GCSF	160 Rabbits: pneumonia sepsis and rGCSF. Prospective, randomized, controlled.	Significantly greater survival in those with sepsis induced leukopenia.		*(122)*
Immunoglobulin	Prospective, randomized, controlled. 55 patients with septic shock.	Significant improvement in survival.		*(123)*
Immunoglobulin	Systematic review of 27 studies in neonates, children and adults with sepsis or septic shock.	Polyclonal immunoglobulin reduces mortality in adults with sepsis or septic shock.		*(124)*

of newer starch solutions that have similar colloidal effects to HAS but with reduced adverse effects usually associated with starches, may make the use of these fluids more attractive.

3.7.2. Extracorporeal Membrane Oxygenation (ECMO)

Patients with refractory hypotension who fail to respond to adequate volume loading and high doses of inotropes are very likely to die. Recent improvements in technology have led to the widespread availability of extracorporeal cardiac-assist devices for patients who have severe myocardial or pulmonary dysfunction unresponsive to conventional therapy. Several reports have suggested that successful treatment of the reversible myocardial dysfunction in sepsis can be achieved using ECMO ***(93–96)***. In children with sepsis, survival is less likely compared with the other usual indications for ECMO (37% survival in children with sepsis vs 52% with other causes of cardiorespiratory failure) ***(94)***. One study of 12 children with meningococcal septic shock and a predicted mortality of 72% showed a 33% mortality when treated with ECMO ***(95)***. However, the criteria for selection of these patients included children with pulmonary failure as well as children with myocardial failure and therefore newer modes of ventilatory therapy may have been equally beneficial. The invasiveness of ECMO, together with the increased risk of adverse effects in patients with sepsis, do not make ECMO an attractive treatment option for patients with septic shock ***(94)***. However, there is no doubt that in desperation its use may be lifesaving.

3.7.3. Steroids

There is some evidence that the use of high-dose glucocorticoid adjunctive therapy in children with meningococcal meningitis may be beneficial. Use of steroids in *Haemophilus influenzae* meningitis and pneumococcal meningitis has been associated with a reduction in neurological sequelae, particularly nerve deafness, and possibly mortality ***(97,98)***. Although the data alluding to meningococcal meningitis are sparse, it is unlikely that significant differences exist between the pathophysiology of meningococcal meningitis and other causes of bacterial meningitis.

Recent studies of meningococcal and other forms of septic shock have demonstrated abnormalities of control of adrenal corticosteroid secretion over the course of illness ***(99–101)***. Although it is rare to have severe adrenal insufficiency on admission, a relative deficiency of adrenal steroid secretory function has been demonstrated in meningococcal disease, often associated with resistance to high doses of inotropes, suggesting that replacement doses of corticosteroids may be beneficial in some patients with meningococcal disease and refractory shock ***(101)***.

The use of high doses of glucocorticoids in adults with septic shock has been demonstrated in several studies to be associated with a higher mortality in those patients treated with steroids compared with controls ***(102)***.

4. Conclusion

The publication of the human genome will lead to massive advances in genomics and proteomics in the coming decade. The possibilities for individualized drug treatment of patients with sepsis, related to their genotype, will become reality. Already, certain genotypes that determine host response have been associated with more severe meningococcal disease ***(72,103,104)***. New technology may soon allow bedside testing of patient's genotypes to allow targeted therapy of even the sickest patient. It is probable that many new agents will be shortly developed based on the unravelling of the host/pathogen interaction. However, until this time we must utilize currently available therapies to the best of our knowledge.

Despite huge advances, our treatment of meningococcal disease remains as antibiotics, fluids, and crude methods of organ support. Only with the widespread acceptance that properly conducted trials can and must be carried out in critically ill children, can we hope to improve the current situation.

There have been only two large properly controlled phase III studies in children with meningococcal septicemia. Although these and the many adult studies to date have not demonstrated a significant survival advantage, there is much that can be learned from these unsuccessful studies that is relevant to the design of future sepsis trials. There is now no obvious reason why all children with meningococcal septicemia cannot be enrolled in double-blind, placebo-controlled studies to evaluate new treatments. These studies should be large enough to minimize random error and avoid type II error (or false-negative result). Definitions for the target population should be explicit, reproducible, and include illness severity scores. Protocols for both the use of the investigational agent, and conventional treatment should be standardized. Outcomes should be clinically relevant and pre-defined, and should include measures of both benefit and harm. In addition, the analysis of results should be carried out both on evaluable patients and on intention to treat. Finally, a health-economic evaluation of the implications of the introduction of ever-increasingly expensive therapies is now mandatory. Only in this way will we be likely to further influence the unacceptably high mortality rate of meningococcal septicemia, with the added advantage of limiting the widespread use of extremely expensive new therapies that have been insufficiently evaluated.

Appendix

Terminology for Sepsis in Adults

Adapted from **ref. *125***.

Systemic Inflammatory Response Syndrome

2 or more of the following:
Temperature >38°C or <36°C
Heart rate >90 beats/min
Respiratory rate >20 breaths/min
White blood call count >12,000/mm^3, <4,000/mm^3 or >10% of immature cells

Sepsis

SIRS plus documented evidence of infection (i.e., a positive culture)

Severe Sepsis

Sepsis associated with organ dysfunction, abnormal perfusion, or hypotension. Evidence of abnormal perfusion includes, but is not limited to:
Metabolic acidosis (usually lactic)
Oliguria
Abnormal mental status

Septic Shock

Sepsis-induced hypotension despite fluid resuscitation plus evidence of abnormal organ perfusion.

Terminology for Sepsis and Sepsis Syndrome in Infants and Children

Adapted from **ref. *126***.

Sepsis

Clinical suspicion of infection and evidence of systemic response to infection (tachycardia, tachypnoea, hyperthermia, or hypothermia[a])

Sepsis Syndrome

Sepsis plus evidence of altered organ perfusion with at least one of the following: acute change in mental status,[b] oliguria, hyperlactemia and hypoxemia.

Septic Shock

Sepsis syndrome with hypotension that is responsive to i.v. fluids or pharmacologic intervention.[c]

Refractory Septic Shock

Sepsis syndrome with hypotension that lasts for >1 h and does not respond to i.v. fluids or pharmacologic intervention and requires vasopressor support.

Multi-Organ Failure

Any combination of disseminated intravascular coagulation, acute respiratory distress syndrome, acute renal failure, hepatobiliary dysfunction and central nervous system dysfunction. (associated with the acute illness).

References

1. American Academy of Pediatrics, Committee on Drugs (1995) Guidelines for the ethical conduct of studies to evaluate drugs in pediatric populations. *Pediatrics* **95,** 287.
2. Platt, M. (1997) Child Health statistical review. *Arch. Dis. Child.* **77,** 542–548
3. Steven, N. and Wood, M. (1995) The clinical spectrum of meningococcal disease, in "Meningococcal Disease" (Cartwright, K. A. V., ed.), John Wiley and Sons, Chichester, UK, pp. 177–205.
4. Opal, S. M. and Cross, A. S. (1999) Clinical trials for severe sepsis: Past failures and future hopes. *Infect. Dis. Clin. North Amer.* **13,** 285–299.
5. Rowell, M. and Zlotkinm S. (1997) The ethical boundaries of drug research in pediatrics. *Pediatr. Clin. North Amer.* **44,** 27–40.
6. Brandtzaeg, P., Kierulf, P., Gaustad, P., Skulberg, A., Bruun, J. N., Halvorsen, S., et al. (1989) Plasma endotoxin as a predictor of multiple organ failure and death in systemic meningococcal disease. *J. Infect. Dis.* **159,** 195–204.
7. Mehta, N., Nadel, S., Booy, R., Galassin,. R., Morrisson, A., and Levin, M. (2000) Reduction in case fatality rate for meningococcal disease associated with improved healthcare delivery. *Pediatr. Res.* **47(4),** 271A.
8. Pollack, M. M., Alexander, S. R., Clarke, N., Ruttimann, U. E., Tesselaar, H. M., and Bachulis, A. C. 1991. Improved outcomes from tertiary center pediatric intensive care: a statewide comparison of tertiary and nontertiary care facilities. *Crit. Care Med.* **19,** 150–159.
9. Derkx, B., Wittes, J., McCloskey, R., and the European Paediatric Meningococcal Septic Shock Trial Study Group (1999) Randomized placebo-controlled trial of HA-1A, a human monoclonal antibody to endotoxin, in children with meningococcal septic shock. *Clin. Infect. Dis.* **28,** 770–777.

---

[a]Tachycardia: infant's heart rate >160/min, children's heart rate >150/min;
Tachypnoea: infant's respiratory rate >60/min, children's respiratory rate >50/min;
Hyperthermia: >38°C
Hypothermia: <36°C

[b]A reduction of at least 3 points in baseline Glasgow Coma Score or its modification for children.

[c]Systolic pressure: infants <65 mmHg, children <75 mmHg or <5th percentile for age.

10. Harth, S. and Thong, Y. (1995) Parental perceptions and attitudes about informed consent in clinical research involving children. *Soc. Sci. Med.* **40,** 1573–1577.
11. Nadel, S., Levin, M., and Habibi, P. (1995) Treatment of meningococcal disease in childhood, in *Meningococcal Disease* (Cartwright, K. A. V., ed.), John Wiley and Sons, Chichester, UK, pp. 208–243.
12. Braude, A. I., Douglas, H., and Davis, C. E. (1973) Treatment and prevention of intravascular coagulation with antiserum to endotoxin. *J. Infect. Dis.* **128,** S157.
13. McCabe, W. R. (1972) Immunization with R mutants of S. minnesota. I. Protection against challenge with heterologous gram-negative bacilli. *J. Immunol.* **108,** 601–610.
14. McCabe, W. R., DeMaria, A., Jr., Berberich, H., and Johns, M. A. (1988) Immunization with rough mutants of Salmonella minnesota: Protective activity of IgM and IgG antibody to the R595 (Re chemotype) mutant. *J. Infect. Dis.* **158,** 291–300.
15. Ziegler E. J., McCutchan J. A., Fierer J., Glauser M. P., Sadoff J. C., Douglas, H., and Braude, A. I. (1982) Treatment of gram-negative bacteremia and shock with human antiserum to a mutant Escherichia coli. *N. Engl. J. Med.* **307,** 1225–1230.
16. Warren, H. S., Amato, S. F., Fitting, C., Black, K. M., Loiselle, P. M., Pasternack, M. S., and Cavaillon, J. M. (1993) Assessment of ability of murine and human anti-lipid A monoclonal antibodies to bind and neutralize lipopolysaccharide. *J. Exp. Med.* **177,** 89–97.
17. Chan, B., Kalabalikis, P., Klein, N., Heyderman, R., and Levin, M. (1996) Assessment of the effect of candidate anti-inflammatory treatments on the interaction between meningococci and inflammatory cells in vitro in a whole blood model. *Biotherapy* **9,** 221–228.
18. McCloskey, R. V., Straube, R. C., Sanders, C., Smith, S. M., and Smith, C. R. (1994) Treatment of septic shock with human monoclonal antibody HA-1A. A randomized, double-blind, placebo-controlled trial. CHESS Trial Study Group. *Ann. Intern. Med.* **121,** 1–5.
19. Angus, D. C., Birmingham, M. C., Balk, R. A., Scannon, P. J., Collins, D., Kruse, J. A., et al. (2000) E5 murine monoclonal antiendotoxin antibody in gram-negative sepsis: a randomized controlled trial. E5 Study Investigators. *JAMA* **283,** 1723–1730.
20. Hailman, E., Lichenstein, H. S., Wurfel, M. M., Miller, D. S., Johnson, D. A., Kelley, M., et al. (1994) Lipopolysaccharide (LPS)-binding protein accelerates the binding of LPS to CD14. *J. Exp. Med.* **179,** 269–277.
21. Gazzano-Santoro, H., Parent, J. B., Grinna, L., Horwitz, A., Parsons, T., Theofan, G., et al. (1992) High-affinity binding of the bactericidal/permeability-increasing protein and a recombinant amino-terminal fragment to the lipid A region of lipopolysaccharide. *Infect. Immun.* **60,** 4754–4761.
22. Larrick, J. W., Hirata, M., Zheng, H., Zhong, J., Bolin, D., Cavaillon, J. M., et al. (1994) A novel granulocyte-derived peptide with lipopolysaccharide-neutralizing activity. *J. Immunol.* **152,** 231–240.
23. Giroir, B. P., Quint, P. A., Barton, P., Kirsch, E. A., Kitchen, L., Goldstein, B., et al. (1997) Preliminary evaluation of recombinant amino-terminal fragment of human bactericidal/permeability-increasing protein in children with severe meningococcal sepsis. *Lancet* **350,** 1439–1443.

24. Levin, M., Quint, P. A., Goldstein, B., Barton, P., Bradley, J. S., Shemie, S. D., Yeh, T., Kim, S. S., Cafaro, D. P., Scannon, P. J., Giroir, B. P., and the $rBPI_{21}$ Meningococcal Sepsis Study Group (2000) Recombinant bactericidal/permeability-increasing protein(rBPI21) as adjunctive treatment for children with severe meningococcal sepsis: a randomised trial. *Lancet* **356,** 961–967.
25. Hellman, J. and Warren, H. S. (1999) Antiendotoxin strategies. *Infect. Dis. Clin. N. Amer.* **13,** 371–386.
26. Parker, T. S., Levine, D. M., Chang, J. C., Laxer, J., Coffin, C. C., and Rubin, A. L. (1995) Reconstituted high-density lipoprotein neutralizes gram-negative bacterial lipopolysaccharides in human whole blood. *Infect. Immun.* **63,** 253–258.
27. Pajkrt, D., Doran, J. E., Koster, F., Lerch, P. G., Arnet, B., van der Poll, T., et al. (1996) Antiinflammatory effects of reconstituted high-density lipoprotein during human endotoxemia. *J. Exp. Med.* **184,** 1601–1608.
28. Alpert, G., Baldwin, G., Thompson, C., Wainwright, N., Novitsky, T. J., Gillis, Z., et al. (1992) Limulus antilipopolysaccharide factor protects rabbits from meningococcal endotoxin shock. *J. Infect. Dis.* **165,** 494–500.
29. Fletcher, M. A., McKenna, T. M., Quance, J. L., Wainwright, N. R., and Williams, T. J. (1993) Lipopolysaccharide detoxification by endotoxin neutralizing protein. *Surg. Res.* **55,** 147–154.
30. Roth, R. I., Su, D., Child, A. H., Wainwright, N. R., and Levin, J. (1998) Limulus antilipopolysaccharide factor prevents mortality late in the course of endotoxemia. *J. Infect. Dis.* **177,** 388–394.
31. Gardlund, B., Sjolin, J., Nilsson, A., Roll, M., Wickerts, C. J., Wikstrom, B., and Wretlind, B. (1993) Plasmapheresis in the treatment of primary septic shock in humans. *Scand. J. Infect. Dis.* **25,** 757–761.
32. Hoffmann, J. N., Hartl, W. H., Deppisch, R., Faist, E., Jochum, M., and Inthorn, D. (1995) Hemofiltration in human sepsis: evidence for elimination of immunomodulatory substances. *Kidney Int.* **48,** 1563–1570.
33. Pollack, M. (1992) Blood exchange and plasmapheresis in sepsis and septic shock. *Clin. Infect. Dis.* **15,** 431–433.
34. Aoki, H., Kodama, M., Tani, T., and Hanasawa, K. (1994) Treatment of sepsis by extracorporeal elimination of endotoxin using polymyxin B-immobilized fiber. *Am. J. Surg.* **167,** 412–417.
35. Ronco, C., Bellomo, R., Homel, P., Brendolan, A., Dan, M., Piccinni, P., and La Greca, G. (2000) Effects of different doses in continuous veno-venous haemofiltration on outcomes of acute renal failure: a prospective randomised trial. *Lancet* **356,** 26–30.
36. Reeves, J. H., Butt, W. W., Shann, F., Layton, J. E., Stewart, A., Waring, P. M., and Presneill, J. J. (1999) Continuous plasmafiltration in sepsis syndrome. Plasmafiltration in Sepsis Study Group. *Crit. Care Med.* **27,** 2096–2104.
37. van Deuren, M., Frieling, J. T., van der Ven-Jongekrijg, J., Neeleman, C., Russel, F. G., van Lier, H. J., et al. (1998) Plasma patterns of tumor necrosis factor-alpha (TNF) and TNF soluble receptors during acute meningococcal infections and the effect of plasma exchange. *Clin. Infect. Dis.* **26,** 918–923.

38. Kawata, T., Bristol, J. R., Rossignol, D. P., Rose, J. R., Kobayashi, S., Yokohama, H., et al. (1999). E5531, a synthetic non-toxic lipid A derivative blocks the immunobiological activities of lipopolysaccharide. *Br. J. Pharmacol.* **127,** 853–862.
39. Salkowski, C. A., Detore, G., Franks, A., Falk, M. C., and Vogel, S. N. (1998) Pulmonary and hepatic gene expression following cecal ligation and puncture: monophosphoryl lipid A prophylaxis attenuates sepsis-induced cytokine and chemokine expression and neutrophil infiltration. *Infect. Immun.* **66,** 3569–3578.
40. Waage, A., Brandtzaeg, P., Halstensen, A., Kierulf, P., and Espevik, T. (1989) The complex pattern of cytokines in serum from patients with meningococcal septic shock. *J. Exp. Med.* **169,** 333–338.
41. van der Poll, T. and van Deventer, S. J. H. (1999) Cytokines and anticytokines in the pathogenesis of sepsis. *Infect. Dis. Clin. North Amer.* **13,** 413–426.
42. Bone, R. C., Grodzin, C. J., and Balk, R. A. (1997) Sepsis: a new hypothesis for pathogenesis of the disease process. *Chest* **112,** 235–243.
43. Lowry, S. F., Calvano, S. E., and van der Poll, T. (1995) Measurement of inflammatory mediators in clinical sepsis, in *Clinical Trials for the Treatment of Sepsis* (Sibbald, W. J. and Vincent, J. L., eds.), Springer-Verlag, New York, pp 86–112.
44. Marchant, A., Deviere, J., Byl, B., De Groote, D., Vincent, J. L., and Goldman, M. (1994) Interleukin-10 production during septicaemia. *Lancet* **343,** 707–708.
45. van Deuren, M., van der Ven-Jongekrijg, J., Demacker, P. N., Bartelink, A. K., van Dalen, R., Sauerwein, R. W., et al. (1994) Differential expression of proinflammatory cytokines and their inhibitors during the course of meningococcal infections. *J. Infect. Dis.* **169,** 157–161.
46. Docke, W. D., Randow, F., Syrbe, U., Krausch, D., Asadullah, K., Reinke, P., et al. (1997) Monocyte deactivation in septic patients: restoration by IFN-gamma treatment. *Nat. Med.* **3,** 678–681.
47. Fisher, C. J., Jr, Agosti, J. M., Opal, S. M., Lowry, S. F., Balk, R. A., Sadoff, J. C., et al. (1996) Treatment of septic shock with the tumor necrosis factor receptor:Fc fusion protein. The Soluble TNF Receptor Sepsis Study Group. *N. Engl. J. Med.* **334,** 1697–1702.
48. Parent, C. and Eichacker, P. Q. (1999) Neutrophil and endothelial cell interactions in sepsis. *Infect. Dis. Clin, North Amer.* **13,** 427–447.
49. Hawkins, H. K., Heffelfinger, S. C., and Anderson, D. C. (1992) Leukocyte adhesion deficiency: Clinical and post-mortem observations. *Pediatr. Pathol. Lab. Med.* **12,** 119–130.
50. Eichacker, P. Q., Hoffman, W. D., Farese, A., Danner, R. L., Suffredini, A. F., Waisman, Y., et al. (1992) Leukocyte CD18 monoclonal antibody worsens endotoxemia and cardiovascular injury in canines with septic shock. *J. Appl. Physiol.* **74,** 1885–1892.
51. Friedman, G., Jankowski, S., Shahla, M., Goldman, M., Rose, R. M., Kahn, R. J., and Vincent, J. L. (1996) Administration of an antibody to E-Selectin in patients with septic shock. *Crit. Care Med.* **24,** 229–233.

52. Moncada, S. and Higgs, A. (1993) The L-arginine nitric oxide pathway. *N. Engl. J. Med.* **329,** 2002–2012.
53. Cobb, J. P. and Danner, R. L. (1996) Nitric oxide and septic shock. *JAMA* **275,** 1192–1196.
54. Murad, F. (1996) Signal transduction using nitric oxide and cyclic guanosine monophosphate. *JAMA* **276,** 1189–1192.
55. Avontuur, J. A., Boomsma, F., van den Meiracker, A. H., de Jong, F. H., and Bruining, H. A. (1999) Endothelin-1 and blood pressure after inhibition of nitric oxide synthesis in human septic shock. *Circulation* **99,** 271–275.
56. Baines, P. B., Stanford, S., Bishop-Bailey, D., Sills, J. A., Thomson, A. P., Mitchell, J. A., et al. (1999) Nitric oxide production in meningococcal disease is directly related to disease severity. *Crit. Care Med.* **27,** 1187–1190.
57. Avontuur, J. A., Tutein Nolthenius, R. P., Buijk, S. L., Kanhai, K. J., and Bruining, H. A. (1998) Effect of L-NAME, an inhibitor of nitric oxide synthesis, on cardiopulmonary function in human septic shock. *Chest* **113,** 1640–1646.
58. Parrillo, J. E., Burch, C., Shelhamer, J. H., Parker, M. M., Natanson, C., and Schuette, W. (1985) A circulating myocardial depressant substance in humans with septic shock. Septic shock patients with a reduced ejection fraction have a circulating factor that depresses in vitro myocardial cell performance. *J. Clin. Invest.* **76,** 1539–1553.
59. Hare, J. M. and Colucci, W. S. (1995) Role of nitric oxide in the regulation of myocardial function. *Prog. Cardiovasc. Dis.* **38,** 155–166.
60. Kumar, A., Kosuri, R., Thota, V., et al. (1993) Nitric oxide and cGMP generation mediates human septic serum induced in vitro cardiomyocyte depression. *Chest* **104,** 12S.
61. Kumar, A. and Thora, V. (1995) Tumor necrosis factor impairs epinephrine stimulated cardiomyocyte contractility and cyclic AMP response through a nitric oxide independent mechanism. *Crit. Care Med.* **23,** A148.
62. Cobb, J. P., Natanson, C., Hoffman, W. D., Lodato, R. F., Banks, S., Koev, C. A., et al. (1992) N omega-amino-L-arginine, an inhibitor of nitric oxide synthase, raises vascular resistance but increases mortality rates in awake canines challenged with endotoxin. *J. Exp. Med.* **176,** 1175–1182.
63. Freeman, B. D. and Cobb, J. P. (1998) Nitric oxide synthase as a therapeutic target in sepsis—more questions than answers? *Crit. Care Med.* **26,** 1146–1147.
64. Hollenberg, S. M. (1998) A yellow light for nitric oxide synthase inhibitors in sepsis: Proceed with caution. *Crit. Care Med.* **26,** 815–816.
65. Avontuur, J. A., Biewenga, M., Buijk, S. L., Kanhai, K. J., and Bruining, H. A. (1998) Pulmonary hypertension and reduced cardiac output during inhibition of nitric oxide synthesis in human septic shock. *Shock* **9,** 451–454.
66. Jourdain, M., Tournoys, A., Leroy, X., Mangalaboyi, J., Fourrier, F., Goudemand, J., et al. (1997) Effects of N omega-nitro-L-arginine methyl ester on the endotoxin-induced disseminated intravascular coagulation in porcine septic shock. *Crit. Care Med.* **25,** 452–459.

67. Kiehl, M. G., Ostermann, H., Meyer, J., and Kienast, J. (1997) Nitric oxide synthase inhibition by L-NAME in leukocytopenic patients with severe septic shock. *Intensive Care Med.* **23,** 561–566.
68. Grover, R., Lopez, A., Lorente, J., et al. (1999) Multicenter, randomized, placebo-controlled, double-blind study of the nitric oxide synthase inhibitor 546C88: effect on survival in patients with septic shock. *Crit. Care Med.* **27,** A33.
69. Rosselet, A., Feihl, F., Markert, M., Gnaegi, A., Perret, C., and Liaudet, L. (1998) Selective iNOS inhibition is superior to norepinephrine in the treatment of rat endotoxic shock. *Am. J. Respir. Crit. Care Med.* **57,** 162–170.
70. Perrella, M. A., Hsieh, C. M., Lee, W. S., Shieh, S., Tsai, J. C., Patterson, C., et al. (1996) Arrest of endotoxin-induced hypotension by transforming growth factor beta1. *Proc. Natl. Acad. Sci. USA* **93,** 2054–2059.
71. Brandtzaeg, P. (1995) Pathogenesis of meningococcal infections, in *Meningococcal Disease* (Cartwright, K. A. V., ed.), John Wiley and Sons, Chichester, UK, pp. 177–205.
72. Hermans, P. W., Hibberd, M. L., Booy, R., Daramola, O., Hazelzet, J. A., de Groot, R., and Levin, M. (1999) 4G/5G promoter polymorphism in the plasminogen-activator-inhibitor-1 gene and outcome of meningococcal disease. Meningococcal Research Group. *Lancet* **354,** 556–560.
73. Esmon, C. T., Taylor, F. B., and Snow, R. T. (1991) Inflammation and coagulation: linked processes potentially regulated through a common pathway mediated by protein C. *Thromb. Haemost.* **66,** 160–165.
74. Comp, P. C., Nixon, R. R., Cooper, M. R., and Esmon, C. T. (1984) Familial protein S deficiency is associated with recurrent thrombosis. *J. Clin. Invest.* **74,** 2082–2088.
75. Heyderman, R. S., Klein, N. J., Shennan, G. I., and Levin, M. (1992) Modulation of the anticoagulant properties of glycosaminoglycans on the surface of the vascular endothelium by endotoxin and neutrophils: evaluation by an amidolytic assay. *Thromb. Res.* **67,** 677–685.
76. Gérard, P., Moriau, M., Bachy, A., Malvaux, P., and De Meyer, R. (1973) Meningococcal purpura: report of 19 patients treated with heparin. *J. Pediatr.* **82,** 780–786.
77. Corrigan, J. J. and Jordan, C. M. (1970) Heparin therapy in septicemia with disseminated intravascular coagulation. *N. Engl. J. Med.* **283,** 778.
78. Taylor, F. B., Jr, Chang, A., Esmon, C. T., D'Angelo, A., Vigano-D'Angelo, S., and Blick, K. E. (1987) Protein C prevents the coagulopathic and lethal effects of Escherichia coli infusion in the baboon. *J. Clin. Invest.* **79,** 918–925.
79. Smith, O. P., White, B., Vaughan, D., Rafferty, M., Claffey, L., Lyons, B., and Casey, W. (1997) Use of protein-C concentrate, heparin, and haemodiafiltration in meningococcus-induced purpura fulminans. *Lancet* **350,** 1590–1593.
80. Rintala, E., Seppala, O. P., Kotilainen, P., Pettila, V., and Rasi, V. (1998) Protein C in the treatment of coagulopathy in meningococcal disease. *Crit. Care Med.* **26,** 965–968.
81. Clarke, R. C., Johnston, J. R., and Mayne, E. E. (2000) Meningococcal septicaemia: treatment with protein C concentrate. *Intensive Care Med.* **26,** 471–473.

82. Bernard, G. R., Vincent, J-L., Laterre, P-F., et al. (2001) Efficacy and safety of recombinant human activated protein C for severe sepsis. *N. Engl. J. Med.* **344,** 699–709.
83. Fourrier, F., Chopin, C., Huart, J. J., Runge, I., Caron, C., and Goudemand, J. (1993) Double-blind, placebo-controlled trial of antithrombin III concentrates in septic shock with disseminated intravascular coagulation. *Chest* **104,** 882–888.
84. Baudo, F., Caimi, T. M., de Cataldo, F., Ravizza, A., Arlati, S., Casella, G., et al. (1998) Antithrombin III (ATIII) replacement therapy in patients with sepsis and/or postsurgical complications: a controlled double-blind, randomized, multicenter study. *Intensive Care Med.* **24,** 336–342.
85. Taylor, F. B., Jr, Chang, A., Ruf, W., Morrissey, J. H., Hinshaw, L., Catlett, R., et al. (1991) Lethal E. coli septic shock is prevented by blocking tissue factor with monoclonal antibody. *Circ. Shock.* **33,** 127–134.
86. Creasey, A. A., Chang, A. C., Feigen, L., Wun, T. C., Taylor, F.B., Jr, and Hinshaw, L. B. (1993) Tissue factor pathway inhibitor reduces mortality from Escherichia coli septic shock. *J. Clin. Invest.* **91,** 2850–2856.
87. Goldfarb, R. D., Glock, D., Johnson, K., Creasey, A. A., Carr, C., McCarthy, R. J., et al. (1998) Randomized, blinded, placebo-controlled trial of tissue factor pathway inhibitor in porcine septic shock. *Shock* **10,** 258–264.
88. Zenz, W., Muntean, W., Gallistl, S., Zobel, G., and Grubbauer, H. M. (1995) Recombinant tissue plasminogen activator treatment in two infants with fulminant meningococcemia. *Pediatrics* **96,** 44–48.
89. Aiuto, L. T., Barone, S. R., Cohen, P. S., and Boxer, R. A. (1997) Recombinant tissue plasminogen activator restores perfusion in meningococcal purpura fulminans. *Crit. Care Med.* **25,** 1079–1082.
90. Murakami, J., Ohtani, A., and Murata, S. (1997) Protective effect of T-686, an inhibitor of plasminogen activator inhibitor-1 production, against the lethal effect of lipopolysaccharide in mice. *Jpn. J. Pharmacol.* **75,** 291–294.
91. Cochrane Injuries Group Albumin Reviewers (1998) Human albumin administration in critically ill patients: systematic review of randomised controlled trials. *BMJ* 235–240.
92. Oragui, E. E, Nadel, S., Kyd, P., and Levin, M. (2000) Increased excretion of glycosaminoglycans in meningococcal septicaemia and their relationship to proteinuria. *Crit. Care Med.* **28,** In press.
93. Stewart, D. L., Dela Cruz, T. V., Ziegler, C., and Goldsmith, L. J. (1997) The use of extracorporeal membrane oxygenation in patients with gram-negative or viral sepsis. *Perfusion* **12,** 3–8.
94. Meyer, D. M. and Jessen, M. E. (1997) Results of extracorporeal membrane oxygenation in children with sepsis. The Extracorporeal Life Support Organization. *Ann. Thorac. Surg.* **63,** 756–761.
95. Goldman, A. P., Kerr, S. J., Butt, W., Marsh, M. J., Murdoch, I. A., Paul, T., et al. (1997) Extracorporeal support for intractable cardiorespiratory failure due to meningococcal disease. *Lancet* **349,** 466–469.
96. Beca, J. and Butt, W. (1994) Extracorporeal membrane oxygenation for refractory septic shock in children. *Pediatrics* **93,** 726–729.

97. Lebel, M. H., Freij, B. J., Syrogiannopoulos, G. A., Chrane, D. F., Hoyt, M. J., Stewart, S. M., et al. (1988) Dexamethasone therapy for bacterial meningitis. Results of two double-blind, placebo-controlled trials. *N. Engl. J. Med.* **319,** 964–971.
98. Odio, C. M., Faingezicht, I., Paris, M., Nassar, M., Baltodano, A., Rogers, J., et al. (1991) The beneficial effects of early dexamethasone administration in infants and children with bacterial meningitis. *N. Engl. J. Med.* **324,** 525–531.
99. Hatherill, M., Tibby, S. M., Hilliard, T., Turner, C., and Murdoch, I. A. (1999) Adrenal insufficiency in septic shock. *Arch. Dis. Child.* **80,** 51–55.
100. Riordan, F. A., Thomson, A. P., Ratcliffe, J. M., Sills, J. A., Diver, M. J., and Hart, C. A. (1999) Admission cortisol and adrenocorticotrophic hormone levels in children with meningococcal disease: evidence of adrenal insufficiency? *Crit. Care Med.* **27,** 2257–2261.
101. Briegel, J., Forst, H., Haller, M., Schelling, G., Kilger, E., Kuprat, G., et al. (1999) Stress doses of hydrocortisone reverse hyperdynamic septic shock: a prospective, randomized, double-blind, single-center study. *Crit. Care Med.* **27,** 723–732.
102. Cronin, L., Cook, D. J., Carlet, J., Heyland, D. K., Math, D. K., Lansang, M. A. D., and Fisher, C. J., Jr. (1995) Corticosteroid treatment for sepsis: a critical appraisal and meta-analysis of the literature. *Crit. Care Med.* **23,** 1430–1439.
103. Westendorp, R. G., Langermans, J. A., Huizinga, T. W., Elouali, A. H., Verweij, C. L., Boomsma, D. I., et al. (1997) Genetic influence on cytokine production and fatal meningococcal disease. *Lancet* **349,** 170–173.
104. Nadel, S., Newport, M. J., Booy, R., and Levin, M. (1996) Variation in the tumor necrosis factor-alpha gene promoter region may be associated with death from meningococcal disease. *J. Infect. Dis.* **174,** 878–880.
105. Angus, D. C., Birmingham, M. C., Balk, R. A., Scannon, P. J., Collins, D., Kruse, J. A., et al. (2000) E5 murine monoclonal anti-endotoxin antibody in gram-negative sepsis: a randomised controlled trial. E5 Study Investigators. *JAMA* **283,** 1723–1730.
106. Asai, Y., Nozo, Y., Ikeuchi, T., Narazaki, R., Iwamoto, K., and Watanabe, S. (1999) The effect of Lipid A analog E5531 on fever induced by endotoxin from Escherichia Coli. *Biol. Pharmaceut. Bull.* **22,** 432–434.
107. Haupt, M. T., Jastremski, M. S., Clemmer, T. P., Metz, C. A., and Goris, G. B. (1991) Effect of ibuprofen in patients with severe sepsis: a randomized, double-blind, multicenter study. The Ibuprofen Study Group. *Crit. Care Med.* **19,** 1339–1347.
108. Opal, S. M., Fisherm C. J., Jr., Dhainaut, J. F., Vincent, J. L., Brase, R., Lowry, S. F., et al. (1997) Confirmatory interleukin-1 receptor antagonist trial in severe sepsis: a phase III, randomized, double-blind, placebo-controlled, multicenter trial. The Interleukin-1 Receptor Antagonist Sepsis Investigator Group. *Crit. Care Med.* **25,** 1115–1124.
109. Cohen, J. and Carlet J. INTERSEPT: an international, multicenter, placebo-controlled trial of monoclonal antibody to human tumor necrosis factor-alpha in patients with sepsis. International Sepsis Trial Study Group. *Crit. Care Med.* **24,** 1431–1440.

110. Dhainaut, J. F., Tenaillon, A., Hemmer, M., Damas, P., Le Tulzo, Y., Radermacher, P., et al. (1998) Confirmatory platelet-activating factor receptor antagonist trial in patients with severe gram-negative bacterial sepsis: a phase III, randomized, double-blind, placebo-controlled, multicenter trial. BN 52021 Sepsis Investigator Group. *Crit. Care Med.* **26,** 1963–1971.
111. Soltys, J. and Quinn, M. T. (1999) Modulation of endotoxin and enterotoxin-induced cytokine release by in vivo treatment with beta-(1,6)- branched beta-(1,3)-glucan. *Infect. Immun.* **67,** 244–252.
112. Olszyna, D. P., Pajkrt, D., Lauw, F. N., van Deventer, S. J., and van Der Poll, T. (2000) Interleukin 10 inhibits the release of CC chemokines during human endotoxemia. *J. Infect. Dis.* **181,** 613–620.
113. Opal, S. M., Jhung, J. W., Keith, J. C., Jr., Perlandy, J. E., Parejo, N. A., Young, L. D., and Bhattacharjee, A. (1998) Recombinant human interleukin 11 in experimental Pseudomonas Aeruginosa sepsis in immunocompromised animals. *J. Infect. Dis.* **178,** 1205–1208.
114. Fiorucci, S., Antonelli, E., Migliorati, G., Santucci, L., Morelli, O., Federici, B., and Morelli, A. (1998) TNF-alpha processing enzyme inhibitors prevent aspirin-induced TNF-alpha release and protect against gastric mucosal injury in rats. *Ailment Pharmacol. Ther.* **12,** 1139–1153.
115. Grover, R., Zaccardelli, D., Colice, G., Guntupalli, K., Watson, D., and Vincent, J. L. (1999) An open-label dose escalation study of the nitric oxide synthase inhibitor, N(G)-methyl-L-arginine hydrochloride (546C88), in patients with septic shock. Glaxo Wellcome International Septic Shock Study Group. *Crit. Care Med.* **27,** 913–922.
116. Eisele, B., Lamy, M., Thijs, L. G., Keinecke, H. O., Schuster, H. P., Matthias, F. R., et al. (1998) Antithrombin III in patients with severe sepsis. A randomized, placebo-controlled, double-blind multicenter trial plus a meta-analysis on all randomized, placebo-controlled, double-blind trials with antithrombin III in severe sepsis. *Intensive Care Med.* **24,** 663–672.
117. Pernerstorfer, T., Hollenstein, U., Hansen, J., Knechtelsdorfer, M., Stohlawetz, P., Graninger, W., et al. (1999) Heparin blunts endotoxin-induced coagulation activation. *Circulation* **100,** 2485–2490.
118. de Jonge, E., Dekkers, P. E., Creasey, A. A., Hack, C. E., Paulson, S. K., Karim, A., et al. (2000) Tissue factor pathway inhibitor dose-dependently inhibits coagulation activation without influencing the fibrinolytic and cytokine response during human endotoxemia. *Blood* **95,** 1124–1129.
119. Fein, A. M., Bernard, G. R., Criner, G. J., Fletcher, E. C., Good, J. T., Jr., Knaus, W. A., et al. (1997) Treatment of severe systemic inflammatory response syndrome and sepsis with a novel bradykinin antagonist, deltibant (CP-0127). Results of a randomized, double-blind, placebo-controlled trial. CP-0127 SIRS and Sepsis Study Group. *JAMA* **277,** 482–487.
120. Tani, T., Hanasawa, K., Endo, Y., Yoshioka, T., Kodama, M., Kaneko, M., et al. (1998) Therapeutic apheresis for septic patients with organ dysfunction:

hemoperfusion using a polymyxin B immobilized column. *Artif. Organs.* **22,** 1038–1044.
121. Gillan, E. R., Christensen, R. D., Suen, Y., Ellis, R., van de Ven, C., and Cairo, M. S. (1994) A randomized, placebo-controlled trial of recombinant human granulocyte colony-stimulating factor administration in newborn infants with presumed sepsis: significant induction of peripheral and bone marrow neutrophilia. *Blood* **84,** 1427–1433.
122. Smith, W. S., Sumnicht, G. E., Sharpe, R. W., Samuelson, D., and Millard, F. E. (1995) Granulocyte colony-stimulating factor versus placebo in addition to penicillin G in a randomized blinded study of gram-negative pneumonia sepsis: analysis of survival and multisystem organ failure. *Blood* **86,** 1301–1309.
123. Schedel, I., Dreikhausen, U., Nentwig, B., Hockenschnieder, M., Rauthmann, D., Balikcioglu, S., et al. (1991) Treatment of gram-negative septic shock with an immunoglobulin preparation: a prospective, randomized clinical trial. *Crit. Care Med.* **19,** 1104–1113.
124. Alejandria, M. M., Lansang, M. A., Dans, L. F., and Mantaring, J. B. (2000) Intravenous immunoglobulin for treating sepsis and septic shock. Cochrane Database Syst. Rev. 2, CD001090.
125. American College of Chest Physicians (1992) Definitions for sepsis and organ failure and guidelines for the use of innovative therapies in sepsis. Society for Critical Care Medicine Consensus Conference. *Crit. Care Med.* **20,** 864–875.
126. Jafari, H. S. and McCracken G. H., Jr. (1992) Sepsis and septic shock: a review for clinicians. *Pediatr. Infect. Dis. J.* **11,** 739–748.

34

Studies on the Effect of Neisserial Porins on Apoptosis of Mammalian Cells

Paola Massari and Lee M. Wetzler

1. Introduction

Microorganisms or microbial products have been shown to induce or protect cells from activation-induced cell death or apoptosis *(1–3)*. Induction of apoptosis by some bacterial invaders, like shigella, might aid in spread of the organism *(4)*, whereas inhibition of apoptosis by other microbes might aid in furthering their intracellular survival *(2,3)*. Viral products have been shown to inhibit apoptosis by mimicking anti-apoptotic related proteins (e.g., Bcl2, FLIPS, etc.) *(2,3,5)*. Thus far, most investigators have demonstrated that bacteria either have no effect or induce apoptosis of various cell types, mainly cells that they encounter upon invasion, e.g., epithelial cells, fibroblasts, and so on. Apoptotic cell death is also a key control mechanism of immune responses *(6)*, but, to date, there have not been many investigations into the effect of microbes on apoptosis in immune cells. Dysregulation of immune cells associated with a lack of apoptosis and abnormal Fas-mediated cell death have been associated with immune dysfunction and hyperimmune states *(7)*.

In regards to *Neisseria*, Muller et al. have investigated the effect of intact gonococci on apoptotic events in the HeLa cell human fibroblast cell line. They found that in the absence of sera, organisms and crude preparations of neisserial porin can induce HeLa cell apoptosis as measured by DNA breakdown, Annexin V staining, and morphology *(8)*. On the other hand, our laboratory, using murine B cells and B-cell lines, has found that purified porin lacking any detergent and in the presence of sera, can protect cells from Fas-mediated and staurosporine-mediated cell death as measured by DNA breakdown, lack of mitochondrial depolarization, chromium lysis assays, trypan blue exclusion,

From: *Methods in Molecular Medicine, vol. 67: Meningococcal Disease: Methods and Protocols*
Edited by: A. J. Pollard and M. C. J. Maiden © Humana Press Inc., Totowa, NJ

and so on *(26)*. Interestingly, it appears that this anti-apoptotic effect is owing to a direct interaction of porin with the mitochondrial porin, VDAC, stabilizing the mitochondrial membrane and preventing depolarization and release of cytochrome c *(26)*. This activity of the mitochondria makes it one of the key control points of cellular apoptosis *(9)*. The main difference between these two results is the fact that: 1) Muller et al. used serum-free conditions and serum starvation is a known inducer of apoptosis *(10,11)*; 2) their porin preparation had significant amounts of detergent, which can be cytotoxic to the HeLa cells; and 3) there were differences in the porins and cell types used in the two studies. The significance of the differences in these findings is still being investigated.

This chapter will list methods of measuring the effect of neisserial porin (and other bacterial products) on various parameters associated with apoptosis including: 1) cell viability by trypan blue exclusion, 2) DNA breakdown by propidium iodide (PI) staining and by gel electrophoresis, and 3) mitochondrial depolarization. Some representative figures will be included describing experiments performed with purified meningococcal PorB, formed into proteosomes and lacking all detergent *(12)*. The breadth of this chapter and the subject of this book does not allow us to discriminate between the findings of the two groups listed earlier, but various investigators can use their own products and these methods to determine their apoptosis-protective or -inducing ability.

2. Materials

2.1. Strains of Mice

The following strains of mice have been used for purification of splenic B cells:

1. C3H/HeJ (*see* **Note 1**).
2. C57 black mice.

2.2. Cells

The following cell types have been used:

1. Jurkat cells (human T lymphocyte cell line, ATCC, Cat. no. TIB-152).
2. CH-12 RMC cells (murine B-cell lymphoma, from Dr. R. Corley, Boston University School of Medicine, Boston, MA).
3. HeLa cells (human adenocarcinoma, ATCC Cat. no. CCL-2).
4. Murine splenic B cells, obtained from C3H/HeJ and C57 black mice by standard protocol (*see* Ch. 15, in Meningococcal Vaccines, edited by A. J. Pollard and M. C. J. Maiden, Humana Press) *(23,25)*.

2.3. Culture Media

1. Bacterial culture medium:
   a. Neisserial liquid medium (*see* Delvig et al., Meningococcal Vaccines, edited by A. J. Pollard and M. C. J. Maiden, Humana Press) containing isovitalex supplement (BBL / Fisher B11876).
2. Cell-culture media:
   a. RPMI 1640 (Bio-Whittaker, supplied in 500-mL bottles, Cat. no. 12-702F). The complete RPMI 1640 medium is supplemented with 2.0 m*M* L-glutamine (Bio-Whittaker, Cat. no. 17-605E, supplied in 100-mL bottles), 0.05 m*M* 2-mercaptoethanol (2-ME, Sigma, Cat. no. M-7522, supplied in 100 mL bottles, 14.3 *M* stock), 100 m*M* HEPES (Sigma, Cat. no. H-0887, supplied in 100-mL bottles), 100 U/mL penicillin, 100 mg/mL streptomycin (Bio-Whittaker, cat. No. 17-602E, supplied in 100-mL bottles) and 10% fetal bovine serum (v/v) (FBS, Sigma, Cat. no. F7524, supplied in 500-mL bottles). High concentration stock of 2-ME is prepared (0.0143 *M* in sterile dd H_2O) and stored at 2–8°C. The complete RPMI 1640 medium is used for CH-12 RMC B-cell line and murine splenic B cells.
   b. RPMI 1640 supplemented with 2.0 m*M* L-glutamine, 100 U/mL penicillin, 100 mg/mL streptomycin, and 5% FBS is used for Jurkat T-cell line.
   c. DMEM (Bio-Whittaker, supplied in 500-mL bottles, Cat. no. 12-604F) supplemented with 2.0 m*M* L-glutamine, 100 U/mL penicillin, 100 mg/mL streptomycin, and 10% FBS is used for HeLa cell line.
   d. Trypsin-Versene mixture (Bio-Whittaker, Cat. no. 17-161E, supplied in 100-mL bottles).

2.4. Buffered Solutions and Reagents

2.4.1. Buffered solution:

1. NaAcetate solution, pH 4.0 (Sigma, Cat. no. S1492). High concentration stock solution is prepared in ddH_2O.
2. $CaCl_2$ solution, (Sigma, Cat. no. C5670). High-concentration stock solution is prepared in ddH_2O.
3. Tris solution, pH 8.0 (Sigma, Cat. no. T3038). High-concentration stock solution is prepared in ddH_2O.
4. Ethylene diamine tetraacetic acid (EDTA) solution (Sigma, Cat. no. E5134). High-concentration stock solution is prepared in ddH_2O.
5. Sodium dodecyl sulfate polyacrylamide gel electrophoresis (SDS-PAGE) running buffer, prepared as a 10X stock solution containing 144 g of glycine (Sigma, Cat. no. G7403), 30 g of Tris, and 10 g of SDS (Sigma, Cat. no. L6026) per liter of solution.
6. Acrylamide gel destaining solution, containing 10% (v/v) acetic acid (Sigma, Cat. no. A9967), 40% (v/v) ethanol.
7. Phosphate-buffered solution, pH 8.0, containing 93.2 mL of 0.1 *M* Na_2HPO_4, (Sigma, Cat. no. S0876) and 6.8 mL of 0.1 *M* NaH_2PO_4, (Sigma, Cat. no. S3139).

8. Phosphate-buffered saline (PBS, Sigma-Fluka, Cat. no. 79378, supplied in 1000-mL bottles).
9. TBE buffer, prepared as a 10X stock solution containing 108 g of Tris base, 55 g of boric acid (Sigma, Cat. no. B6768) and 8.3 g of EDTA per liter of solution.
10. Agarose gel loading dye, prepared as 10X stock solution containing 15% Ficoll (Sigma, Cat. no. F-2637), 0.2% bromophenol blue (Sigma, Cat. no. B-0126), 0.2% xylene cyanol FF (Kodak, Cat. no. T-1579) and 0.1% SDS (Sigma, Cat. no. L-4390), in ddH_2O.
11. Trypan blue (Fluka, Cat. no. 93590) % in 0.81% NaCl (Sigma) and 0.09% KCl (Sigma, Cat. no. P-4504).

2.4.2. Reagents

1. 2,dimercaptoethanol (Sigma, Cat. no. M3148).
2. Zwittergent 3-14 (Z3-14) (Calbiochem, Cat. no. 693017).
3. Ethanol (Sigma, Cat. no. 21142, supplied in 2-L bottles). 20–80% solutions are prepared in ddH_2O.
4. DEAE resin (BioChemika, Cat. no. T30473).
5. CM sepharose resin (Sigma Cat. no. CCL6B100).
6. Sephacryl S-300 resin (BioChemika, Cat. no. 84937).
7. Acrylammide solution (National Diagnostics, Cat. no. EC890).
8. Coomassie brilliant blue, (Sigma, Cat. no. B1131) 0.4% solution, prepared in destaining solution (as in **Subheading 2.4.1., item 7**).
9. D-octyl-glucoside (Sigma, Cat. no. O9882).
10. DMSO (Sigma, Cat. no. D-8779, supplied in 100-mL bottles).
11. Staurosporine (Sigma, Cat. no. S4400). High concentration (1 m*M*) stock solution is prepared in sterile DMSO.
12. Rhodamine 123 (Molecular Probes, Cat. no. R-302). High concentration (1 m*M*) stock solution is prepared in sterile DMSO.
13. Propidium iodide (Molecular Probe, Cat. no. P-3566, supplied in 10 mL solution in ddH_2O).
14. Rnase A (Sigma, Cat. no. R6513), prepared as 10 mg/mL stock solution in ddH_2O. Stored below 0°C.
15. Proteinase K (Sigma, Cat. no. P8044), prepared as 20 mg/mL stock solution in ddH_2O. Stored below 0°C.
16. Agarose (Biorad, Cat. no. 162-0133).
17. Ethidium bromide (Sigma, Cat. no. E-8751) 5 mg/mL in ddH_2O.

3. Methods

Neisserial porins are the major outer-membrane component and can be isolated from organisms utilizing a method originally developed by Blake and Gotschlich ***(13)*** with subsequent modifications ***(14,15)***. Gonococcal porin (Por or Protein I in older nomenclature, two types, PIA or PIB of one allele) can be isolated from strains that lack the reduction modifiable protein (Rmp or Protein III in older nomenclature *(16)*. Meningococci contain two porins in two different alleles, PorA (class 1 protein in older nomenclature) or PorB (class 2 or 3 protein in older nomenclature). They also contain a reduction modifiable protein (RmpM), termed class 4 protein in older nomenclature). Strains have been genetically modified to allow purification of either PorA or PorB without contamination by the other porin of by RmpM *(17–19)*. This method will discuss the purification of PorB from a meningococcal strain lack both RmpM and PorA. Similarly, this method can be used to purify meningococcal PorA from strains lacking PorB and RmpM. The reason for isolating these proteins from strains lacking Rmp and other porins is to improve the purity of the subsequent porin preparation.

3.1. Neisserial Porin Purification

1. Grow 6–12 L of *N. meningitidis* culture in neisserial liquid media until mid-log phase at 37°C *(15)*.
2. After 10 h centrifuge the culture for 15 min at 1500*g* at 4°C and resuspend pellets of organisms in an equal volume of 1 *M* NaAcetate, pH 4.0, with 1 m*M* 2,dimercaptopropanol.
3. Add 6 volumes of 5% zwittergent 3-14 (Z3-14) in 0.5 *M* $CaCl_2$ to the bacterial pellet and stir for 1 h.
4. Add ethanol to a concentration of 20% (v/v), for precipitation of DNA and nuclear and cellular fragments (*see* **Note 2**).
5. After centrifugation (as in **Subheading 3.1., item 2**), collect the supernatant and precipitate the total protein content with 80% (v/v) ethanol.
6. After an overnight incubation at 4°C , centrifuge the solution at 12,000*g* for 30 min at 4°C and resuspend the crude Por preparation obtained in 50 m*M* Tris, pH 8.0, with 10 m*M* EDTA and 5% Z3-14.
7. The solution is centrifuged again (as in **Subheading 3.1., item 6**) and then subjected to chromatography purification on two ion-exchange columns, a DEAE resin column followed by a CM sepaharose resin column in tandem.
8. Precipitate the protein present in the flow through by the addition of ethanol to a concentration of 80% (v/v). Resuspend the precipitate in as small a volume as possible of 50 m*M* Tris, pH 8.0, with 10 m*M* EDTA and 5% Z3-14.
9. Centrifuge this solution (as in **Subheading 3.1., item 6**) and load the resuspended pellet on a on a gel-filtration molecular sieve column, Sephacryl S-300. Collect 10-ml fractions and analyze by SDS-PAGE to determine the fractions containing purified Por, which are then pooled and used in further experiments.

3.2. Proteosomes Formation

Proteosomes, pure protein micelles, are prepared from purified Por in order to remove the detergent *(12)*.

1. Precipitate the chromatographically purified Por the addition of 80% (v/v) ethanol. Wash the precipitate once with 70% ethanol and then resuspend in a solution

containing the dialyzable detergent 10% D-octyl glucoside (w/v) in 10 m*M* HEPES, pH 7.2, to a concentration of 1 mg of Por per mL.

2. Dialyze the solution against 4 L of 10 m*M* phosphate buffer, pH 8.0, with multiple changes of the dialyzing buffer to remove any remaining detergent. The pure proteosomes appear as an oily precipitate.
3. Determine the protein concentration by any standard assay (i.e., coomassie blue, Pierce BCA assay, etc.). Using this procedure to purify Por and form proteosomes allows for minimal LPS contamination, less than 0.01% as demonstrated by Limulus lysate assays or silver staining of gels.

3.3. N. meningitidis *Porin PorB Protective Effect on Cell Survival upon Induction of Apoptosis with Staurosporine*

1. Culture the cells (as in **Subheadings 2.2., items 1–4**) at a concentration of 5 × 10^5 per mL in 24-wells plates and incubate them for 24 h with medium alone, or with medium containing 10 μg/mL of PorB proteosomes.
2. After 24 h, add staurosporine at a final concentration of 1 μ*M* for induction of apoptosis *(26)*.
3. 24 h later, harvest samples of cells and stain with a 0.2% trypan blue solution (*see* **Note 3**). Incubate the cells for 10 min and count a minimum of 100 cells for each sample. Assays were performed in triplicate.
4. Calculate the percentage of dead cells as a ratio between the number of dye-retaining cells (non viable) and total number of cells per mL, as determined using a hemacytometer (**Fig. 1**).

3.4. N. meningitidis *Porin PorB Protective Effect on DNA Degradation Induced by Staurosporine*

3.4.1. Hypodiploid DNA Content

1. Culture cells (as in **Subheading 3.3., steps 1** and **2**) *(26)*. Harvest cells and wash once with cold PBS followed by a second wash in PBS containing 2% FBS.
2. Resuspend the cells in 300 μL of the same buffer and permeabilize with 750 μL of ice-cold ethanol for 10 min at 4°C (*see* **Note 4**).
3. Centrifuge permeabilized cells at 1500*g* at 4°C for 5 min, wash once with cold PBS and centrifuge again.
4. Resuspend the pellets in 300 μL of PBS containing 50 μg/mL PI and 0.5 mg/mL RnaseA and incubate for 20 min in the dark. After a final wash with PBS containing 2% FBS, determine the hypo-diploid DNA content by flow cytometry (**Fig. 2**).

3.4.2. DNA Laddering

1. Harvest cells (as in **Subheading 3.4.1., step 1**) and wash once with cold PBS.
2. Cell pellets were then resuspended in DNA loading buffer solution containing 1% SDS, 0.5 mg/mL Rnase A, and 5 mg/mL proteinase K and loaded on a 2% agarose gel (*see* **Note 5**).

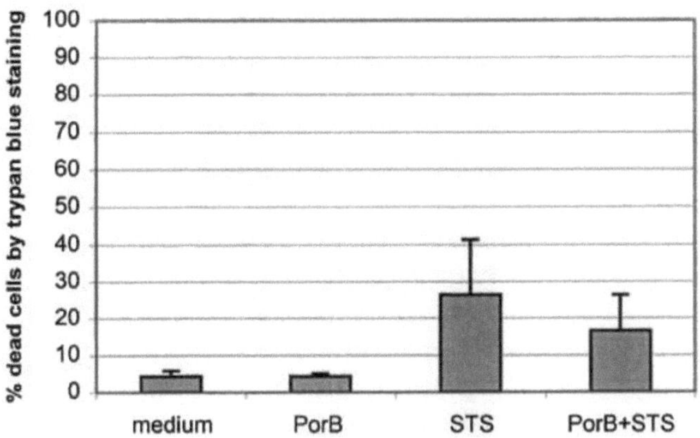

Fig. 1. PorB does not affect viability per se, and protects from cells death induced by staurosporine (STS) treatment.

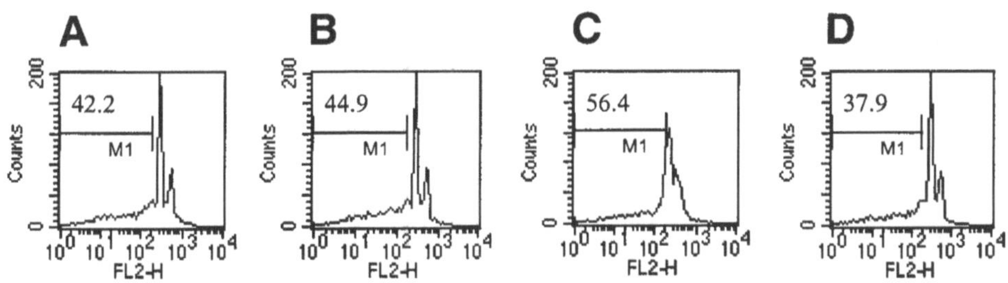

Fig. 2. Percent of cells containing hypodiploid DNA owing to the protective effect of PorB on staurosporine-induced apoptosis, measured as propidium iodide fluorescence of cells treated with medium for 24 h **(A)**, PorB for 24 h **(B)**, STS for 24 h **(C)**, and PorB for 24 h plus STS for additional 24 h **(D)**.

3. DNA laddering was visualized by ethidium bromide fluorescence on a standard ultraviolet (UV) transilluminator (**Fig. 3**).

3.5. N. meningitidis *Porin PorB Effect on Apoptotic Mitochondrial Membrane Potential ($\Delta\Psi_m$) Loss Induced by Staurosporine*

1. Incubate the cells (as in **Subheadings 3.3., steps 1** and **2**) *(26)* with 5 μg/mL of rhodamine 123 (*see* **Note 6**) for 30 min at 37°C.
2. Wash the cells once in cold PBS, resuspend in 300 μL of PBS containing 2% FBS and immediately analyzed by flow cytometry (*see* **Note 7**) (**Fig. 4**).
3. Gating was used to exclude cellular debris associated with necrosis.

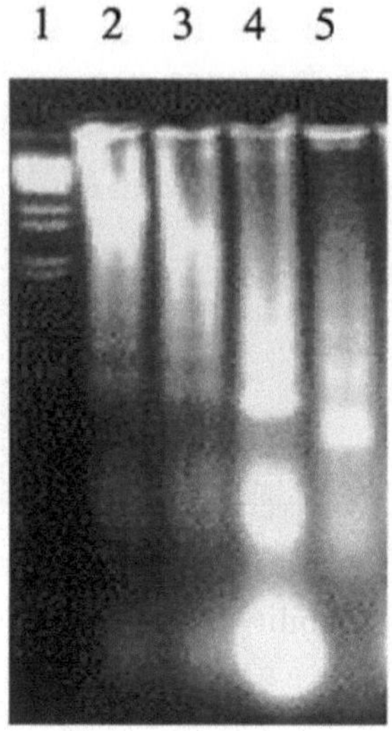

Fig. 3. Protection of apoptotic induced DNA laddering by PorB. Lane 1, DNA marker; lane 2, medium control; lane 3, PorB; lane 4, STS; lane 5, PorB + STS.

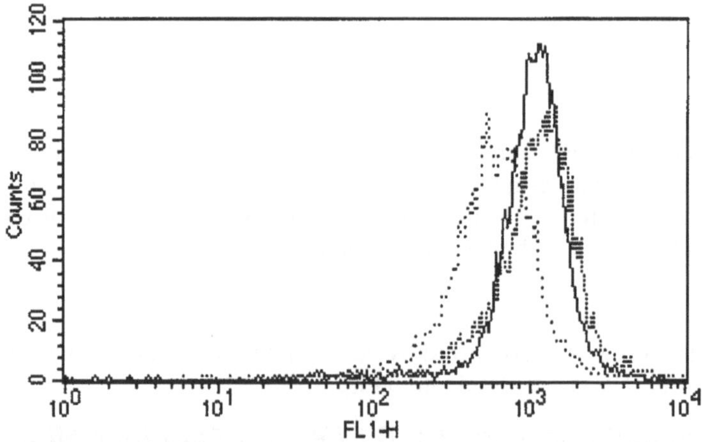

Fig. 4. Protection from $\Delta\Psi_m$ loss induced by staurosporine owing to PorB incubation, measured as rhodamine 123 fluorescence. Solid line, medium control. Dotted line, STS 24 h. Dashed line, PorB 24 h, and STS 24 h.

4. Notes

1. This strain of mice has been shown to LPS hyporesponsive due to three specific defects in the cytoplasmic portion of the LPS co receptor Toll-Like Receptor 4 (TLR4) ***(20–22)***. TLR4 is essential for transduction of a signal upon binding of LPS to its receptor CD14 ***(20,22)***. The mitogenic response of cells from mice with defective TLR4 (such as this strain or strain B10SnCCR) responds extremely poorly to LPS. However, they can respond to other immune stimulators such as tumor necrosis factor (TNF), interferon (IFN), interleukin (IL)1, and so on and to other mitogens whose activity is not dependent on TLR like ConA, PHA, lipopeptides, Muramyldipeptide, and, significantly for this chapter, Por ***(23,25)***.
2. Prior to and when precipitating proteins with ethanol at this stage, water-bath sonication can help with improved purity of the porin preparation.
3. A cell-permeable dye which is rapidly expelled by live cells and only retained in dead cells.
4. It is advisable to resuspend the cells very carefully, to obtain complete permeabilization of all the cells.
5. It is preferably to freeze the samples at –20°C and successively centrifuge them at high speed for 10 min before running them on agarose gel, owing to the viscosity of the whole-cell preparations.
6. Lipophilic cations such as rhodamine 123 (rh123) are transported into the mitochondria in accordance with the mitochondrial membrane potential, and concentrate within the mitochondrial matrix of electrically unaltered mitochondria.
7. It is advisable to not let the cells sit on ice for more than 1 h before fluorescence-activated cell sorter (FACS) analysis.

Reference

1. Chen, Y. and Zychlinsky, A. (1994) Apoptosis induced by bacterial pathogens. *Microb. Pathog.* **17,** 203–212.
2. Barry, M. and McFadden, G. (1998) Apoptosis regulators from DNA viruses. *Curr. Opin. Immunol.* **10,** 422–430.
3. Tschopp, J., Irmler, M., and Thome, M. (1998) Inhibition of fas death signals by FLIPs. *Curr. Opin. Immunol.* **10,** 552–558.
4. Zychlinsky, A. and Sansonetti, P. J. (1997) Apoptosis as a proinflammatory event: what can we learn from bacteria-induced cell death? *Trends. Microbiol.* **5,** 201–204.
5. Ploegh, H. L. (1998) Viral strategies of immune evasion. *Science* **280,** 248–253.
6. Scaffidi, C., Kirchhoff, S., Krammer, P. H., and Peter, M. E. (1999) Apoptosis signaling in lymphocytes. *Curr. Opin. Immunol.* **11,** 277–285.
7. Nagata, S. and Suda, T. (1995) Fas and Fas ligand: lpr and gld mutations. *Immunol. Today* **16,** 39–43.
8. Muller, A., Gunther, D., Naumann, M., Meyer, T. F., and Rudel, T. (1999) Neisserial porin (PorB) causes rapid calcium influx in target cells and induces apoptosis by the activation of cysteine proteases. *EMBO J.* **18,** 339–352.

9. Kroemer, G., Zamzami, N., and Susin, S. A. (1997) Mitochondrial control of apoptosis. *Immunol. Today* **18,** 44–51.
10. Kulkarni, G. V. and McCulloch, C. A. (1994) Serum deprivation induces apoptotic cell death in a subset of Balb/c 3T3 fibroblasts. *J. Cell Sci.* **107(Pt.5),** 1169–1179.
11. Simm, A., Bertsch, G., Frank, H., Zimmermann, U., and Hoppe, J. (1997) Cell death of AKR-2B fibroblasts after serum removal: a process between apoptosis and necrosis. *J. Cell Sci.* **110(Pt.7),** 819–828.
12. Wetzler, L. M., Blake, M. S., Barry, K., and Gotschlich, E. C. (1992) Gonococcal porin vaccine evaluation: comparison of Por proteosomes, liposomes and blebs isolated from *rmp* deletion mutants. *J. Infect. Dis.* **166,** 551–555.
13. Blake, M. S. and Gotschlich, E. C. (1982) Purification and partial characterization of the major outer membrane protein of *Neisseria gonorrhoeae. Infect. Immun.* **36,** 277–283.
14. Lytton, E. J. and Blake, M. S. (1986) Isolation and partial characterization of the reduction-modifiable protein of *Neisseria gonorrhoeae. J. Exp. Med.* **164,** 1749–1759.
15. Wetzler, L. M., Blake, M. S., and Gotschlich, E. C. (1988) Characterization and specificity of antibodies to protein I of *Neisseria gonorrhoeae* produced by injection with various protein I—adjuvant preparations. *J. Exp. Med.* **168,** 1883–1897.
16. Wetzler, L. M., Gotschlich, E. C., Blake, M. S., and Koomey, J. M. (1989) The construction and characterization of *Neisseria gonorrhoeae* lacking protein III in its outer membrane. *J. Exp. Med.* **169,** 2199–2209.
17. Guttormsen, H. K., Wetzler, L. M., and Naess, A. (1993) Humoral immune response to the class 3 outer membrane protein during the course of meningococcal disease. *Infect. Immun.* **61,** 4734–4742.
18. Klugman, K. P., Gotschlich, E. C., and Blake, M. S. (1989) Sequence of the structural gene (*rmpM*) for the class 4 outer membrane protein of *Neisseria meningitidis*, homology to gonococcal protein III and *Escherichia coli* OmpA, and construction of meningococcal strains that lack class 4 protein. *Infect. Immun.* **57,** 2066–2071.
19. Tommassen, J., Vermeij, P. Struyvé, M., Benz, R., and Poolman, J. T. (1990) Isolation of *Neisseria meningitidis* mutants deficient in class 1 (Por A) and class 3 (Por B) outer membrane proteins. *Infect. Immun.* **58,** 1355–1359.
20. Poltorak, A., He, X., Smirnova, I., Liu, M. Y., Huffel, C. V., Du, X., et al. (1998) Defective LPS signaling in C3H/HeJ and C57BL/10ScCr mice: mutations in Tlr4 gene. *Science* **282,** 2085–2088.
21. Sultzer, B. M., Castagna, R., Bandekar, J., and Wong, P. (1993) Lipopolysaccharide nonresponder cells: the C3H/HeJ defect. *Immunobiology* **187,** 257–271.
22. Takeuchi, O., Hoshino, K., Kawai, T., Sanjo, H., Takada, H., Ogawa, T., et al. (1999) Differential roles of TLR2 and TLR4 in recognition of gram-negative and gram-positive bacterial cell wall components [In Process Citation]. *Immunity* **11,** 443–451.
23. Wetzler, L. M., Ho, Y., and Reiser, H. (1996) Neisserial porins induce B lymphocytes to express costimulatory B7-2 molecules and to proliferate. *J. Exp. Med.* **183,** 1151–1159.

24. Snapper, C. M., Rosas, F. R., Kehry, M. R., Mond, J. J., and Wetzler, L. M. (1997) Neisserial porins may provide critical second signals to polysaccharide-activated murine B cells for induction of immunoglobulin secretion. *Infect. Immun.* **65,** 3203–3208.
25. 1994. In vitro assays for lymphocyte function, in *Current Protocols in Immunology* (Coligan, J. E., Kruisbeek, A. M., Margulies, D. H., Shevach, E. M., and Strober, W., eds.), John Wiley and Sons, New York, pp. 3.0.1–3.19.7
26. Massari, P., Ho, Y., and Wetzler, L. M. (2000) *Neisseria meningitidis* porin PorB interacts with mitochondria and protects cells from apoptosis. *PNAS.* **97(16),** 9070–9075

35

Molecular Recognition Mechanisms of Meningococci

Identifying Receptor-Ligand Pairs Involved in Microbe-Host Interactions

Mumtaz Virji and Laura Serino

1. Introduction

Neisseria meningitidis is a human specific pathogen and resides primarily in the nasopharynx of its host. The molecular-recognition mechanisms that operate at the host-microbe interface to impart such precise host/tissue specificity are not fully defined. Given the host muco-cilliary clearance mechanisms, an obvious prerequisite for colonization is the ability of bacteria to make firm and rapid contact with the nasopharyngeal mucosa. The specificity for the niche indicates that one or more meningococcal adhesins have evolved an exquisite level of affinity for particular target molecules. They also exhibit considerable structural and phase modulations that aid in immune evasion. These properties have been exploited to derive distinct phenotypes for investigations on the mechanisms of adhesion. The in vitro investigations that use cell cultures of human origin or "humanized" cells (created by transfection of animal cells with human DNA) have identified a number of receptors targeted by meningococci. Detailed examination of the molecular mechanisms of bacterial ligation with the receptors will clarify the basis of tissue specificity and tropism and provide information that may lead to novel strategies to control the disease. We will describe some of the methods we have implemented over the years for such investigations.

From: *Methods in Molecular Medicine, vol. 67: Meningococcal Disease: Methods and Protocols*
Edited by: A. J. Pollard and M. C. J. Maiden © Humana Press Inc., Totowa, NJ

1.1. Generation of Distinct Adhesive Phenotypes and Control of Phenotypic Variation

Meningococcal outer membrane is often, but not always, covered with a negatively charged capsule, a polymer that has the property of minimizing recognition of underlying bacterial antigens by host immune system. In addition, sialylation of lipopolysaccharides (LPS) adds to the negative charge of the surface with a similar effect. Both may also be expected to influence the interactions of outer-membrane adhesins with their cognate receptors. Furthermore, as is well-known, phase and antigenic variations occur at high frequencies in a large number of surface molecules of meningococci including the adhesins pili, Opa, and Opc. Therefore, it becomes imperative that bacterial phenotype is carefully examined when studying molecular mechanisms of adhesion—at least with respect to the known surface components. The frequent antigenic/phase variation in meningococcal ligands (rates as high as 1/500 have been observed for pili, Opa, etc.) also makes it necessary to apply strict handling procedures of any isolated strains, variants, or mutants. One advantage of phase variation is that isolates with distinct surface characteristics can be obtained with relative ease. Coupled with the fact that some of the adhesins affect bacterial colony morphology, this knowledge can help isolation of adhesion variants. Although in capsulate phenotypes this method is of limited use, in acapsulate phenotypes it has been useful for isolation of pilus and opacity protein variants *(1,2)*. Other methods have used adhesive-cell surfaces or phagocytic cells for derivation of variants with distinct characteristics. For example, to select an invasive phenotype from a blood isolate (invariably capsulate and inefficient at invasion under most culture conditions), endothelial cells may be infected with the bacteria and incubated for several hours. Then the extracellular bacteria can be eliminated by selective methods and intracellular bacteria isolated. This may yield, for example, acapsulate, L8 LPS (asialylated), Opc-expressing phenotype because, in asialylated phenotype, Opc is an extremely efficient invasin for human endothelial cells—the cell entry being achieved via integrins in the presence of serum *(3)*. Alternately, phagocytic cells may be used in the absence of opsonins to selectively eliminate acapsulate adhesive bacteria. Those that survive phagocytic killing are likely to be capsulate or they may be acapsulate that have no Opa proteins. We used one such strategy to identify the meningococcal ligand for CEACAM1 (CarcinoEmbryonic Antigen related Cell Adhesion Molecule-1; *[4]*), a human cell receptor for neisserial Opa proteins identified in our laboratory by the use of transfection technology *(5,6)*. Opa-expressing variants were repeatedly isolated from predominantly Opa-deficient cultures by selection of adhesive bacteria on CEACAM-expressing target cells (**Fig. 1**). Opa proteins were subsequently

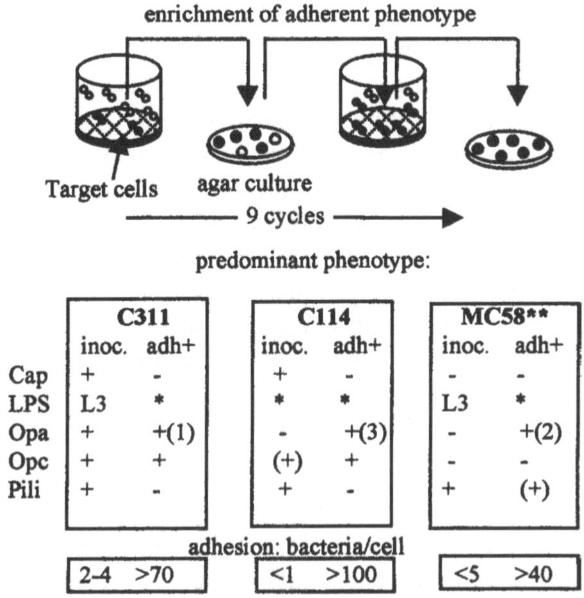

Fig. 1. Derivatives of meningococci isolated by selection on target cells expressing CEACAM receptors. Three distinct meningococcal strains were used to establish the identity of the ligand that recognized human CEACAM1 (CD66a). Inoculated (inoc.) and adherent (adh+) derivatives of each strain are shown. Primary isolates of strains C311 and C114 were not strongly adherent because of the presence of sialylated LPS (L3 immunotype) and/or capsule. C114 and MC58 derivative used were also lacking Opa proteins. After the enrichment procedure for adhesive phenotype, the derivatives of each strain were found to lack surface sialic acids (i.e., were noncapsulated and contained nonsialylated L8 LPS immunotype). In addition, they either retained or gained the expression of one or more Opa proteins (numbers shown in parenthesis). Phenotypic analysis was carried out by dot immunoblotting using MAbs as described in the text. Opa expression was established by Western blotting using MAb B33. Note that pilus expression was either lost or reduced during this procedure.

*LPS showed no reactivity with MABSM82 (*see* **Note 1**).

**The derivative of MC58 used contained mutations in capsule and *Opc* genes.

confirmed as CEACAM-binding ligands by co-precipitation methods described in **Subheading 3.2.3.**

Selection of naturally occurring variants has enabled us to gain considerable understanding of the interplay between the surface polysaccharides and adhesins *(7)*. In addition, specific mutations can be created in genes encoding the ligands of interest. Deletion-insertion constructs containing kanamycin or other antibiotic-resistance genes have been used widely. However, if multiple ligands have to be mutated (for example to obtain acapsulate, nonsialylated LPS derivative that has no Opa proteins), one soon runs out of suitable selection markers. In this case, the use of a mixture of phase variants and mutants is inevitable. It is important to note that growth on selective media can sometimes result in altered phenotypes, e.g., in our hands, selection on kanamycin resulted in predominantly L8 LPS phenotype from a starting culture expressing L3 LPS. One final point to note is that pilus expression (not necessarily pilin expression) is readily lost by nonselective subculture on agar ***(8)***. This method can be used to derive nonpiliated bacteria but, as indicated earlier, the observation also points to the caution required in handling meningococcal cultures and unnecessary repeated subcultures should be avoided.

1.2. Searching for Target Molecules

The search for host-cell receptors targeted by meningococci has accelerated with advances in cell and molecular biology and with the availability of cloned cDNA encoding surface receptors of human cellular origin. In addition, other direct biochemical and immunochemical approaches (co-precipitations, ligand/receptor overlay) have also helped in identifying or confirming the identity of receptor-ligand pairs, and will be described.

1.3. Getting Closer to Understanding Tissue Tropism

When a family of variable molecules such as Opa proteins target a single receptor, the question arises as to how receptor specificity is determined and maintained in the face of structural changes that dominate the surface-exposed regions of Opa proteins. In addition, while maintaining the overall specificity for CEACAMs, distinct Opa proteins also exhibit preference for certain subsets of the CEA family, which comprises a number of related receptors ***(4)***. Using a range of Opa variants together with transfected target cells expressing distinct members of the CEA family, truncated receptor constructs or site-directed mutants of receptors, the molecular basis of receptor specificity and tissue tropism can be addressed ***(5,6,9)***. Procedures that can be used to derive such reagents have been described in detail in **ref. *10***.

1.4. Models for Studying Cellular Interactions

The ease with which transformed cell lines can be cultured and their longevity make them a popular choice for studying cellular interactions. Cell lines such as Chang conjunctiva epithelial cells or HEP-2 laryngeal carcinoma cells have been used often in meningococcal studies. However, it is important to bear in mind that many transformed cell lines may have altered receptor repertoires compared with their normal counterparts. It is well-documented that

CEACAM molecules are upregulated in certain cancers, whereas they are downregulated in others ***(11)***. In addition, some primary cells such as human umbilical vein endothelial cells (HUVECs) and certain epithelial cell lines may not express some receptors under in vitro conditions unless stimulated to do so by treatment with cytokines. Experiments have demonstrated that both HUVECs and Chang cells express receptors for meningococcal pili, but there is a paucity of CEACAM expression. The latter can be upregulated by cytokines such as TNF ***(12)***. For CEACAM studies, we have tended to use lung carcinoma cells such as A549 or colonic carcinoma cells such as HT29 and Caco-2; all of which express several CEACAM molecules.

Other in vitro constructed models include humanised cells of animal origin. These have been used for identification of receptors and examination of targeting and signaling mechanisms via a particular molecule. Several animal cell lines have proved useful for transfection with human cDNA encoding receptors of interest. In the absence of Opc (that targets receptors on untransfected cells) meningococci do not bind to Chinese hamster ovary (CHO) or African green monkey kidney (COS) cells, which can therefore be used for transfection with Opa and pilus receptors.

2. Materials

2.1. Bacterial Strains

Many of the meningococcal isolates in our collection were obtained from Manchester Public Health Laboratories. Several strains were also donated by Dr. John Heckels, Professor Jon Saunders, and Dr. Mark Achtman.

2.2. Reagents

1. HBHI: brain-heart infusion (BHI) agar supplemented with 10% (v/v) heated horse blood. Horse blood (TCS Cat. No. HBO35) is heated at 100°C for 45 min and then centrifuged at 3000*g* for 30 min. The clear extract is added to autoclaved BHI.
2. PBSB: Sterile Dulbecco's phosphate-buffered saline (PBS) (Sigma Cat. no. D-8537) containing 0.9 m*M* $CaCl_2$ and 0.5 m*M* $MgCl_2$ (Sigma Cat. no. D-8662). Stored at 4°C.
3. BSA block: 3% (w/v) bovine serum albumin (BSA) (Sigma Cat. no. A-2058) in PBS containing 0.05% (v/v) Tween-20 (Sigma Cat. no. P-1379) and 0.05% sodium azide (Sigma Cat. no. S-2002). Prepared in bulk and stored at 4°C.
4. Milk block: 5% (w/v) Skim milk powder in PBS containing 0.05% (v/v) Tween-20 and 0.05% sodium azide. Prepared in bulk and stored at 4°C.
5. 1% BSA-PBST (diluent for antibodies): 1% (w/v) BSA in PBS containing 0.05% (v/v) Tween-20 and 0.05% sodium azide. Prepared in bulk and stored at 4°C.
6. TBS (Tris-buffered saline): 0.05 *M* Tris-HCl, 0.15 *M* NaCl, pH 7.6, autoclaved and stored at room temperature.

7. NaCl-Tween: 0.9% (w/v) NaCl and 0.05% (v/v) Tween-20. 10X stock (9% NaCl, 0.5% Tween-20) stored at room temperature; diluted in distilled water as required.
8. AP buffer (Alkaline phosphatase [AP] substrate buffer): 100 m*M* Tris base, 100 m*M* NaCl, and 5 m*M* $MgCl_2$ adjusted to pH 9.5 with HCl. Autoclaved sterile stocks prepared in bulk and stored at room temperature.
9. AP Substrates: 5-Bromo-4-chloro-3-indolylphosphate (BCIP) (Sigma Cat. no. B-8503): 50 mg/ml in N,N-dimethylformamide (DMF); Nitro Blue Tetrazolium (NBT) (Sigma Cat. no. N-6876): 50 mg/mL in 70% (v/v) DMF. Stored at –20°C. For use, add 3.3 µL BCIP and 6.6 µL NBT to 1 mL AP buffer just before use.
10. Secondary antibodies for immunoblotting and immunofluorescence: goat anti-mouse IgG conjugated to AP (Sigma Cat. No A-3688); goat anti-mouse IgG conjugated to tetramethylrhodamine isothiocyanate (TRITC) (Sigma Cat. no. T-5393); goat anti-human Ig Fc conjugated to AP (Sigma Cat. no. A-9544); rabbit anti-rat IgG conjugated to fluorescein isothiocyanate (FITC) (Sigma Cat. no. F-1763).
11. Primary mouse monoclonal antibodies (MAbs) against meningococci: SM1 (against Class I pili; ***[13]***; AD211 and U101 (against Class II pili; ***[14–15]***), B306 (against Opc protein; ***[16]***); B33 (against Opa proteins; ***[17]***); anti-capsular antibodies against distinct capsule types ***[18]***; SM82 (anti-LPS, ***[19]***) (*see* **Note 1**).

    All antibodies are diluted in 1% BSA-PBST containing 0.05% sodium azide (unless used in the presence of viable target cells).
12. Protein A coupled to sepharose CL-4B (Sigma Cat. no. P-3391): 1 g of resin suspended in 10 mL PBS containing 0.05% sodium azide, stored at 4°C. Wash 3 times with PBS as required before use.
13. OG solubilization buffer: 200 m*M* n-octyl β-D glucopyranoside (OG) (Sigma Cat. no. O-8001) in 50 m*M* Tris-HCl, pH 7.4, containing 1 m*M* each of $CaCl_2$ and $MgCl_2$.
14. Protease inhibitors: 1 m*M* phenylmethylsulfonylfluoride (PMSF) (Sigma Cat. no. P-7525), 1 µ*M* E-64 (Sigma Cat. no. E-3132), 1 µ*M* pepstatin A (Sigma Cat. no. P-4265), 100 µ*M* EDTA (BDH Cat. no. 10093).
15. Freezing medium for bacteria: 1% (w/v) Proteose Peptone or Nutrient Broth containing 10% (v/v) glycerol. Autoclaved stocks stored at 4°C.
16. 1% SDS-NaOH (solubilization buffer): 1% sodium dodecyl sulphate (SDS) in 0.1 *M* NaOH. Stored in suitable plastic containers at room temperature.

2.3. Target Cells

1. HUVECs: isolated routinely from umbilical cords as required.
2. Human epithelial cell lines: Chang (conjunctiva), HEP-2 (laryngeal), A549 (lung), HT29 and Caco-2 (colonic), etc: available from ECACC or ATCC (*see* **Note 2**).
3. CHO cells: available from ECACC (Ref. No. 85050302).
4. African green monkey kidney cells (COS-1): available from ECACC (Ref. No. 880311701).

2.4. Media for Eukaryotic Cells

Many of the tissue culture-grade materials can be obtained from Sigma. All media use tissue culture-grade water.

1. HUVECs: Endothelial Cell Growth Medium (EGM) (Clonetics Cat. no. CC-3124) (containing Endothelial Cell Basal Medium [EBM] [CC-3121], Bovine Brain Extract [BBE] 3 mg/mL [CC-4092], hEGF 10 mg/mL, Hydrocortisone 1 mg/mL [CC-4035], fetal bovine serum [FBS] [CC4101), gentamicin 50 mg/mL, and amphotericin-B 50 μg/mL [CC-4081]).
2. COS, Caco-2, HT29: DMEM: (Sigma Cat. no. D-5546).
3. Chang, Hep-2: Medium 199 (Sigma Cat. no. M-2154).
4. CHO: Ham's F10 (Sigma Cat. no. N-6013).
5. Hanks' balanced Salt Solution (HBSS): (Sigma Cat. no. H-9269) for washing cells.
6. FBS: (GibcoBRL Cat. no. 10106-169).
7. Growth media (other than EGM) are supplemented with 2 m*M* glutamine (Sigma G7513) and 10% FBS. 50 U/mL penicillin and 50 μg/mL streptomycin (Sigma P-0906) may be added.
8. Freezing medium: Growth medium supplemented with 10% (v/v) dimethyl sulphoxide (DMSO) (Sigma Cat. no. D-2650) and 20% FBS.
9. Infection medium: Medium 199 supplemented with 2% FBS.

2.5. Other Tissue Culture-Related Items

1. Trypsin/EDTA (Sigma T-4174).
2. Gelatin (Sigma G-1393).
3. Collagenase (Sigma C-5138).
4. Chloroquine (Sigma C-6628): 10 m*M* in TBS.
5. DEAE Dextran (Sigma D-9885): 10 mg/mL in TBS.
6. Paraformaldehyde: 2% (w/v) in PBSB, pH 7.4.

2.6. Disposable Plasticware

1. Sterile pipets and other standard tissue-culture materials.
2. 96-well Cell-culture plates (Costar Cat. no. 3595).
3. 24-well Cell-culture plates (Costar Cat. no. 3524).
4. 25 cm^2 and 75 cm^2 Tissue-culture flasks (Corning Cat. no. 25100 and 25110).
5. Blotting trays for nitrocellulose strips (BIORAD Cat. no. 170-3902).

2.7. Equipment

Tissue-culture facilities and equipment for safe handling of meningococci including:

1. Class II Microbiological Satefy Cabinets.
2. 5% CO_2 incubators.

3. Microscopes: Inverted phase contrast with fluorescence attachment and a camera attached to a special port or other cell-imaging accessories; dissection-type microscope with sub-stage lighting for examination of bacterial cultures.
4. Centrifuges.
5. Spectrophotometer.
6. Colony Counter.
7. SDS-PAGE and Western blotting apparatus:
   a. XCell II™ Mini Cell (NOVEX Cat. no. E10001).
   b. Mini Trans Blot Cell (BioRad Cat. no. 170-3939).
   c. 10% Bis-Tris Gels (NOVEX Cat. no. NP0303).
   d. Dot Blotter Hybri-dot® Manifold (Bethesda Research laboratories Cat. no. 1050MM).
   e. PROTRAN® Nitrocellulose Transfer Membrane (Schleicher & Schuell Cat. no. 10401196).
   f. Nitrocellulose disks (0.45 μm) (Sartorius Cat. no. 11306-85-K).

Information on the suppliers of tissue culture-related equipment can be found in **ref.** ***(20)***.

3. Methods

All studies on meningococci are performed under suitable safety conditions.

3.1. Isolation of Distinct Bacterial Phenotypes

3.1.1. Culture Conditions

Meningococci are grown routinely on HBHI at 37°C in 5% CO_2 (v/v) in air. Frozen stocks are generally established after a minimum number of subcultures.

Bacteria are frozen in 10% glycerol broth and stored in liquid nitrogen. For experiments, aliquots are scraped out (using sterile flat metal spatulas) from frozen culture stocks, inoculated on agar plates, and cultures used after 16–18 h of growth.

3.1.2. Preparation of Bacterial Suspensions

1. Grow the strain of interest overnight on HBHI agar plates at 37°C in 5% CO_2.
2. Make a suspension of the bacteria in 2 mL PBSB. Remove large bacterial aggregates by centrifugation at 150*g* for 1 min. Without disturbing the pellet, remove the homogeneous suspension into a sterile tube.
3. Solubilize an aliquot of the suspension (10–50 μL) in 1 mL of 1% SDS-NaOH and measure the nucleic acid content by determining the absorbance of the solution at 260 nm (A_{260}).
4. For *N. meningitidis* strains, A_{260} of 1.8 corresponds to a bacterial density of *c.* 1 × 10^9 colony-forming units (cfu)/mL in our laboratory.

3.1.3. Isolation of Phase Variants by Colony Immunoblotting

This method utilizes MAbs that recognize the native ligand of interest (*see* **Note 1**).

1. Prepare bacterial suspensions as above (**Subheading 3.1.2.**).
2. Adjust the bacterial density using PBSB and plate out a small volume (50–200 μL) on 3–4 plates to obtain *c.* 1000 colonies per plate.
3. After overnight growth at 37°C in 5% CO_2, count the colonies (if phase switch rates need to be determined) and then lift them onto nitrocellulose disks. A second colony lift can be carried out from the same plates if required, following 3–4 h incubation of the agar plates to allow regrowth of colonies. Return plates to the incubator.
4. Leave the filters to air dry for 20–30 min prior to soaking in Milk block for 2 h at room temperature.
5. Wash off the blocking solution with NaCl-Tween and incubate with the required primary antibody (*see* **Note 3**) for 1 h at room temperature.
6. After 4 washes in NaCl-Tween, the binding of the antibody is detected by incubating the filters for 1 h with alkaline phosphatase-conjugated secondary antibodies at dilutions recommended by the manufacturer and verified in the laboratory.
7. After 4 washes in NaCl-Tween, colony blots are developed using NBT-BCIP substrates (*see* **Subheading 2.2.**) in AP buffer.
8. The variant with the required phenotype (e.g., pilin-expressing phenotype in a nonpiliated parent culture) can be identified by the use of MAb (e.g., SM1) and is isolated from the original plate the next day and picked with a fine plastic loop or needle for subculturing. This single colony isolate is normally frozen in 2 vials containing 10% glycerol broth.
9. Complete characterization of the isolate with respect to other surface structures is then carried out on bacterial suspensions prepared from overnight cultures grown from frozen stocks (*see* **Note 4**).

3.1.4. Isolation of Distinct Phenotypes by Selection on Target Cells

Tissue-culture conditions (*see* **Subheading 3.2.1.**).

3.1.4.1. Isolation of Internalized Bacteria (e.g., Selection for Cap$^-$, "Asialylated" Phenotypes)

1. Culture host cells (HUVECs or Chang epithelial cells) in 24-well tissue-culture plates. Each well should contain 0.5–1 mL of the appropriate growth medium.
2. If growth media have been supplemented with antibiotics, remove the medium, and wash the cells three times with HBSS.
3. Inoculate two or more monolayers with bacterial suspension in 0.5 mL of infection medium at the infection ratio of 200–500 bacteria per target cell.

4. Incubate for 3 h and then wash the cells twice with HBSS to remove excess nonadherent bacteria.
5. Add 500 µL gentamicin (200 µg/mL) in the infection medium to each well and incubate for 1.5 h at 37°C to eliminate any extracellular bacteria. The gentamicin treatment has been found to be effective against numerous *N. meningitidis* strains (*see* **Note 5**).
6. After the incubation time, wash off the gentamicin (3 washes with HBSS) and permeabilize the cells by adding 150 µL of 1% saponin (it permeabilizes target cells without affecting the bacterial viability). After 10 min mix the contents of the well with a pipet and plate aliquots (10→100 µL) onto HBHI agar plates. A preliminary experiment will be necessary to determine the level of invasion so that appropriate dilutions of the suspension can be plated to obtain reasonable numbers of colonies on a plate.
7. Analyze the resulting bacterial cultures by colony immunoblotting as described earlier. In addition, several colonies can be subcultured to establish frozen stocks, which then allow in depth analysis of their phenotypic nature.

3.1.4.2. Isolation of Adherent/Nonadherent Phenotype by Selection on Target Cells

*3.1.4.2.1. Adherent/Cell-Associated Phenotype (**Fig. 1**)*

1. Culture target cells (e.g., transfected CHO cells expressing CEACAM molecules) in 24-well culture plates and infect as above (*see* **Subheading 3.1.4.1.**)
2. After a 2–3 h attachment period, remove unattached bacteria by repeated washings (4–5 times).
3. Adherent (cell-associated) bacteria are released by the addition of 1% saponin. These bacteria are grown overnight on HBHI agar plates and used to infect fresh monolayers the following day.
4. Repeat this procedure several times (3–9 times).
5. Phenotypic characterization of the cell-associated derivatives and the parental phenotype are determined by immunoblotting.

This procedure was used to identify Opa as a ligand for CEACAMs *(5)*. It can also be used to obtain piliated bacteria from nonpiliated cultures using HUVECs, for example.

3.1.4.2.2. Non-Adherent Phenotype

Non-adherent bacteria can be enriched by recycling on a number of monolayers on the same day. It involves transfer of bacterial suspension from infected wells to fresh target monolayers allowing for 1–2 h attachment period to remove adherent phenotypes. These methods yield “enriched” cultures that can be used to isolate single “clonal” derivatives (*see* **Subheading 3.1.3.**).

3.1.5. Isolation of Mutants by Allelic Replacement

In order to construct insertion mutants in the gene of interest, a kanamycin (*kan*) antibiotic cassette is inserted in the gene-coding sequence.

1. Digest the plasmid harboring the *kan* resistance cassette, pUC4kan (Pharmacia) with *Eco*RI, *Bam*HI, or *Pst*I to yield a 1.3 kb fragment containing the kan resistance gene.
2. Insert a neisserial DNA uptake sequence (10 bp 5′GCCGTCTGAA-3′) at the 3′end of the gene-coding sequence.
3. Linearize the resulting plasmid by digestion with *Eco*RI and transform into the meningococcal strain by the standard plate method.
4. Grow piliated bacterial cultures overnight.
5. Lift a few bacterial colonies (8–10) from the plate and spread over a small area (*c.* 1–2 cm^2) on a fresh agar plate and incubate for 3–4 h at 37°C in 5% CO_2.
6. Add *c.* 10 μg of plasmid DNA (in a 5–10 μL aliquot) and mix with the bacteria on the agar surface.
7. After a 4 h-incubation, select for transformed cells on HBHI plates containing 100 μg/mL kanamycin to identify transformants in which a double cross-over event has replaced the wild-type gene with the inactivated gene containing the *Kan* cassette. Purify the *Kan*-resistant colonies and confirm the presence of the *Kan* cassette either by polymerase chain reaction (PCR) or by Southern blotting.

3.1.6. Maintenance of Selected Phenotype

Once a clone of interest is obtained from the initial isolate (parent strain), a stock clonal culture is established and maintained as frozen glycerol stock in liquid nitrogen. Experiments are carried out on overnight cultures (16–18 h growth) set up from the glycerol stocks.

3.2. Identification of Receptors on Target Cells

3.2.1. Tissue-Culture Conditions

1. Endothelial cells. Isolation and culture conditions for HUVECs are similar to those described elsewhere (*see* Chapter 37). Briefly, endothelial cells are obtained from umbilical veins by collagenase treatment and cultured in EGM medium. Cells from passages 1–3 are normally seeded in gelatin-coated culture plates and used 2–3 d after reaching confluency.
2. Other cell lines. Cell lines are maintained as frozen stocks in liquid nitrogen. They are cultured in the appropriate media described in **Subheading 2.4.** For experiments, cells are seeded in tissue-culture plates at 30–50% confluency and used when they have reached the desired confluency (*see* **Note 6**).

3.2.2. Identification of Receptors by Transient Transfection of Mammalian Cells

COS-1 cells are transfected with cDNA molecules subcloned into the expression vectors CDM8 or πH3M using the DEAE Dextran method ***(21)***.

1. Trypsinize confluent monolayers from one 25 cm^2 flask and seed into 96- or 24-well plates as required.
2. Incubate in a CO_2 incubator until cells have reached *c.* 75% confluency.

3. Prepare transfection solution: (DNA is normally used at 1 μg/well [96-well plates] and 6 μg/well [24-well plates] and all volumes can be adjusted according to particular requirements).
   a. 10–15 μg of DNA from the desired construct is dissolved in 150 μL TBS.
   b. Add this solution to a double volume (300 μL) of 10 mg/mL DEAE-Dextran solution in TBS.
   c. Add 6.5 mL DMEM + 5% FBS to this mixture to a final volume of 7 mL and add chloroquine (70 μL of 10 m*M* stock) to a final concentration of 100 μ*M*. This DMEM transfection medium should finally contain *c.* 5% FBS, 400 μg/mL DEAE Dextran, 1–2 μg/mL of DNA, and 100 μ*M* chloroquine.
4. Wash the cell cultures with DMEM medium without serum and add DMEM transfection medium (600 μL/well in 24-well plate and 100 μL/well in 96-well plates).
5. Incubate the plates for 2–4 h at 37°C.
6. Remove the medium and replace with DMEM containing 10% DMSO for 1–2 min at room temperature.
7. Wash the cells three times with DMEM and incubate overnight with DMEM containing 10% FBS.
8. On the next day, change the medium with DMEM containing 10% FBS and allow the cells to grow for 2–3 d.
9. Receptor expression by transfected cells can be monitored by antibody labeling and immunofluorescence microscopy (**Fig. 2**).

3.2.2.1. Bacterial Adherence to Transfected Cells

1. Bacterial suspension is prepared as described in **Subheading 3.1.2.** and the density adjusted to obtain 1–2 × 10^8/mL in the infection medium.
2. To a monolayer of transfected cells add bacterial suspension to obtain an infection ratio of approx 100–200 bacteria per target cell.
3. Incubate at 37°C for 3 h, then wash away unbound bacteria (**Subheading 3.1.4.2.**).
4. Fix the monolayers with 2% paraformaldehyde solution for 30 min prior to detection by immunolabeling (*see* **Note 7**).

3.2.2.2. Immuno-fluorescence Detection of Adherent Bacteria and Expressed Receptor

1. Wash the fixed monolayers three times with distilled water or PBS and block nonspecific sites for 1 h or more with BSA block.
2. Incubate the fixed monolayers with the specific MAbs to cellular receptors and bacteria (e.g., mouse MAb against LPS or anti-capsular antibody and rat or rabbit anti-receptor antibody), diluted in 1% BSA-PBST for 1 h. Wash 3 times in NaCl-Tween.
3. Add a secondary antibody conjugated to TRITC (e.g., goat anti-mouse IgG) or FITC (e.g., rabbit anti-rat IgG or goat anti-rabbit IgG) to detect specific binding of the primary MAbs to bacteria and receptors, respectively (*see* **Note 8**).

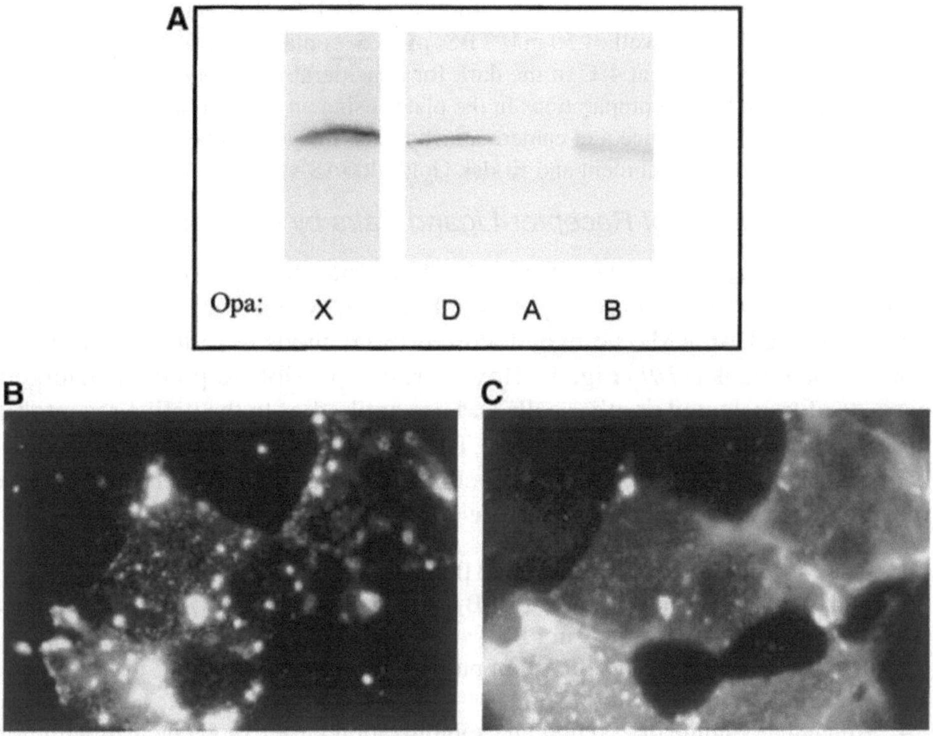

Fig. 2. The effect of ligand affinity on co-precipitation and receptor targeting. **(A)** Western blot showing different amounts of Opa proteins of meningococcal strains MC58 (OpaX) and C751 (Opa A, B and D) co-precipitated with CEACAM1. Opa proteins of meningococci exhibit differences in their affinity for CEACAM1. This determines the efficiency with which they are co-precipitated with CEACAM receptors from octyl glucoside extracts. If receptors and ligands are pre-solubilized in the detergent, the efficiency of co-precipitation of the pair is reduced further. Therefore, it is desirable to let receptor-ligand pairs ligate prior to extraction with the detergent as described in the text. Immunofluorescence micrographs showing receptor expression **(C)** and adherence of capsulate OpaX-expressing meningococci **(B)** to COS cells transiently transfected with cDNA encoding CEACAM1. High-affinity OpaX is effective to some extent even in the presence of capsule, especially when the target cells express the receptor at high density. **(B)** and **(C)** represent the same field. Bacteria were detected with mouse anti-capsular MAb followed by TRITC conjugated anti mouse antibody and the receptor with the rat MAb YTH71.3 (Serotec) followed by FITC-labeled anti-rat antibody.

4. Incubate the plates at room temperature in the dark for 1 h, wash 4X with NaCl-Tween. Add 50 μL/well of 50 m*M* TBS, pH 8.5, containing 0.05% sodium azide. Plates can be stored at 4°C in the dark for considerable periods.
5. Examine the labeled preparations in the plates using an appropriate inverted microscope with fluorescence and camera attachments. Images can be recorded using an ordinary camera attachment and Kodak Gold (400ASA) or a similar film.

3.2.3. Identification of Receptor-Ligand Pairs by Co-precipitation

Once a receptor is identified, the bacterial ligand involved can be co-precipitated from detergent lysates of bacteria. We have used soluble receptors such as CEACAM1-Fc manufactured by methods described in transfection protocol books ***(10)*** (**Fig. 3**). However, it is possible to produce detergent extracts of transfected or other cells and use antibodies to the native receptor in order to affinity purify the receptor. The following method can be used for bacterial ligands that are soluble in octyl glucoside. Other detergents may be more suitable in some cases (*see* **Note 9**).

1. Grow the bacteria overnight on HBHI agar plates at 37°C in 5% CO_2.
2. Make a bacterial suspension in PBSB (*see* **Subheading 3.1.2.**), adjust to obtain a density of 1×10^{10} cfu/mL in PBSB.
3. To 100 μL (10^9 cfu), add 100 μL of purified receptor (1–5 μg) and mix gently for 1–2 h at room temperature.
4. Add equal volume of 200 m*M* OG solubilization buffer supplemented with protease inhibitor cocktail for 2 h at 4°C.
5. Remove insoluble material by centrifugation at 10,000*g* for 20 min at 4°C.
6. If using receptor-Fc constructs, precipitate the receptor-ligand complexes by incubating for 1 h with protein A-sepharose (50–100 μL of 100 mg/mL slurry). If using the native receptor, add protein A-sepharose complexed to anti-receptor antibody. Prepare the latter by incubating protein A-sepharose (50–100 μL of 100 mg/mL slurry) with 200–400 μg/mL antibody for 45 min. Wash 1X to remove unadsorbed antibody.
7. Collect protein A-sepharose by centrifugation at maximum speed in a microcentrifuge for 1 min and wash 3 times with 1 mL of 50 m*M* OG solubilization buffer and 3 times with 1 mL PBS.
8. Carefully remove PBS in the final step by using a fine pipet tip and resuspend the pellets in an equal volume of 2X SDS-PAGE dissociation buffer. Heat the samples at 100°C for 5 min.
9. Analyze the samples by SDS-PAGE using 10% polyacrylamide gels and detect by silver-staining (Amersham Silver Enhancement kit) and/or Western blotting (**Figs. 2** and **3**).
10. Control lanes should contain material from a parallel experiment carried out preferably using control receptors prepared in a similar manner to the test receptor.

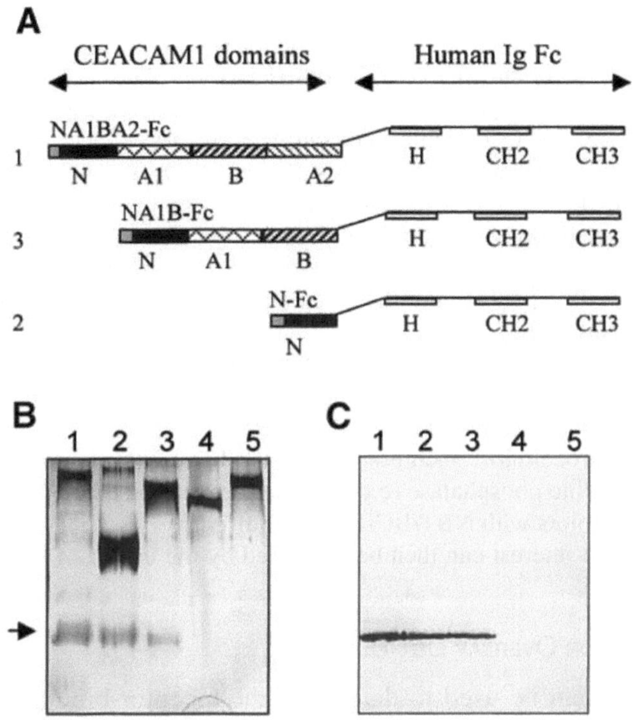

Fig. 3. Co-precipitation and overlay studies to define CEACAM-Opa interactions. **(A)** Diagramatic representation of the structures of Fc chimeric constructs of CEACAM1 used in experiments. **(B)** SDS-PAGE and **(C)** Western blot demonstrating co-precipitation of meningococcal ligand and soluble CEACAM1-Fc chimeric constructs from meningococcal lysates prepared in octyl glucoside. Tracks (1–5 in B and C are identical): Tracks 1, 2, 3: CEACAM1-Fc (constructs 1, 2, 3 shown in A) track 4: CD14-Fc and track 5: CD31-Fc. Silver-stained gel (B) shows receptor molecules (High Mr bands tracks 1–5) and a single common protein (Mr *c*.35 K, arrow) in tracks 1–3 only. The N-domain of the receptor was sufficient to co-precipitate the protein (track 2). The 35K protein reacted with the anti-Opa MAb B33 in Western blots (C), establishing its identity as Opa protein.

11. Any unique molecules found in the test sample can be identified by further electrophoresis and excision from gels and sequencing or immunoblot analysis with panels of MAbs.

3.2.4. Receptor/Ligand Overlay

3.2.4.1. Receptor Overlay Western Blots

These can be used to identify bacterial ligands interacting with a given receptor *(5)*. Whole-cell lysates of bacteria are first subjected to electrophoretic separation under mild, nondenaturing conditions. Purified receptors are then overlaid and receptor binding detected.

1. Grow the strain of choice overnight on HBHI agar plates at 37°C in 5% CO_2.
2. Prepare a bacterial suspension in PBSB at *c.* 2 × 10^{10} cfu/mL and dilute with an equal volume of 200 m*M* OG solubilization buffer to prepare extracts. Approximately 10^8 – 5 × 10^8 cfu equivalent per track was sufficient for Opa/CEACAM studies *(5)*.
3. Incubate for 1 h at 37°C with gentle mixing.
4. Centrifuge at 10,000*g* for 20 min at 4°C.
5. Decant the supernatant and apply required volumes per lane to 10% polyacrylamide gels without subjecting the lysates to heat and under nonreducing conditions (*see* **Note 10**).
6. Transfer the proteins onto nitrocellulose membranes and block overnight at 4°C.
7. Incubate the membranes with the appropriate soluble receptor-Fc chimeric molecule (2–10 μg/mL) diluted in 1% BSA-PBST.
8. Wash the nitrocellulose membranes and incubate with anti-Fc antibody conjugated to alkaline phosphatase (e.g., goat anti-human Ig Fc-AP conjugated).
9. Develop the blots with NBT/BCIP in AP buffer.
10. The ligand of interest can then be identified by the use of MAbs or sequencing from gels.

3.2.4.2. Receptor Overlay Dot-Blots

This method can be used to determine the receptor-binding properties of various isolates and large numbers of bacteria can be screened simultaneously. It can also be used to determine the features of a receptor (adhesiotopes) required by a ligand for efficient interactions. Receptor analogs, truncated constructs, and mutants have been utilized ***(9,21)***.

1. Prepare bacterial suspensions in PBSB to obtain 2–5 × 10^9 cfu/mL.
2. Apply 3 μL volumes onto nitrocellulose strips or use dot-blotting apparatus and add 25 μL PBS containing equivalent cfu/well of the dot-blotting manifold. Nitrocellulose strips are cut to fit into blotting trays.
3. Block in Milk block for 2 h (room temperature) or 16 h (4°C).
4. Overlay with purified receptor (10–50 n*M*) and detect as above (**Subheading 3.2.4.1.**) (**Fig. 3**; *see* **Note 11**).

3.2.4.3. Ligand Overlay

This procedure is an alternative procedure to receptor overlay and has been used to determine the relative binding of variants to truncated receptor constructs and mutants ***(5)***.

1. Apply 3 μL of the purified chimeric soluble receptors (50–200 n*M*) onto nitrocellulose strips.

2. Block nonspecific sites using 3% BSA-PBST.
3. Remove the block and apply bacterial suspensions (*c.* 5 × 10^8–10^9 cfu/mL) diluted in 1% BSA-PBST. Distinct variants or strains expressing distinct Opa proteins, for example, can be compared by testing several strips in parallel.
4. Remove unbound bacteria by washing the strips 4X in NaCl-Tween.
5. Detect the binding of the bacteria to the receptor by probing with an antibody directed against a bacterial antigen (e.g., using anti-LPS MAb).
6. Detect the antibody binding by using an alkaline phosphatase-conjugated secondary antibody and develop as described earlier.
7. Appropriate controls should include strips with receptors incubated with nonadherent variants as well as those not exposed to bacteria (*see* **Note 12**).

3.2.4.4. Quantification of Dot-Blot Analysis

Experiments should be performed in triplicates. The levels of reactivity can then be determined by scanning the dot-blots and performing densitometric analysis using the NIH Scion Image program available from the NIH web site. Relative color intensity can be expressed by plotting the curve areas in arbitrary units.

4. Notes

1. The MAb SM1 reacts with all Class I pili-expressing strains of meningococci tested to date. The MAbs AD211 and U101 together react with the vast majority of Class II pili-expressing isolates. The epitopes of the latter two MAbs may occur individually or simultaneously on Class II pili. B306 is a broadly cross-reacting anti-Opc MAb. The latter three antibodies were provided by Dr. Mark Achtman. These antibodies are effective in detecting their respective antigens on native as well as denatured ligands. The MAb B33 that recognizes all Opa proteins was provided by Dr. Claudia Lammel. It is directed against a buried epitope in the native protein and can only be used with the denatured antigen, for example in Western blots. However, it may be used for immunodotblotting if the ligand is first denatured. SM82 can be used for detection of L3/L9 LPS immunotype but when LPS is sialylated the antibody reactivity is lost. SM82 does not bind to L8 immunotype that lacks the terminal lactoneotetraose required for sialylation. It can be used to differentiate L8 and L3 immunotypes as well as sialylated and nonsialylated L3/L9 immunotypes *(7)*. Thus serogroup B strain MC58 expressing L3 immunotype that intrinsically sialylates its LPS may contain a proportion of LPS that is not sialylated and is recognized by SM82. Similarly, serogroup A strain C751 that expresses L9 LPS but does not intrinsically sialylate its LPS, will be recognized by SM82. However, when C751 is grown on cytidine monophosphate N-acetyl neuramininc acid (CMP-NANA) a substrate required for sialylation, SM82 reactivity is lost as C751 utilizes CMP-NANA and sialylates its LPS *(2,7)*. Anti-capsular antibodies recognizing serogroups A, B, C, and so on were provided by Dr. Wendell Zollinger.

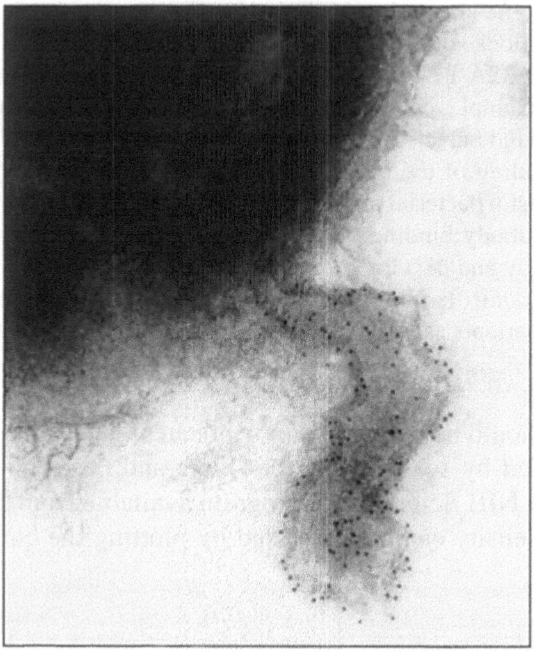

Fig. Fig. 4. Pilin+ phenotype of strain C751. Immunoelectron microscopy of a nonpiliated meningococcal isolate showing pilin monomers located in the outer membrane some of which can be seen extruding from the bacterial surface. The pilins were labeled with SM1 and protein A conjugated to 5-nm gold particles.

2. Most cell lines are available from either European Collection of Animal Cell Cultures (ECACC) or American Type Culture Collection (ATCC). The web sites offer details on cell lines and culture conditions.
   ECACC web site: http://www.camr.org/ecacc.htm
   ATCC web site: http://www.atcc.org
3. Antibody concentrations: For immunoblotting, MAbs supplied as ascites are used at 1 : 1000–1 : 5000 dilutions as a rule but higher dilutions can be used for some antibodies and should be established in the laboratory. For immunofluorescence, MAbs are used at 1 : 200–1 : 500 dilutions.
4. Use of MAbs for isolation of piliated bacteria.

   Although pilin isolates will undoubtedly be pilus−, the isolates expressing pilin may or may not produce assembled pili. Pilin may be incorporated into outer-membrane and will react with all the available antibodies against pili. (**Fig. 4**). In this case, pilin does not mediate bacterial adherence and does not support efficient transformation. Electron microscopic examination is necessary to confirm the piliation status of an isolate. SM1, AD211, and U101 recognize both pilin monomers and assembled pili.

For the isolation of piliated bacteria, a better strategy may be to select on target cells (*see* **Subheading 3.1.4.2.1.**)

5. When gentamicin survival assay is used to obtain "internalized" phenotype, it is necessary to carry out a control experiment to establish that the bacteria isolated were truly internalized. This is necessary because in some situations, e.g., when bacteria tend to form large clumps on target cell surface, many may escape the action of gentamicin. The following control experiment will establish if survivors have escaped the antibiotic action by cell entry or via other means. Host cells are pre-incubated with 2 μg/mL cytochalasin D (CD) in infection medium for 30 min prior to infection with bacteria. CD is present throughout the infection period at 1 μg/mL. Pre-treatment with CD prevents cytoskeletal activity and bacteria usually remain externally adherent to the target cells. The subsequent gentamicin treatment should effectively eliminate all bacteria. If a significant number survives, then the assay cannot be used to study internalization or to isolate an invasive phenotype.
6. For adhesion and invasion experiments, all monolayers are used at confluency. For transfection experiments, sub-confluent monolayers are used.
7. For receptor immunolocalization, it is important to maintain immunoreactivity of antigenic epitopes of the target receptor, therefore the choice of fixative is important. Paraformaldehyde preserves cell morphology and immunoreactivity of most antigens and has been used widely for such applications. In contrast, organic solvents destroy many antigenic epitopes but they may expose buried epitopes and can be useful in some cases.
8. For double-labeling experiments in co-localization studies, it is necessary to choose antibodies carefully to ensure no undesirable cross-reaction occurs. Suitable pre-adsorbed antibodies are available from many manufacturers.
9. For co-precipitation, antibodies against the receptor may be required. Those directed against the cytoplasmic domain are most useful but others that bind to sites on the receptor not targeted by bacteria can also be used. It should be noted that receptor-ligand complexes of low affinity or sensitive to minor conformational changes may not stay intact in the presence of detergents (*see* **Fig. 2**) or anti-receptor antibodies.
10. Nonreducing gel conditions employ normal gels but the sample buffer does not contain mercaptoethanol and samples are not heated prior to loading on gels.
11. If a receptor is present at limiting dilutions, it may be "mopped up" by high-affinity ligands when both high- and low-affinity ligands are present on the same nitrocellulose strip. It is therefore advisable to make sure that receptor is present in excess and distinct ligands should be tested on separate strips also to verify their receptor-binding properties.
12. In ligand-overlay experiments, the use of unnecessarily high numbers of bacteria may produce high "background" staining; since phase variants present in any control nonadherent culture may be drawn to the receptor, which acts as an affinity concentrator.

Acknowledgments

The work in MV's laboratory is currently supported by grants from the Medical Research Council, the National Meningitis Trust and the Spencer Dayman Meningitis Laboratories. MV is an MRC Senior Fellow. Some studies on CEACAM1 were done in collaboration with Dr. Suzanne Watt.

References

1. Virji, M., Alexandrescu, C., Ferguson, D. J. P., Saunders, J. R., and Moxon, E. R. (1992) Variations in the expression of pili: the effect on adherence of *N. meningitidis* to human epithelial and endothelial cells. *Mol. Microbiol.* **6,** 1271–1279.
2. Virji, M., Makepeace, K., Ferguson, D. J. P., Achtman, M., and Moxon, E. R. (1993) Meningococcal Opa and Opc proteins: their role in colonisation and invasion of human epithelial and endothelial cells. *Mol. Microbiol.* **10,** 499–510.
3. Virji, M., Makepeace, K., and Moxon, E. R. (1994) Distinct mechanisms of interaction of Opc-expressing meningococci at apical and basolateral surfaces of human endothelial cells; the role of integrins in apical interactions. *Mol. Microbiol.* **14,** 173–184.
4. Beauchemin, N., Draber, P., Dreksler, G., Gold, P., Gray-Owm, S., Grant, F., et. al. (1999) Redefined nomenclature for members of the Carcinoembryonic Antigen family. *Exp. Cell Res.* **252,** 243–249.
5. Virji, M., Watt, S. M., Barker, S., Makepeace, K., and Doyonnas, R. (1996) The N-domain of the human CD66a adhesion molecule is a target for Opa proteins of *Neisseria meningitidis* and *Neisseria gonorrhoeae. Mol. Microbiol.* **22,** 929–939.
6. Virji, M., Makepeace, K., Ferguson, D. J. P., and Watt, S. M. (1996) Carcinoembryonic antigens (CD66) on epithelial cells and neutrophils are receptors for Opa proteins of pathogenic *Neisseriae. Mol. Microbiol.* **22,** 941–950.
7. Virji, M., Makepeace, K., Peak, I. R. A., Ferguson, D. J. P., Jennings, M. P., and Moxon, E. R. (1995) Opc- and pilus- dependent interactions of meningococci with human endothelial cells: molecular mechanisms and modulation by surface polysaccharides. *Mol. Microbiol.* **18,** 741–754.
8. Virji, M. Makepeace, K., Peak, I., Payne, G., Saunders, J. R., Ferguson, D. J. P., and Moxon, E. R. (1995) Functional implications of the expression of PilC proteins in meningococci. *Mol. Microbiol.* **16,** 1087–1097.
9. Virji, M., Evans, D., Hadfield, A., Grunert, F., Teixeira, A. M., and Watt, S. M. (1999) Critical determinants of host receptor targeting by *Neisseria meningitidis* and *Neisseria gonorrhoeae*: identification of Opa adhesiotopes on the N-domain of CD66 molecules. Mol. Microbiol. 34, 538-551.
10. Challis, R. A. J. (ed.) (1987) *Methods in Molecular Biology: Receptor Signal Transduction Protocols, vol. 83. Humana Press, Totowa, New Jersey.*
11. Hammarstrom, S. (1999) The carcinoembryonic antigen (CEA) family: structures, suggested functions and expression in normal and malignant tissues. *Semin. Cancer Biol.* **9,** 67–81.

12. Majuri, M. L., Hakkarainen, M., Paavonen, T., and Renkonen, R. (1994) Carcinoembryonic antigen is expressed on endothelial cells. A putative mediator of tumor cell extravasation and metastasis. *Apmis* **102,** 432–438.
13. Virji, M., Heckels, J. E., and Watt, P. J. (1983) Monoclonal antibodies to gonococcal pili: studies on antigenic determinants on pili from variants of strains P9. *J. Gen. Microbiol.* **129,** 1965–1973.
14. Wang, J. F., Morelli, G., Bopp, M., Kusecek, B., and Achtman, M. (1991) Clonal and antigenic analyses of *Neisseria meningitidis* bacteria belonging to the ET37 complex isolated from Mali and elsewhere, in *Proceedings of the Seventh International Pathogenic Neisseria Conference* (Achtman, M., Kohl, P., Marchal, C., Morelli, G., Seiler, A., and Thiesen, B., eds.), Walter de Gruyter, Berlin, pp. 141–146.
15. Achtman, M., Kusecek, B., Morelli, G., Eickmann, K., Wang, J. F., Crowe, B., et al. (1992) A comparison of the variable antigens expressed by clone IV-1 and subgroup III of *Neisseria meningitidis* serogroup A. *J. Infect. Dis.* **165,** 53–68.
16. Achtman, M., Neibert, M., Crowe, B. A., Strittmatter, W., Kusecek, B., Weyse, E., et al. (1988) Purification and characterization of eight class 5 outer membrane protein variants from a clone of *Neisseria meningitidis* serogroup A. *J. Exp. Med.* 168, 507–525.
17. Lammel, C., Karu, A. E., and Brooks, G. F. (1988) Antigenic specificity and biological activity of a monoclonal antibody that is broadly cross reacting with gonococcal protein IIs, in: *Gonococci and Meningococci* (Poolman, J. T., Zanen, H. C., Meyer, T. F., Heckels, J. E., Makela, P. R. H., Smith, H., et al., eds.), Kluwer Academic Publishers, Dordrecht, pp. 737–743.
18. Zollinger, W. D., Boslego, J., Froholm, L. O., Ray, J. S., Moran, E. E., and Brandt, B. L. (1987) Human bactericidal antibody response to meningococcal outer membrane protein vaccines. *Antonie van Leeuwenhoek* **53,** 403–411.
19. Virji, M. and Heckels, J. E. (1988) Nonbactericidal antibodies against *Neisseria gonorrhoeae*: evaluation of their blocking effect on bactericidal antibodies directed against outer membrane antigens. *J. Gen. Microbiol.* **134,** 2703–2711.
20. Harrison, M. A. and Rae, I F., eds. (1997) *General Techniques of Cell Culture*, Cambridge University Press, Cambridge, UK.
21. Watt, S. M., Fawcett, J., Murdoch, S. J., Teixeira, A. M., Gschmeissner, S. E., Hajibagheri, N. M. A. N., and Simmons, D. L. (1994) CD66 identifies the biliary glycoprotein (BGP) adhesion molecule: cloning, expression, and adhesion functions of the BGPc splice variant. *Blood* **84,** 200–210.

36

Experimental Nasopharyngeal Colonization by *Neisseria meningitidis* using Explant Organ Culture

Robert C. Read and Linda Goodwin

1. Introduction

This chapter will describe the use of organ cultures of human nasopharyngeal mucosa to study the interaction of *Neisseria meningitidis* with this complex tissue. Colonization of nasopharyngeal mucosa is the first step in the pathogenesis of meningococcal disease. Supporting evidence for this is the correlation between the prevalence of community carriage and the occurrence of meningococcal disease *(1)*. During nonepidemic periods, the baseline prevalence of nasopharyngeal carriage of meningococci is 5–10% but is considerably higher in certain populations such as military personnel *(2)*, and in households of cases *(3)*. There are a number of influences on the acquisition of meningococcal carriage; these include smoking *(4)* but not season *(5)*. It is possible that coincident viral infections may affect acquisition of meningococcal carriage *(6,7)*. There is good evidence that genetic factors are involved, as some individuals appear resistant to acquisition of carriage, while others chronically or intermittently carry *N. meningitidis (8)*. Carriage of the organism also appears to be associated with secretor status *(9)*. The precise site within the nasopharynx that *Neisseria meningitidis* colonizes and invades is not known. However, during natural carriage, the organism can be isolated both from the rhinopharynx and from the throat *(10)*.

Organ culture is culture of pieces of tissue derived from animals or humans. It permits the study of the interaction of *Neisseria meningitidis* with tissue that has physiologically relevant cellular and matriceal components. Viable organ cultures of upper-respiratory mucosa have many relevant functional characteristics: they have the "normal" population of human epithelial cells and leuko-

From: *Methods in Molecular Medicine, vol. 67: Meningococcal Disease: Methods and Protocols*
Edited by: A. J. Pollard and M. C. J. Maiden © Humana Press Inc., Totowa, NJ

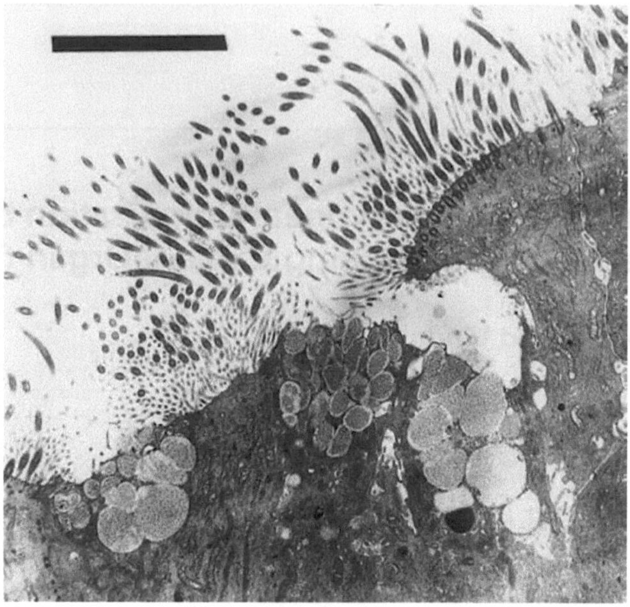

Fig. 1. Transmission electron micrograph showing normal pseudostratified ciliated epithelium derived from human nasal turbinate. Ciliated epithelial cells are interspersed with goblet cells, one of which has discharged its contents. Bar, 15 μm.

cytes, they will secrete mucus, produce periciliary fluid, and contain a population of beating cilia. The disadvantages of human organ-culture systems are that the tissue is inevitably resected from patients with coincident disease, and the experiments involved are usually labor-intensive. Unlike experiments with monolayers of transformed cells, which can often be completed in a single day, the replicates required to smooth out biological variation among donors of explants means that a series of experiments may take several months.

The constituents of the epithelium and its underlying mucosa vary according to the site within the upper-respiratory tract. The anterior nares are lined by stratified squamous keratinizing epithelium. The remainder of the respiratory tract is lined by ciliated, pseudostratified, columnar cells interspersed with occasional mucus-secreting cells (shown in **Fig. 1**) except at the following sites:

1. A small zone of stratified epithelium below the pharyngeal fornix,
2. Nonkeratinizing squamous epithelium in the oropharynx,
3. The anterior surface of the epiglottis and the upper half of its posterior surface,
4. The upper half of the aryepiglottic folds, and
5. The vocal cords.

The midline pharyngeal tonsil is located on the dorsal wall of the nasopharynx and is covered mainly by pseudostratified columnar cells. It may become quite large in childhood and together with lymphoid tissue near the auditory orifices, constitutes the adenoids. At the trachea, the stratified squamous epithelium covering the vocal cords becomes ciliated pseudostratified columnar. Submucosal glands are numerous and are found wherever there is cartilage within the airway wall. The pseudostratified columnar epithelium that lines the conducting airways is made up of eight distinct cell types: basal, ciliated, mucus, serous, clara, dense core granulated (DCG), special type, and brush ***(11)***. The relative frequency of these cells at the different airway levels has not been investigated extensively in humans ***(12)***. There are intense collections of lymphoid tissue within the tonsils and adenoids. Overlying these areas, the epithelium tends to be relatively sparsely ciliated compared to other parts of the upper-respiratory tract. Mucus originates mainly from goblet cells as globules that gradually coalesce. In addition to trapping inhaled bacteria, mucus has direct antibacterial activity; it contains some secretory IgA, lysosyme, transferrin, lactoferrin, and immunoglobulin.

Upper-respiratory tract organ cultures can be derived from nasal turbinates (the mucosa that overlies the scroll bones within the nasopharynx), the adenoids (an area within the nasopharyngeal vault in which epithelium-covered lymphoid tissue projects into the lumen), or tonsils. Nasal turbinates are usually resected for nonallergic nasal obstruction such as nasal septal deviation. However, adenoids and tonsils are normally resected in patients who have had chronic infection of these tissues. Tissue is dissected into conveniently-sized explants and maintained in culture medium in such a way that the mucosal surface is exposed and available for interaction with bacteria. Organ cultures can be maintained in suspension in culture medium ***(13)***, or can be immersed in medium but embedded in a solid phase, e.g., agar, such that their mucosal surface is oriented appropriately ***(14,15)***. Alternatively, organ cultures can be maintained so that their mucosal surfaces are not immersed in medium, but are exposed to humidified air. Whether the organ cultures are immersed in medium or cultured with an "air-interface" appears to alter the behavior of some pathogens with the surface of the explant; for example, *Haemophilus influenzae* appears to adhere with greater affinity to mucus in an air-interface model ***(16)***.

Bacterial interaction with explants can be measured in a number of ways. The simplest measurement is to count viable bacteria in association with homogenates of the tissue. By immersing explants in a bactericidal solution (such as antibiotic or sodium taurocholate) prior to homogenization, some estimate of the organisms that have penetrated the tissue of the explant can be made. Microscopy can be conducted after fixation using light, fluorescence, or electron microscopy (EM). EM

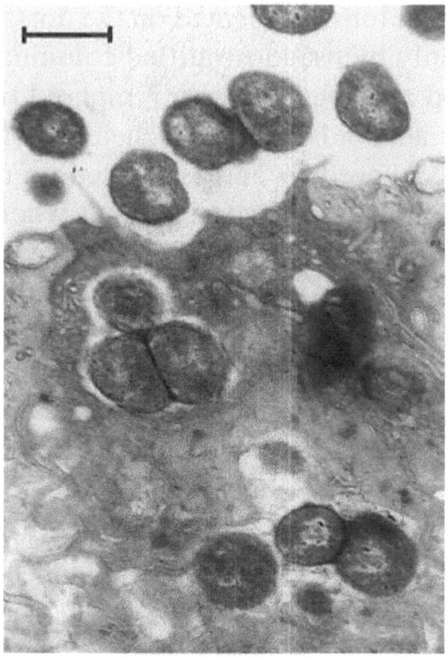

Fig. 2. Transmission electron microscopy showing epithelial-cell entry of group B *N. meningitidis* after infection of nasal turbinates for 24 hours. Meningococci are seen within membrane-bound vesicles of a nonciliated cell. Bar, 500 nm.

has the advantage that it can provide useful information on the tropism of bacteria for individual cell types and more accurate identification of bacteria.

A number of groups have studied the interaction of *Neisseria meningitidis* with human airway mucosa. Using adenoids, Stephens et al. showed that meningococci attached selectively to nonciliated columnar cells, and during this process microvilli of nonciliated cells elongated and surrounded the organisms. Meningococci appeared to undergo parasite-directed endocytosis and were later observed in subepithelial tissues adjacent to lymphoid tissue ***(17)***. Using nasal turbinates, Read et al. showed that there was little association of *N. meningitidis* with secreted mucus and that endocytosis into nonciliated cells is observed in only a minority of explants (**Fig. 2**). Meningococci that have penetrated the basement collagen membrane were seen dividing within macrophages ***(18)***. Some meningococcal virulence determinants have been studied in these systems. Rayner et al. ***(19)***, using human adenoids, showed that meningococcal infection caused epithelial damage, loss of ciliated epithelium, and ciliary disorganization, which was greatest with piliated variants of the group B strain MC58. Pili increased adherence of meningococci to nonciliated cells. This group also showed that there was very little adherence of *Neisseria* to mucus. Stephens et al. investigated the effect of loss of the ($\alpha2\rightarrow8$)-linked polysialic acid capsule on adherence of *N. meningitidis* to the surface of human adenoids and found that noncapsulate strains were more adherent to the surface of the adenoid mucosa. Both the wild-type and noncapsulate strain were internalized by the adenoid mucosa. They noted that capsulate meningococci were internalized in large vacuoles and nonciliated epithelial cells, whereas noncapsulate meningococci appeared not to be internalized within membrane-bound vesicles ***(20)***. Read et al. ***(21)*** investigated the effect of co-infection with influenza virus B on subsequent attachment of *N. meningitidis* to the surface of nasal turbinate mucosa. Influenza virus did not increase association of an ET-5 strain (K454) with the mucosa even when the explants were pre-treated with the virus for 7 d prior to superinfection with *N. meningitidis*.

New technologies are now available for the investigation of *Neisseria* gene expression and selection during penetration of human nasopharyngeal mucosa. The relatively simple techniques of organ culture described here will be increasingly useful over the next few years as we employ new molecular tools to elucidate further the pathogenesis of this disease.

2. Materials

2.1. Organ Culture

1. Tissue samples are obtained from patients undergoing surgery by ENT surgeons (*see* **Note 1**). Informed consent is required from the patient for the ex vivo tissue to be used.
2. Tissue-culture medium: Minimal Essential Medium (MEM; Gibco, UK) contains Earle's salts, calcium, L-glutamine, and phenyl red; Medium 199 (M199) (Flow Laboratories, UK) contains Earle's salts, 20 m*M* HEPES (N-2-hydroxyethylpiperazine-N′-2-ethanesulphonic acid buffer), calcium and magnesium with glutamine, but without phenyl red. This medium contains higher concentrations of amino acids and vitamins than MEM. Phosphate-buffered saline (PBS): (0.6 *M* Na_2HPO_4, 0.6 *M* Kh_2PO_4, NaCl, 0.9% [w/v]). Antibiotics used to sterilize commensal flora include penicillin (50 U/mL), streptomycin (50 μg/mL), and gentamicin (50 μg/mL) in combination. These are generally added to MEM or M-199.
3. Petri-dishes: organ cultures are conducted in 3-cm petri-dishes. For interface models, a 3-cm petri-dish is placed inside a 5-cm petri-dish (Sterilin, UK).
4. Electrophoretic agar (1%) is used to immobilize tissue in petri-dishes (No.1; Oxoid, UK).
5. Irrigation of air-interface explants can be conducted using strips of sterile filter paper (e.g., No. 1, Whatman, UK) or dialysis membrane.
6. Miscellaneous equipment required includes a thermostatic waterbath, microcentrifuges, a pH meter with 5% CO_2 in air, UV spectrophotometer, scalpels and plastic microbiological loops, and a Class II microbiological hood.

2.2. Homogenization and Viable Counting

1. Homogenization is conducted by us using a one-shot cell disrupter (Warwick Instruments, UK), which exerts a pressure of 10 psi across the tissue. After use, sterilization is conducted using 70% methylated spirits followed by rinsing in sterile PBS. Viable counting of homogenates requires Eppendorf tubes and PBS or Mueller-Hinton Broth as diluent.

2.3. Fixation for Histology and EM

1. For preparation of paraffin-embedded tissue, tissue can be fixed in 10% formalin for 24 h.
2. For fixation for immunofluorescence, tissue can be lightly fixed in 1% paraformaldehyde (pH 7.0–8.0).
3. For transmission EM and scanning EM, tissue is fixed in 2.5% glutaraldehyde and 2% formaldehyde in 0.04 *M* sodium cacodylate with 5% sucrose and a 0.05% CaCl.

2.4. Cutting and Preparation of Sections for Light Microscopy

1. Dehydration of fixed tissues conducted with ethanol at a range of concentrations from 70–100% tissue is embedded in paraffin wax at 56°C.
2. Tissue is cut using a standard microtome (e.g., Slee 550, Mainz, Germany).
3. Staining for conventional histology uses hematoxylin and eosin (Surgipath, UK).
4. For immunofluorescence, sections on slides are flooded with primary antibody (affinity chosen depends upon the microbial target; for meningococcal immunofluorescence, anticapsular, anti-Porin, or anti-TBP antibodies can be used) at a concentration of 1:20 in PBS, for 15 min. Secondary antibody, which again depends on the species in which the primary antibody is made (good examples are goat anti-rabbit conjugated to FITC or Cy3), at a concentration of 1:20 in PBS containing 5% blocking serum (serum from the species of the secondary antibody, e.g., goat).

2.5. Preparation for Transmission EM

1. Fixed tissue is placed in buffer (0.04 *M* sodium cacodylate buffer with 5% sucrose and 0.05% CaCl).
2. Osmium tetroxide is prepared at 1.3% from a stock 2% solution.
3. Resin is prepared using a combination of resin 48 g, HWO 52 g and BDMA 1.78 g together with an accelerator (benzyl dimethylamine).
4. 2% Uranyl acetate is prepared in 50% ethanol.
5. Propylene oxide is prepared in a 1:1 mixture with resin (all materials available from TAAB Lab Equipment, Aldermaston, UK).

2.6. Preparation for Scanning EM

1. For critical point drying solutions of acetone and 100% ethanol at equal concentrations are made.
2. Sputter-coating is conducted with a commercial sputter-coater (e.g., TAAB 300-S).

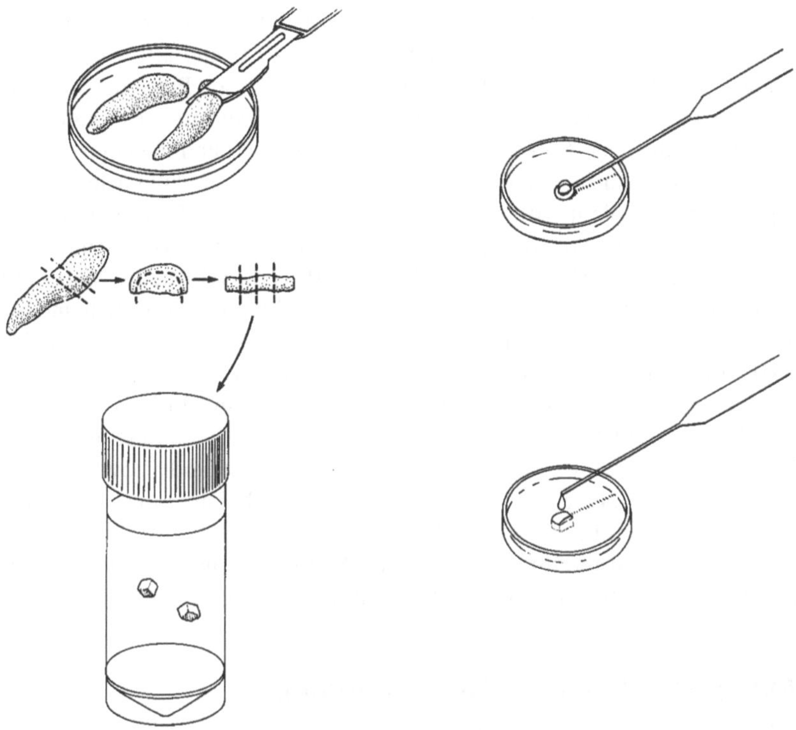

Fig. 3. Dissecting nasal turbinates for organ culture. Cubes of mucosa are produced by cutting a section of the turbinate, trimming away submucosal tissue followed by cutting mucosa into cubes of approximate dimensions of 4 × 4 × 4 mm.

3. Methods

3.1. Preparation of Organ Cultures (*see* Fig. 3)

1. Transport the mucosal tissue to the laboratory in MEM with antibiotics. Dissect the tissue to produce convenient-sized explants (e.g., 4 × 4 mm).
2. Cut nasal turbinates in cross-sections, and then place each half-moon shaped section on its side. Trim the epithelium away from the underlying cartilage and the supporting connective tissue. Turn the strips of mucosa on their side and cut into cubes which have an epithelium on one surface. This process is usually conducted in a 10-cm Petri dish containing MEM with antibiotics. Transfer cubes of tissue to a universal container containing MEM with antibiotics. Examine the explants with a dissecting microscope to ensure that they have ciliary activity (observed as a "shimmering" at the edge of the explant). Place the tissue in MEM without antibiotics and incubate at 37°C for at least 4h prior to use.
2. Maintain the explant in a 3-cm petri dish containing the tissue submerged in MEM or M199. In order to position the explant so that its epithelial surface projects

upwards and is continually available for interaction with bacteria, embed the explant in a seat of 1% agar. Warm the agar to 40°C and allow to cool. At temperatures less than 37°C, 1% electrophoretic agar will set. Place the agar within the 3-cm Petri dish while molten and then position the tissue cut-surface downwards in the center of the agar. Carefully add additional agar around the edge of the explant to ensure that cut surfaces are not available for interaction with bacteria.

3. To produce an explant with an air-interface place a 3-cm Petri dish inside a 5-cm petri dish with a strip of filter paper across the inner Petri dish so that it can bathe the explant with MEM (7 ml) from the outer Petri dish. Place explants cut-surface downwards onto the filter paper in the centre of the inner Petri dish and place 1% molten agar around the explant to fix in position. Irrigate the tissue with 200 μL of MEM until it is ready for inoculation with bacteria.
4. Grow *N. meningitidis* cultures up to mid-log phase in Muller-Hinton broth and wash 3 times in PBS. Prepare 1×10^7 cfu of the experimental strain in 100 μL of PBS, and drop carefully onto the center of the explant, and allow the infection to proceed. If an immersed model is being used, simply bathe the explant in its seat of agar in 1×10^7 cfu in 3 mL of MEM.
5. Over the course of the infection, remove the tissue from the Petri dish, immerse in 3 changes of PBS, and then either homogenize for viable counting or fix for microscopy.

3.2. Homogenization and Viable Counting

1. To homogenize tissue, place the explant in the chamber of the one-shot cell disrupter together with 1 mL of Muller-Hinton broth to obtain a suspension. Hold the probe in place while the disruption cycle (20 s) proceeds. Remove the cup, and aspirate the contents of the capsule into an Eppendorf. Dilutional counting can then be conducted.
2. To estimate the number of bacteria that have penetrated the tissue, immerse the explants in 0.25% sodium taurocholate (bile salts) for 30 s (*see* **Note 7**). Immediately wash the tissue through two changes of PBS in a universal container prior to homogenisation in the one-shot cell disrupter. This concentration of sodium taurocholate kills a suspension of 10^7 *Neisseria meningitidis* within 30 s. Explants that have been treated with sodium taurocholate and then washed and homogenized exhibit no bactericidal activity against *N. meningitidis*, which suggests that this substance, as expected, does not enter this mucosal tissue.

3.3. Preparation of Tissue for Histology

1. To produce frozen sections (useful for immunofluorescence) snap-freeze tissue in liquid nitrogen. Cut sections with a cryostat set at –20°C. This has to be conducted under category 2 conditions.
2. For paraffin wax-embedded tissue, dehydrate formalin-fixed tissue using graded alcohol immersions of 2 h each at 70, 95, and 100%. Place the tissue in paraffin wax at 56°C over 2 h and then embed in fresh wax. Cut suitable sections with a microtome.

3.4. Transmission EM

1. Following fixation of tissue, remove fixative and replace with buffer and leave until it is ready for further processing. Conduct the processing in a fume cabinet. Remove the buffer and replace with osmium tetroxide and roll tissue for 1 h. Remove osmium tetroxide and replace with 50% ethanol in distilled water. Roll the tissue for 15 min. Remove the ethanol and stain the tissue with 2% uranyl acetate. Replace this again with 50% ethanol and continue the dehydration through graded ethanols. Replace 100% ethanol with propylene oxide for 15 min (this is a carcinogen and great care must be taken in handling material at this stage). Place the tissue in a 1:1 propylene oxide/resin mixture and leave in a fume cabinet overnight in embedding moulds. Take care to exclude air from the resin. Orientate the moulds containing the tissues using an orange stick for cutting. Following embedding cut 5 or 6 1 μ sections from the central portion of each specimen, stain with toluene blue, and examine by light microscopy. Sections containing appropriately oriented epithelium can then be selected and placed on a 300 mesh carbon-coated copper grid (Agar Scientific) for examination by TEM.

3.5. Preparation for Scanning EM

1. Process the fixed explant through gentle buffer washes, 1% osmium tetroxide (in identical buffer) for 1 h, dehydrate through graded ethanols to acetone, and conduct critical point drying in CO_2. Mount the tissue on aluminium stubs, and then sputter-coat with gold using the SEM 300-S sputter-coater.
2. Examine stubs with mounted tissue in an appropriate scanning electron microscope. Set the center of each specimen at 0° tilt, increase magnification to 2.5 K and examine the features of the surface in a box pattern. This can be done using a screen graticule. Calculate the percentage of the surface of the mucosa that is ciliated, nonciliated, covered with normal mucosa or covered with extruded or stripped (damaged) mucosa. *N. meningitidis* can usually be easily identified because of its characteristic shape and it is possible to describe the numbers of bacteria associated with particular surface characteristics (*see* **Fig. 4**).

4. Notes

1. Middle or inferior turbinates are generally approx 5-cm maximum length and usually contain cartilage unless a submucosal resection has been conducted. Human adenoids are usually obtained from children and are rarely resected intact but consist of strands of friable tissue. Human tonsils are usually quite foul, very bloody, and difficult to handle because of the tendency of the tissue to collapse on cutting. In the case of nasal turbinates, the tissue is not always suitable for organ culture. Sometimes the tissue has obvious severe bruising and/or pus. This material is clearly unsuitable. A good piece of tissue will have a salmon pink color and be relatively smooth. Note that the anterior tip of a turbinate usually has squamous epithelium and this should be dissected away. With adenoids, it can be very difficult to orientate the tissues so that the epithelial surface can be

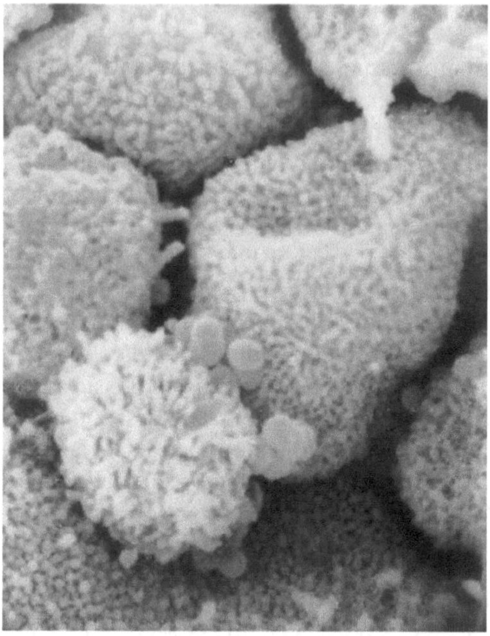

Fig. 4. Scanning electron micrograph of *Neisseria meningitidis* is adherent to the surface of turbinate mucosa. Cell junctions of the nonciliated cells are separating, and some meningococci are seen between cells.

placed upwards in the preparation. Epithelial surfaces can be identified using a dissecting microscope and ciliary activity can be seen. They tend to be a different color to the adventious tissue, but in diseased tissue it can be very difficult to tell the difference between the two. In our hands, with both the agar-embedded model and the air-interface model, control tissue will retain some ciliary activity for at least 7 d. However, we have noted by this time that there is some loss of integrity on histology. "Normal" histology is usually retained for at least 48 h of culture. We tend to use our tissue immediately unless the experiment requires more prolonged periods of culture.

2. The inoculum size of *N. meningitidis* is critical. We use inocula of 1×10^6 cfu or 1×10^7 cfu. With lower inocula than this, the meningococcus does not always succeed in these models.
3. We have found a wide difference in the success of *N. meningitidis* between tissues derived from different human hosts. In fact, there can be almost a 1,000-fold difference in the recovered bacteria between one host and another during experimental infections, but there is consistent retrieval within-host. Therefore, to power the study, we usually require at least six different donors per series of experiments, though obviously this depends on the study that is being done.

Typically, we will compare a wild-type organism with a mutant, though more than two comparators will require at least 10 different donors for statistical power. A typical turbinate will yield between 15 and 20 explants only, which limits the size of the experiments you can perform.

4. Careful preparation for histology and EM is critical. Rough handling of the fixed explant at any stage will result in stripping of the epithelium. Care should be taken that the explants are not rolled violently during the preparation steps, and that air is excluded from tubes containing the explants. A recent trick that we have used is to immerse tissue in plasma and then add clot activator so that the tissue can then be fixed and processed inside a protective clot.
5. Scanning microscopy of explants infected with *Neisseria* can be difficult, but the experienced eye can easily tell the difference between *N. meningitidis* and other objects such as epithelial blebs and mucous globules. Immunogold labeling of bacteria has been surprisingly difficult as only a small percentage of the organisms seem to become coated with the marker.
6. Transmission EM is also labor-intensive; because the sections are only 1-μm thin, you do not always cut through a section containing *N. meningitidis*. We were only able to identify meningococci by TEM in 40% of infected explants, whereas we were able to show them in 100% using SEM *(18)*. Therefore with TEM, we generally take multiple cuts at various points through the center portion of the specimen in order to capture meningococci and quantify the interactions. The organisms can usually be seen on the toluene blue-stained sections, in case you wish to choose ultrathin sections for photography.
7. An alternative method of estimating internalization of meningococci into the tissue is to bathe the tissue in an antibiotic that penetrates tissue poorly (e.g., gentamicin), prior to homogenizing tissue for viable counting of bacteria. To estimate the concentration of antibiotic required to do this, the Minimum Bactericidal Concentration (MBC) of the experimental strains should be measured, in addition to the minimum length of time required for 100% kill of bacteria in suspension.

Acknowledgment

We are grateful to the Wellcome Trust, the Ralph Sutcliffe Fund, and the National Meningitis Trust for supporting our work.

References

1. Broome, C. V. (1986) The carrier state: *Neisseria meningitidis. J. Antimicrob. Chemother.* **18(suppl. A),** 25–34.
2. Riordan, T., Cartwright, K., Andrews, N., Stewart, J., Burris, A., Fox, A., et al. (1998) Acquisition and carriage of meningococci in marine commando recruits. *Epidemiol. Infect.* **121,** 495–505.
3. Greenfield, S. and Feldman, H. (1967) Familial carriers and meningococcal meningitis. *N. Engl. J. Med.* **277,** 497–502.
4. Stewart, J. M., Cartwright, K. A., Robinson, P. M., and Noah, N. D. (1989) Effect of smoking on meningococcal carriage. *Lancet* **865,** 723–725.

5. Greenwood, B. M., Blakeborough, I. S., Bradley, A. K., Wali, S., and Whittle, H. C. (1984) Meningococcal disease in season in sub-Saharan Africa. *Lancet* **839,** 1339–1342.
6. Olcen, P., Kjellander, J., Danielsson, D., and Lundquist, B. L. (1981) Epidemiology of *Neisseria meningitidis*; prevalence and symptoms from the upper respiratory tract in family members of patients with meningococcal disease. *Scand. J. Infect. Dis.* **13,** 105–109.
7. Young, L. S., LaForce, F. M., Head, J. J., Feeley, J. C., and Bennett, J. V. (1972) A simultaneous outbreak of meningococcal and influenza infections. *N. Engl. J. Med.* **287,** 5–9.
8. Rigg, G. (1934) Studies of meningococcal infection; the carrier problem. *J. Exp. Med.* **59,** 553.
9. Blackwell, C. C., Weir, D. M., James, V. S., Todd, W. T., Banatvala, N., Chaudhuri, A. K., et al. (1990) Secretor status, smoking and carriage of *Neisseria meningitidis*. *Epidem. Infect.* **104,** 203–209.
10. Olcen, P., Kjellander, J., Danielsson, D., and Lundquist, B. L. (1979) Culture diagnosis of meningococcal carriers: yield from different sites and influence of storage in transport medium. *J. Clin. Pathol.* **32,** 1222–1225.
11. Jeffery, P. K. and Corrin, B. (1984) Structural analysis of the respiratory tract, in *Immunology of the Lung and Upper Respiratory Tract* (Bienenstock, J., ed.), Raven Press, New York, pp. 1–27.
12. Jeffery, P. K and Reid, L. (1975) New observations of rat epithelium: a quantitative and electron microscopic study. *J. Anat.* **120,** 295–320.
13. Farley, M. M., Stephens, D. S., Mulks, M. H., Cooper, M. D., Bricker, J. V., Mirra, S. S., and Wright, A. (1986) The pathogenesis of IgA protease-producing and non-producing *Haemophilus influenza* on human nasopharyngeal organ cultures. *J. Infect. Dis.* **154,** 752–759.
14. Read, R. C., Wilson, R., Rutman, A., Lund, V. J., Todd, H. C., Brain, A. P., et al. Interaction of non-typable *Haemophilus influenzae* with human respiratory mucosa in vitro. *J. Infect. Dis.* **163,** 549–558.
15. Read, R. C., Rutman, A., Jeffery, P. K., Lund, V. J., Brain, A. P., Moxon, E. R., Cole, P. J., and Wilson, R. (1992) Interaction of capsulate *Haemophilus influenzae* with human airway mucosa *in vitro*. *Infect. Immun.* **60,** 3244–3252.
16. Jackson, A. D., Cole, P. J., and Wilson, R. (1996) Comparison of *Haemophilus influenzae* type B infection of human respiratory mucosa organ cultures maintained with an “air-interface” or submerged in medium. *Infect. Immun.* **64,** 2353–2355.
17. Stephens, D. S., Hoffman, L. H., and McGee, Z. A. (1983) Interaction of *Neisseria meningitidis* with human nasopharyngeal mucosa: attachment and entry into columnar epithelial cells. *J. Infect. Dis.* **148,** 369–376.
18. Read, R. C., Fox, A., Miller, K., Gray, T., Jones, N., Borrow, R., Jones, D. M., and Finch, R. G. (1995) Experimental infection of human nasal mucosal explants with *Neisseria meningitidis*. *J. Med. Microbiol.* **42,** 353–361.

19. Rayner, C. F. J., Dewar, A., Moxon, E. R., Virji, M., and Wilson, R. (1995) The effect of variations in the expression of pili on the interaction of *Neisseria meningitidis* with human nasopharyngeal epithelium. *J. Infect. Dis.* **171,** 113–121.
20. Read, R. C., Goodwin, L., Parsons, M. A., Silcocks, P., Kaczmarski, E. B., Parker, A., and Baldwin, T. J. (1999) Co-infection with influenza B virus does not affect association of *Neisseria meningitidis* with human nasopharyngeal mucosa in organ culture. *Infect. Immun.* **67,** 3082–3086.
21. Stephens, D. S., Spellman, P. A., and Swartley, J. S. (1993) Effect of the ($\alpha 2 \rightarrow 8$)-linked polysialic acid capsule on adherence of Neisseria meningitidis to human mucosal cells. *J. Infect. Dis.* **167,** 475–479.

37

Invasion of the Central Nervous System by *Neisseria meningitidis*

Colin Tinsley and Xavier Nassif

1. Introduction

Neisseria meningitidis is an extracellular pathogen responsible for septicemia and meningitis. The occurrence of meningitis requires that bacteria cross the blood-brain barrier (BBB) and induce an inflammatory response within the subarachnoid space. The mechanisms that lead to the development of cerebrospinal fluid (CSF) pleocytosis once bacteria have reached the CSF have been studied using several animal models. These mechanisms are similar among extracellular pathogens responsible for meningitis (i.e., *Haemophilus influenzae* type b, *Streptococcus pneumoniae*, and *N. meningitidis*). The *in situ* production of cytokines is the primary event leading to transmigration of leucocytes through the BBB ***(1–4)***.

The BBB is one of the tightest barriers in the body, and few bacterial pathogens are able to breach this barrier; this strongly suggests that these pathogens have developed specific attributes responsible for this step. Two factors play a synergistic role in bacterial invasion of the CSF: 1) high levels of bacteremia, and 2) the ability of the meningococcus to interact specifically with the components of the BBB. For each of the steps of pathogenesis major virulence factors have been described. The polysaccharide capsule plays an essential role in the bloodstream survival and the pili are essential in mediating interaction of the bacteria with the BBB. The role of pilus-mediated adhesion in promoting the crossing of the BBB in patients has been well-established. However the precise mechanisms by which pilus mediated adhesion is responsible for the crossing of the BBB are unidentified, and other bacterial attributes that are likely to be involved in this step remain to be looked at. This highlights the

From: *Methods in Molecular Medicine, vol. 67: Meningococcal Disease: Methods and Protocols*
Edited by: A. J. Pollard and M. C. J. Maiden © Humana Press Inc., Totowa, NJ

need for suitable models permitting the study of these steps. We will describe here two different groups of techniques used for the study of these two aspects of central nervous system (CNS) invasion: the bloodstream survival and the crossing of the BBB. The former relies essentially on the use of the infant rat model, and the latter on in vitro models.

1.1. In vitro Model

1.1.1. The Blood-Brain Barrier

The aim of these in vitro models is to provide a tool that mimics the interaction of *N. meningitidis* with the components of the BBB. An understanding of the potentials and limitations of the model requires firstly a brief review of the major characteristics of the BBB.

The barrier between the blood and the brain parenchyma is formed differently by the endothelial cells and at the choroidal plexus. The brain endothelial cells differ from those in most peripheral capillaries in two important respects. Firstly they undergo a very slow rate of fluid-phase uptake as assayed by the translocation of tracer molecules such as horseradish peroxidase *(5)*. This limits the amount of transcellular flux. Secondly the surfaces of contact between the cells of the brain capillaries are sealed by tight junctions, which limits the amount of paracellular flux. The walls of the blood vessels on the surface of the brain demonstrate a very significant barrier to the movement of ions because their electrical resistance is at least 1500 Ωcm^2 *(6)*. Hence it is the combination of the limited paracellular and transcellular movement of molecules and ions that accounts for the existence of the barrier. However the BBB is now recognized as more than an impermeable barrier; indeed these endothelial cells are very similar to polarized cells. The reason that endothelial cells in the brain become different from those in the periphery is not fully understood, but it is clear that astrocytes influence the development of the altered permeability of these endothelial cells *(7)*.

The other components of the BBB are the choroidal plexuses. These are the major site of CSF synthesis and are located in the ventricles *(8)*. These are leaflike structures in the CSF with a central core of blood vessels covered by epithelium. The endothelial cells in the choroidal plexus are fenestrated and have a peripheral structure. The BBB in this region is formed by tight junctions at the ventricular surface of the epithelial cells, which form a true polarized epithelium identical to that found in the kidney. These epithelial cells produce the CSF, which has a very high turnover rate, being replaced entirely every 4–6 h.

The understanding of the crossing of the BBB by a bacterial pathogen requires the localization of the site of entry into the CSF: is it the choroidal plexus or the meningeal capillaries? (It is theoretically unlikely that an extracellular pathogen such as *N. meningitidis* would enter the CSF by traveling inside leukocytes.) In addition, clinical observations argue against such a route because fulminant meningococcemia is often accompanied by an infection of the CSF before an inflammatory response, or leukocytes, are observed in the CSF. To determine the anatomical structure where the crossing of the barrier takes place, an animal model reproducing the human disease should be used. The only animal model in which *N. meningitidis* have been shown to invade the meninges is the infant rat ***(9)***. The intraperitoneal injection of meningococci is followed by a bacteremia and subsequently by invasion of the CSF. However the specificity of the crossing of the BBB in infant rats is questionable, because *N. meningitidis* is only known to interact specifically with cells of human origin. Recently using material obtained from a patient who died early during the course of a fulminant meningococcemia, *i.e.*, at a time when *N. meningitidis* were crossing the BBB, numerous *N. meningitidis* were seen strongly adhering to the endothelial cells of both the capillaries of the choroidal plexuses and the meninges ***(10)***, suggesting that both structures could be traversed by *N.* meningitidis to invade the CSF.

Though considerable progress has been made in our understanding of its anatomy and physiology, a major difficulty in the study of the crossing of the BBB by a pathogen remains the lack of a suitable in vitro model mimicking this barrier. The ideal model would use a brain endothelial cell line, and a choroidal epithelial cell line, which make tight junctions in vitro. Some cell lines are available, but none has the ability to form tight junctions ***(11,12)***. More sophisticated models have been developed but they are laborious and also have the drawback of using animal cells, and consequently are not very useful in the study of the meningococcus, which would require human material. On the other hand, it is apparent that the BBB, both at the level of the endothelium and the choroid plexus, shows many of the characterisitics of polarized epithelium, a more readily acheivable model. Hence studies performed with tight junction-forming epithelial cells, for example T84 epithelial cells, may yield information shedding light on the mechanisms of entry into the CSF ***(13)***.

1.1.2. Advantages and Limitations of the T84 Model

This model allows the study of the interaction of meningococci with a monolayer of cells forming tight junctions, this being a hallmark of the cells of the BBB. Using this model, it has been shown that *N. meningitidis* is capable of traversing such a monolayer without altering the integrity of the tight junctions ***(14,15)***. No bacteria are seen between the cells, and furthermore no loss of electrical resistance is observed and there is no delocalization of the proteins classically associated with tight junctions (e.g., ZO1 and E-cadherin). On the other hand, confocal microscopy and electron microscopy (EM) have demonstrated the presence of bacteria inside the cells. This suggests that meningococci cross a tight junction-forming monolayer using the transcellular route, and may therefore transcytose through such a monolayer. However one cannot exclude the possibility that this organism may be able to cross using the paracellular route without destroying the junctions. Initially, the adhesion of *N. meningitidis* is localized, resulting in the formation of clumps of bacteria on the apical surface of the monolayer. The bacteria then spread onto the surface of the cells as the clumps disappear and are replaced by a monolayer of meningococci covering the cells, a diffuse adherence in contrast to the initial localized adherence. At this stage, bacteria adhere intimately and firmly to the apical membrane, and in some places are found to be intracellular. Pilus-mediated adhesion is probably most critical during the first step of localized adherence. At the diffuse adherence step, the bacteria have lost their pili and are intimately attached to the cells. There is evidence that PilT, a cytoplasmic, nucleotide binding protein, involved in pilus retraction, is required for the dispersion of the bacteria in moving from the localized to the diffuse adherence pattern, to induce the loss of piliation, and allow the subsequent intimate attachment ***(16)***. Many questions still remain, and this model may therefore be used to address the cellular mechanisms involved in this trancytosis as well as the screening of various bacterial mutants deficient in this process.

In using this model, one should always keep in mind that T84 are not derived from the human brain. However, as mentioned earlier, this is a relatively easy in vitro model to set up in order to study the tanscytosis of a bacterial pathogen through a monolayer of human cells. Models for studying the interaction of *N. meningtidis* with various human endothelial cells are available and will be reviewed in Chapter 37.

1.2. In Vivo Model

1.2.1. Description of the Model

The procedure is based on the infant rat model of infection by *Escherichia coli* ***(17)***, adapted for *N. meningitidis* ***(9,18)***. The bacteria are injected intraperitoneally and the course of infection can be established by determining the number of bacteria in the blood and the CSF at various time points. The major question concerning this model is that this organism has not been shown to interact with rat cells and therefore the crossing of the BBB by the bacteria in infant rats may not result from a specific interaction of the bacteria with the cellular barrier, as in the human disease, but from the ability of the bacteria to induce a sustained bacteremia. Whether or not this model can measure the specific interaction of meningococci with the BBB, it is suitable to assess the ability of the bacteria to multiply in the bloodstream. The endpoint measured in this model depends on the inoculum, but it can be either the mortality at 24, 48, or even 72 h, the number of bacteria in the blood or in the CSF at several time points, or alternatively one may score the number of rats that have bacteria in the CSF after 24 h, especially when low inocula are used. For comparison between mutants, the latter are more sensistive than the assessment of the mortality, and the number of rats having positive CSF cultures at 24 h correlates with the ability of the bacteria to survive in the bloodstream.

The virulence of different strains in the model varies and it is neccessary to start by performing a calibration of the system. This involves inoculation of different doses of the strain and the definition of the minimum quantity of the wild-type strain neccessary to induce a sustained bacteremia. The outcome of the infection is also dependent on the strain of rat used, and consistent results may be obtained by using litters of inbred rats. A litter of 10 pups is sufficient for the determination of the minimum infectious dose. When comparing strains, e.g., to test the effect of mutation of a gene, the number of rats used is the minimum that will give statistically significant results.

1.2.2. Advantages and Limitations of the Infant Rat Model

Though the properties of the infant rat model are not very clearly defined, the bacteremia caused by the meningococcus is probably dependent partly on its ability to scavange iron and to resist the nonspecific immunity of the infant rat. In this respect, acapsular strains are nonvirulent in the infant rat model, in keeping with the capsule's known role in protection against host immunological defenses. Furthermore, the addition of exogenous, specific anti-meningococcal antibody results in the clearance of the infection and this has been proposed as the basis for a comparison of meningococcal antigens as potential vaccine components, screening monoclonal antibodies (MAbs) for their ability to rescue the rats from infection by meningococci ***(9)***.

It remains to be determined whether the model can be used to study pathogenic properties of *N. meningitidis* other than the resistance to serum bactericidal activity. The unanswered questions, as with the yet imperfectly defined in vitro models of meningococcal-host interactions, underline the fact that progress in understanding of the pathogenesis of meningococcal disease is achieved in parallel with developments in the models, which in the future may benefit from transgenic animals expressing human cellular receptors specific for the meningococcus.

2. Materials

2.1. T84 Model

2.1.1. Quantification of the Interaction with and Penetration of a Cellular Monolayer

1. Cell line: T84 (ATCC).
2. Culture medium: 1:1 Dulbecco's minimal essential medium (DMEM): Ham's F12 medium (Gibco-BRL Life Technologies), supplemented with 10% fetal

bovine serum (FBS), 200 m*M* L-glutamine, 100 U/mL penicillin, 100 μg/mL streptomycin, 0.25 μg/mL amphotericin B.
3. Infection medium: As culture medium but without the addition of antibiotics.
4. Tissue-culture trays (Falcon).
5. Transwell premeable supports (Costar).
6. Millicell-ERS resistance meter (Millipore).
7. GCB-agar plates (per liter): GCB medium base (Difco) 36 g. Sterilize by autoclaving, then add Kellogg's supplements and ferric nitrate ***(19)*** immediately before pouring plates. Kellogg supplement 1 is (per 100 mL): glucose 40 g, L-glutamine 1 g, thiamine 2 mg, and is added at a final concentration of 1%. Supplement 2 is 12.3 m*M* $Fe(N0_3)_3$ and is added at 0.1%.

2.1.2. Immunomicroscopic Investigations of the Interaction of Nm with Cellular Monolayers

1. METM: 50 m*M* MES, 3 m*M* EGTA, 5 m*M* $MgCl_2$, 0.5% Triton X100, pH 7.4.
2. Examples of antibodies and stains are listed in **Table 1**.
3. Microscopic mounting medium: Moviol (Sigma).
4. EM fixing solution: 0.1 *M* sodium cacodylate, pH 7.2, 0.1 *M* sucrose, 5 m*M* $CaCl_2$, 5 m*M* $MgCl_2$, containing 1.25% glutaraldehyde and 1.25% paraformaldehyde.

2.2. In Vivo Model

1. Mother and litter of infant rats (inbred Lewis rats), 4 d old at the time of the experiment (*see* **Note 3**).
2. GCB-agar plates: Prepared as described in **Subheading 2.1.1.**
3. GC-phosphate liquid medium (per L): Proteose peptone #3 (Difco) 5.0 g, K_2HPO_4 (anhydrous) 4.0 g, KH_2PO_4 (anhydrous) 1.0 g, NaCl 5.0 g. The solution is sterilized by autoclaving and Kellogg's supplements and ferric nitrate (*see* GCB-agar plates in **Subheading 2.1.1.**) are added before use.

3. Methods

3.1. The T84 Model

T84 are human polarized epithelial cells ***(20)***. Several human epithelial cell lines have the ability to form tight junctions in vitro. However T84 are preferred because they have the ability to form tight junctions having an electrical resistance similar to that observed in the BBB. The polarization allows us to define an apical and basolateral surface of cells grown on permeable membrane supports and to study the directional movement of meningococci across the monolayers.

3.1.1. Quantification of the Interaction with and Penetration of a Cellular Monolayer

1. Grow cells at 37°C under 5% CO_2 in T84 culture medium.
2. For experimental assays resuspend the cells in preheated infection medium (*see* **Note 1**) and seed onto permeable supports of 0.33 cm^2 (Transwells) placed in the wells of a tissue-culture tray, at a density of 5×10^5 per well.
3. After 4 d growth, assess the formation of tight junctions by measuring the transepithelial resistance (TER) using a Millicell-ERS resistance meter. Monolayers

Table 1
Immunocytochemical Stains and Antibodies

Component	Antibody or stain	Producer
Bacteria	Ethidium bromide, 0.1 μg/mL	
	Antibody to meningococcal antigens	Noncommercial sources
F-actin	Phalloidin-alexa488 conjugate	Molecular Probes, Eugene, OR.
Tubulin	Anti-α tubulin MAb	Amersham Life Science Products, Bucks, UK
Cell adhesion molecules	Anti-PECAM-1	R&D Systems, Abingdon, UK
	Anti-ICAM-1	R&D Systems
	Anti-CD44h	R&D Systems
	Anti-CD46	Serotec, Oxford, UK
Tight junctions	Rabbit anti-Z01	Zymed Labs, San Francisco, CA
Adherence junctions	Anti-VE cadherin	Immunotech, Marseilles, France
Focal adhesion plaques	Anti-paxillin	Transduction Labs, Lexington, KY
	Anti-h-vinculin	Sigma
	Secondary antibodies to Ig:	
	Anti-rabbit-rhodamine conjugate	Jackson ImmunoResearch Labs, West Grove, PA
	Anti-rabbit-Cy3 conjugate	Jackson ImmunoResearch Labs
	Anti-mouse-Cy5 conjugate	Jackson ImmunoResearch Labs

641

are ready to be used when the TER has reached between 500 and 2000 ohm.cm^2, which resistivity should be achieved within 5 d after seeding (*see* **Note 2**).

4. Harvest the bacteria from GCB-agar plates after overnight growth at 37°C in a humid atmosphere containing 5% CO_2 and dilute into the infection medium to give around 5 × 10^4 bacteria per mL. This can typically be achieved by making a 1/1000 dilution of a suspension of OD_{600} of 0.1, but should be determined experimentally for each strain.
5. Before the assay, remove the medium from both compartments of the transwell. Refill the lower chamber with fresh, sterile medium, and the upper one with with 5 × 10^4 bacteria in 1 mL. Leave the bacteria in contact with the cells for 1 h, then remove the supernatant and gently wash the Transwells three times with 1 mL of PBS and replace with new infection medium. Every hour from this time until the times chosen for the measurements of adhesion and invasion (typically 4, 9, and 24 h) transfer the Transwell supports to a new well containing infection medium and wash the cells in the upper compartment to avoid an excessive growth of nonadhesive meningococci.
6. To assay the degree of adhesiveness of the bacteria to the cells, remove the supernatant containing unattached bacteria and wash the transwells three times with PBS to remove nonadherent bacteria. Transfer the transwell to a new tissue culture well containing 1mL of 1% saponin in PBS. Scrape the transwells with a pipet tip to suspend the cells, vortex to dissociate the bacteria. Plate serial dilutions of the supernatant and cell-associated fractions onto GCB-agar plates in order to enumerate the bacteria.
7. To quantify bacterial internalization, remove the supernatant containing unattached bacteria, wash the transwells three times with PBS, then add fresh infection medium containing gentamicin (150 μg/mL), an impermeant antibiotic, in order to kill external bacteria. After 60 min of incubation at 37°C remove the medium and wash the monolayer twice with PBS. Lyse the cells by incubation at room temperature for 15 min in 1 mL of 1% saponin in PBS in order to liberate the internalized bacteria. Adherence and internalization may be expressed either simply as numbers of bacteria or as a ratio with respect to the number of supernatant bacteria at 1 h.
8. To study the crossing of the monolayer by meningococci follow the procedure above, and after 8 h of incubation transfer the Transwells into a new tissue-culture well containing fresh medium in the lower compartment and incubate at 37°C for one h. Measure the number of bacteria crossing the membrane during this hour by enumeration of the CFU in the medium of the lower chamber at 9 h after infection. Contuinue to wash the upper chamber every hour then perform the same measurement for the 24th h. Verify the integrity of the cell monolayer by determination of the TER at 9 and 24 h after infection.

3.1.2. *Immunomicroscopic Investigations of the Interaction of* N. Meningitidis *with Cellular Monolayers*

In order to investigate more closely the interaction of the bacteria with the monolayers, immunofluorescence microscopy may be performed in order to visualize for example the retraction of the meningococcal pili or the relocalization of cellular proteins. A sufficient variety of fluorochrome-conjugated antibodies are available to allow the simultaneous visualization of several different mammalian cellular components (*see* **Table 1** in materials section for examples). Bacterial components are visualized by indirect immunofluorescence using a primary anti-bacterial antibody, and bacterial cells may also be revealed by staining directly with ethidium bromide.

1. Grow T84 cells as described in **Subheading 3.1.1.** and infect with *N. meningitidis* for the appropriate length of time.
2. Wash the cells six times with PBS then stabilize the cytoskeleton by incubation with cold METM for 5 s, followed by fixation with 2.5% paraformaldehyde for 20 min. Wash the cells with PBS, neutralize with 0.1 *M* glycine for 5 min, then permeabilize with 0.5% triton X100 in PBS for 1 min. Before staining, saturate the preparations in PBS containing 0.2% gelatin. Use the same buffer for dilution of all immunological reagents.
3. Incubate the samples with the appropriate dilution of antibody or antiserum (either follow the supplier's recommendations or test antibodies to determine the optimum dilutions) for 30 min at room temperature. After three washes in PBS reveal the bound antibody with the appropriate anti-species fluorochrome-conjugated antibody. For a list of some immunological stains, *see* **Table 1**.
4. Excise the filters with the labeled cell monolayers and attached bacteria, place on a microscope slide in mounting medium, and seal under a coverslip with nail varnish.
5. Observe directly by immunofluorescence microscopy. In order to study the samples in greater detail, a confocal laser-scanning microscope may be used. Alternatively, after fixation and embedding, the samples may be stained and investigated by EM.

3.2. The In Vivo Model

The virulence of different strains in the model varies and it is neccessary to start by performing a calibration of the system in order to define of the minimum quantity of the wild-type strain neccessary to induce a sustained bacteremia or to kill half of the rats.

3.2.1. Definition of the Properties of the Meningococcal Strain (see **Note 4**).

1. Grow *N. meningitidis* on GCB-agar plates overnight in a humid atmosphere containing 5% carbon dioxide.
2. Resuspend the bacteria in pyrogen-free 0.9% NaCl to an OD_{600} of 1.0, then dilute serially 10-fold to give suspensions of optical density (OD) 0.1 and 0.01. Depending on the strain of meningococcus, these will contain around 2×10^8, 2×10^7, and 2×10^6 bacteria per millilitre.

3. Mark the infant rats for subsequent identification, with an indelible marker pen, on both their backs and abdomens. The infant rats will be glabrous at this stage but may begin to grow hair during the course of the experiment.
4. Anaesthetize the rats with diethyl ether, then inject them intraperitoneally (iP) with 100 μL of the bacterial suspensions (*see* **Note 5**). For example, 3 rats may be inoculated with the suspension of OD600 of 1.0, 4, with that of 0.1 and 3 with that of 0.01. Enumerate the bacteria in the suspensions used for inoculation by plating serial dilutions onto GCB-agar plates.
5. At time points of 1, 3, 6, 9, and 24 h post-infection, make a small nick is the infant rats' tail veins and remove samples of blood (5 μL) with a micropipet. Dilute immediately in tubes containing 495 μL of GC-phosphate for subsequent enumeration.
6. Bacterial load in the CSF may be measured during the experiment ***(18)***, but this is more easily achieved after killing the animals, for example at 24 h after infection. Kill the rats by iP injection of phenobarbital, then the remove the skin from the nape of the neck and the back of the head. Puncture the cisterna magna by inserting a hypodermic needle, avoiding the small blood vessels, and withdraw (typically) 10–15 μL of CSF (*see* **Note 6**). Dilute a portion of this sample 10-fold into GC-phosphate for subsequent analysis of bacterial counts.

3.2.2. Comparison of the Virulence of Mutant Strains

After the characteristics of the bacterial and rat strains have been determined, comparison of the virulence of bacterial mutants may be undertaken.

Inject half of each litter with the wild-type and half with the mutant bacteria. To study the growth in the blood and the lethality of infection, inject the quantity of bacteria, which in the case of the wild-type would kill about 50% of the infant rats within 24 h. For investigation of the crossing into the CSF, it is better to decrease the dose so that about 90% remain alive for 24 h, and in this case the experiment may be continued further to 48 h, sacrificing half the rats at 24 h and the remaining animals after 2 d.

4. Notes

4.1. The T84 Model

1. All manipulations involving the live T84 cells must be performed using media preheated to 37°C. Prolonged exposure to low temperatures, for example during washing, may destroy the integrity of the monolayer.
2. Before and during the experiment, the integrity of the monolayer should be checked by examination (phase contrast) with a binocular microscope. Failure to reach the required TER may be caused by contamination, notably with mycoplasma, which are not visible by routine microscopic observation of the monolayer. If such an infection is suspected, the bacteria may be visualized by staining the cells with ethidium bromide, and confirmed by culture on specialized

medium (e.g., from Difco). The best course of action is to discard all solutions and to start again with fresh cells.

During the course of the experiments, meningococci should be visible first, with difficulty, as single diplococci, then as clumps of bacteria, often demonstrating a "twitching" motility. Later in the experiment, the clumps spread to form a layer of bacteria covering infected cells.

4.2. In Vivo Model

3. Consistent results may be obtained by using a large number of outbred rats or a smaller number (1 or 2 litters of 10) of inbred rats. The rats, a mother and her litter, are placed in their cage at least 24 h before the experiment in order to give them time to acclimatize to their new surroundings, and are chosen such that the infants will be between 4 and 5 d old at the start of the experiment.
4. The virulence of most strains of *N. meningitidis* in this model is significantly increased by passage in the infant rat. Hence, for comparison of mutants with a wild-type strain, it is recommended first to pass the wild-type bacteria twice in the model, selecting those bacteria most capable of survival in the animal. Use this rat-adapted strain for making mutants to investigate, for example, the effects of deletion of a gene.
5. Anaesthesis of the infant rats is performed in a large glass jar, containing a wad of cotton soaked in diethyl ether and well-separated from the animals themselves. The animals must be anaesthetized before injection of the bacteria, otherwise muscular contractions will eject the inoculum. Injection of the bacterial suspension is best performed using a 1-mL hypodermic syringe and a 25-gauge needle.
6. Because the blood may contain substantial numbers of bacteria, it is important to avoid contamination of the CSF sample. If, during the taking of CSF, any contamination with blood is noticed as a red coloration in the CSF visible at the surface, the needle must be withdrawn and no further liquid taken. However significant contamination may occur without being visible, and for this reason the potential contamination should be noted by counting the number of red cells using a malassez cell. In any case, the relative numbers of bacteria in the two compartments should indicate whether the results can be explained by contamination of the CSF with blood or if there has been a real crossing of the BBB, which may be accompanied by a clearance of bacteria from the blood.

References

1. Saukkonen, K., Sande, S., Cioffe, C., Wolpe, S., Sherry, B., Cerami, A., and Tuomanen, E. (1990) The role of cytokines in the generation of inflammation and tissue damage in experimental gram-positive meningitis. *J. Exp. Med.* **171,** 439–448.
2. Quagliarello, V. J., Wispelwey, B., Long Jr., W. J., and Scheld, W. M. (1991) Recombinant human interleukin-1 induces meningitis and blood-brain barrier injury in the rat. *J. Clin. Invest.* **87,** 1360–1366.

3. Tuomanen, E., Tomasz, A., Hengstler, B., and Zak, O. (1985) The relative role of bacterial cell wall and capsule in the induction of inflammation in pneumococcal meningitis. *J. Infect. Dis.* **151,** 535–540.
4. Burroughs, M., Prasad, S., and Tuomanen, E. (1991) Peptidoglycan derived from lysis of *Haemophilus influenzae* induces blood-barrier permeability independant leukocytosis, in *Programs and Abstracts of the 31st Interscience Conference on Antimicrobial Agents and Chemotherapy*, American Society for Microbiology, Washington, D.C.
5. Reese, T. S. and Karnovsky, M. J. (1967) Fine strutural localization of a blood-brain barrier to exogenous peroxidase. *J. Cell. Biol.* **34,** 207–217.
6. Butt, A. M., Jones, H. C., and Abbott, N. J. (1990) Electrical resistance across the blood-brain barrier in anaesthetized rats: a developmental study. *J. Physiol.* **429,** 47–62.
7. Janzer, R. C. and Raff, M. C. (1987) Astrocytes induce blood-brain barrier barrier properties in endothelial cells. *Nature* **325,** 253–256.
8. Levine, S. (1987) Choroid plexus: target for systemic disease and pathway to the brain. *Lab. Invest.* **56,** 231–233.
9. Saukkonen, K., Abdillahi, H., Poolman, J. T., and Leinonen, M. (1987) Protective efficacy of monoclonal antibodies to class 1 and class 3 oter membrane proteins of *Neisseria meningitidis* B:15:P1.16 in infant rat infection model: new prospects for vaccine development. *Microb. Path.* **3,** 261–267.
10. Pron, B., Taha, M. K., Rambaud, C., Fournet, J. C., Pattey, N., Monnet, J. P., et al. (1997) Interaction of *Neisseria meningitidis* with the components of the blood-brain barrier correlates with an increased expression of PilC. *J. Infect. Dis.* **176,** 1285–1292.
11. Durieu-Trautmann, O., Bourdoulous, S., Roux, F., Bourre, J. M., Strosberg, A. D., and Couraud, P. O. (1993) Immortalized rat brain microvessel endothelial cells: II. Pharmacological characterization. *Adv. Exp. Med. Biol.* **331,** 205–210.
12. Prud'homme, J. G., Sherman, I. W., Kirkwood, M. L., Moses, A. V., Stenglein, S., and Nelson, J. A. (1996) Studies of *Plasmodium falciparum* (human Malaria) cytoadherence using immortalized human brain endothelial cells. *Int. J. Parasitol.* **26,** 647–655.
13. Tuomanen, E. (1996) Entry of pathogens into the central nervous system. *FEMS Microbiol. Rev.* **18,** 289–299.
14. Merz, A. J., Rifenbery, D. B., Grove Arvidson, C., and So, M. (1996) Traversal of a polarized epithelium by pathogenic *Neisseriae*: facilitation by type IV pili and maintenance of epithelial barrier function. *Mol. Med.* **2,** 745–754.
15. Pujol, C., Eugene, E., de Saint Martin, L., and Nassif, X. (1997) Interaction of *Neisseria meningitidis* with a polarised monolayer of epithelial cells. *Infect. Immun.* **65,** 4836–4842.
16. Pujol, C., Eugene, E., Marceau, M., and Nassif, X. (1999) The meningococcal PilT protein is required for induction of intimate attachment to epithelial cells following pilus-mediated adhesion. *Proc. Natl. Acad. Sci. USA* **96,** 4017–4022.

17. Bortulossi, R., Ferrieri, P., and Wannamaker, L. W. (1978) Dynamics of *Escherichia coli* infection and meningitis in infant rats. *Infect. Immun.* **22,** 480–486.
18. Saukkonen, K. (1988) Experimental meningococcal meningitis in the infant rat. *Microb. Pathog.* **4,** 203–211.
19. Kellogg, D. S. J., Peacock, W. L., Deacon, W. E., Brown, L., and Pirkle, C. I. (1963) *Neisseria gonorrhoeae*. I. Virulence genetically linked to clonal variation. *J. Bacteriol.* **85,** 1274–1279.
20. Madara, J. L. and Dharmsathaphorn, K. (1985) Occluding junctions structure-function relationships in a cultured epithelial monolayer. *J. Cell. Biol.* **101,** 2124–2133.

38

Interactions of Meningococci with Endothelium

Robert S. Heyderman and Nigel J. Klein

1. Introduction

The vascular endothelium forms an essential barrier against invasion by *Neisseria meningitidis* from the nasopharynx into the circulation and against meningococcal invasion from the bloodstream into the brain. In previous chapters, there has therefore been considerable emphasis on techniques designed to investigate the mechanisms underlying meningococcal interactions with epithelial and endothelial surfaces. The vascular endothelium is also a major target for the host inflammatory response to meningococcal infection and indeed the ensuing endothelial damage underlies many of the clinical manifestations associated with this condition ***(1,2)***. For this reason, our work has focused on understanding the cellular and molecular consequences of meningococcal-endothelial interactions.

A number of previous studies have provided important clues as to how meningococci cause endothelial damage (reviewed in ***1,2***). Of particular significance are the histological studies of meningococcal disease, which showed that cutaneous lesions not only contained large numbers of organisms associated with the vascular endothelium but also demonstrated the presence of inflammatory cells, particularly polymorphonuclear neutrophils (PMN) ***(3)***. Initially it became apparent from our studies that bacteria alone rarely cause marked endothelial disruption but in the presence of inflammatory cells, bacterial structure was a critical determinant of endothelial-cell injury ***(4)***. Furthermore, we established that both endothelial and leukocyte activation is required to cause maximal endothelial damage ***(4,5)***. More recently we have investigated the mechanisms by which the meningococcus initiates this endothelial dysfunction ***(6–10)***. Our studies show that: 1) meningococci are potent inducers of

From: *Methods in Molecular Medicine, vol. 67: Meningococcal Disease: Methods and Protocols*
Edited by: A. J. Pollard and M. C. J. Maiden © Humana Press Inc., Totowa, NJ

endothelial adhesion molecules, particularly CD62E, which are necessary for leukocyte attachment to the vascular wall; 2) adherent meningococci induce greater expression of adhesion molecules and pro-coagulant activity than nonadherent organisms; 3) meningococci activate leukocytes, leading to changes in adhesion molecule expression, including the beta2 integrin CD11b/CD18, and facilitating attachment to the vascular endothelium; and 4) the combination of stimulated neutrophils adherent to activated endothelial cells causes disruption of the endothelial cell-associated extracellular matrix (ECM), leading to hemostatic and hemodynamic dysfunction.

In this chapter we will concentrate on the methods that can be applied to study the consequences of meningococcal-endothelial interactions. In our in vitro studies we have used monolayers of human umbilical vein endothelial cells (HUVEC) as a model of the post-capillary venule. We will detail below the methods that we have employed to assess changes in ECM expression, tissue-factor procoagulant activity and cell adhesion molecule expression in response to *N. meningitidis* and a range of other inflammatory stimuli ***(4,7,9,11–13)***. These experiments have been conducted with a range of clinical and laboratory generated mutant strains of *N. meningitidis*, which are described elsewhere ***(4,7,9,14)***. We will also set out the immunocytochemical methods that can be applied to tissues such as skin biopsies and post-mortem material from patients with meningococcal disease to explore meningococcal endothelial interactions in vivo.

2. Materials

All general chemicals not detailed below were purchased from either BDH (Poole, Dorset, UK) or Sigma (Poole, Dorset, UK) and were high purity grade.

2.1. Endothelial-Cell Culture (see Notes 1–3*)*

1. Collagenase: 0.1% collagenase Type II (Cat. no. 17101-015; Life Technologies, Paisley, UK) is made up in Dulbecco's modified Eagle medium (DMEM), without pyruvate, with 4500 mg/mL glucose and 0.04M HEPES (Cat. no. 41965-039; Life Technologies).
2. Fetal calf serum: (FCS) from Life Technologies (Cat. no. 10106-169) is heat-inactivated at 56°C for 30 min prior to use.
3. Wash medium: RPMI 1640 with HEPES (Cat. no. 42402-016; Life Technologies) containing 4 μg/mL gentamicin (Roussel, Dublin, Ireland).
4. Endothelial Primary Culture Medium: MCDB 131 medium (Cat. no. 10372-019; Life Technologies) supplemented with bovine brain extract (Cat. no. cc-4092 Clonetecs), endothelial growth factor (EGF; cc-4107 Clonetecs), hydrocortisone (Cat. no. cc-4035 Clonetecs), 2 m*M* L-glutamine (Cat. no. 25030-024; Life Technologies), 1% penicillin, and streptomycin (Cat. no.15070-022; Life Technologies) and 20% FCS.

5. Endothelial Sub-Culture Medium: Following passage, and at least 48 h before each experiment we use RPMI 1640 medium with 25 m*M* HEPES Buffer (Cat. no. 10372-019; Life Technologies, Paisley, UK) supplemented, 20% FCS, and 2 m*M* L-glutamine.
6. Cord Dissection Instruments: forceps (Cat. no. 406/0072/04 and 406/0073/04), Spencer Wells clamps (Cat. no. 406/0056/01) and strong dialysis tubing clamps (Cat. no. 275/1271/00) were purchased from BDH. Disposable plastic quills were purchased from Avon Medicals Ltd, Reditch, Worcs.
7. Trypsin-EDTA solution X10 (Cat. no. 35400-027; Life Technologies).

2.2. Endothelial ECM Expression

1. Glass Bond (Loctite, Welwyn Garden City, Herts, UK).
2. IgG1 mouse monoclonal antibody (MAb) raised against the human fibronectin cell attachment fragment (clone 3E3 from Chemicon, Harrow, Middx, UK; Cat. no. MAb 88916).
3. Fluorescein isothiocyanate (FITC)-labeled goat anti-mouse IgG $F(ab')_2$ (Cat. no. F0479; DAKO, Cambridge, UK).
4. Gold conjugated poly-l-lysine (Cationic gold) and silver enhancer were from Biocell Research Laboratories.
5. Vector shield mounting medium (Cat. no. H-1000; Vector Laboratories, Peterborough, UK).
6. Heparinase II (Cat. no. H6512) and III (EC 4.2.2.8; Cat. no. H8891) were obtained from Sigma.

2.3. Endothelial Procoagulant Activity

1. Barbitone-buffered saline (BBS): 6 m*M* sodium diethyl barbiturate, pH 7.35.
2. Soniprep 150 probe sonicator (MSE, Scientific Instruments, Crawley, Sussex).
3. Water bath.
4. Inosithin 0.5 mg/mL in BBS (Associated Concentrates, New York).
5. Human pooled plasma prepared in house from 10 healthy adult volunteers (*see* **Note 4**).
6. Rabbit-brain thromboplastin as Manchester reagent from Manchester Comparative Reagents Ltd., (Stockport).
7. Murine monoclonal anti-tissue factor (TF) antibody IgG1 (Cat no. 4509) from American Diagnostica, Greenwich, CT).

2.4. Endothelial Adhesion-Molecule Expression

1. Puck's A saline (Cat. no. P 2917; Sigma).
2. Wash medium: PBS plus 5% FCS plus 0.02% Na azide.
3. Antibodies: mouse MAbs to human ICAM-1 (CD54; clone 84H10; Cat. no. MCA532), CD62E (clone 1.2B6; Cat. no. MCA883) and VCAM-1 (CD 106; clone 1.G11B1; Cat. no. MCA907) were obtained from Serotec (Oxford, UK). Mouse MAbs to human CD31 (Cat. no. MO823) and irrelevant control antigens were obtained from DAKO (High Wycombe, UK).

4. Goat anti-mouse F $(ab')_2$ phycoerythrin conjugate (Cat. no. F0480; DAKO).
5. Formal saline (BDH).
6. Flow cytometer such as the FACSCALIBUR (Becton Dickinson) and appropriate software such as Cell Quest (Becton Dickinson).

2.5. Endothelial Function in Tissue Sections

1. Protease XXIV (HK053-5K; BioGenix Laboratories, San Ramon, CA).
2. Antigen retrieval citrate buffer at pH 6.0 (HDS05, SD Supplies, Aylesbury, UK).
3. Antibodies: mouse MAbs against CD31 (Cat. no. MO823), CD68 (clone PG-M1; Cat. no. M0876), and neutrophil elastase (clone NP57; Cat. no. M0752) from DAKO. For antibodies against cellular adhesion molecules, *see* **Subheading 2.4.**
4. Primary antibody-binding detection kits: Vector (Universal detection kit, Cat. no. PK-6200; plus DAB Substrate Kit, Cat. no. SK-4100) or DAKO Envision+ System, Peroxidase (Mouse; Cat. no. K4006).
5. Mayer's haemalum (Cat. no. 35060 4T; BDH).
6. DPX mountant (Distrene 80, Dibutyl Phalate and Xylene) (Cat. no. 36029 2F; BDH).

3. Methods

3.1. Endothelial Cell Culture

We use methods based on the original descriptions by Gimbrone and Jaffe *(15,16)*. In view of the changes in cell morphology/function over time and passage number, we always use HUVECs from the first subculture passage and within 72 h of reaching confluence. Poorly growing cells or cultures with a significant number of fibroblast-like cells are not used.

3.1.1. Primary Culture (see **Notes 5** and **6**)

1. Collect umbilical cords in sterile bottles containing RPMI wash medium (*see* **Note 7**).
2. Inspect the cords for damage and extrude the blood from the vessels between gloved fingers (*see* **Note 8**).
3. Wipe the cord clean of blood and remove areas of damage.
4. Cut off one end of the cord to reveal a clean surface, identify the umbilical vein, dilate with forceps, and cannulate with a plastic quill. Secure the quill in the vein with strong cotton thread. Clamp holes in the cord carefully with forceps.
5. Using a syringe, flush the vein through with wash medium to remove any remaining blood and to dilate the vein. Clamp the distal end of the cord with a dialysis tubing clamp.
6. Infuse 10–20 mL of 0.1% collagenase type II in DMEM into the vein. Clamp the quill using forceps and leave a syringe in place to seal the end.
7. Incubate the cord at 37°C for 8–12 min depending on the batch of collagenase.
8. Collect the digest in a 50-mL conical centrifuge tube containing 2 mL of heat-inactivated FCS and gently flush the vein with a further 20–30 mL of wash medium to remove any remaining nonadherent cells.

9. Sediment the cells at 190 g at 22°C for 10 min. Discard the supernatant and resuspend the cells in 5 mL of primary culture medium (*see* **Note 9**).
10. Seed the collagenase digests into 25 cm^2 tissue-culture flasks and incubate at 37°C in 5% CO_2 (*see* **Note 10**).

3.1.2. HUVEC Sub-Culture (see **Notes 11** *and* **12***)*

1. Wash confluent HUVEC monolayers in the 25 cm^2 flasks with sterile PBS to remove nonadherent cells and the culture medium (the high concentrations of serum and calcium in the medium may interfere with the passage procedure).
2. Passage the cells with trypsin-EDTA to either 24-well, flat-bottom, tissue-culture plates or to gelatinized 13-mm coverslips in 24-well, flat-bottom plates in RPMI culture medium.

3.2. Endothelial ECM Expression (see **Note 13***)*

3.2.1. ECM Staining (see **Notes 14** *and* **15***)*

1. Wash confluent HUVEC monolayers grown on gelatinized coverslips in 24-well, tissue-culture plates in fresh medium.
2. Incubate with the appropriate stimulus (e.g., neutrophils, endotoxin, or cytokines, or live organisms) in the absence of antibiotics (*see* **refs. *4,5,12***). Control cells incubated with culture medium alone are included in each experiment.
3. On completion of stimulation, wash the confluent HUVEC monolayers three times with wash medium.
4. Fix in cold methanol (–20°C) for 10 min and then wash in PBS.
5. Mount the coverslips onto glass slides using Glass Bond.
6. Stain the monolayer with the primary anti-FN (fibronectin) antibody for 1 h.
7. Wash with PBS.
8. Detect primary antibody binding by incubating with FITC-labeled goat anti-mouse IgG for 30 min.
9. Wash in PBS.
10. Visualize anionic sites (heparan sulphate) with a 5 nm gold conjugated poly-l-lysine probe diluted 1:100 in PBS without calcium or magnesium, pH 1.2 for 60 min.
11. Wash with deionized water and develop with a silver enhancer for 15 min (or until the intensity of stain is optimal) at room temperature.
12. Mount the coverslips in mounting medium for visualization and photography with a fluorescent microscope.

3.2.2. Removal of Glycosaminoglycans Component of the ECM (GAGs) by Enzyme Treatment (see **Note 16***)*

1. Wash live HUVEC monolayers grown on glass coverslips in wash medium.
2. Incubate with 5 U/mL of heparinase II or III in culture medium for 4 h.
3. Fix in cold methanol as before.
4. Stain the ECM as in **Subheading 3.2.1.**

3.2.3. ECM Staining in the Absence of Cells

1. Treat confluent HUVEC monolayers grown on glass coverslips with either 2 *M* urea or 0.1 *M* ammonium hydroxide ***(17,18)***.
2. Once the cells lift off or lyse, respectively, wash with PBS and fix with cold methanol as before.
3. Stain the ECM as in **Subheading 3.2.1.**

3.3. Endothelial Procoagulant Activity (see **Notes 17** and **18***)*

1. Wash HUVEC monolayers grown on 24-well tissue-culture plates in fresh medium.
2. Incubate in duplicate with the appropriate stimulus (e.g., live organisms, endotoxin, or cytokines) for 6 h in the absence of antibiotics. Control cells incubated with culture medium alone are included in each experiment.
3. At the completion of the incubation, discard the cell supernatants and freeze the tissue-culture plate with the monolayers *in situ* at –70°C until required for assay.
4. On the day of assay, thaw the tissue-culture plates at room temperature, and add 500 μL of BBS added to each well.
5. Sonicate the cells using a Soniprep 150 probe sonicator at 10 mA for 10 s.
6. Measure total cellular procoagulant activity (PCA) by a one stage unactivated partial thromboplastin time (UPTT) following relipidation with inosithin (*see* **Note 19**):
   a. solublize the inosithin (0.5 mg/mL) in BBS at 37°C for 2 h (this can be stored at 4°C for up to 2 wk).
   b. Relipidate the apoprotein by mixing 50 μL of sonicate with 50 μL of normal pooled plasma and 50 μL of inosithin at 37°C for 3 min in a glass tube ***(19)***.
   c. Recalcify the relipidated mixture with 50 μL of 25 m*M* calcium chloride at 37°C, mixing the solution by tilting the glass tube regularly from vertical to near horizontal, in and out of the water bath ***(20)***.
   d. Measure the time to clot formation.
   e. Express the results as mean PCA units (MU) derived from standard curves generated with rabbit-brain thromboplastin where a UPTT of 25 s = an arbitrary value of 10,000 MU.
7. Confirm the specificity of the PCA detected by neutralization with monoclonal anti-TF antibody.

3.4. Endothelial Adhesion-Molecule Expression

1. Wash confluent HUVEC monolayers grown on 24-well tissue-culture plates in fresh medium.
2. Incubate with the appropriate stimulus (e.g., live organisms, endotoxin, or cytokines) in the absence of antibiotics (*see* **ref.** *7*). Control cells incubated with culture medium alone are included in each experiment.
3. Wash HUVEC with Puck's A saline and then remove immediately.
4. Harvest HUVEC monolayers by incubation in 0.5 mL Puck's A saline at room temperature for 5–10 min (until cell just begin to round up).

5. Gently dislodge endothelial cells from the plate by gentle mechanical scraping with a wide-bore plastic Pasteur pipet and then remove to plastic FACS tubes (max 8 wells at a time).
6. Add 1 mL of wash medium per tube and centrifuge cells at 190*g* for 5 min.
7. Remove supernatant by tipping the FACS tube to the vertical and blotting excess medium from the rim with absorbent paper.
8. Add 20 μL of appropriately diluted primary antibody (e.g., anti- ICAM-1, CD62E, and VCAM-1). Include an irrelevant isotype matched antibody to control for nonspecific binding of antibodies.
9. Resuspend cell pellet and antibody gently.
10. Incubate at room temperature for 15 min.
11. Add 2 mL of wash medium.
12. Centrifuge cells at 190*g* for 5 min and then remove supernatant as before.
13. Add 20 μL of appropriately diluted secondary antibody (e.g., goat anti-mouse $F(ab)_2$ phycoerythrin conjugate).
14. Repeat **steps 8–11**.
15. Resuspend in 500 μL of 1% formal saline.
16. Analyze staining by flow cytometry using Cell Quest software. Identify endothelial cells by their forward-scatter and side-scatter position and by expression of CD31. For each sample, collect 5000 within the endothelial gate (*see* **Fig. 1.**).

3.5. Endothelial Function in Tissue Sections (see **Note 20***)*

Immunohistochemistry is performed by established methods *(21)* using either the peroxidase labelled avidin-biotin technique or a novel polymer-based peroxidase technique (see below). All incubations were performed in a humidified chamber at room temperature.

1. Dewax 4-μm paraffin sections from the appropriate tissue in xylene (incubate 3 times 2–3 min each) and 100% ethanol (incubate 3 times 2–3 min each) to water.
2. Incubate in 3% hydrogen peroxide for 5 min to quench endogenous peroxidase activity.
3. Antigen-retrieval: not required for all antigens, should be optimized for new antigens:
   Protease digestion: incubate with 0.025% protease XXIV and 0.025% $CaCl_2$ in Tris-HCl, pH 7.2–7.6 for 5–10 min (*see* **Note 22**).
   OR
   Heat-induced target retrieval: immerse the slides in retrieval buffer and heat in a microwave (95–99°C) for 10–20 min and then allow to cool for an equal amount of time.
4. Wash in PBS-Tween 20 (0.05%), remove excess buffer using absorbent paper and then block slides with either 10% serum from the species from which the secondary antibody is taken or skimmed milk. Incubate for 10 min at room temperature (*see* **Note 21**).
5. Wash and then overlay the section with 40 μL of the appropriate antibody for 1 h at room temperature.

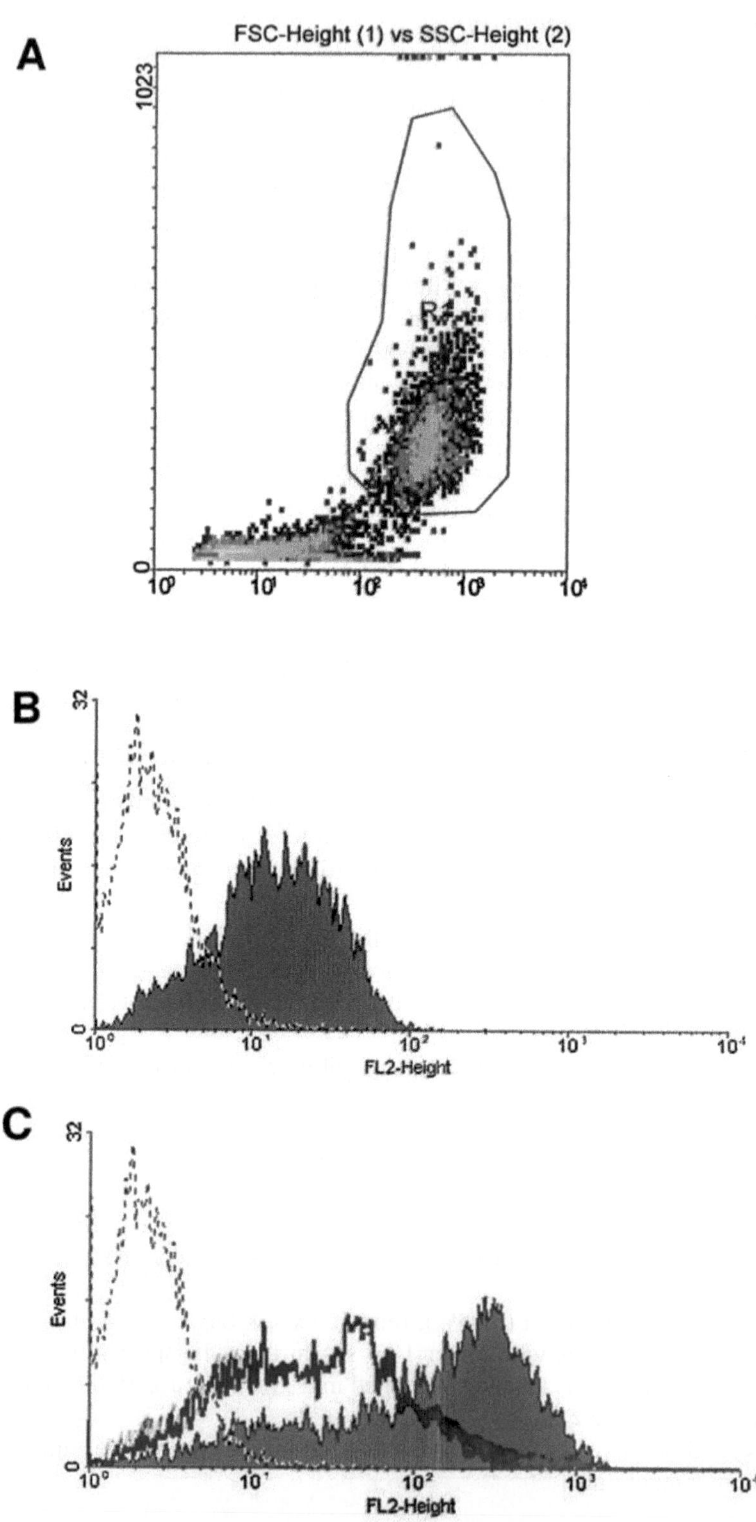
A
FSC-Height (1) vs SSC-Height (2)
1023
0
R1
B
32
Events
0
FL2-Height
C
32
Events
0
FL2-Height

6. Wash as before and then visualize primary antibody binding using either an avidin/ biotin horse radish peroxidase commercial kit or an enzyme-conjugated polymer horseradish peroxidase commercial kit (*see* **Note 23**).
7. Wash in tap water.
8. Counterstain with Mayer's haemalum for 3–5 min and then dip into a suitable bluing agent (tap water or 37 m*M* ammonia).
9. Dehydrate in ethanol, clear in xylene, and mount in DPX in a fume chamber (*see* **Fig. 2**).

4. Notes

1. Sterile plasticware and glassware are used throughout.
2. Collagenase and FCS may be stored in aliquots at –20°C.
3. Endothelial cells are very serum-dependent, requiring 20% serum by volume for incubation periods longer than a few hours. We have used a variety of media including DMEM, RPMI 1640, and Iscove's MEM. We have found that MCDB 131 provides the optimum yield. However, in view of the numerous growth factors, HUVEC cultures should be grown in RPMI 1640 sub-culture medium at least 48 h before each experiment.
4. The subjects are venesected using a 23-gauge needle into 3.8% sodium tri-citrate. The blood is centrifuged at 1200*g* for 10 min at 4°C. The plasma is pooled, aliquoted, snap-frozen in liquid nitrogen, and then stored at –70°C. Clotting times checked at regular intervals did not vary between aliquots, nor over the time of storage (up to 18 mo).
5. All media should be warmed to 37°C in a water bath or incubator before use.
6. Despite the high risk of contamination of the cords by maternal vaginal and skin flora, we have had few problems with infection. In the summer months fungal contamination has occurred. Anti-fungal agents such as amphotericin are not been employed as they often only suppress the organism rather than clear it from the culture. Contaminated cultures should be discarded immediately.
7. Successful recovery of endothelial cells may be achieved up to 48 h after delivery. Cords from known HIV- or Hepatitis virus B-infected mothers are not used. All manipulations and subsequent cell culture are performed using a strict aseptic technique in a class II cabinet.

Fig. 1. *(previous page)* Endothelial flow cytometry showing CD31 and ICAM-1 (CD54) expression in response to purified endotoxin. Confluent HUVEC were stimulated with 100 ng/mL of *E. coli* 0111:B4 LPS for 6 h. **(A)** Gating of the endothelial-cell population based on forward- and side-scatter characteristics; **(B)** CD31 expression (shaded area) in comparison to staining with an irrelevant isotype matched control (dashed line) in resting HUVEC (there was no effect with endotoxin); and **(C)** ICAM-1 (CD54) expression in resting cells (solid line), LPS-stimulated cells (shaded area) in comparison to staining with an irrelevant isotype-matched control (dashed line).

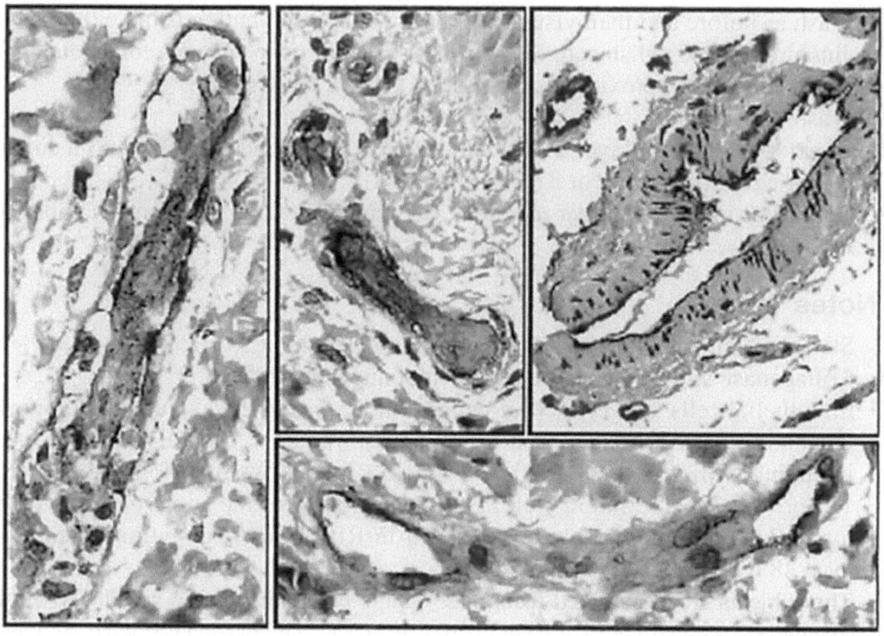

Fig. 2. Immunohistochemical staining of CD31 in formalin-fixed, paraffin-embedded skin. Endothelial staining with anti-CD31 antibody following heat-induced target retrieval. A range of different-sized blood vessels are shown with little or no nonspecific staining elsewhere. (Photographs courtesy of Dr. S. Faust.)

8. The speed of the procedure is critical for the viability of the isolated HUVECs. All cell handling is performed with large-bore pipets and kept to a minimum. Care should be taken not overfill the vein as this has a tendency to cause the vessel wall to rupture. With experience, the technique produced healthy primary cultures from 80–90% of cords.
9. Collagenase treatment of the cords yields a small white pellet that is occasionally contaminated with red blood cells (RBCs). Although great emphasis was placed on removing all traces of red cells before collagenase treatment in the original descriptions of this method ***(15,16)***, this does not seem to either affect the efficacy of the collagenase or the eventual purity of the primary culture.
10. Visualization of the collagenase digests by phase contrast microscopy reveals single endothelial cells, HUVECs in sheets, RBCs, and occasionally fibroblasts and smooth-muscle cells. The fibroblasts and smooth-muscle cells are particularly prominent if the collagenase is left in contact with the vein for too long; however, they do not persist in these cultures. Although over 90% of the endothelial cells derived by collagenase digestion are thought to be viable, only 20–50% adhere to the plastic. It has been estimated that an innoculum of at least 3×10^5 viable cells is required to achieve confluence. The HUVECs sediment

and adhere to the plastic flasks within 2–6 h, at which point excessive RBC contamination can be removed. The cells that are adherent to the plastic form small clusters, which gradually coalesce to form monolayers in 24–72 h.
11. Gelatin is prepared as a 10% solution in sterile water by autoclaving. This solidifies when stored at 4°C. Gelatinize sterile glass coverslips by incubation in 24-well plates with approx 250 μL of pre-warmed gelatin solution at 37°C for at least 2 h. Remove excess gelatin by washing twice with warm wash medium.
12. Endothelial cells can be easily recognized by their cobblestone appearance on phase contrast microscopy. The endothelial nature of the cells can be confirmed by their positive staining for von Willebrand's Factor (vWF; DAKO, Cat. no. A0082), showing characteristic cytoplasmic Weibel-Palade bodies and positive staining for CD31.
13. More precise quantification of fibronectin (FN) may be undertaken by cellular enzyme-linked immunosorbent assay (ELISA) as described in Daromola et al ***(6)***.
14. All incubations were performed in a humidified chamber at room temperature.
15. FN and heparan sulphate integrity is assessed semi-quantitatively by scoring the presence or absence of staining in 10 high-power microscopic fields. If the fibrillar pattern of staining is seen in 8 or more fields, the coverslip is given a score of three; 5–7 fields scores 2; 2–4 fields scores 1, and staining in 1 field or less scores 0.
16. Used to distinguish GAGs and fibronectin staining and to establish the nature of the GAGs detected (*see* **refs. *11,12***).
17. HUVEC TF expression in response to endotoxin is maximal between 4–6 h ***(22)***, decreasing to baseline within 48 h.
18. Experiments in which live meningococci are employed should be carried out in the microbiology laboratory, employing a Class I cabinet where there is a danger of aerosols. Prior to assay, the cells are thawed at room temperature and the wells incubated overnight in BBS containing 10% penicillin/streptomycin solution at 37°C and then re-frozen to ensure that all the meningococci are dead. The safety of this method of bacterial killing has been verified.
19. Pre-warm all reagents including the sonicates to 37°C.
20. All sections should be mounted on poly-L-lysine coated slides.
21. The blocker should be restricted to the wet region of the slide by surface tension alone; if you have trouble use a hydrophobic marker to restrict the blocker and subsequent antibodies.
22. There are a variety of different enzymes available for this purpose from companies such as BioGenix Laboratories, DAKO and Vector.
23. In general, DAB should be developed for 5–10 min but this may depend on the level of the antigen.

Acknowledgments

We would like to thank Dr. Saul Faust, Miss Odile Harrison, Dr. Alick Stevens, Dr. Garth Dixon, and Dr. James Greening for their expert help and advice in the preparation of this chapter.

References

1. Brandtzaeg, P. (1995) Pathogenesis of meningococcal disease, in *Meningococcal Disease* (Cartwright, K., ed.), John Wiley and Sons, Chichester, UK, pp. 71–114.
2. Heyderman, R. S. and Habibi, P. (2000) Meningococcal infections of the skin, in *Textbook of Paediatric Dermatology* (Harper, J., Oranje, A., and Prose, N., eds.), Blackwell Science, Oxford, pp. 384–394.
3. Soto, M. N., Langer, B., Hoshino-Shimizu, S., and de Brito, T. (1976) Pathogenesis of cutaneous lesions in acute meningococcemia in humans: light, immunofluorescent, and electron microscopic studies of skin biopsy specimens. *J. Infect. Dis.* **133,** 506–514.
4. Klein, N. J., Ison, C. A., Peakman, M., et al. (1996) The influence of capsulation and lipooligosaccharide structure on neutrophil adhesion molecule expression and endothelial injury by *Neisseria meningitidis. J. Infect. Dis.* **173,** 172–179.
5. Klein, N. J., Levin, M., Strobel, S., and Finn, A. (1993) Degredation of glycosaminoglycans and fibronectin on endotoxin-stimulated endothelium by adherent neutrophils: relationship to CD11b/CD18 and L-selectin expression. *J. Infect. Dis.* **167,** 890–898.
6. Daramola, O. A., Heyderman, R. S., Klein, N. J., Shennan, G. I., and Levin, M. (1997) Detection of fibronectin on the surface of human endothelial cells by enzyme-linked immunosorbent assay (ELISA): enzymatic degradation by activated plasminogen. *J. Immunol. Methods* **202,** 67–75.
7. Dixon, G. L. J., Heyderman, R. S., Kotovicz, K., et al. (1999) Endothelial adhesion molecule expression and its inhibition by recombinant bactericidal/permeability increasing protein ($rBPI_{21}$) is influenced by the capsulation and LOS structure of *Neisseria meningitidis. Infect. Immun.* **67,** 5626–5633.
8. Heyderman, R. S., Ison, C. A., Peakman, M., Levin, M., and Klein, N. J. (1999) Neutrophil response to *Neisseria meningitidis*: inhibition of adhesion molecule expression and phagocytosis by recombinant bactericidal/ permeability-increasing protein ($rBPI_{21}$). *J. Infect. Dis.* **179,** 1288–1292.
9. Heyderman, R. S., Klein, N. J., Ison, C. A., et al. (1997) The induction of human endothelial tissue factor expression by *Neisseria meningitidis. Microb. Pathog.* **22,** 265–274.
10. Peters, M. J., Dixon, G., Kotowicz. K. T., et al. (1999) Circulating platelet-neutrophil complexes represent a subpopulation of activated neutrophils primed for adhesion, phagocytosis and intracellular killing. *Br. J. Haematol.* **106,** 391–399.
11. Klein, N., Shennan, G., Heyderman, R., and Levin, M. (1992) Alteration in glycosaminoglycan metabolism and surface charge on human umbilical vein endothelial cells induced by cytokines, endotoxin and neutrophils. *J. Cell Sci.* **102,** 821–832.
12. Klein, N. J., Shennan, G. I., Heyderman, R. S., and Levin, M. (1993) Detection of glycosaminoglycans on the surface of human umbilical vein endothelial cells using gold conjugated poly-l-lysine with silver enhancement. *J. Histochem. Biochem.* **25,** 291–298.
13. Heyderman, R. S., Klein, N. J., Daramola, O. A., and Levin, M. (1995) Modulation of the endothelial procoagulant response to lipopolysaccharide and tumour

necrosis factor-α *in vitro*: evaluation of new treatment strategies. *Inflamm. Res.* **44,** 275–280.
14. Hammerschmidt, S., Birkholz, C., Zähringher, U., et al. (1994) Contribution of genes from the capsule gene complex (cps) to lipooligosaccharide biosynthesis and serum resistance in *Neisseria meningitidis. Mol. Microbiol.* **11**, 885–896.
15. Jaffe, E. A., Nachman, R. L., Becker, C. G., and Minick, C. R. (1973) Culture of human endothelial cells derived from umbilical veins. *J. Clin. Invest.* **52,** 2745–2756.
16. Gimbrone, M. A., Cotran, R. S., and Folkman, J. (1974) Human vascular endothelium in culture: growth and DNA synthesis. *J. Cell. Biol.* **60,** 673–684.
17. Klotz, S. A. and Maca, R. D. (1988) Endothelial cell contraction increases Candida adherence to exposed extracellular matrix. *Infect. Immun.* **56,** 2495–2498.
18. Liotta, L. A., Lee, C. W., and Morakis, D. J. (1980) New method for preparing large surfaces of intact human basement membrane for tumor invasion studies. *Cancer Lett.* **11,** 141–152.
19. Gonmori, H. and Takeda, Y. (1976) Properties of human tissue thromboplastins from brain, lung, arteries and placenta. *Thromb. Haemost.* **36,** 90–103.
20. Dacie, J. V. and Lewis, S. M. (1990) *Practical Haematology*, 7th ed. Churchill Livingstone, Edinburgh.
21. Heyderman, E. (1979) Immunoperoxidase technique in histopathology: applications, methods and controls. *J. Clin. Pathol.* **32,** 971–978.
22. Colucci, G., Balconi, G., Lorenzet, R., Pietra, A., and Locati, D. (1983) Cultured human endothelial cells generate tissue factor in response to endotoxin. *J. Clin. Invest.* **71,** 1893–1896.

39

A Promoter Probe Plasmid Based on Green Fluorescent Protein

A Strategy for Studying Meningococcal Gene Expression

Steven A. R. Webb, Paul R. Langford, and J. Simon Kroll

1. Introduction

Many bacterial genes are regulated in an environment-responsive fashion, and from the perspective of a pathogen, the host represents just another environment. Many genes that contribute to virulence are differentially expressed in response to host environments that they encounter during colonization and invasion *(1)*. Recognition of this has led to the development of selection or reporter systems that utilize the increased activity of promoters during growth in vivo to identify genes that are selectively expressed during infection, and, thus, may contribute to the infection process *(2–5)*. One of these techniques, differential fluorescence induction *(2,3)*, involves the use of a promoter-probe plasmid that utilizes a variant of green fluorescent protein (GFP) as its reporter. The technique has been used successfully to identify novel *Salmonella typhimurium* genes that are selectively expressed following exposure to acid environments *(3)* and during infection of macrophages *(2)*. GFP reporter systems have also been used to evaluate in vivo gene expression in other organisms including *Staphylococcus aureus (6)*, *Listeria monocytogenes (7)*, and *Mycobacterium marinum (8)*. This chapter describes the use of the GFP-promoter-probe plasmid, pJSK411, which is suitable for the evaluation of differential gene expression in *Neisseria meningitidis* (**Fig. 1**).

The principle behind a promoter-probe plasmid that uses GFP is the same as for other reporter genes, such as luciferase or β-galactosidase. The plasmid

From: *Methods in Molecular Medicine, vol. 67: Meningococcal Disease: Methods and Protocols*
Edited by: A. J. Pollard and M. C. J. Maiden © Humana Press Inc., Totowa, NJ

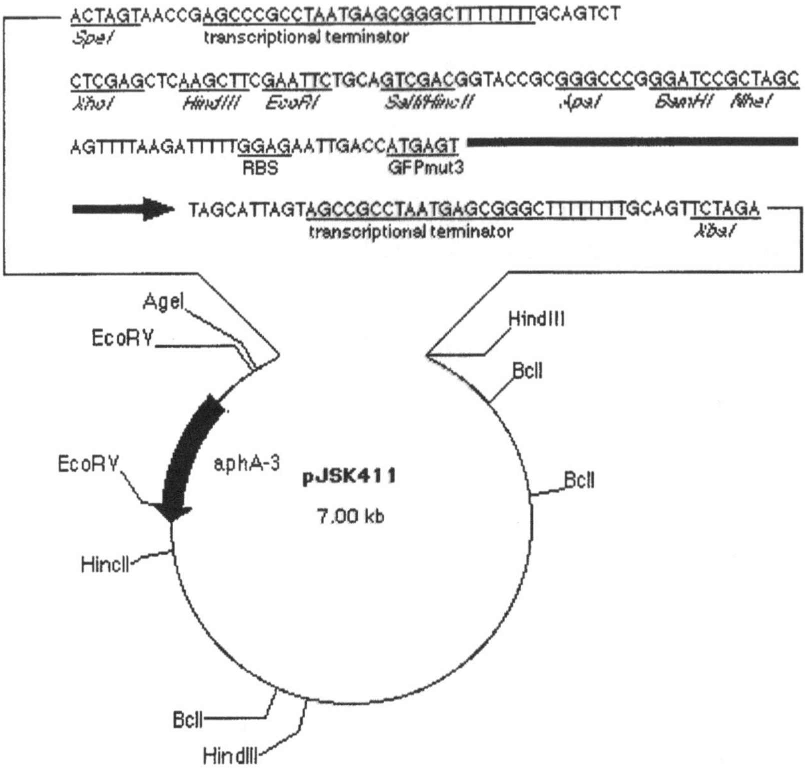

Fig. 1. Map of pJSK411 demonstrating restriction sites within the multiple cloning site. The binding site for the 401US primer overlies the *Xho*I site and the 411DS primer binding site lies within the coding region of GFPmut3.

contains a cloning site, into which DNA of known or unknown sequence, but which may contain a promoter, is positioned immediately upstream of a promoterless reporter gene. The utility of a promoter-probe plasmid arises from production of the reporter molecule being dependent on the activity of the promoter in response to changes in environmental conditions. In the most favorable case, the expression of the reporter gene will reflect the pattern of expression of the gene(s) normally transcribed by the promoter. Inferences about the pattern of gene expression can then be made for any environment in which the reporter gene product can be accurately quantified.

Ideally a promoter-probe plasmid has a broad host range, allowing cloning and other genetic manipulations to be carried out in *Escherichia coli* before the construction is moved into the organism of interest. pJSK411 fulfills this criterion, having been constructed using the broad host-range plasmid pMGC18.1

as its base replicon *(9)*. pMGC18.1 is a derivative of the conjugative plasmid pLES2 *(10)*, in which the β-lactamase gene has been replaced with a kanamycin-resistance cassette, and can be conjugated into strains of *N. meningitidis* from S17-1 λ *pir* strains of *E. coli (11)*. As a reporter, pJSK411 contains a variant GFP gene encoding GFPmut3: a brighter, more soluble, and fluorescence-activated cell sorter (FACS)-optimized variant of wild-type GFP *(12)*. GFP offers several advantages compared with other reporter genes. It does not appear to alter the growth or virulence properties of bacteria; detection by its fluorescence does not require the addition of other substrates; and only a short lag-time occurs between onset of transcription and detection of signal *(12–14)*. The major limitations of GFP are its long half-life, which limits its capacity to detect downregulation of gene expression, and a potentially nonlinear relationship between the rate of transcription and the magnitude of fluorescence signal *(15)*. GFP-mediated fluorescence can be detected using ultraviolet (UV) microscopy, fluorimetry, and flow cytometry.

2. Materials

2.1. Amplification, Purification, and Verification of Putative Promoter Region

1. Qiagen Genomic-tip System (Qiagen, Cat. no. 10243).
2. Oligonucleotide primers. These are specific for each putative promoter region. We have chosen routinely to incorporate a terminal *Eco*R I site (5′- GCGCGGATCC. . . .-3′) or *Xho*I site (5′-AGCCGCTCGAG. . . .-3′) in the upstream primer sequence, and a terminal *Bam*HI site (5′-GCGCGGATCC. . . .-3′) in the downstream primer. Primers are designed to have broadly similar annealing temperatures so that multiple polymerase chain reactions (PCR) can be performed using the same thermal cycling conditions.
3. Tbr DNA polymerase (DyNAzym II DNA polymerase, Flowgen, cat. no. D5-3026) and 10X optimized buffer (Flowgen, Cat. no. D5-3026), 25 mM dNTP solution, derived by mixing each of the four individual 100 m*M* dNTP solutions (Pharmacia, Cat. no. 27-2035-01).
4. 1% agarose gel for electrophoresis.
5. GeneClean III kit (Anachem, Cat. no. 1001-600) or QIAEX gel extraction kit (Qiagen, Cat. no. 20021) with Qiavac 6S (Qiagen, Cat. no. 19503).
6. Restriction enzymes and appropriate buffers as determined by sequence of putative promoter region.

2.2. Cloning and Verification of Promoter Regions in pJSK411 in DH5α

1. *Eco*RI (Roche, Cat. no. 1175084) or *Xho*I (Roche, Cat. no. 0899194) and *Bam*HI (Roche, Cat. no. 0567604), One-Phor-All Buffer PLUS (Pharmacia, Cat. no. 27-0901-02).

2. Quick Flow Maxi Kit (Hybaid, Cat. no. RY14020) or Qiagen Plasmid Giga Kit (Qiagen, Cat. no. 12191).
3. *Eco*RI (Roche, Cat. no. 1175084), 10X buffer H (Roche), *Xho*I (Roche, Cat. no. 0899194), 10X buffer H (Roche), 10X One-Phor-All Buffer PLUS (Pharmacia, Cat. no. 27-0901-02), 1% agarose gel, GeneClean III kit or (Anachem, Cat. no. 1001-600) or QIAEX gel-extraction kit (Qiagen, Cat. no. 20021) with Qiavac 6S (Qiagen, Cat. no. 19503).
4. *Bam*HI (Roche, Cat. no. 0567604).
5. Calf-intestinal phosphatase (Promega, Cat. no. M1821), 10X One-Phor-All Buffer PLUS (Pharmacia, Cat. no. 27-0901-02).
6. T4 DNA ligase (Promega, Cat. no. M1801), 10X One-Phor-All Buffer PLUS (Pharmacia, Cat. no. 27-0901-02), 10 m*M* ATP (Pharmacia, cat. no 27-2056-01).
7. Competent DH5α cells (purchased from Life Technologies (Cat. no. 18258-012), or prepared in house), 14-mL Falcon tubes (Marathon, Cat. no. 2059), Luria-Bertani agar plates ***(16)***, Luria-Bertani broth ***(16)***, supplemented SOC media ***(16)***, kanamycin (Sigma, Cat. no. K4000), 50-mL skirted tubes (Merck, Cat. no. 91051), glycerol (Sigma, Cat. no. G-6279).
8. Wizard Plus Minipreps DNA Purification System (Promega, Cat. no. A1330) or QIAprep 8 Miniprep Kit (Qiagen, Cat. no. 27142) with Qiavac 6S (Qiagen, Cat. no. 19503).
9. Oligonucleotides 411US (5′-GCAGTCTCTCGAGCTCAAGCTT-3′) and 401DS (5′-CCTCTCCACTGACAGAAAA-3′), Red Hot Taq (Advanced Biotech, Cat. no. AB-0406-B), 10X Red Hot Taq buffer (Advanced Biotech, Cat. no. AB-0406-B), 25 m*M* dNTP solution, derived by mixing each of the four individual 100 m*M* dNTP solutions (Pharmacia, Cat. no. 27-2035-01), 25 m*M* magnesium chloride (Advanced Biotech, Cat. no. AB-0406-B), 2% agarose-gel electrophoresis.

2.3. Transfer of Defined Promoter Fusions into N. meningitidis *Strains*

1. Competent *E. coli* S17-1 λ*pir* cells, Luria-Bertani agar plates ***(16)***, Luria-Bertani broth ***(16)***, supplemented SOC media ***(16)***, kanamycin (Sigma, Cat. no. K4000), 50-mL skirted tubes, glycerol (Sigma, Cat. no. G-6279).
2. Nalidixic acid resistant *N. meningitidis* recipient strain.
3. Luria-Bertani broth ***(16)***, kanamycin (Sigma, Cat. no. K4000), Mueller-Hinton broth media (Oxoid, Cat. no. CM405), Vitox (Oxoid, Cat. no. SR0090A).
4. Nalidixic acid (Sigma, Cat. no. N4382), Mueller-Hinton broth media (Oxoid, Cat. no. CM405), GC agar (Oxoid, Cat. no. CM367), Vitox (Oxoid, Cat. no. SR0090A), 250-mL conical flask.
5. 0.45 μ*M* nitrocellulose filters (Millipore, Cat. no. HAWP02500), GC agar (Oxoid, Cat. no. CM367), Vitox (Oxoid, Cat. no. SR0090A).
6. Kanamycin (Sigma, Cat. no. K4000), nalidixic acid (Sigma, Cat. no. N4382), 50-mL skirted tubes (Merck, Cat. no. 91051), Mueller-Hinton broth media (Oxoid, Cat. no. CM405), Vitox (Oxoid, Cat. no. SR0090A).

7. Wizard Plus Minipreps DNA Purification System (Promega, Cat. no. A1330), *Bam*HI (Roche, Cat. no. 0567604), buffer B (Roche).
8. 401US and 411 DS oligonucleotide primers (Red Hot Taq) Advanced Biotech, Cat. no. AB-0406-B), 10X Red Hot Taq buffer (Advanced Biotech, Cat. no. AB-0406-B), 25 m*M* dNTP solution, derived by mixing each of the four individual 100 m*M* dNTP solutions (Pharmacia, Cat. no. 27-2035-01). Restriction enzymes and appropriate buffers as determined by sequence of putative promoter region.

2.4. Evaluation of GFP Expression from Meningococci by UV Microscopy and Flow Cytometry

1. Facsfix comprising a solution of 2% formaldehyde (BDH, Cat. no. 10113 6C) and 2% glucose (Sigma, Cat. no. G-5400) in phosphate-buffered saline (PBS; Sigma, Cat. no. D8537), propidium iodide (Sigma, Cat. no. P-4170).
2. Round-bottom 6-mL Falcon Tubes, (Marathon, Cat. no. F2054), micro-facs tubes (Luckham, Cat. no. LP/2).

3. Methods

3.1. Amplification, Purification, and Verification of Putative Promoter Region

1. Extract chromosomal DNA from a half to a full plate of the meningococcal strain of interest using the Qiagen Genomic-tip System and resuspend in approx 1 mL of water.
2. Identify putative promoter regions from annotated genome sequence, with particular emphasis being placed on transcriptional organization. Design suitable primers for amplification of putative promoter regions (*see* **Notes 1–4**). A 5′ extension that includes an *Eco*RI site is incorporated into upstream primers, and a 5′ extension that includes an *Bam*HI site is incorporated into the downstream primer. If an *Eco*RI or a *Bam*HI site is located within the amplified region, alternative restriction sites need to be incorporated into the primers. These sites are incorporated into the primers so as to facilitate subsequent cloning into the corresponding restriction sites in pJSK411 (**Fig. 1**).
3. The components for 100 μL of PCR mix are 100 pmol each of the upstream and downstream primers, 2 μL of 25 m*M* dNTP, 10 μL of 10X DyNAzyme optimized buffer, 0.5 or 1.0 U of DyNAzyme, 1 μL meningococcal chromosomal DNA solution, and molecular biology-grade water to the final volume (*see* **Note 5**). Depending on the number of targets being amplified, a master mix strategy can be employed (*see* **Note 6**). Various PCR conditions have been used depending on the thermal cycler used, but a successful schedule for experiments using a DNA Engine Thermal Cycler is: 94°C for 5 min followed by 30 cycles of 94°C for 30 s, between 42–48°C for 30 s, and 72°C for 90 s. A final extension is carried out at 72°C for 10 min.
4. Resolve PCR products using 1% agarose-gel electrophoresis and excise products corresponding to the predicted size from the gel.

5. Purify PCR products from the agarose gel using either a GeneClean III kit, or, when a large number of samples have been generated, using a QIAEX gel extraction kit, which can process up to 48 samples in parallel (*see* **Note 6**).
6. Check for correct PCR amplification of the desired DNA fragment by a restriction digest using an enzyme that is predicted from the target sequence to lie within the amplified fragment (*see* **Note 7**). The identity of occasional fragments that do not have a suitable internal restriction site can be verified by sequencing.

3.2. Cloning and Verification of Promoter Regions in pJSK411 in DH5α

1. Prepare PCR products for cloning by double digestion with restriction endonucleases at sites incorporated into the PCR primers (e.g., *Eco*RI and *Bam*HI), typically undertaken using a total volume of 20 μL with a final concentration of 2X One-Phor-All Buffer PLUS. A master mix can be used for large-scale preparations. Digests are performed at 37°C for 2–3 h, after which the enzymes are heat-inactivated by holding at 85°C for 30 min.
2. Prepare pJSK411 vector from DH5α by use of the Quick Flow Maxi Kit or the Qiagen Plasmid Giga Kit. We have used a 5000-mL culture volume for the large-scale preparation of pJSK411.
3. **Steps 3–6** describe the preparation of vector for cloning (*see* **Note 8**). Digest the vector with *Eco*RI for 2 h at 37°C, typically in 100 μL reactions containing 80 μL of pJSK411 plasmid preparation, 1X buffer H, and 100 U of enzyme. Resolve this reaction using 1% agarose-gel electrophoresis and excise the linearized product, which runs at 7.0 Kb. Purify this product using the GeneClean III and resuspend in 100 μL of water.
4. Digest this linearized product with *Bam*HI using 25 μL reactions comprising 18 μL of resuspended product, 5 μL of One-Phor-All Buffer PLUS (2X), and 20 U of *Bam*HI. This reaction proceeds for 2 h at 37°C, and the restriction enzyme is then heat-inactivated by exposure to 85°C for 30 min.
5. Phosphatase the termini of the double digested plasmid by the addition of 24 μL of water and 1 μL of calf intestinal phosphatase to each reaction (final concentration of One-Phor-All Buffer PLUS is now 1X). Incubate the reaction mix for 15 min at 37°C, 15 min at 56°C, and then cool to 4°C for 5 min. A further 1 μL of calf intestinal phosphatase enzyme is added, and the same incubation process is repeated. Heat-inactivate the phosphatase by incubation at 85°C for 15 min. Evaluate each batch of prepared vector prior to use in large-scale cloning (*see* **Note 9**). Small amounts of *Eco*RI linearized plasmid and nonphosphatased but double-digested plasmid should be retained for use as controls.
6. Ligate PCR products containing putative promoter regions (**step 1**), in a directed fashion, into the prepared vector (**step 5**). Typically, mix 2 μL of prepared vector with 10 μL of prepared insert (which contains 2 μL of One-Phor-All Buffer PLUS), 2 μL of 10 m*M* ATP, 1 μL of T4 DNA ligase, and 5 μL of water. If different volumes of insert are used, the volumes of water and/or One-Phor-All

Buffer PLUS should be adjusted so that final concentration of buffer is 1X (*see* **Note 10**). Master mix solutions can be used for large scale preparation (*see* **Note 6**). Incubate this reaction overnight at 14°C and then heat-inactivate the ligase by incubation at 65°C for 20 min. Control experiments containing single *Eco*RI digested vector (for ligase), and double-digested but non-phosphatased vector (for phosphatase) should be conducted in parallel.

7. Transform competent DH5α cells with ligation reactions (*see* **Note 11**). We normally add 10 μL of ligation mix to 40 μL of competent cells on ice. Incubate this mixture for 30 min at 4°C, expose to heat shock of 37°C for 90 s, and then cool to 4°C for 5 min. Add each transformation mixture to 1 mL of supplemented SOC media in a 14-mL Falcon tube, and place in a shaking incubator at 180 RPM for 1.5 h. Transfer this culture to a 2-mL Eppendorf tube, centrifuge at 14,000*g* for 2 min, and resuspend the bacterial pellet in 60 to 100 μL of residual media. Plate the resupended bacteria onto Luria-Bertani agar plates containing 50–75 μg/mL of kanamycin, which are then incubated overnight at 37°C. The average recovery of transformants is in the range of 10–100 colonies per plate. A control transformation using intact pJSK411 should be conducted to confirm adequate competence of the DH5α cells.
8. Sub-culture potential transformant colonies in 10 mL of Luria-Bertani broth containing 50–75 μg/mL of kanamycin. Store an aliquot of 1 mL of culture at –70°C following the addition of 200 μL of sterile 80% glycerol. The remaining culture volume is used for plasmid purification using either the Wizard Plus Minipreps DNA Purification System kit or the QIAprep 8 Miniprep kit with the Qiavac 6S system which allows up to 48 plasmid extractions to be performed in parallel (*see* **Note 6**). Resuspend extracted plasmid in 50 μL of water. The yield of plasmid extraction at this stage is not important.
9. Confirm the successful incorporation of an insert by a PCR approach using the 401US and 411DS primers which correspond to sequence on either side of the cloning region of pJSK411. The reaction mix consists of 100 pmol of 401US and 411DS primers, 5 μL of Red Hot Taq DNA polymerase buffer, 4 μL of 25 m*M* magnesium chloride, 1 μL of 25 m*M* dNTPs, 0.5 μL of Red Hot Taq DNA polymerase, 1 μL of plasmid prepared from potential transformants, and water to a total of 50 μL. PCR conditions suitable for use in a DNA Engine Thermal Cycler are: 94°C for 5 min, then 30 cycles of 94°C for 45 s, 50°C for 45 s, and 72°C for 1 min, with a further extension period of 10 mins at 72°C. Estimate the size of PCR products by electrophoresis using 2% agarose gel. Successful incorporation of an insert results in a fragment that is 135 b.p. larger than the original fragment cloned, whereas vector-alone religation produces a PCR product of 190 b.p. in size (*see* **Note 6**).

3.3. Transfer of Defined Promoter: Fusions into N. meningitidis *Strains*

1. Purified plasmid that has been demonstrated to contain an appropriate insert (**Subheading 3.2.**) is used to transform competent *E. coli* S17-1 λ*pir* cells (*see*

Note 11) *(11)*. Add 5 μL of plasmid solution to 40 μL of competent cells, which are incubated and plated out using the protocol described in **Subheading 3.2.** Average recovery in our hands has been in the range of 100 to several thousand colonies. A single colony is selected (without further evaluation). Sub-culture this colony in 2 mL of Luria-Bertani broth containing 50–75 μg/mL of kanamycin. Store 1 mL of this culture at –80°C after supplementation with glycerol to 20%, and the remaining 1 mL is used for a conjugation reaction with the recipient meningococcal strain.

2. Generate a nalidixic acid-resistant strain, which acts as the recipient strain for conjugation reactions (*see* **Notes 12** and **13**).
3. The method of conjugation of plasmid into *N. meningitidis* strains is based on previously described methods *(9,17)*. Culture *E. coli* S17-1 *λpir* donor strains in overnight broth culture, resuspend at 1:100 dilution in Mueller-Hinton broth supplemented with Vitox, and incubate without shaking for 1.5 h at 37°C in 5% CO_2.
4. Culture the nalidixic acid-resistant recipient meningococcal strain on a Vitox supplemented GC plate, and harvest from plates into 50 mL of prewarmed Mueller-Hinton broth to a cell density of ca. 2×10^6 CFU/mL. Incubate this sub-culture without shaking for 2 to 4 h at 37°C with 5% CO_2, in a 250-mL flask, which allows a high surface-to-volume ratio.
5. Mix approx 10^7 recipient meningococcal cells (1 mL) and 10^6 donor cells (100 μL) in a 2-mL Eppendorf tube. Centrifuge this mixture at 14,000*g* for 2 min, and resuspend in 100–200 μL of the supernatant. Pipet this resuspension on to a 0.45-μ*M* filter placed on a GC agar plate supplemented with Vitox, which is then incubated for 3–5 h.
6. Scrape and/or vortex the filters using 3–5 mL of Mueller-Hinton media in a 50-mL skirted tube. Remove the filter and centrifuge the suspension at 3000*g* for 10 min, resuspend in 100–200 μL of the supernatant, and then plate onto GC agar supplemented with Vitox, and containing nalidixic acid (20 μg/mL) and kanamycin (100 μg/mL).
7. Incubate these plates overnight and select single colonies for further evaluation. Colonies may not appear until up to 18 h after plating. In our hands, average recovery of transconjugants has ranged from 10 to several hundred colonies per plate. A donor *E. coli* strain and the recipient meningococcal strain should be plated on selective GC plates to ensure that no breakthrough growth is possible.
8. Sub-culture a single potential transconjugant colony by streaking to confluence on to a GC agar plate supplemented with Vitox and containing kanamycin (100 g/mL) and nalidixic acid (20 μg/mL). A sample scraped from this plate should be resuspended in Mueller-Hinton broth with 20% glycerol and stored at –80°C pending confirmation of successful conjugation.
9. Verify successful conjugation by plasmid extraction and demonstration of intact plasmid, combined with PCR using 401US and 411DS primers followed by a restriction digest using the same enzyme that was used to confirm initial successful amplification of the PCR product from chromosomal DNA.

10. Extract plasmid from potential transconjugant colonies by use of the Wizard Plus Minipreps DNA Purification System using about half a plate of meningococci as substrate (*see* **Note 14**). Resupend plasmid in approx 50 μL of water. Demonstrate the presence of intact plasmid by digestion of 20 μL of resuspended plasmid with *Bam*HI, determining the size of linearized product using 1% agarose gel electrophoresis.
11. If appropriately sized plasmid is present, undertake a PCR reaction using 100 pmol of 401US and 411DS primers, 5 μL of Red Hot Taq DNA polymerase buffer, 4 μL of 25 m*M* magnesium chloride, 1 μL of 25 m*M* dNTPs, 0.5 μL of Red Hot Taq DNA polymerase, 1 μL of plasmid prepared from potential transconjugants, and water to a total of 50 μL. PCR conditions suitable for use in a DNA Engine Thermal Cycler are: 94°C for 5 min, then 30 cycles of 94°C for 45 s, 50°C for 45 s, and 72°C for 1 min, with a further extension period of 10 min at 72°C.
12. Divide the PCR into two samples and digest one sample with the same restriction enzyme that was used to verify the original putative promoter region (**Subheading 3.1.**). We have found that most restriction enzymes are sufficiently active in Red Hot Taq buffer for purification or buffer exchange not to be necessary.
13. Resolve digested and undigested PCR products using 2% agarose-gel electrophoresis and compare the observed with expected sizes. We have never observed plasmid instability in an MC58 background, nor chromosomal incorporation of the construction. About 1 in 30–50 constructions will be found to be incorrect at this stage owing to the occurrence of a deletion, which in our experience has always occurred within the *E. coli* S17-1 *λpir* cells. This has necessitated repeat transformation of *E. coli* S17-1 *λpir* cells using plasmid derived from DH5α cells. This deletion has not been observed to occur for the same plasmid during repeat construction and we believe it to be a random, rather than a construct-specific, event (*see* **Note 15**).

3.4. Evaluation of GFP Expression from Promoter: Reporter Fusions

1. Meningococcal cells are fixed using 1:1 Facsfix and stained using 1:1000 of 1 mg/mL of propidium iodide. This fixation and staining technique is suitable irrespective of the environment from which meningococci have been isolated. Fixed cells should be kept at 4°C, and analysis performed within 3–4 d (*see* **Note 16**).
2. Cells can be examined using UV microscopy, for which filter sets suitable for examination of fluorescein isothiocyanate fluorophores are used.
3. The GFP signal can be quantitated, and the effects of environmental conditions explored, using flow cytometry. We have experience with evaluation of differential expression associated with iron-restriction, heat-shock, hyperosmolar states, growth in acidic conditions, and growth in anticoagulated fresh human blood. We have assessed fluorescence using a FACSCalibur cytometer (Becton-Dickinson) using Cellquest software (Becton-Dickinson).
4. Transfer fixed and propidium iodide stained cells into 6 mL round-bottom Falcon Tubes or micro-facs tubes (*see* **Note 17**). The flow cytometer settings used have varied but reasonable starting points are as follows: FSC (channel EO2, log

scale), SSC (log scale, amplification = 556, threshold =398), FL1-H (log scale, amplification = 674), and FL3-H (log scale amplification = 705). Use low flow rates at all times.

5. Use the following plots during routine analysis: FL3-H histogram (accepting all events but gating propidium-stained events: this distinguishes cells [propidium stains nucleic acids] from debris); FSC vs SSC dot plot (accepting all propidium-stained events, based on the FL3-H gate but gating on a defined region within the dot-plot: this serves to ensure that cells of equal size and clumpiness are compared); and FL1-H histogram (accepting all propidium-stained events that are located within the defined FSC vs SSC gated area: variation in cell size and clumping can occur between samples and the FL1-H signal increases with increasing FSC and SSC signal. Thus gating serves to prevent confounding of the FL1-H signal that would otherwise occur). The mean FL1-H fluorescence of the population of gated events can be calculated by Stats option (within the Cellquest software) and represents the quantified GFP expression.
6. Control experiments using wild-type meningococci and meningococci containing pJSK411 (*see* **Note 18**) should be undertaken in each environment assessed, to ensure that any changes in FL1-H signal do not arise as a direct consequence of the environment on bacterial autofluorescence. The maximum change in fluorescence that we have observed for these control strains is 10% of baseline.
7. **Figure 2** shows the 4.7-fold increase in fluorescence detected from meningococci harboring a pJSK411 construction containing the inducible *groES/EL* promoter before and after a 5-h incubation in whole blood (*see* **Notes 19** and **20**).

4. Notes

1. For a given putative promoter region, the downstream primer should be designed so that the amplified fragment terminates within the ribosome binding site of the first gene in a transcriptional unit. Location more 3′, within the coding region of the gene of interest, should generally be avoided as it may lead to the additional creation of a translational fusion as well as the desired transcriptional fusion. The location of the upstream primer is to some extent arbitrary, but should extend at least 300–400 b.p. upstream from the location of the downstream primer. Design oligonucleotide primers so that the annealing temperature of the binding portion of the primer is in the range of 55–65°C.
2. In the absence of direct experimental evidence establishing promoter activity in particular DNA regions, their identification simply by using genome data is to a considerable extent arbitrary. The accuracy with which regions likely to contain a promoter are identified improves with experience. An alternative to the directed approach we have adopted would, of course, be to construct a bank of random chromosomal fragments cloned in pJSK411, and then to use cycles of FACS analysis to identify clones that demonstrate differential GFP expression. We have not pursued this approach because of difficulties associated with performing flow cytometry with live meningococci.

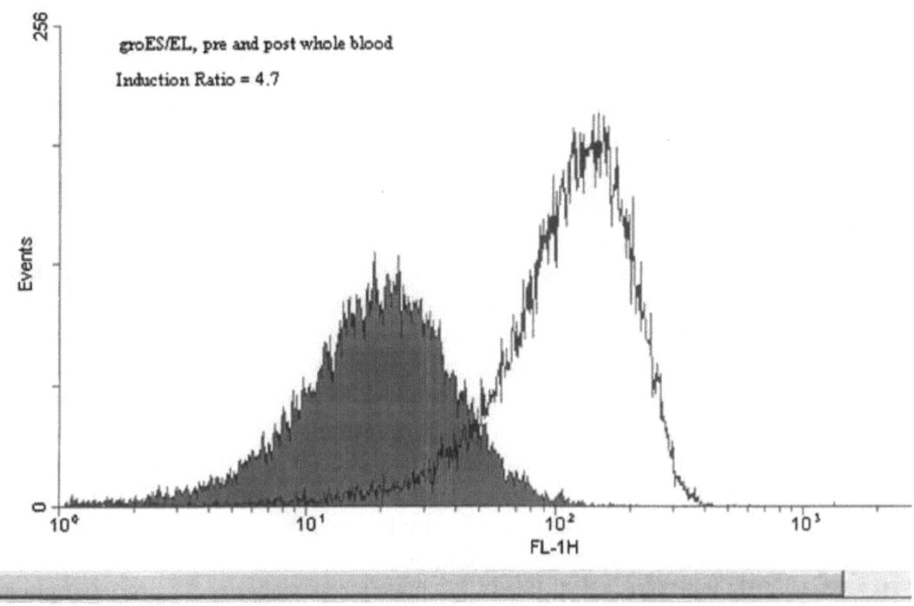

Fig. 2. FL1-H histogram obtained using the described gating strategy derived from MC58 cells containing pJSK411 : groES/EL (which contains the cloned promoter for the *groES/EL* heat-shock operon) immediately after exposure to whole blood (shaded curve) compared with cells that have been exposed to whole blood for 5 h (open curve).

3. For large-scale amplification of putative promoter regions, we purchase oligonucleotides that have been packaged in 96-well plates by the manufacturer. This facilitates the use of a multi-channel pipet for high-throughput PCR, which is then conducted in thin-wall 96-well PCR plates (Thermofast 96, Advanced Biotechnology, AB-0700).
4. Initially we did not screen potential promoter primers for mispriming against other regions of the genome. As a result we had some problems with false priming, especially when primers were inadvertently located within repeat regions. We would recommend careful selection of primers to minimize this problem.
5. High-fidelity PCR amplification of putative promoter regions is essential as single base-pair substitutions may alter function. In this regard, we have found Tbr to be the most reliable high-fidelity DNA polymerase.
6. For high-throughput work, many of the steps described (including PCR of putative promoter regions, check internal digests, digests of terminal restriction sites, ligation of promoter fragments into pJSK411, confirmatory plasmid extractions, and confirmatory PCR reactions) can be performed in 48- or 96-well formats. DNA manipulations are undertaken in thin-wall plates, plasmid extractions using the QIAprep 8 Miniprep Kit with Qiavac 6S, and gel purifications using the

QIAEX Gel Extraction Kit. The use of these techniques substantially reduces the marginal cost and effort of constructing additional promoter fusions. We have not, however, been able reliably to perform transformation reactions in multi-well plates, and have continued to do these in individual Eppendorf tubes.

7. In our experience, the use of restriction endonuclease digestion at a single previously identified internal site to produce fragments of the expected size has been an adequately reliable test for successful amplification of a target sequence.
8. The vector, pJSK411, does not allow selection for, or identification of, successful incorporation of a cloned insert, but the technique outlined in **Subheading 3.2., steps 2–5** results in an acceptably low rate of vector-alone religation.
9. Evaluate each batch of prepared vector prior to its use in large-scale cloning by determining the rate of background religation of 5 μL of vector solution (in the absence of a suitably prepared insert) and by determining the optimal concentration of vector (we test with 1, 2, and 5 μL) for cloning in the presence of a suitably prepared insert. A background religation rate of more than 1 or 2 colonies per plate should prompt a further round of digestion with *Bam*HI. In the absence of any selection system, large-scale cloning is critically dependent on minimal rate of background vector alone religation.
10. The use of One-Phor-All Buffer PLUS at different stages of the processing serves to minimize the need for repurification of DNA and buffer changes. We have found ligation to occur with high efficiency when performed in 1X One-Phor-All Buffer PLUS, although the addition of ATP to the reaction mix is critical.
11. We made *E. coli* DH5α cells competent by a modification of standard methods as follows. One mL of an overnight culture of *E. coli* is diluted into 100 ml of Luria-Bertani media, and incubated for a further 2–3 h. This culture is placed on ice for 5 min, then centrifuged at 2500 rpm for 10 min at 4°C, and then resuspended in 40 mL of "transformation buffer I," which contains 30 m*M* potassium acetate, 100 m*M* rubidium chloride, 10 m*M* calcium chloride, 50 m*M* manganese (II) chloride, and 15% glycerol. After holding for 5 min on ice, this suspension is centrifuged at 2500 rpm for 10 min at 4°C, and then resuspended in 4 mL of "transformation buffer II," which contains 10 m*M* MOPS, 75 m*M* calcium chloride, 10 m*M* rubidium chloride, and 15% glycerol, with the pH adjusted to 6.5 with potassium hydroxide. Following a further 15 min on ice, this suspension is aliquoted into 40–400 μL samples and stored at –70°C. Alternatively, we have purchased competent DH5α cells from Life Technologies (Cat. no. 18258-012).
12. To facilitate selection of transconjugants, the recipient meningococcal strain is made nalidixic acid-resistant. This is achieved by one-step mutation. Parent meningococcal strains are cultured overnight on Vitox-supplemented GC agar plates. Bacteria from these plates are resuspended in 10 mL of Vitox-supplemented Mueller-Hinton broth, to a starting optical density (OD) at 600 nm of approx 0.2. This resuspension is held in a shaking incubator at 37°C for 8–10 h. At this point a further 10 mL of Vitox-supplemented Mueller-Hinton broth is added, together with nalidixic acid to a final concentration of 10 μg/mL, and culture is continued overnight. The following morning the culture is centrifuged for 10 min at 3000*g*, and the pellet is resuspended in

100–200 µL of residual medium. Bacteria are plated on Vitox-supplemented GC agar plates containing nalidixic acid 20 µg/mL. Single colonies are sub-cultured and confirmed as meningococci by colony morphology and gram-stain.

13. We have successfully conjugated pJSK411 into serogroup B and serogroup C *N. meningitidis* (strains MC58 [B], 8013 [C], and a capsule-deficient mutant of MC58 *[9,18]*). Satisfactory transfer and performance of the plasmid and reporter system should be established experimentally for other strains.
14. Although the Wizard Plus Minipreps DNA Purification System, and the Quick Flow Midi Kit (Hybaid, Cat. no. RY 13050), are designed for use with *E. coli*, we have found them useful for the extraction of plasmid from meningococci. The only cautionary note is that if bacteria are frozen in resuspension buffer, subsequent lysis of cells that occurs on thawing results in substantial contamination of plasmid DNA with chromosomal DNA.
15. Although we have observed occasional instability of the plasmid during growth in *E. coli* S17-1 *λpir* cells, we have not observed instability within the meningococcal strains that we have used. Neither the presence of the plasmid, or GFP expression, has any measurable effect on the rate of growth in shaking broth culture, and the plasmid is stable in the absence of kanamycin-selective pressure for at least 4 sub-cultures.
16. GFP is relatively stable at 4°C but degrades over 24–48 h at room temperature. We have performed satisfactory flow cytometric analysis as long as 72 h after sample preparation.
17. Microfacs tubes have the advantage of being capable of being placed in a 96-well microtiter plate, which facilitates the use of a multi-channel pipet for high-throughput screening.
18. A transcriptional attenuator is located upstream from the multiple cloning site of pJSK411. We (and others) have demonstrated transcription through the transcriptional attenuator if a strong promoter is cloned upstream from the attenuator. However, the background rate of GFP expression in the absence of a cloned promoter in pJSK411 is low. Western blots and flow cytometry demonstrate low levels of expression of GFPmut3 from pJSK411. The mean fluorescence of MC58 bearing pJSK411 is 10–20% greater than the background level of autofluorescence observed from wild-type meningococci.
19. Although we have observed unequivocal induction of GFP expression from some constructions in different environmental models, there is a potential difficulty in deciding the minimum level of change in fluorescence, which should be interpreted as evidence of induction. Our limited experience in evaluating the same construction repeatedly under the same inducing conditions suggests to us that an increase in mean fluorescence more than 50% above baseline is likely to be reproducible and experimentally significant.
20. Our interest in the use of GFP in meningococci has been predominantly as a reporter gene for evaluation of gene expression. However, innately fluorescent meningococci have obvious application for the tracking of bacteria during their interaction with cells and tissues. Several stable high-expressing

meningococcal promoters have been identified that appear to be suitable for this purpose.

Acknowledgments

This work was supported by a grant to J.S.K. from the Meningitis Research Foundation. S.A.R.W. was generously supported by an Amy and Athelstan Saw and P.F. Sobotka Fellowships from the University of Western Australia.

References

1. Mekalanos, J. J. (1992) Environmental signals controlling expression of virulence determinants in bacteria. *J. Bacteriol.* **174,** 1–7.
2. Valdivia, R. H. and Falkow, S. (1997) Fluorescence-based isolation of bacterial genes expressed within host cells. *Science* **277,** 2007–2011.
3. Valdivia, R. H. and Falkow, S. (1996) Bacterial genetics by flow cytometry: rapid isolation of *Salmonella typhimurium* acid-inducible promoters by differential fluorescence induction. *Mol. Microbiol.* **22,** 367–378.
4. Mahan, M. J., Slauch, J. M., and Mekalanos, J. J. (1993) Selection of bacterial virulence genes that are specifically induced in host tissues. *Science* **259,** 686–688.
5. Heithoff, D. M., Conner, C. P., Hanna, P. C., Julio, S. M., Hentschel, U., and Mahan, M. J. (1997) Bacterial infection as assessed by in vivo gene expression. *Proc. Natl. Acad. Sci. USA* **94,** 934–939.
6. Cheung, A. L., Nast, C. C., and Bayer, A. S. (1998) Selective activation of sar promoters with the use of green fluorescent protein transcriptional fusions as the detection system in the rabbit endocarditis model. *Infect. Immun.* **66,** 5988–5993.
7. Freitag, N. E. and Jacobs, K. E. (1999) Examination of *Listeria monocytogenes* intracellular gene expression by using the green fluorescent protein of *Aequorea victoria. Infect. Immun.* **67,** 1844–1852.
8. Barker, L. P., Brooks, D. M., and Small, P. L. (1998) The identification of *Mycobacterium marinum* genes differentially expressed in macrophage phagosomes using promoter fusions to green fluorescent protein. *Mol. Microbiol.* **29,** 1167–1177.
9. Nassif, X., Puaoi, D., and So, D. (1991) Transposition of Tn*1545*-Δ 3 in the pathogenic neisseriae: a genetic tool for mutagenesis. *J. Bacteriol.* **173,** 2147–2154.
10. Stein, D. C., Silver, L. E., Clark, V. L., and Young, F. E. (1983) Construction and characterization of a new shuttle vector, pLES2, capable of functioning in *Escherichia coli* and *Neisseria gonorrhoeae. Gene* **25,** 241–247.
11. Simon, R., Priefer, U., and Puhler, A. (1983) A broad host range mobilization system for in vivo genetic engineering: transposon mutagenesis in Gram-negative bacteria. *Biotechnology* **1,** 784–791.
12. Cormack, B. P., Valdivia, R. H., and Falkow, S. (1996) FACS-optimized mutants of the green fluorescent protein (GFP). *Gene* **173,** 33–38.
13. Valdivia, R. H. and Falkow, S. (1998) Flow cytometry and bacterial pathogenesis. *Curr. Opin. Microbiol.* **1,** 359–363.

14. Valdivia, R. H., Hromockyj, A. E., Monack, D., Ramakrishnan, L., and Falkow, S. (1996) Applications for green fluorescent protein (GFP) in the study of host-pathogen interactions. *Gene* **173,** 47–52.
15. Misteli, T. and Spector, D. L. (1997) Applications of the green fluorescent protein in cell biology and biotechnology. *Nature Biotechnol.* **15,** 961–964.
16. Sambrook, J., Fritsch, E. F., and Maniatis, T. (1989) *Molecular Cloning: A Laboratory Manual.* Cold Spring Harbor Laboratory Press, Cold Spring Harbor, NY.
17. Seifert, H. S. and So, M. (1991) Genetic systems in pathogenic Neisseriae. *Methods Enzymol.* **204,** 342–357.
18. Virji, M., Makepeace, K., Peak, I. R., Ferguson, D. J., Jennings, M. P., and Moxon, E. R. (1995) Opc- and pilus-dependent interactions of meningococci with human endothelial cells: molecular mechanisms and modulation by surface polysaccharides. *Mol. Microbiol.* **18,** 741–754.

40

Signature-Tagged Mutagenesis

S. Bakshi, Y.-H. Sun, R. Chalmers, and C. M. Tang

1. Introduction

Signature-tagged mutagenesis (STM) was originally developed by David Holden while studying the filamentous fungus *Aspergillus fumigatus*. In attempts to define virulence determinants for this pathogenic fungus, candidate factors were selected by reference to previous circumstantial evidence and knowledge of the pathophysiology of the disease. Genes encoding candidate virulence determinants were isolated, disrupted, and the resulting mutants tested in animal models of disease. This strategy was, however, unsuccessful as none of the candidate genes proved to have a role in pathogenesis, highlighting the limitations of using preconceptions to identify pathogenicity determinants. Large-scale genetic approaches had been used to investigate the behavior of pathogenic microbes in tissue culture-based experiments, but such assays do not reflect the diversity of environments experienced by bacteria in a host. At that time, the major limitation to performing genetic screens using complex systems, such as animal models, was that only a single mutant could be assessed in a single assay; STM was devised to circumvent this key stumbling block. By labeling each mutant with a unique DNA sequence tag, it became possible to differentiate individual mutants from each other within a pool ***(1)***. A single animal could then be infected with a mixed population of mutants and attenuated strains be identified by their inability to establish infection. Therefore, the essential benefit of STM is that it allows genetic screens to be performed using complex models of pathogenesis so that the advantages of mutational analysis can be combined with biologically relevant assays. Rather than applying STM to *A. fumigatus*, David Holden's group decided to first address *Salmonella typhimurium* pathogenesis to establish proof-in-principle

From: *Methods in Molecular Medicine, vol. 67: Meningococcal Disease: Methods and Protocols*
Edited by: A. J. Pollard and M. C. J. Maiden © Humana Press Inc., Totowa, NJ

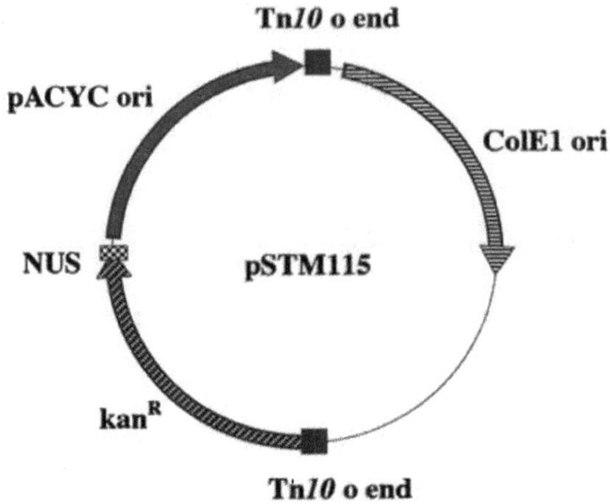

Fig. 1. Map of pSTM115. The plasmid contains the 70 bp outside ends of Tn*10* flanking the kanamycin-resistance marker (kan^R), a copy of *Neisseria* DNA uptake sequences (NUS), and the origin of replication (ori) from pACYC184. The backbone of the plasmid is derived from pBluescript (Stratagene) from which the β-lactamase gene has been deleted.

of STM. The work led to the isolation of previously characterized virulence genes and the identification of an entirely novel 40 kb pathogenicity island that had eluded investigators in the field ***(2)***. STM has now been successfully applied to a wide range of bacterial ***(3–8)*** and fungal pathogens ***(9)***.

S. typhimurium was chosen for the original work on STM for two reasons. First, there are excellent genetic systems available for this bacterium, and second, there is a well-characterized animal model of invasive salmonellosis. This emphasises that the requirements for performing an effective STM screen are: 1) the ability to generate libraries of insertional mutations in the organism of interest, and 2) having a biologically relevant assay(s) for screening the mutants. These constraints mean that STM may not be applicable to all pathogenic microbes. In this chapter, we will outline the potential pitfalls of performing STM on *Neisseria meningitidis* and the ways in which these problems can be circumvented. Particular emphasis will be given to constructing libraries of insertional mutants in *Neisseria* spp.; the suitability of models for studying *N. meningitidis* pathogenesis is dealt with elsewhere in this book. We also describe some technical refinements to the STM methodology that may be helpful.

Difficulties in constructing libraries of insertional mutants in *N. meningitidis* and *N. gonorrhoeae* have hampered the study of pathogenesis in these bacteria. A number of mutagenesis protocols have been described, but each has significant shortcomings. The transposons Tn*916* and Tn*1545-Δ3* have been successfully introduced into *Neisseria* spp. by conjugation ***(10,11)***, but the range of isolates that are susceptible to mutagenesis with these transposons and the diversity of insertions obtained are limited. Both are large genetic elements that are difficult to manipulate. Furthermore, in Tn*916* and Tn*1545-Δ3*, the genes encoding the transposases are located within the transposon ends and these elements are therefore potentially unstable. Indeed, Tn*1545-Δ3* insertions are known to be unstable in *N. gonorrhoeae* ***(12)***. Despite these problems, Tn*916* has been successfully employed to characterize genes that contribute to lipopolysaccharide (LPS) ***(13)*** and capsule biosynthesis in an isolate of *N. meningitidis* ***(14)***.

Shuttle mutagenesis was devised to take advantage of the natural competence of *Neisseria* spp. for DNA uptake and its efficient system of homologous recombination ***(15)***. In this approach, fragments of *Neisseria* genomic DNA are ligated into vectors in *Escherichia coli* and modified by transposon mutagenesis. The mutated fragments are then re-introduced into *Neisseria* by transformation. The first description of shuttle mutagenesis was based on Tn3 ***(15)*** and subsequently the use of Tn*1721* derivatives was reported ***(16)***. There are two principal problems encountered with this method. Firstly, the numerous restriction:modification systems active in *Neisseria* spp. ***(17)*** lead to unrepresentative isolation of genomic DNA in *E. coli* (C. Tang and I. Mehr, unpublished data), especially when large genomic fragments (3–4 kb) are ligated into high-copy number vectors as in shuttle mutagenesis. This problem is compounded when the mutated, but incorrectly modified, alleles are transferred back into *Neisseria*. Secondly, there are several loci in *N. meningitidis* that confer a high frequency of transformation to DNA sequences, often two orders of magnitude greater than for DNA fragments of similar length ***(18)***. For this reason, a previous attempt to use shuttle mutagenesis for *N. meningitidis* STM was unsuccessful ***(18)***.

In insertion : duplication, small fragments of *Neisseria* DNA are ligated into a suicide vector in *E. coli*. Once the plasmid is transferred into *Neisseria*, a single cross-over event leads to a gene-disruption event. Although this method is subject to the same constraints as shuttle mutagenesis, the problems may be less marked as smaller fragments of genomic DNA (usually <1 kb) are used. Insertion : duplication has been successfully employed for *Streptococcus pneumoniae* STM ***(19)*** and this may be a feasible, albeit labor-intensive, strategy for *Neisseria* spp.. A major advantage of this approach is that recovery of the integration site is simple. The integrated plasmid undergoes spontaneous excision from the chromosome and can be simply recovered in *E. coli*.

The principle of modifying genomic DNA from a target organism in vitro prior to its transfer back into the original host is straightforward. Systems for in vitro transposition have been described using the purified components of the Tn7 ***(20)*** and mariner ***(21)*** transposons for the mutagenesis of transformable bacterial pathogens such as *Haemophilus influenzae* and *S. pneumoniae*. Our recent work has taken advantage of the well-characterized in vitro behavior of Tn*10* ***(22)*** and we have applied this method to the mutagenesis of *Neisseria* spp. The advantages of this approach are that it circumvents restriction:modification systems and yields a high frequency of transformation (~800 transformants/μg of DNA).

2. Materials

2.1. Stock Solutions

1. 50 mg/mL chloramphenicol.
2. 50 mg/mL ampicillin.
3. 10 mg/mL ribonuclease A (Sigma).
4. 0.5 *M* ethylene diamine tetracetic acid (EDTA), pH 8.0, (BDH Ltd.).
5. Phenol:chloroform:isoamyl alcohol (PCI, 25:24:1).
6. Chloroform:isoamyl alcohol (CI, 24:1).
7. 10 m*M* Tris-HCl, pH 8.0, 2 m*M* EDTA (TE) (BDH Ltd.).

2.2. Purification of the Transposase

1. Buffer A: 25 m*M* TES/NaOH pH 7.5, 1 m*M* EDTA pH 8.0, 10 m*M* dithiothreitol (DTT) (Sigma).
2. 3 *M* ammonium sulphate/buffer A.
3. Triton X-100, electrophoresis grade (Fischer Scientific).
4. Triton X-100, reduced (Sigma).
5. Isopropyl β-D-thiogalactopyranoside (IPTG) (Sigma).
6. Phenylmethylsulfonylfluoride (PMSF) (Sigma).
7. Luria Broth (LB) (Life Technologies Ltd.).

2.3. Transposition Reactions

1. Dilution buffer: Buffer A containing 3 *M* LiCl and 25% (v/v) ethanol.
2. 1.5% glycerol.
3. 10 m*M* DTT.
4. 250 μg/mL bovine serum albumen (BSA) Ultrapure (Boehringer Mannheim).
5. 200 μg/mL tRNA.

2.4. Repair Reactions

1. 5X Repair buffer: 25 m*M* Tris-HCl, pH 8.0, 33 m*M* NaCl, 6.6 m*M* $MgCl_2$, 2 m*M* DTT, 1 m*M* adenosine triphosphate (ATP) (Pharmacia Biotech).
2. 0.5 m*M* each dNTP (PE Applied Biosystems).
3. T_4 DNA Ligase (Life Technologies Ltd.).
4. T_4 DNA Polymerase (Life Technologies Ltd.).

2.5. Labeling of Tags

1. 50 m*M* $MgCl_2$, Life Technologies Ltd.
2. 200 μ*M* dNTPs.
3. 10 m*M* Tris-HCl, pH 7.6, 50 m*M* KCl.
4. Taq DNA Polymerase (Life Technologies Ltd.).

2.6. Plasmid Dot Blots

1. Whatmann 3M paper.
2. 0.5 *N* NaOH, 1.5 *M* NaCl.
3. 1.5 *M* NaCl, 0.5 *M* Tris-HCl pH, 7.6.
4. 4. 20X SSC.

2.7. Extraction of Genomic DNA

1. 10% sodium dodecyl sulfate (SDS).
2. 20 mg/mL proteinase K.
3. 5 *M* NaCl.
4. 10% hexadecyltrimethyl ammonium bromide in 0.7 *M* NaCl (CTAB).
5. Isopropanol.
6. 70% ethanol.

3. Methods

3.1. Purification of the Transposase Enzyme

3.1.1. Induction of Transposase Enzyme

E. coli BL21 (DE3)/pLysS ***(23)*** is used for transposase expression. Plasmid pNK2853 is a pET-3a derivative with the transposase gene of IS*10*-Right ***(24)*** under the control of a bacteriophage T7 promoter ***(25)***.

1. Transform *E. coli* BL21 (DE3)/pLysS with pNK2852 and select on LB agar containing ampicillin and chloramphenicol.
2. Streak out 10 colonies onto LB agar ± 1 m*M* IPTG; lack of growth on IPTG indicates high level expression of the transposase.
3. Select the colony with the greatest difference in growth, with and without IPTG, for expression of transposase and use to inoculate 5 mL of LB with antibiotics.
4. Grow the culture to mid-log phase and dilute repeatedly until it reaches a volume of 500 mL; use 25 mL of this culture to inoculate each of twelve 500-mL cultures in 2-L Erlenmeyer flasks and incubate with shaking at 200 rpm.
5. When the cultures reach an optical density $(OD)_{600}$ of 0.3–0.6, induce transposase expression by adding IPTG to a final concentration of 1 m*M*.
6. Incubate for 1 h.
7. Harvest the cells by centrifugation at 5,000*g* for 15 min, then wash by re-suspension in 100 mL of Buffer A and re-centrifuge.

8. Re-suspend the cells in an equal weight of Buffer A, and store in liquid nitrogen until use. All subsequent steps are carried out at 0–4°C.

3.1.2. Purification of the Enzyme

1. Prepare an extract by re-suspending 5 g of frozen cells (2.5 g wet weight of original cell pellet) in 25 mL Buffer A.
2. Make the extract up to 2 m*M* for PMSF and bring to 50 mL with Buffer A containing 10% (w/v) Triton X-100.
3. Incubate the extract for 30 min, then centrifuge at 23,000*g* for 10 min.
4. Discard the supernatant and re-suspend the pellet in 10 mL of Buffer A by gentle pipetting, then make up to 80 mL with the same buffer.
5. Repeat centrifugation and re-suspension three more times and finally re-suspend the pellet in 25 mL of Buffer A.
6. Pass the sample through a French press four times at 12,000 p.s.i.
7. Centrifuge the sample at 39,000*g* for 30 min and save the supernatant. In this step, transposase bound to sheared DNA remains in the supernatant, and the pellet is discarded.
8. Make up the supernatant to 0.25 *M* ammonium sulphate by adding 3 *M* ammonium sulphate/buffer A and immediately mix by inversion. Precipitation of transposase occurs rapidly and is allowed to continue overnight.
9. Collect the precipitate by centrifugation at 10,000*g* for 30 min and discard the DNA-containing supernatant.
10. Re-suspend the pellet thoroughly in 0.75 mL of Buffer A (final volume of 1.1 mL) by vigorous pipetting.
11. Add an equal volume of 4 *M* NaCl/100 m*M* Triton X-100 in Buffer A and mix rapidly; the buffer composition is now identical to the gel-filtration buffer.
12. Incubate the suspension for 1 h and centrifuge at 23,000*g* for 30 min.
13. Save the transposase-containing supernatant.
14. Pass the solubilized transposase through a Millex-GV4 filter (12 mm^2; 0.22-μm pore size) and apply 200 μL aliquots to a Superose 12 column (1 cm × 30 cm) which has been pre-equilibrated with 2 *M* NaCl/50 m*M* Triton X-100 in Buffer A. This step removes some minor protein contaminants and some high molecular weight non-protein contaminants.
15. Using a flow rate of 0.25 mL per min, collect 0.25-mL fractions.
16. Monitor the column eluate by absorbance at 280 nm to identify the fractions containing transposase.
17. Analyze the fractions by sodium dodecyl sulfate polyacrylamide-gel electrophoresis (SDS-PAGE).
18. Pool the four peak fractions containing transposase and store immediately at –70°C.

3.2. Plasmid Donor for In Vitro Transposition

We have constructed a plasmid donor, pSTM115, for in vitro transposition of *Neisseria* (**Fig. 1**). The plasmid has a number of properties that make it suitable for

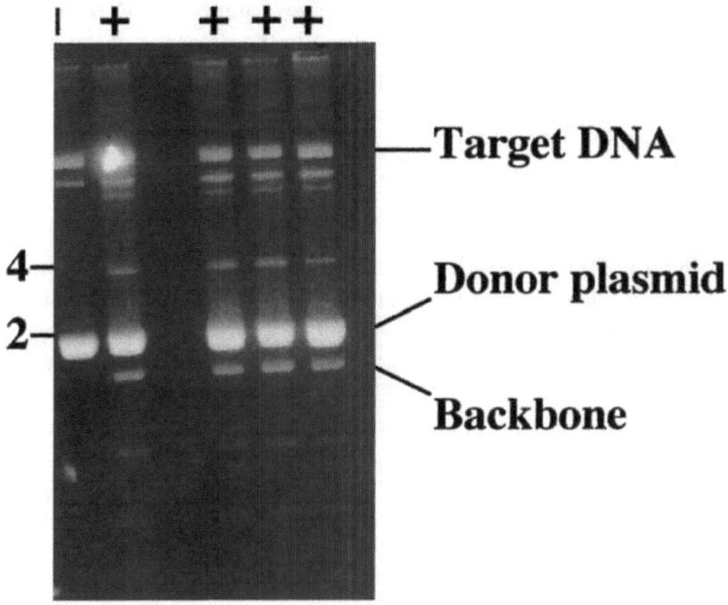

Fig. 2. Transposition reactions. Transposition reactions fractionated by electrophoresis on a 1.1% agarose gel, stained with ethidium bromide, and visualized by UV transillumination. Reactions containing transposase are indicated by +;– shows the products of a reaction from which transposase was excluded. In the presence of the transposase, the transposon is excised from the donor plasmid, pSTM115, resulting in the appearance of the plasmid backbone. The positions of a 1 kb DNA ladder are indicated.

Neisseria mutagenesis, and contains: 1) the gene encoding resistance to kanamycin from Tn*903* for selection in *Neisseria* spp. and *E. coli*, 2) *Neisseria* DNA uptake sequences ***(26)***, 3) the origin of replication from pACYC184 to facilitate the isolation of sequences flanking the transposon insertion site, and 4) a unique *Bam*HI site for ligating in signature tags, all flanked by the minimal 70 bp outside ends of Tn*10* required for efficient excision and integration by the transposase. Furthermore, the cryptic Tn*10* recognition site and the β-lactamase gene have been deleted from the backbone of the plasmid.

3.3. Transposition Reactions

1. First dilute the transposase in a buffer containing high salt in ethanol. This is necessary to activate the protein before it is added to the reaction mixture; if transposase is added directly to the reaction mixture, little or no activity is detected. The activation effect is dependent upon high salt concentration and the presence of organic solvent in the dilution mixture (*see* **Note 1**).

2. Combine caesium chloride-purified *Neisseria* genomic DNA (15 μg) with the plasmid donor (5 μg) in a 600 μL volume in the presence of the purified altered target specificity (ATS) Tn*10* transposase ***(27)***.
3. Incubate for 18 h at 30°C.
4. Stop the reaction by the addition of EDTA (final concentration, 2 m*M*).
5. Extract the products once with PCl.
6. Precipitate in ethanol.
7. Collect the DNA by centrifugation.
8. Re-suspend in 30 μL ddH_2O.
9. Analyze an aliquot by agarose-gel electrophoresis to confirm that transposition has occurred (**Fig. 2**).
10. Tn*10* leaves a 9 bp gap at the 5′ ends of insertion sites ***(28)***. To repair the products, use T_4 DNA polymerase (10 U) and T4 DNA ligase (10 U).
11. Incubate 15 μL DNA from transposition reactions in 300 μL repair buffer at 22°C for 90 min.
12. Clean by extraction with PCI and Cl, then precipitate the DNA with ethanol.
13. Transform *N. meningitidis* with the modified, repaired DNA by standard methods.

Southern analysis of 40 transformants from each of two separate transposition reactions demonstrated that each transformant arises from the single integration of the transposon at a distinct site (**Fig. 3A**). Furthermore, the insertion site is stable during the course of infection of infant rats inoculated by the intraperitoneal route (**Fig. 3B**).

3.4. Detection of Signature Tags

In STM, the profile of mutants in the inoculum is compared with those recovered from the animal. Mutants that fail to establish sustained infection are designated as attenuated. Bacterial DNA is extracted from mutants in the inoculum and from those mutants recovered from animals using the CTAB method ***(29)*** (*see* **Note 5**).

1. Amplify tags from chromosomal DNA (100 ng) in the presence of dNTPs (200 μmol each) and 1.5 m*M* $MgCl_2$ with primers NG13 (5′-ATCCTACAACC TCAAGCT-3′) and NG14 (5′-ATCCCATTCTAACCAAGC-3′) using cycling conditions as follows: an initial denaturation step of 94°C for 5 min, followed by 20 cycles of 94°C for 30 s, 50°C for 45 s, and 72°C for 10 s. As only 80 bp products are being amplified, brief extension times can be used.
2. Fractionate products from the first round by agarose-gel electrophoresis.
3. Purify using the Qiaquick gel-extraction method (Qiagen) (*see* **Note 4**).
4. To label PCR products, perform a second "hot" PCR (20 μL volume) using 5 μL of 825 nM [$^{32-}$P]-dCTP and the same cycling conditions as for the first round.
5. To separate the constant flanking regions of the tags from the central, variable regions, digest the PCR products with a restriction enzyme that recognizes a site

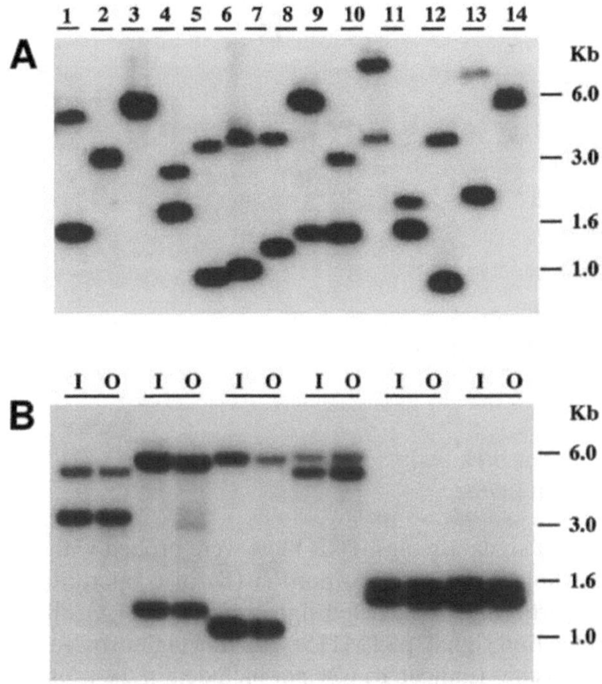

Fig. 3. Southern analysis of *N. meningitidis* mutants. Southern hybridization of *N. meningitidis* mutants obtained by in vitro Tn*10* mutagenesis. Genomic DNA was digested with *Cla*I restriction enzyme, separated by gel electrophoresis, and fragments transferred to nylon membranes. The blots were probed with the kan^R cassette from pSTM115. There is a single *Cla*I restriction site within the kan^R cassette and therefore, a single integration of the transposon generates two hybridizing bands. In **(A)**, 14 mutants obtained from a single transposition were analyzed. Each mutant contains a single, distinct insertion of the transposon. **(B)** shows the hybridization patterns obtained from mutants inoculated (I) intraperitoneally into 5-d-old infant rats, and from mutants recovered from the systemic circulation at 20 h (O). The same hybridization results are observed for both the input and output bacteria indicating that the site of insertion is stable during the course of experiments. The positions of a 1 kb DNA ladder are shown.

at the junction between the two regions. Add a mixture containing the restriction enzyme, buffer, and water to the labeled PCR products (final volume, 200 μL). Incubate the digest in a thermal cycler at 37°C for 2 h.

6. Denature for 5 min at 94°C prior to addition to the hybridisation buffer.
7. Apply plasmid DNA or PCR products to membranes using a dot-blot apparatus (Biorad) (*see* **Notes 2** and **3**).
8. Transfer the membranes to Whatmann 3M paper soaked in 0.5 N NaOH, 1.5 *M* NaCl for 5 min, then to 3 *M* Whatmann paper soaked with neutralization buffer

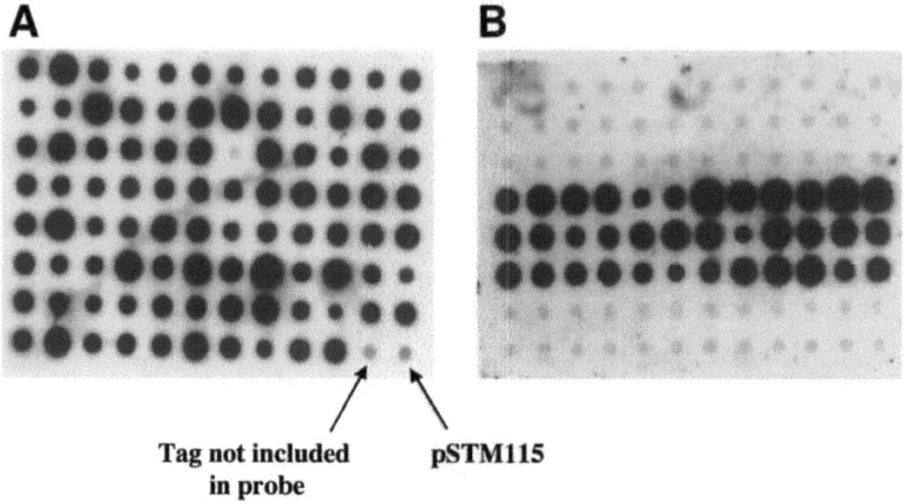

Fig. 4. Selection of signature tags. PCR blots were probed with tags amplified and labeled from the whole **(A)** or from a portion **(B)** of a microtiter plate. The wells contain pSTM115 harboring pre-selected signature tags. In (A), all but one of the tags give a good hybridization signal. pSTM115 without a tag (arrowed) is used as control; the tag in another plasmid (indicated) was not included in the probe. In (B), only tags in the middle three rows of the microtiter dish were used to generate the probe. No cross-hybridization is detected with tags in other sections of the plate.

(1.5 *M* NaCl, 0.5 *M* Tris-HCl, pH 7.6) for 5 min, and finally to paper containing 2X SSC for 5 min.

9. Air-dry the membranes for 10 min at 80°C.
10. Fix the DNA by UV cross-linking.
11. Carry out hybridizations as described previously ***(30)***.

4. Notes

1. Chemicals generally need to be of the best quality available for in vitro transposition. The following are detailed because their purity may affect the results: BSA ultrapure, Boehringer Mannheim; Triton X-100 electrophoresis grade, Fischer Scientific; Triton X-100 reduced, Sigma Chemical Company.
2. In work with *S. typhimurium,* a pool of random tags was used to construct the library. However, a third of all mutants were found to carry tags that could not be amplified ***(1)***. Therefore, all the mutants had to be screened prior to animal experiments to ensure they contained functioning tags. An alternative strategy is to pre-select tags before constructing the library (**Fig. 4**) ***(3)***. Plasmid dot blots or PCR blots, rather than colony blots, can then be used in hybridizations, thereby

increasing the sensitivity of detection. However, the principal drawback is that if pools of 96 mutants are to be screened, mutagenesis must be performed independently 96 times.

3. To save time and expense, tags can be amplified by PCR and applied to blots. If, however, tags are amplified with the same primers used for the cold and hot PCRs, primer-to-primer annealing leads to unacceptable levels of background hybridization (H. Crooke, personal communication). Therefore, primers annealing to sequences outside the signature tags should be designed. It is also necessary to estimate the amount of PCR product that gives the optimal signal-to-noise ratio in trial hybridizations. PCR products of differing lengths may be observed (data not shown). The variation results from some plasmids carrying multiple tags, though this has no adverse effect on experiments.
4. First-round PCR products can be purified using the Qiaquick PCR purification method (Qiagen) rather than by gel extraction. Ten µL of the 40 µL eluate is added to hot PCRs. To ensure that tags have been correctly amplified, an aliquot of the PCRs is examined by agarose-gel electrophoresis. It is helpful to perform a control reaction in which all of the components of PCR are included except for Taq polymerase to differentiate specific products from primers and/or RNA present in the target DNA.
5. For *E. coli* and *N. meningitidis*, we have used a rapid method for DNA extraction. In brief, a 10 µL loop of bacterial cells is harvested from a plate and re-suspended in 200 µL TE. A 20 µL aliquot of the suspension is then added to an equal volume of 0.25 *M* KOH and heated to 100°C for 5 min to lyse the cells. The solution is spun briefly, and 20 µL of 0.25 *M* HCl is added to neutralize the solution. The mixture is then buffered with 20 µL of 0.5 *M* Tris-HCl, pH 7.6, and diluted with 540 µL of ddH_2O. The debris is allowed to settle and 300 µL of the supernatant is transferred to a fresh tube and treated with RNAse (3 µL of a 10 mg/mL stock). Five µL of this DNA is then used in cold PCRs.

   Using the simplifications outlined in **Notes 4** and **5**, it is possible to isolate DNA from bacteria recovered on a plate in the morning and perform hybridizations later on the same day.

5. Summary

Several caveats should be considered when performing STM screens. Firstly, STM may not detect mutants with important functional defects that can be complemented by other mutants in the inoculum. Secondly, when establishing a screen for attenuated mutants, it is necessary to ensure that all fully virulent mutants can "survive" the assay, and that none are lost through stochastic events. It may therefore be necessary to inoculate animals with a high total dose, resulting in an overwhelming infection. Despite these limitations, STM has proved a powerful tool for identifying genes that are required during pathogenesis, and has been applied to the study of numerous pathogens in diverse environments. More recently, tagging mutagenesis has been used to analyze the growth rate of strains under a variety of growth conditions in the laboratory *(31)*. Future studies will doubtless see the application of STM to understanding the biology of an ever-expanding range of microbial diseases and also for the systematic analysis of gene function in organisms for which whole genome sequences are available.

Acknowledgments

We are grateful to Microscience Ltd. for supporting research in our laboratory. Helen Crooke, David Holden, Richard Moxon, and Jacqui Shea have provided advice and helpful discussions. CMT is an MRC Clinician Scientist. Research in R.C.'s laboratory is supported by the Royal Society and the Wellcome Trust.

References

1. Hensel, M., Shea, J. E., Gleeson, C., Jones, M. D., Dalton, E., and Holden, D. W. (1995) Simultaneous identification of bacterial virulence genes by negative selection. *Science* **269,** 400–443.
2. Shea, J. E., Hensel, M., Gleeson, C., and Holden, D. W. (1996) Identification of a virulence locus encoding a second type III secretion system in *Salmonella typhimurium. Proc. Natl. Acad. Sci. USA* **93,** 2593–2597.
3. Mei, J. M., Nourbakhsh, F., Ford, C. W., and Holden, D. W.. (1997) Identification of *Staphylococcus aureus* virulence genes in a murine model of bacteraemia using signature-tagged mutagenesis. *Mol. Microbiol.* **26,** 399–407.
4. Chiang, S. L. and Mekalanos, J. J. (1998) Use of signature-tagged transposon mutagenesis to identify *Vibrio cholerae* genes critical for colonization. *Mol. Microbiol.* **27,** 797–805.
5. Darwin, A. J. and Miller V. L. (1999) Identification of *Yersinia enterocolitica* genes affecting survival in an animal host using signature-tagged transposon mutagenesis. *Mol. Microbiol.* **32,** 51–62.
6. Edelstein, P. H., Edelstein, M. A., Higa, F., and Falkow, S. (1999) Discovery of virulence genes of *Legionella pneumophila* by using signature tagged mutagenesis in a guinea pig pneumonia model. *Proc. Natl. Acad. Sci. USA* **96,** 8190–8195.
7. Zhao, H., Li, X., Johnson, D. E., and Mobley, H. L. (1999) Identification of protease and rpoN-associated genes of uropathogenic *Proteus mirabilis* by negative selection in a mouse model of ascending urinary tract infection. *Microbiology* **145,** 185–195.
8. Camacho, L. R., Ensergueix, D., Perez, E., Gicquel, B., and Guilhot, C. (1999) Identification of a virulence gene cluster of *Mycobacterium tuberculosis* by signature-tagged transposon mutagenesis. *Mol. Microbiol.* **34,** 257–267.
9. Cormack, B. P., Ghori, N., and Falkow, S. (1999) An adhesin of the yeast pathogen *Candida glabrata* mediating adherence to human epithelial cells. *Science* **285,** 578–582.

10. Kathariou, S., Stephens, D. S., Spellman, P., and Morse, S. A. (1990) Transposition of Tn916 to different sites in the chromosome of *Neisseria meningitidis*: a genetic tool for meningococcal mutagenesis. *Mol. Microbiol.* **4,** 729–735.
11. Nassif, X., Puaoi, D., and So, M. (1991) Transposition of Tn*1545*-delta 3 in the pathogenic *Neisseriae*: a genetic tool for mutagenesis. *J. Bacteriol.* **173,** 2147–2154.
12. Crooke, H., Griffiss, J. M., John, C. M., Lissenden, S., Bramley, J., Regan, T., et al. (1998) Characterization of a sialyltransferase-deficient mutant of *Neisseria gonorrhoeae* strain F62: instability of transposon Tn1545 delta3 in gonococci and evidence that multiple genetic loci are essential for lipooligosaccharide sialylation. *Microb. Pathog.* **25(5),** 237–252.
13. Kahler, C. M., Carlson, R. W., Rahman, M. M., Martin, L. E., and Stephens, D. S. (1996) Two glycosyltransferase genes, *lgtF* and *rfaK,* constitute the lipooligosaccharide ice (inner core extension) biosynthesis operon of *Neisseria meningitidis*. *J. Bacteriol.* **178,** 6677–6684.
14. Swartley, J. S. and Stephens, D. S. (1994) Identification of a genetic locus involved in the biosynthesis of N- acetyl-D-mannosamine, a precursor of the (alpha 2→8)-linked polysialic acid capsule of serogroup B *Neisseria meningitidis*. *J. Bacteriol.* **176,** 1530–1534.
15. Seifert, H. S. and So, M. (1991) Genetic systems in pathogenic *Neisseriae*. *Methods Enzymol.* **204,** 342–357.
16. Kahrs, A. F., Bihlmaier, A., Facius, D., and Meyer, T. F. (1994) Generalized transposon shuttle mutagenesis in *Neisseria gonorrhoeae*: a method for isolating epithelial cell invasion-defective mutants. *Mol. Microbiol.* **12,** 819–831.
17. Stein, D. C., Gunn, J. S., Radlinska, M., and Piekarowicz, A. (1995) Restriction and modification systems of *Neisseria gonorrhoeae*. *Gene* **157,** 19–22.
18. Claus, H., Frosch, M., and Vogel, U. (1998) Identification of a hotspot for transformation of *Neisseria meningitidis* by shuttle mutagenesis using signature-tagged transposons. *Mol. Gen. Genet.* **259,** 363–371.
19. Polissi, A., Pontiggia, A., Feger, G., Altieri, M., Mottl, H., Ferrari, L., and Simon, D. (1998) Large-scale identification of virulence genes from *Streptococcus pneumoniae*. *Infect. Immun.* **66,** 5620–5629.
20. Gwinn, M. L., Stellwagen, A. E., Craig, N. L., Tomb, J. F., and Smith, H. O. (1997) *In vitro* Tn7 mutagenesis of *Haemophilus influenzae* Rd and characterization of the role of *atpA* in transformation. *J. Bacteriol.* **179,** 7315–7320.
21. Akerley, B. J., Rubin, E. J., Camilli, A., Lampe, D. J., Robertson, H. M., and Mekalanos, J. J. (1998) Systematic identification of essential genes by *in vitro* mariner mutagenesis. *Proc. Natl. Acad. Sci. USA* **95,** 8927–8932.
22. Chalmers, R. M. and Kleckner, N. (1994) Tn*10*/IS*10* transposase purification, activation, and *in vitro* reaction. *J. Biol. Chem.* **269,** 8029–8035.
23. Studier, F. W., Rosenberg, A. H., Dunn, J. J., and Dubendorff, J. W. (1990) Use of T7 RNA polymerase to direct expression of cloned genes. *Methods Enzymol.* **185,** 60–89.
24. Halling, S. M. and Kleckner, N. (1982) A symmetrical six-base-pair target site sequence determines Tn*10* insertion specificity. *Cell* **28,** 155–163.

25. Haniford, D. B., Chelouche, A. R., and Kleckner, N. (1989) A specific class of IS10 transposase mutants are blocked for target site interactions and promote formation of an excised transposon fragment. *Cell* **59,** 385–394.
26. Elkins, C., Thomas, C. E., Seifert, H. S., and Sparling, P. F. (1991) Species-specific uptake of DNA by gonococci is mediated by a 10-base-pair sequence. *J. Bacteriol.* **173,** 3911–3913.
27. Bender, J. and Kleckner, N. (1992) IS*10* transposase mutations that specifically alter target site recognition. *EMBO J.* **11,** 741–750.
28. Morisato, D. and Kleckner, N. (1984) Transposase promotes double strand breaks and single strand joints at Tn*10* termini *in vivo. Cell* **39,** 181–190.
29. Ausubel, F. M., Brent, R., Kingston, R. E., Moore, D. E., Seidman, J. G., Smith, J. A., and Struhl, K. (eds.) (1991) *Current Protocols in Molecular Biology*. Green Publishing Associates, NY.
30. Holden, D. W., Kronstad, J. W., and Leong, S. A. (1989) Mutation in a heat-regulated hsp70 gene of *Ustilago maydis. EMBO J.* **8,** 1927–1934.
31. Winzeler, E. A., Shoemaker, D. D., Astromoff, A., Liang, H., Anderson, K., Andre, B., et al. (1999) Functional characterization of the *S. cerevisiae* genome by gene deletion and parallel analysis. *Science* **5429,** 901–906.

Index

G

M

Q

R

MIX
Papier aus verantwortungsvollen Quellen
Paper from responsible sources
FSC® C105338

If you have any concerns about our products,
you can contact us on
ProductSafety@springernature.com

In case Publisher is established outside the EU,
the EU authorized representative is:
Springer Nature Customer Service Center GmbH
Europaplatz 3, 69115 Heidelberg, Germany

Printed by Libri Plureos GmbH
in Hamburg, Germany